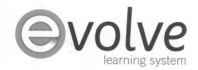

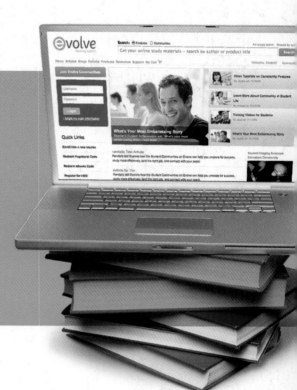

RESPIRATORY CARE ANATOMY and PHYSIOLOGY

Foundations for Clinical Practice

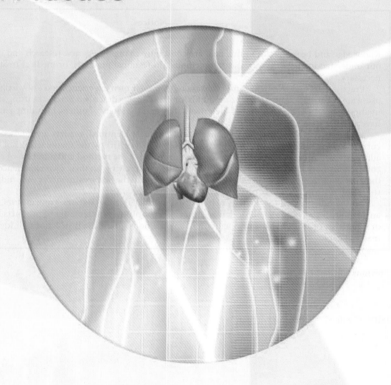

THIRD EDITION

WILL BEACHEY, PhD, RRT, FAARC

Professor and Director
Respiratory Therapy Program
St. Alexius Medical Center and The University of Mary
Bismarck, North Dakota

ELSEVIER

3251 Riverport Lane
St. Louis, Missouri 63043

RESPIRATORY CARE ANATOMY AND PHYSIOLOGY:
FOUNDATIONS FOR CLINICAL PRACTICE, Third Edition   ISBN: 978-0-323-07866-5
Copyright © 2013 by Mosby, an imprint of Elsevier Inc.
Copyright © 2007, 1998 by Mosby, Inc., an affiliate of Elsevier Inc.

Notices

Knowledge and best practice in this field are constantly changing. As new research and experience broaden our understanding, changes in research methods, professional practices, or medical treatment may become necessary.

Practitioners and researchers must always rely on their own experience and knowledge in evaluating and using any information, methods, compounds, or experiments described herein. In using such information or methods they should be mindful of their own safety and the safety of others, including parties for whom they have a professional responsibility.

With respect to any drug or pharmaceutical products identified, readers are advised to check the most current information provided (i) on procedures featured or (ii) by the manufacturer of each product to be administered, to verify the recommended dose or formula, the method and duration of administration, and contraindications. It is the responsibility of practitioners, relying on their own experience and knowledge of their patients, to make diagnoses, to determine dosages and the best treatment for each individual patient, and to take all appropriate safety precautions.

To the fullest extent of the law, neither the Publisher nor the authors, contributors, or editors, assume any liability for any injury and/or damage to persons or property as a matter of products liability, negligence or otherwise, or from any use or operation of any methods, products, instructions, or ideas contained in the material herein.

Previous editions copyrighted

ISBN: 978-0-323-07866-5

Content Manager: Billie Sharp
Content Development Specialist: Betsy McCormac
Publishing Services Manager: Julie Eddy
Project Manager: Jan Waters
Design Direction: Paula Catalano

Printed in China

Last digit is the print number: 9 8 7 6 5 4 3 2 1

For Gabriela and Delaney, my curious, smart, beautiful granddaughters who inject a spurt of life into everything they do.

Contributors

Elizabeth A. Hughes, PhD, RRT, AE-C
Associate Professor
Respiratory Therapy Department
School of Health Sciences
University of Mary and St. Alexius Medical Center
Bismarck, North Dakota

Christine K. Sperle, MEd, RRT, AE-C
Assistant Professor and Director of Clinical Education
Respiratory Therapy Department
School of Health Sciences
University of Mary and St. Alexius Medical Center
Bismarck, North Dakota

S. Gregory Marshall, PhD, RRT, RPSGT, RST
Associate Professor and Chair
Texas State University-San Marcos
College of Health Professions
Department of Respiratory Care
San Marcos, Texas

Reviewers

Robert L. Joyner, Jr., PhD, RRT, FAARC
Associate Dean
Henson School of Science & Technology
Director Respiratory Therapy Program Salisbury University
Salisbury, Maryland

Richard B. Wettstein, MMed, cTTS, RRT
Assistant Professor
University of Texas Health Science Center at San Antonio
San Antonio, Texas

Kenneth A. Wyka, MS, RRT, AE-C, FAARC
Center Manager and Respiratory Care Patient Coordinator
Anthem Health Services
Queensbury, New York

Preface

The term *respiratory care* in the title of this book refers to more than a specific healthcare profession or the care of patients with lung disease. It refers to the responsibility of a multidisciplinary patient care team and to the restoration of normal integrated function by all organ systems that play a part in tissue oxygenation, acid-base regulation, and fluid balance. Delivery of effective respiratory care requires a deep understanding of the physiology and pathophysiology of the lungs, heart, vascular system, and kidneys. This book is addressed to all members of the healthcare team who care for patients with heart and lung ailments.

The main audience for this book is respiratory therapy students, but the book is also written for practicing healthcare professionals, whether they are respiratory therapists, critical care nurses, physical therapists, medical students, or resident physicians. The intent is to give readers a physiological foundation to support clinical practice.

A major goal is to make clear the physiological mechanisms that underpin various therapeutic, diagnostic, and monitoring procedures. Although this book presents basic anatomy of the pulmonary, cardiovascular, and renal systems, it focuses mainly on explanations of physiological processes. The subject matter is set in a clinical context, not only to make it relevant to practicing healthcare professionals, but also to help students learn how to think like clinicians.

FEATURES

This book retains the characteristic features of the first and second editions, which are aimed at helping readers think critically about concepts in a clinical context. Each chapter begins with the same pattern:
- Learning objectives
- Chapter outline
- Key terms (defined in context)

Important features that stimulate critical thought and place the content in the clinical setting include:
- Concept questions (open-ended discussion questions that require more from the student than selecting an answer on a multiple choice question)
- Clinical focus boxes (clinical scenarios that apply the subject matter to the clinical situation, showing the students the practical importance of understanding physiological concepts)

Each chapter ends with a section called "Points to Remember" to help students reflect on key concepts in the chapter.

NEW TO THIS EDITION

The scope and depth of the subject matter is expanded to provide the reader with a broader, more comprehensive knowledge base. A new chapter has been added along with several new and revised Clinical Focus scenarios. All chapters have been revised and updated, including a number of the illustrations. The arrangement of the chapters has been changed at the end of the book for better continuity.

A new Chapter 15, Physiology of Sleep-Disordered Breathing, is aimed at clarifying the physiological mechanisms that underlie sleep-disordered breathing (SDB) and its treatment. Basic anatomical considerations and neural control of sleep are covered, as well as the physiological bases for the diagnosis and treatment of the various forms of SDB, and the cardiovascular consequences of untreated disease.

Student Workbook and Online Evolve Learning Resources

- An accompanying **workbook** is available, which includes diagrams, illustrations, case studies, and open-ended and multiple choice questions.
- **Online student Evolve resources** include **answers to the concept questions** in the textbook and **answers to the questions in the workbook.**

LEARNING ENHANCEMENTS

Each chapter begins with a chapter outline, learning objectives, and a list of key terms. A bulleted list of "Points to Remember" appear at the end. Bolded key terms throughout the text are defined in context rather than in a separate glossary. Open-ended concept questions are interspersed throughout the text to help students reflect on what they have learned, and to foster critical thought and discussion. Clinical focus boxes situate the subject matter in a clinical context to help students adopt modes of thinking used by practicing clinicians and to connect theory with practice. The appendixes contain helpful tables and definitions of terms and symbols. Derivations of some of the more complex equations appear in Appendix III.

To accommodate differing faculty expectations and individual reader needs regarding the scope and depth of study, a detailed multilevel table of contents is provided. Students, instructors, and other readers can use the table of contents to easily identify content areas of interest. A detailed index allows the reader to further identify and find more specific information.

EVOLVE RESOURCES

Evolve is an interactive teaching and learning environment designed to work in coordination with *Respiratory Care Anatomy and Physiology: Foundations for Clinical Practice, third edition.* The Evolve site features electronic resources for instructors that include answer keys to text Concept Questions and to workbook questions; a Test Bank of questions using NBRC exam-style multiple choice questions with answers referencing textbook page numbers; and a chapter-by-chapter PowerPoint slide presentation. Instructors may use Evolve to provide an Internet-based course component that reinforces and expands the concepts presented in class. Evolve may be used to publish the class syllabus, outlines, and lecture notes; set up "virtual office hours" and e-mail communication; share important dates and information through the online class calendar; and encourage student participation through chat rooms and discussion boards. Evolve allows instructors to post exams and manage their grade books online (http://evolve.elsevier.com/Beachey/RespiratoryAP/). For more information, visit or contact an Elsevier sales representative.

Instructor Online Evolve Teaching Resources

- **PowerPoint slide presentations** for each chapter, which can be edited as desired
- An **image collection** for each chapter, which can be used to create new PowerPoint slides
- A **question test bank** for each chapter containing multiple choice and true-false questions
- **Answers** for the question test bank, concept questions, and workbook.

Acknowledgements

I am profoundly thankful to my faculty colleagues, Elizabeth A. Hughes, PhD, RRT, AE-C and Christine K. Sperle, MEd, RRT, AE-C for their revision and updating of Chapter 16, *Fetal and Newborn Cardiopulmonary Physiology*, and for authoring the accompanying workbook. I am also sincerely grateful to S. Gregory Marshall, PhD, RRT, RPSGT, RST for his contribution of Chapter 15, *Physiology of Sleep-Disordered Breathing*, and to Ruben D. Restrepo, MD, RRT, FAARC for developing and authoring the web-based resources for this book. Finally, I owe a debt of thanks to my managing editor, Billie Sharp, and my development editor, Betsy McCormac, for their kindness, flexibility, and extreme patience with me in putting the third edition together.

Will Beachey, PhD, RRT, FAARC

Contents

APPENDICES

INDEX

THE RESPIRATORY SYSTEM

CHAPTER 1

The Airways and Alveoli

OBJECTIVES

After reading this chapter, you will be able to:
- Differentiate between the structures of the upper and lower airways
- Describe how the upper and lower airways differ in their ability to filter, humidify, and warm inspired gas
- List the goals of artificial airway humidification when natural humidification mechanisms are bypassed
- Describe what keeps the large cartilaginous airways and small noncartilaginous airways patent
- Explain why the larger upper airways normally present more resistance to airflow than the smaller lower airways

- Identify the difference between conducting airways and the respiratory zones of the lung
- Describe how the various lung clearance mechanisms function and interact
- List the optimal conditions for effective mucociliary lung clearance
- Explain the way in which various abnormal physiological processes impair the effectiveness of lung clearance mechanisms

KEY TERMS

acinus
acute respiratory distress syndrome
alveoli
apnea
atelectasis
bronchioles
bronchospasm
canals of Lambert
carina
dead space
edema
emphysema
eosinophils
epiglottis
epiglottitis
glottis (rima glottidis)
hypoxemia
interstitium

intrapulmonary shunt
intubation
isothermic saturation boundary (ISB)
laryngospasm
larynx
mucokinesis
mucosa
parenchyma
pharynx
pores of Kohn
respiration
stridor
terminal bronchioles
tracheostomy
turbinates
ventilation
ventilator-associated pneumonia (VAP)

The main function of the lungs is to bring atmospheric gases into contact with the blood. The process of moving gas in and out of the lungs (**ventilation**) and moving oxygen and carbon dioxide between air and blood (**respiration**) requires an elaborately designed, complex organ system. This design must allow efficient operation with minimal work and maintain adequate reserves to accommodate heavy demand. At the same time, the lung must protect itself from the numerous contaminants prevalent in the environment. Knowledge of lung and chest wall architecture is essential for understanding how therapeutic procedures affect abnormal respiratory function.

THE AIRWAYS

The conducting airways connect the atmospheric air with the gas-exchange membrane of the lungs. These airways do not participate in gas exchange but simply provide the pathway by which inspired air reaches the gas-exchange surface. In transit to this surface, inspired gas is warmed, humidified, and filtered by the upper airways.

Upper Airways

The upper airways consist of the nose, oral cavity, **pharynx**, and **larynx** (Figure 1-1). The larynx marks the transition between the upper and lower airways.

Nose

The nose is mainly an air-conditioning and filtering device. Although the resistance to airflow through the nose is greater than resistance through the mouth, most adults breathe through the nose at times of rest. High nasal resistance from swollen mucous membranes and rapid breathing from exercise usually cause people to switch to mouth breathing. Specialized

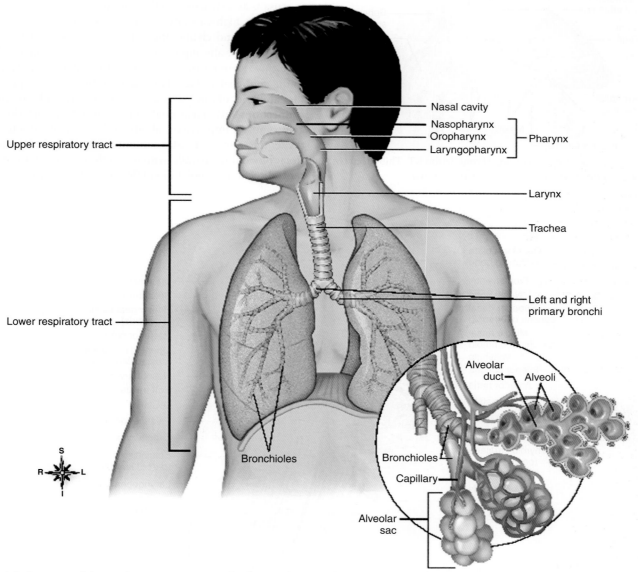

Figure 1-1 Structure of the respiratory system. Note the division between the upper and lower respiratory tracts. (From Patton KT, Thibodeau GA: *Anatomy & physiology*, ed 7, St. Louis, 2010, Mosby.)

structures in the nose increase its airflow resistance, but these structures are necessary for the nose to accomplish its filtering, warming, and humidifying functions.

The cartilaginous anterior portion of the nasal septum divides the nasal cavity into two channels called nasal fossae. The vomer and ethmoid bones form the posterior septum (Figure 1-2). The two nasal fossae lead posteriorly into a common chamber (the nasopharynx) through openings called choanae. The nasal septum is often deflected to one side or the other, more often to the left than the right,[1] possibly making the passage of a catheter or artificial airway through this

side difficult. Three downward-sloping, scroll-shaped bones called conchae project from the lateral walls of the nasal cavity toward the nasal septum. The conchae create three irregular passages—the superior meatus, middle meatus, and inferior meatus (Figure 1-3). Because they create turbulence, the conchae are also called **turbinates**. The convoluted design of the turbinates greatly increases the surface area of the nasal cavity. The maxillary bone forms the anterior three fourths of the nasal cavity floor, called the hard palate (see Figure 1-3). Cartilaginous structures form the posterior fourth, called the soft palate. Palatal muscles close the posterior openings of the nasal cavities during swallowing or coughing, isolating the nasal cavities from the oral cavity.

Squamous, nonciliated epithelium lines the anterior third of the nose; pseudostratified, ciliated columnar epithelium interspersed with many mucus-secreting glands covers the posterior two thirds, including the turbinates. This mucus-secreting epithelium is called the respiratory **mucosa**. Immediately under the mucosa is an extensive capillary network adjoining a system of still deeper, high-capacity vessels. These deep vessels can dilate or constrict and change the volume of blood that flows into the capillaries, altering the mucosa's thickness. The capillaries have tiny openings or fenestrations that allow water transport to the epithelial surface. These fenestrations are not present in the capillaries of lower airways. Countercurrent blood flow and connections between arterial and venous vessels (arteriovenous anastomoses) improve the ability of the nasal mucosa to adjust the temperature and water content of inspired air. Warm arteriolar blood flows parallel with but in the opposite (countercurrent) direction of cooler blood flowing in the venules, lessening

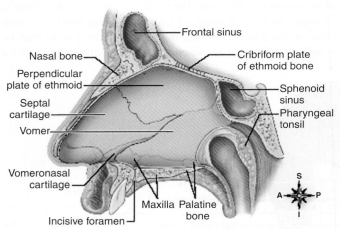

Figure 1-2 The bony nasal septum. (From Patton KT, Thibodeau GA: *Anatomy & physiology*, ed 7, St. Louis, 2010, Mosby.)

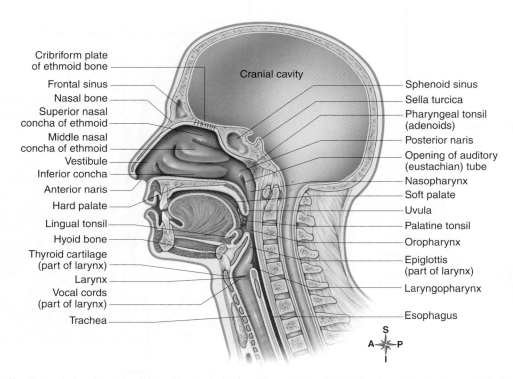

Figure 1-3 The nasal cavity and pharynx viewed from the medial side. (From Patton KT, Thibodeau GA: *Anatomy & physiology*, ed 7, St. Louis, 2010, Mosby.)

the mucosa's heat and water-vapor loss. Arteriovenous anastomoses and countercurrent blood flow are not present in airways below the larynx.[2]

The main functions of the nose are the humidification, heating, and filtering of inspired air. As inspired air passes over the richly vascular epithelial surface (made larger by the presence of the turbinates), its temperature and water content increase rapidly. The turbinates disrupt the incoming airstream and create swirling, chaotic flow, increasing the chances that tiny airborne particles will collide with and adhere to the sticky mucous layer covering the nasal epithelium. Nasal secretions contain immunoglobulins and inflammatory cells, which are the first defense against inspired microorganisms. The nose is so efficient as a filter that most particles larger than 5 μm in diameter do not gain entry to the lower airways.[3]

By the time inspired air reaches the nasopharynx, it gains considerable water vapor and heat. Exhaled air cools as it leaves the nose, causing water vapor to condense on its structures, which humidifies the subsequent inspired air.

CONCEPT QUESTION 1-1

Compared with breathing through the nose, how does breathing strictly through the mouth affect humidification, warming, and filtering of inspired air?

The process of **intubation** involves the insertion of an artificial airway or endotracheal tube through the nose or mouth and into the trachea (Figure 1-4), which means the air-conditioning function of the nose is lost, and unmodified cool, dry gas directly enters the trachea. This places a heavy burden on the tracheal mucosa, which is not designed to accommodate cool, dry gases.

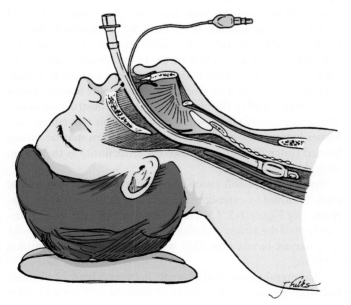

Figure 1-4 An oral endotracheal tube in position. The inflated cuff at the tip of the tube isolates the lower trachea and airways from the pharynx. (From Barnes TA: *Core textbook of respiratory care*, ed 2, St Louis, 1994, Mosby.)

CONCEPT QUESTION 1-2

In what way is the upper airway mucosa superior to the tracheal mucosa in accommodating cool, dry gases?

Connected to the nasal cavities are several empty airspaces within the skull and facial bones called paranasal sinuses. These sinuses are lined with a mucus-secreting epithelium, continuous with the epithelium of the nasal cavities. Mucus from the sinuses drains into the nasal cavity through openings located beneath the conchae. The sinuses are symmetrically paired and located in the frontal, ethmoid, sphenoid, and maxillary bones. Inflammation and infection may swell the membranes lining the sinuses, impairing drainage and increasing sinus cavity pressure. Chronic sinus infections provide a source of bacteria-laden secretions that are sometimes aspirated into the lower respiratory tract, potentially causing lower respiratory infections.

Pharynx

The pharynx is the space behind the nasal cavities that extends down to the larynx (see Figure 1-1). The term pharynx stems from the Greek word meaning "throat." The nasopharynx is the portion behind the nasal cavities that extends down to the soft palate. The oropharynx, the space behind the oral cavity, is bounded by the soft palate above and the base of the tongue below. The laryngopharynx is the space below the base of the tongue and above the larynx.

As inspired gas abruptly changes its direction of flow at the posterior nasopharynx, inhaled foreign particles collide with and adhere to the sticky mucous membrane. Lymphatic tissues in the nasopharynx and oropharynx provide an immunological defense against infectious agents. These tissues include the pharyngeal (adenoid), palatine, and lingual tonsils (see Figure 1-3). These tissues may become inflamed and swollen and may interfere with nasal breathing especially in children owing to their smaller airways; chronic inflammation of the tonsils may warrant surgical removal.

The eustachian tubes, also called auditory tubes, connect the middle ear with the nasopharynx (see Figure 1-3). These tubes allow pressure equalization between the middle ear and atmosphere. Inflammation and excessive mucus production in the nasopharynx may block the eustachian tubes and hinder the pressure-equalizing process; this can momentarily impair hearing and cause pain, especially during abrupt changes in atmospheric pressure. Children younger than 3 years of age are especially susceptible to this condition because their eustachian tubes are small and easily occluded; artificial pressure-equalizing tubes, also known as myringotomy tubes, are sometimes placed through the ear's tympanic membrane (eardrum) to create an alternate route for pressure equalization.

CONCEPT QUESTION 1-3

Why may a throat infection lead to a middle-ear infection (otitis media)?

Endotracheal Tubes, Drying of Secretions, and Humidification Goals

You are called to the bedside of a patient who is mechanically ventilated through an endotracheal tube. The pressure required to inflate the lungs is so great that the high-pressure alarm is sounding, cutting short the delivery of each breath. You notice that there are no water droplets condensed on the inner surface of the ventilator's inspiratory tube. You also notice that heated wires are incorporated into the wall of the inspiratory tubing. You pass a suction catheter down through the endotracheal tube to remove any secretions that might be present, and you meet considerable resistance as you try to advance the catheter. The secretions are thick and difficult to remove when you apply suction.

Discussion

Mechanical ventilation in the critical care setting requires placement of an endotracheal tube into the trachea. Bypassing the upper airway in this manner would introduce cool, dry gas directly into the lower trachea unless heat and artificial humidity are supplied to the endotracheal tube. Otherwise, the mucous membrane of the lower airways, which is not designed to warm and humidify incoming gas, would lose water to the incoming gas, and secretions would thicken and become immobile. Secretions could then accumulate and partially or completely block some of the airways or, as in the case described, accumulate inside the endotracheal tube and partially block inspiratory gas flow.

The heated wires incorporated into the ventilator's inspiratory tubing are designed to prevent gas from cooling on its way to the patient, which reduces water condensation and accumulation in the tubing. However, if the wires heat the gas enough to evaporate all of the condensed water, the relative humidity decreases to less than 100%. The lower trachea and airways beyond the endotracheal tube tip lose water to the incoming gas through evaporation, which dehydrates and thickens airway secretions. The presence of even a slight amount of condensation inside the inspiratory tubing means that the inspired gas is 100% saturated with water vapor. Total absence of condensation means the gas is probably less than 100% saturated, increasing the likelihood of thickened secretions and endotracheal tube obstruction. Inspired gas exits the tip of an endotracheal tube about 2 cm above the carina. The goal of humidification in mechanical ventilation is to duplicate the heat and humidity conditions that would normally exist at this point in the nonintubated trachea: approximately 32°C to 34°C and 100% relative humidity[17] (see Figure 1-10).

The oropharynx and laryngopharynx accommodate food and air and are lined with nonciliated, stratified squamous epithelium. The laryngopharynx, also called the hypopharynx, separates the digestive and respiratory tracts. Proper function of sensory and motor nerves innervating the pharyngeal musculature is crucial in preventing food and liquid aspiration into the respiratory tract. The pharyngeal reflex has its sensory component in the ninth cranial (glossopharyngeal) nerve and its motor component in the tenth cranial (vagus) nerve. This reflex arc is responsible for the gag and swallowing reflexes.

Deeply unconscious persons sometimes lose the pharyngeal and laryngeal reflexes and aspirate foreign material into their lungs. In such individuals, an artificial airway (endotracheal tube) with an inflatable cuff may be inserted orally or nasally through the larynx and into the trachea. After it is in place, the cuff is inflated to form a seal between the tracheal wall and tube to minimize aspiration of pharyngeal contents (see Figure 1-4). However, even if the cuff is properly inflated, pharyngeal secretions eventually migrate past the cuff into the lower airway, For this reason, mechanically ventilated patients, in whom endotracheal intubation is required, are susceptible to the development of lung infections, or **ventilator-associated pneumonia (VAP)**; the longer the duration of mechanical ventilation, the greater the risk of VAP. Normal pharyngeal muscle tone prevents the base of the tongue from falling back and occluding the laryngopharynx, even in a person who is supine and asleep. Deep unconsciousness may relax pharyngeal muscles enough to allow the base of the tongue to rest against the posterior wall of the pharynx, occluding the upper airway; this is called soft tissue obstruction and is the most common threat to upper airway patency. If the head droops forward, the oral cavity and pharynx-larynx axis form an acute angle that may partially or completely obstruct the upper airway (Figure 1-5). Partial upper airway obstruction produces a low-pitched snoring sound as inspired air vibrates the base of the tongue against the posterior wall of the pharynx. Complete obstruction causes strong inspiratory efforts without sound or air movement. Soft tissues between the ribs and above the sternum may be sucked inward (intercostal and suprasternal retractions) as the person struggles to inhale.

Both forms of soft tissue upper airway obstruction can be easily removed by extending the neck and pulling the chin anteriorly (see Figure 1-5, *C*). This maneuver pulls the tongue forward out of the airway and aligns the oral and nasal cavities with the pharynx-larynx axis. This is sometimes called the sniffing position.

Pharyngeal anatomy plays a role in the incidence of obstructive sleep **apnea** (OSA),[4] as do pharyngeal reflexes and muscle tone. The normal pharynx narrows during sleep, greatly increasing upper airway resistance. Abnormal enlargement of soft tissues can further narrow or occlude the airway, and repetitive cessations of breathing (apnea) may occur during sleep.

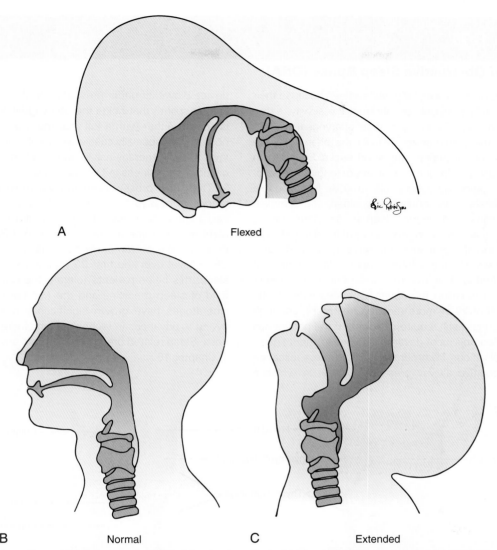

A   Flexed

B   Normal   C   Extended

Figure 1-5 Head position affects airway patency. **A,** A flexed head may occlude the airway. **B,** The normal position of the head and neck. **C,** An extended head aligns the oral cavity and pharynx with the trachea, opening the airway and facilitating intubation. (Modified from Scanlan CL, Spearman CB, Sheldon RL: *Egan's fundamentals of respiratory care,* ed 6, St Louis, 1995, Mosby.)

Larynx

The larynx is a cartilaginous, cylindrical structure that acts as a valve on top of the trachea. The larynx is sometimes called the voice box because it contains the vocal cords that control the size of the opening into the trachea (**glottis [rima glottidis]**). The main cartilage of the larynx in the middle of the neck is the thyroid cartilage, sometimes called the Adam's apple, which is easily palpable in men.

The larynx lies at the level of the fourth through sixth cervical vertebrae in men and is located higher in women and children. The top portion of the larynx is a complex triangular box that is flat posteriorly and composed of an intricate network of cartilages, ligaments, and muscle (Figure 1-6). A mucous membrane continuous with the mucous membrane of the pharynx and trachea lines the interior of the larynx. Nine cartilages (three paired and three unpaired) and many muscles and ligaments form the larynx. The unpaired **epiglottis** is a thin, flat, leaf-shaped cartilage above the glottis. The lower end of the epiglottis

(a long, narrow stem) is attached to the thyroid cartilage. From this attachment, it slants upward and posteriorly to the base of the tongue, where its upper free end is broad and rounded (see Figures 1-3 and 1-6). A vascular mucous membrane covers the epiglottis. The lower base of the tongue is attached to the upper epiglottis by folds of mucous membrane, forming a small space (the vallecula) between the epiglottis and tongue (Figure 1-7). The vallecula is an important landmark used during the insertion of a tube into the trachea (intubation).

Besides speech, the major function of the larynx is preventing the lower airway from aspirating solids and liquids during swallowing and breathing. The epiglottis does not seal the airway during swallowing.[5] Instead, the upward movement of the larynx toward the base of the tongue pushes the epiglottis downward, which causes it to divert food away from the glottis and into the esophagus. The free portion of the upper epiglottis in an adult lies at the base of the tongue, but in a newborn it lies much higher, behind the soft palate. This position of the upper epiglottis helps

Treatment of Obstructive Sleep Apnea (OSA)

Individuals with OSA stop breathing while asleep because their pharyngeal soft tissues repetitively obstruct the airway, either partially or completely. Sleep decreases pharyngeal muscle tone, increasing the tendency to obstruct the pharyngeal airway, especially in obese people with short necks. People with receding lower jaws (retrognathia) or large tongues (macroglossia) are also especially susceptible to OSA. Most people with OSA are obese, snore loudly during sleep, and complain of daytime sleepiness and fatigue. Sleep studies performed in diagnostic laboratories for sleep-related breathing disorders are required to confirm the presence and severity of OSA. OSA severity is determined by the number of apneas (absent airflow) and hypopneas (reduced airflow) that occur per hour of sleep; this measurement is called the apnea-hypopnea index (AHI). Generally, an AHI of 20 or more requires treatment, although an AHI of only 5 might still require treatment if the patient has heart failure and complains of daytime sleepiness and fatigue.

The most efficacious treatment of OSA is the application of continuous positive airway pressure (CPAP), in which a

device blows air under pressure into the nostrils; this acts as an "air splint" that holds the pharyngeal airway open.[4] CPAP is applied either with a full face mask or directly through the nostrils with specially cushioned nasal prongs called "nasal pillows." CPAP therapy has been shown to substantially reduce daytime drowsiness in OSA patients.

The CPAP pressure required for most patients with OSA ranges from 6 to 12 cm H_2O. Sleep studies usually require two nights—one night to document the AHI and another night to determine the optimal level of CPAP. Modern CPAP devices have a "ramp" feature that gradually increases the CPAP level over the first 30 minutes as the patient tries to sleep; this helps patients tolerate the procedure better. The field of sleep medicine and the number of diagnostic sleep laboratories have grown significantly over the last decade owing to advances in technology and increased public awareness. Sleep related breathing disorders are discussed in detail in Chapter 15.

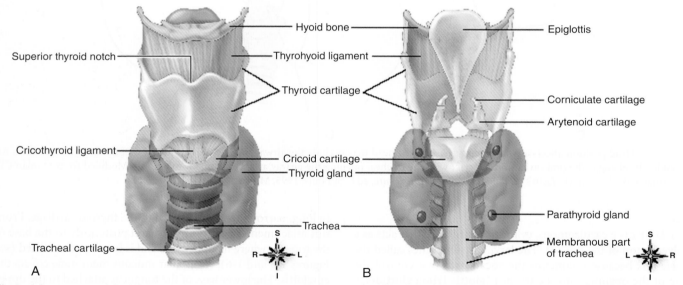

Figure 1-6 Anatomy of the larynx. **A,** Anterior view. **B,** Posterior view. (From Patton KT, Thibodeau GA: *Anatomy & physiology*, ed 7, St. Louis, 2010, Mosby.)

to account for preferential nose breathing in newborns and why it is difficult to achieve effective deposition of inhaled aerosolized medications in the lower airways of a newborn.[6]

The vascular mucous membrane covering the epiglottis may become swollen and enlarged if inflamed by infectious agents or mechanical trauma. A swollen epiglottis may severely obstruct or occlude the laryngeal air passage of a small newborn. Inflammation of the epiglottis (**epiglottitis**) is a life-threatening emergency in infants and requires immediate placement of an artificial airway by skilled medical personnel.

The thyroid cartilage is the largest of all laryngeal cartilages, enclosing the main cavity of the larynx anteriorly (see Figure 1-6). The lower epiglottis attaches just below the notch on its inside upper anterior surface.

The cricoid cartilage, just below the thyroid, is the only complete ring of cartilage that encircles the airway in the larynx or trachea. The cricothyroid ligament connects the cricoid and thyroid cartilages (see Figure 1-6). The cricoid limits the endotracheal tube size that can pass through the larynx. The cricoid ring is the narrowest portion of the upper airway in an

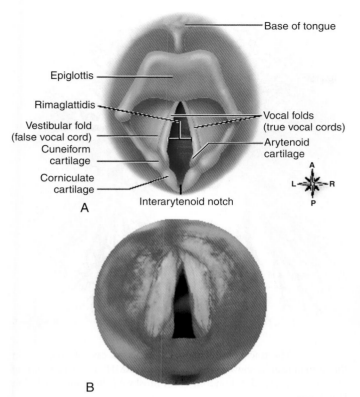

Base of tongue
Epiglottis
Rimaglattidis
Vestibular fold
(false vocal cord)
Cuneiform
cartilage
Corniculate
cartilage
Vocal folds
(true vocal cords)
Arytenoid
cartilage
Interarytenoid notch
A
B

Figure 1-7 Vocal cords, epiglottis, and glottis. **A,** Vocal cords viewed from above. **B,** Photographic view of the same structures. (*A,* from Patton KT, Thibodeau GA: *Anatomy & physiology,* ed 7, St. Louis, 2010, Mosby. *B,* Custom Medical Stock Photo Inc.)

infant. Inside the larynx, the vocal cords lie just above the cricoid cartilage.

The membranous space between the thyroid and cricoid cartilages, the cricothyroid membrane (see Figure 1-6), is sometimes the puncture site for an emergency airway opening when structures above it are occluded. A longer term surgical opening into the airway (**tracheostomy**) is generally located 1 to 3 cm below the cricoid cartilage.

The remaining cartilages (arytenoid, corniculate, and cuneiform) are paired. These cartilages are in the lumen of the larynx and serve as attachments for ligaments and muscles (see Figure 1-6). The arytenoids are attachment points for vocal ligaments that stretch across the lumen of the larynx and attach to the thyroid cartilage.

The vocal folds consist of two pairs of membranes that protrude into the lumen (inner cavity) of the larynx from the lateral walls (see Figures 1-3 and 1-7). The upper pair is called the false vocal cords; the lower pair is called the true vocal cords because only these folds play a part in vocalization. The true vocal folds form a triangular opening between them that leads into the trachea below. This opening is called the rima glottidis, or glottis (see Figure 1-7).

The vocal cords' ability to open and close the airway is essential for generating and releasing high pressure in the lung during a cough (an extremely important lung defense mechanism). Artificial airways such as endotracheal and tracheostomy tubes render a cough ineffective because they prevent the vocal cords from sealing the airway.

The vocal cords are wider apart during quiet inspiration than expiration. During deep inspiration, the vocal cords offer little airflow resistance. The glottis is the narrowest part of the adult larynx. Swelling (edema) of the vocal cords increases resistance to airflow, especially in an infant. Glottic and subglottic **edema** secondary to viral infections, also known as croup, is a common cause of upper airway obstruction in infants and young children. During inspiration, croup causes a characteristic high-pitched crowing sound called **stridor**. This sound is created by high-velocity air flowing through a narrowed glottis.

The laryngeal mucous membrane is composed of stratified squamous epithelium above the vocal cords and pseudostratified columnar epithelium continuous with the mucosa of the trachea below the vocal cords. Branches of the tenth cranial (vagus) nerve provide motor innervation for all intrinsic muscles of the larynx through the recurrent laryngeal nerve.

CLINICAL FOCUS 1-3

Seriousness of Airway Edema in Adults and Young Children

A 2-year-old boy is brought to the emergency department at 2:00 AM by his parents. The parents state that their son had been well until last evening. At that time, he complained of having a sore throat, experiencing pain while swallowing, and feeling hot. Later that night, his breathing became more rapid and labored. The parents then brought their son to the emergency department.

The boy arrives in the following condition: he is quiet, he is sitting upright and leaning forward and drooling, and he appears to be anxious. His temperature, heart rate, and respiratory rate are increased. He is reluctant to respond to questions; his voice sounds muffled. A lateral soft tissue x-ray of the neck shows that the epiglottis at the base of the tongue is extremely large and balloon-shaped, the classic "thumb" sign characteristic of epiglottitis. Is this a life-threatening problem for this child?

Discussion

The airway diameter of a small child is approximately half the diameter of an adult. Any amount of mucous membrane swelling in the child's airway narrows the diameter more than the same amount of swelling in the adult airway. One sign of upper airway swelling in children is stridor during inspiration. Stridor is caused by air vibrating as it moves through the narrowed glottis. In an adult, this swelling merely causes hoarseness and perhaps a sore throat. The same swelling nearly closes the smaller airway of a child. Drooling and muffled speech are more serious signs because they mean the epiglottis is so swollen that it prevents swallowing. Epiglottitis in a young child is a life-threatening emergency. A physician skilled in pediatric intubation must place an endotracheal tube into the trachea immediately to protect the airway from complete obstruction. This tube must remain in place until all signs of swelling subside.

This nerve passes downward around the aorta and returns upward to the larynx. Intrathoracic disease or surgery may injure this nerve, causing partial or complete paralysis of the vocal cords. Paralyzed vocal cords move to the midline, increasing airway resistance.[7] Sensory innervation of the larynx is also supplied by the vagus nerve except for the sensory nerves of the anterior surface of the epiglottis, which are supplied by the ninth cranial (glossopharyngeal) nerve. The laryngeal reflex, which has sensory and motor components in the vagus nerve, causes the vocal cords inside the larynx to close the tracheal opening (**laryngospasm**). Laryngospasm occurs if anything except air enters the trachea. Drowning victims often have little water in their lungs because of laryngospasm.

CONCEPT QUESTION 1-4

Why may removing an endotracheal tube (extubation) cause laryngospasm?

Lower Airways

The lower airways (airways below the larynx) divide in a pattern known as dichotomous branching, in which each airway divides into two smaller "daughter" airways. Each division or bifurcation gives rise to a new generation of airways. The branches of the trachea and bronchi resemble an inverted tree—hence the term "tracheobronchial tree" (Figure 1-8).

Trachea and Main Bronchi

The trachea begins at the level of the sixth cervical vertebra and in an adult extends for about 11 cm to the fifth thoracic vertebra. It divides there into the right and left mainstem bronchi, one for each lung (Figure 1-9). The point of division is called the **carina**. Inspired air becomes 100% saturated with water vapor and is warmed to body temperature (37° C) after it passes through two or three airway subdivisions below the carina[8]; the point at which this occurs is known as the **isothermic saturation boundary** (**ISB**) (Figure 1-10). Above the ISB, the temperature and humidity of gas in the airways fluctuates, decreasing with inspiration and increasing with exhalation. Below the ISB, gas temperature and humidity remain constant at body temperature and 100% relative humidity. Cold air or mouth breathing moves the ISB deeper into the airways but never by more than a few generations.

The anterior (ventral) part of the trachea is formed primarily by 8 to 20 regularly spaced, rigid, horseshoe-shaped cartilages. Stretched across the open posterior ends of the tracheal cartilages, the ligamentous membrane forms a flat dorsal surface contacting the esophagus (see Figures 1-6, *B*, and 1-9). This membrane contains horizontally oriented smooth muscle, the trachealis. Contraction of the trachealis pulls the ends of the horseshoe-shaped cartilages closer together, slightly narrowing the trachea and making it more rigid. Rigidity of the trachea is important for preventing collapse from external pressure, especially during vigorous coughing. Coughing exerts a collapsing force only on the part of the trachea inside the thoracic cavity, the part below about the sixth tracheal cartilage.[7] Above this level, the trachea is outside the thorax and not influenced by intrathoracic pressure.

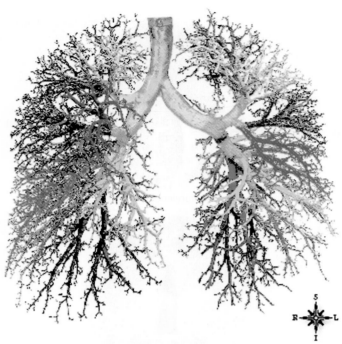

Figure 1-8 The tracheobronchial tree. A plastic cast of airspaces in the human lung is shown. (From McMinn RMH et al: *Color atlas of human anatomy*, ed 3, London, 1993, Mosby-Wolfe, Courtesy Ralph Hutchings.)

At the carina, the right mainstem bronchus angles only 20 to 30 degrees away from the midline, forming a more direct continuation of the trachea than the left mainstem bronchus. The left mainstem bronchus breaks away more sharply, forming a 45- to 55-degree angle with the vertical tracheal midline (see Figure 1-9). The left bronchus is smaller in diameter than the right but twice as long.

CONCEPT QUESTION 1-5

Foreign material aspirated into the trachea is more likely to enter which main bronchus? Why?

If an endotracheal tube is inserted too far during the process of intubation, its tip is more likely to enter the right bronchus than the left. If this occurs, the left lung cannot be ventilated, which the clinician can detect by using a stethoscope to compare the intensity of breath sounds between left and right sides of the chest while manually ventilating the lung. Diminished breath sounds on the left side of the chest in this context are associated with right mainstem bronchial intubation. It is a standard procedure to listen to breath sounds with a stethoscope (auscultation) immediately after intubation.

The cartilage of the mainstem bronchi resembles the cartilage of the trachea initially, except that cartilage completely surrounds the bronchi at their entry point into the lung tissue, and the posterior membranous portion disappears. As the bronchi continue to branch, the cartilage becomes more irregular and discontinuous, no longer encircling the airway in complete sections (see Figure 1-9).

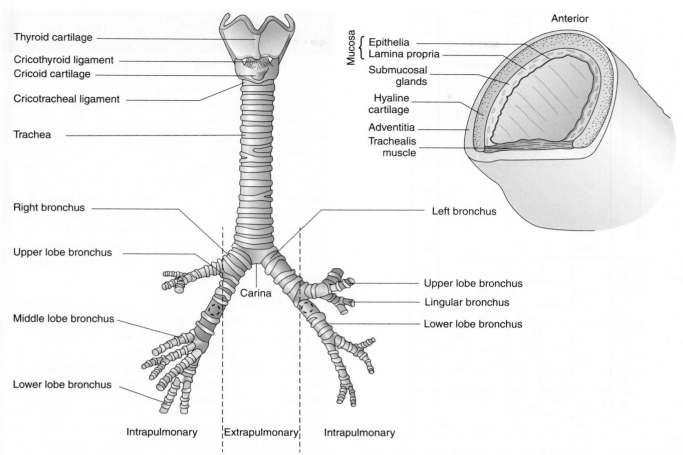

Figure 1-9 The trachea and mainstem, lobar, and segmental bronchi. The extrapulmonary-intrapulmonary boundary marks the point at which the mainstem bronchi penetrate the lung tissue. (Modified from Kacmarek et al: *Egan's fundamentals of respiratory care*, ed 10, St. Louis, 2012, Mosby.)

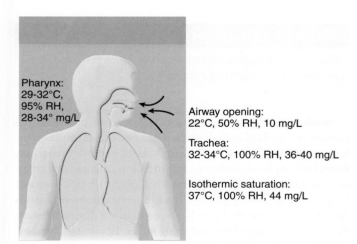

Figure 1-10 Normal temperature and humidity of inspired gas during spontaneous breathing at different points along the respiratory tract. *RH,* Relative humidity.

Conducting Airway Anatomy

All airways down to the level just before **alveoli** first appear are called conducting airways (Figure 1-11). No gas exchange between air and blood occurs across airway walls; they serve merely to conduct air to the alveoli—the gas-exchange surface of the lung. Beginning with the trachea, each of these conducting airways undergoes dichotomous branching until 23 to 27 subdivisions are formed.

The mainstem bronchi divide to form lobar bronchi, which undergo several divisions to form segmental and subsegmental bronchi. Segmental bronchial anatomy (Figure 1-12) is the basis for the application of chest physical therapy, in which a person is positioned for gravitational drainage of secretions from the various lung segments. Chest physical therapy is a respiratory therapy modality often used in treating lung diseases that produce large quantities of airway secretions.

Beyond the third generation of airway divisions, the bronchi enter the **parenchyma**, the essential supportive tissue composing the lung. Elastic fibers of the parenchyma surround and attach to the airways; their natural recoil forces act as tethers that hold the airways open during forceful exhalation. These tethering forces also limit the degree to which smooth muscle contraction (**bronchospasm**) can narrow the airway; diseases that weaken parenchymal recoil forces make the airways prone to more severe narrowing or collapse, especially during exhalation. The natural elastic recoil forces of the lung are extremely important in keeping the small, noncartilaginous airways open.

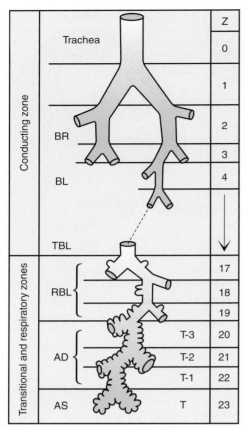

Figure 1-11 Branching of the conducting and terminal airways. Alveoli first appear in the respiratory bronchioles, marking the beginning of the respiratory or gas-exchange zone. *BR*, Bronchus; *BL*, bronchiole; *TBL*, terminal bronchiole; *RBL*, respiratory bronchiole; *AD*, alveolar duct; *AS*, alveolar space; *Z*, order of airway division. (Modified with permission from Springer Science+Business Media: Morphometry of the human lung, 1963, Weibel ER, Berlin, Springer-Verlag. Courtesy Ewald R. Weibel.)

The conducting airway subdivisions produce approximately 1 million terminal tubes at the level where alveoli (the gas-exchange units) first appear (see Figure 1-11). This enormously expansive branching gives rise to a massive increase in the cross-sectional area of the airways from the trachea (3 to 4 cm^2) to the alveolar surface (approximately 50 to 100 m^2—half the area of a tennis court—or about 40 times the surface area of the body).

A complex engineering design is required to distribute air uniformly and rapidly through millions of tubes of various lengths and diameters without creating too much frictional resistance to air movement. The design of the tracheobronchial tree is so efficient that an airflow rate of 1 L per second, commonly achieved during a resting inspiration, requires a pressure difference of less than 2 cm H_2O between the trachea and alveoli.

The volume of conducting airway gas must be relatively small so that most of the inhaled breath can contact the gas-exchange membrane. The volume of this gas (including the upper airways) is only about 150 mL in the average adult compared with a total inhaled volume per breath of about 500 mL. Because the conducting airways do not participate in gas exchange, they are called the anatomical **dead space**.

Absent Breath Sounds after Intubation

A 58-year-old man experiencing full cardiac arrest arrives in the emergency department. You insert an endotracheal tube into his trachea and ventilate the lungs with a hand-operated bag-and-valve device. You notice that a lot of pressure is required to put air into the patient's lungs. You also observe that the right and left sides of the chest do not rise evenly during ventilation. With your stethoscope, you auscultate the patient's chest and hear air entering the right lung but not the left lung. Based on your findings, you withdraw the endotracheal tube slightly and now hear equal breath sounds on both sides. You secure the endotracheal tube and ventilate the patient's lungs effectively.

Discussion

If you insert an endotracheal tube too far into the trachea, the tube may enter the right mainstem bronchus because it is more in line with the trachea than the left mainstem bronchus (see Figure 1-9). All air must then enter only the right lung, which explains why the inflation pressure was high when you first ventilated the patient's lungs. This also accounts for the unequal chest movement and lack of breath sounds from the left lung during ventilation. Proper positioning of the endotracheal tube is crucial to ensure equal ventilation to both lungs. Observing chest movement and listening to breath sounds are important initial ways to check for proper positioning of the endotracheal tube; proper placement is definitively confirmed with a chest x-ray film.

CONCEPT QUESTION 1-6

What general effect does endotracheal intubation have on the volume of anatomical dead space?

Bronchioles are airways less than 1 mm in diameter that contain no cartilage in their walls. Their patency depends on the tethering retractile forces of the lung's elastic parenchymal tissue. Bronchial and bronchiolar smooth muscle is oriented in a circular, spiral fashion, facilitating airway narrowing when it contracts (Figure 1-13). Strong smooth muscle contractions or spasms may nearly collapse the bronchioles, especially if disease weakens the lung's opposing elastic tethering forces. In contrast, tracheal smooth muscle is transversely oriented between the two ends of its horseshoe-shaped cartilages (see Figures 1-6, *B*, and 1-9).

At the nineteenth or twentieth generation, the **terminal bronchioles** divide to form several generations of respiratory bronchioles, marking the beginning of the respiratory, or gas-exchange, zone (see Figures 1-11 and 1-13). The respiratory bronchioles are tubes containing thin, saclike pouches called alveoli in their walls. Alveoli are the gas-exchange membranes that separate air from pulmonary capillary blood. Alveolar ducts open into

CLINICAL FOCUS 1-5

Airway Anatomy and Drainage of Lung Secretions

The chest radiograph of your patient with CF reveals an area of **atelectasis** in the right middle lobe of the lung; mucous plugging of the airway is suspected. In addition, your patient has a noisy, moist-sounding cough that produces thick secretions. Auscultating the patient's chest with your stethoscope, you hear moist, bubbling sounds (rhonchi) over the right middle lobe.

You decide to use gravitational drainage to help mobilize the patient's secretions. With the help of Figure 1-12, decide which position would best drain secretions out of the right middle lobe.

Discussion

In Figure 1-12, the right middle lobe includes the medial and lateral segments, and these lie inferior to (below) the large airways. Therefore, a position in which the patient lies on the left side with the head lower than the feet makes the best use of gravity to move secretions from the right middle lung segments.

Because the right middle lobe bronchus projects in a downward and anterior direction, rolling the patient partly back and propping the back with a pillow aligns the middle lobe bronchus in an even more vertical position. This drainage position allows the patient to cough up secretions more easily and aids in the resolution of pneumonia.

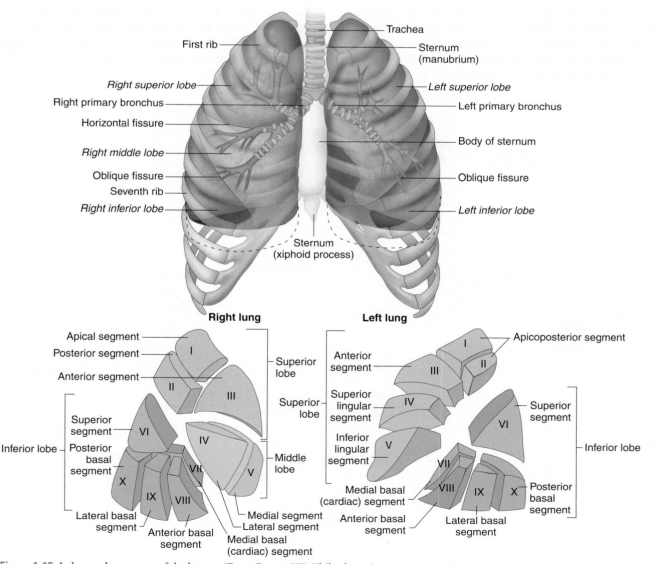

Figure 1-12 Lobes and segments of the lungs. (From Patton KT, Thibodeau GA: *Anatomy & physiology*, ed 7, St. Louis, 2010, Mosby.)

blind terminal units called alveolar sacs and alveoli. The airways beyond the terminal bronchiole are collectively called the **acinus**, which is the functional respiratory unit of the lung (i.e., all alveoli are contained in the acinus) (see Figure 1-13). In other words, each terminal bronchiole gives rise to an acinus.

Collateral air channels called **pores of Kohn** connect adjacent alveoli with one another (see Figure 1-13). The **canals of Lambert** connect terminal bronchioles and nearby alveoli. These collateral air passages make it possible for the acinus supplied by a mucus-plugged bronchiole to receive ventilation from neighboring airways and alveoli.

Sites of Airway Resistance

Dichotomous branching of the airways through many generations creates an enormous increase in the total airway cross-sectional area. Therefore, the velocity of airflow is sharply reduced as inspired gas approaches the alveoli. Flow velocity is so low in small, distal airways that molecular diffusion is the dominant mechanism of ventilation beyond the terminal bronchioles. Airways less than 2 mm in diameter account for only about 10% of total resistance to airflow because of their huge cross-sectional area (Figure 1-14). (Table 1-1 shows the relative size of airway cross sections at different levels.) Although the resistance of a single terminal bronchiole is greater than the resistance of a single lobar bronchus, the cross-sectional

area of all terminal bronchioles combined greatly exceeds the cross-sectional area of all the lobar bronchi combined. For this reason, upper airway resistance is normally much greater than lower airway resistance.

Conducting Airway Histology

A mucus-secreting epithelium (mucosa) lines the lumen of the conducting airways (Figure 1-15). A basement membrane beneath the epithelium separates it from the lamina propria below, which contains smooth muscle, elastic fibers, blood vessels, and nerves. The epithelium and lamina propria constitute the respiratory mucosa. Below the mucosa is the submucosa, which contains numerous mucous glands (submucosal glands) that have ducts leading to the epithelial luminal surface. A connective tissue sheath, the adventitia, surrounds cartilaginous airways and blood vessels. This sheath ends at the bronchioles; their airway walls are in direct contact with the lung parenchyma.

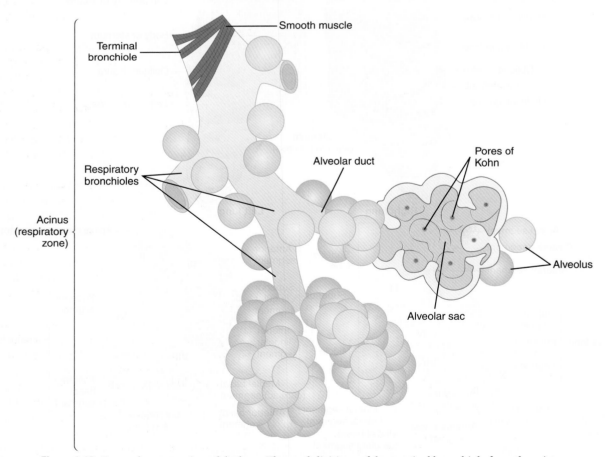

Figure 1-13 Gas-exchange portion of the lung. These subdivisions of the terminal bronchiole form the acinus.

The mucosal epithelium of the trachea and bronchi consists of tall, columnar, ciliated, pseudostratified epithelial cells interspersed with numerous mucus-secreting goblet cells (see Figure 1-15). The goblet cells and submucosal mucous glands secrete mucus onto the ciliated epithelial surface of the airways, forming a mucous blanket that is continually propelled upward in the direction of the pharynx. The submucosal glands contribute the greater volume of mucus; their secretion increases under the influence of parasympathetic nervous stimulation. All epithelial cells are attached to the basement membrane, but not all of them reach the airway lumen, and they appear to be stratified (see Figure 1-15)—hence the term "pseudostratified." Epithelial cells gradually flatten and lose their cilia as they proceed from bronchi to alveoli; cartilage disappears, and goblet cells gradually decrease in number and disappear (see Figure 1-15).

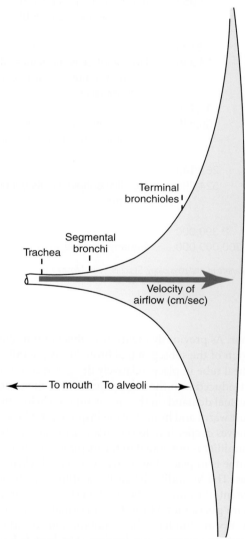

Figure 1-14 Distribution of airway cross-sectional area in the lung. The airways less than 2 mm in diameter collectively form a much larger cross-sectional area than the area formed by larger airways. Flow resistance of small airways is therefore less than flow resistance of large airways. (From Leff AR, Schumaker PT: *Respiratory physiology: basics and applications*, Philadelphia, 1993, Saunders.)

Other Epithelial Cells

Other bronchial epithelial cells include basal cells, serous cells, Kulchitsky cells, brush cells, Clara cells, and intermediate (or undifferentiated) cells. Serous cells may transform to goblet cells if chronically exposed to air pollutants, including cigarette smoke. Cigarette smoke causes all mucous cells to proliferate and spread into the small bronchioles, where they are usually absent. Cigarette smoke also ultimately reduces ciliary activity. Kulchitsky cells are endocrine cells more prominent in newborns than adults and are apparently precursors of carcinoids and small cell bronchogenic carcinomas.[9] Clara cells, found in the terminal and respiratory bronchioles, are nonciliated secretory cells bulging upward into the airway lumen. These cells are normally the sole source of secretions at this level because mucous cells are absent. Their secretions apparently also form part of the alveolar liquid lining. Injury to the epithelium at this level may cause the Clara cells to differentiate into ciliated or mucous cells.[9]

Mucociliary Clearance Mechanism

Each ciliated epithelial airway cell contains about 250 cilia beating about 1300 times per minute, moving the sheet of mucus toward the pharynx at a rate of approximately 2 cm per minute. The cilia have a rapid, forward, propulsive stroke, reaching up high into the viscous gel layer of mucus with their tips and pulling the mucous blanket up the airway. The recovery stroke is slower, and the flexible cilia bend as they are pulled backward (tips down) through the lower, less viscous sol layer of mucus (see Figure 1-15). The gel layer traps microbes and inhaled particles on its sticky surface.

Normal ciliary function and mucous composition are crucial for the effective function of this important lung clearance mechanism, often called the mucociliary escalator. It is the lung's main method for removing microbes and inhaled particles that have gained access to the bronchial tree. The combined actions of the mucociliary mechanism, a functional glottis that prevents aspiration, and an intact cough mechanism are remarkably effective in keeping the lower airways of healthy individuals sterile.[10]

Airway mucus is a viscoelastic, sticky substance; it has an elastic recoil property that facilitates **mucokinesis**, or mucous movement. When cilia pull the sheet of mucus forward, it stretches and then snaps forward in the direction of the pull. If the delicate balance between mucous water content and airway humidity is disrupted, the mucous sheet may become dehydrated, thick, and immobile. Conversely, overhydration causes mucus to become thin and watery, destroying the ciliary propulsive mechanism.

Approximately 100 mL of mucus is secreted per day in normal, healthy people. This volume greatly increases in individuals with acute and chronic airway inflammation. In chronic bronchitis, asthma, pneumonitis, and cystic fibrosis (CF), production of abnormally thick, sticky mucus is increased, impairing ciliary function and mucokinesis. Mucus builds up, partially blocks or plugs airways, and becomes a stagnant breeding ground for infectious microorganisms.

Ciliary disorders also impair mucous transport. Immotile cilia syndrome, also known as ciliary dyskinesia, is a genetic

TABLE 1-1

Subdivisions of the Respiratory Tree

Generation	Name	Diameter (cm)	Length (cm)	Number per Generation	Histological Notes
0	Trachea	1.8	12.0	1	Wealth of goblet cells
1	Primary bronchi	1.2	4.8	2	Right larger than left
2	Lobar bronchi	0.8	0.9	5	3 right, 2 left
3	Segmental bronchi	0.6	0.8	19	10 right, 8 left
4	Subsegmental bronchi	0.5	1.3	20	—
5	Small bronchi	0.4	1.1	40	Cartilage still a component; pseudostratified ciliated columnar respiratory epithelium
↓					
10		0.1	0.5	1020	
11	Bronchioles (primary and secondary)	0.1	0.4	2050	No cartilage; presence of smooth muscle, cilia, and goblet cells
↓					
13		0.1	0.3	8190	
14	Terminal bronchioles	0.1	0.2	16,380	No goblet cells; presence of smooth muscle, cilia, and cuboidal cells
15	Respiratory bronchioles	0.1	0.2	32,770	
16		0.1	0.2	65,540	No smooth muscle; cuboidal cell epithelium; cilia are sparse
↓					
18		0.1	0.1	262,140	
19	Alveolar ducts	0.05	0.1	524,290	No cilia; cuboidal cells become flatter
↓					
23		0.04	0.05	8,390,000	
24	Alveoli*	244	238	300,000,000	Squamous cells

Modified from Weibel ER: Morphometry of the human lung. In Martin DE, Youtsey JW, editors: *Respiratory anatomy and physiology,* St Louis, 1988, Mosby.
*Alveolar dimensions are given in micrometers.

disorder that causes a lack of normal beating activity. People with this syndrome are predisposed to multiple chronic respiratory infections that may eventually cause bronchiectasis, a disease process that weakens and dilates bronchial walls. This disease causes permanent anatomical airway dilations that tend to collect secretions, which become infected, creating further airway damage.

Importance of Humidity. Normally, the upper airways—the nose, pharynx, and trachea—heat and humidify inspired air. However, when an artificial airway such as an endotracheal tube (see Figure 1-4) is in place, these functions are completely bypassed. The addition of supplemental heat and humidity becomes critically important. The temperature of normal room air is about 22° C and has a relative humidity of about 50%, equivalent to a water vapor content of about 10 mg per liter of air (see Figure 1-10). During normal quiet breathing, inspired air warms to body temperature (37° C) and achieves 100% relative humidity soon after it passes the bifurcation of the trachea. Under these conditions, each liter of air contains about 44 mg of water vapor. As previously mentioned, this point in the airway, in the region of the subsegmental bronchi,[8] is the ISB. With an endotracheal tube in place, relatively dry gas at room temperature is introduced into the trachea just above the carina, placing an unusual demand on the airway mucosa below this point, which must warm and humidify the inspired air. Consequently, the ISB moves deeper into lower airway generations. If supplemental humidity is not added to the inspired air when an endotracheal tube is in place, lower airway mucus thickens as water evaporates. The humidity deficit is the difference between the water content of room air (about 10 mg/L) and saturated body temperature gas (about 44 mg/L). Abnormally thick mucus in the lower airways hinders ciliary motion and the efficiency of the mucociliary clearance mechanism. The lung is less able to remove contaminants and becomes susceptible to infections as mucus becomes immobile and consequently builds up. If airways become completely plugged with mucus, their downstream alveoli receive no ventilation and cannot impart oxygen to the blood.

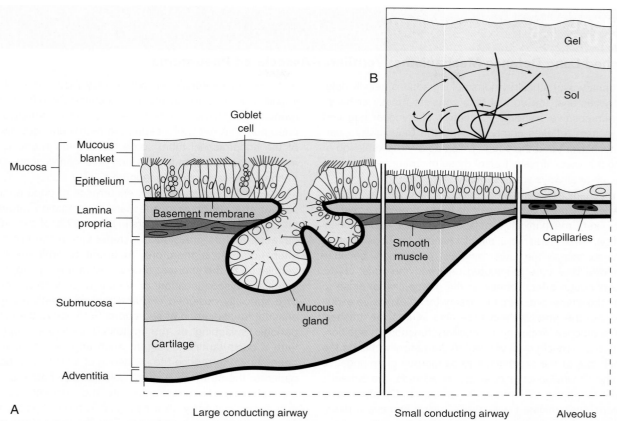

Figure 1-15 A, Respiratory mucosal epithelium. Most airways contain ciliated, pseudostratified columnar epithelium. **B,** Detail of ciliary action. Cilia reach up into the gel mucous layer during the forward propulsive stroke, withdrawing and retracting in the sol layer.

Nonepithelial Cells in the Airway

Inflammation of the lung causes various white blood cells such as **eosinophils** and neutrophils to enter the airways. Allergic asthma, a chronic inflammatory airway disease, is associated with increased eosinophils in airway secretions. Bacterial infections cause neutrophils, sometimes called pus cells, to migrate into the airways where they engulf or phagocytize the bacteria. The resulting cellular debris is a stringy, sticky, purulent (pus-containing) substance that increases mucus viscosity and impairs mucociliary transport.

Mast cells are located on the epithelial surface of the airways and in the airway walls near smooth muscle. Mast cells have granules in their cytoplasm that contain preformed inflammatory agents. These agents include histamine, various prostaglandins, leukotrienes, thromboxane, and platelet-activating factor. Besides increasing the permeability of mucosal epithelium to water, inflammation causes the mucosa to swell and smooth airway muscle to contract (bronchospasm).

Mast cells release their inflammatory agents when activated by a process called immune sensitization, which is common in people who have certain allergies. Inhaled irritants or antigens, such as ragweed pollen, cause the plasma B cells to synthesize immunoglobulin E (IgE), which is an abnormal response to the antigen (Figure 1-16). IgE first binds to specific receptor sites on the mast cell surface, sensitizing the mast cell. The antigen combines with IgE molecules attached to the surface of the

mast cell, which inactivates the antigen. However, in this process, the antigen cross-links two IgE molecules, which causes the mast cell membrane to rupture and release inflammatory agents into the airway tissues (see Figure 1-16). Histamine causes the normally tight, impermeable cell wall junctions of the airway epithelium to open, allowing it to penetrate deeply, breaking down more mast cells and creating more vascular leakage, mucosal swelling, and bronchospasm. Mast cell breakdown, airway inflammation, and subsequent bronchospasm are features of asthma, a condition characterized by chronic airway inflammation and hypersensitivity. Clinical Focus 1-7 discusses asthma and the basis for its pharmacological management.

Epithelial Chloride Channel Regulation and Secretion Viscosity

Water movement into the airway lumen is an osmotic process influenced by epithelial cell membrane secretion of chloride ions.[10] Chloride ions are secreted into the airway through specialized epithelial channels. Positively charged sodium ions follow the negatively charged chloride ions into the airway. Transmembrane secretion of ions provides the osmotic force for water flow into the airway lumen and plays a major role in hydrating the mucus and facilitating normal ciliary function. This mechanism is defective in cystic fibrosis (CF), a disease characterized by thick, immobile airway secretions (see Clinical Focus 1-8).

CLINICAL FOCUS 1-6

Breached Lung Defense Mechanisms: Ventilator-Associated Pneumonia

The oropharynx of a healthy nonsmoking adult is heavily colonized by bacteria; the normal flora consists mostly of harmless gram-positive bacteria. Protective pharyngeal gag and laryngospasm reflexes combined with the mucociliary clearance mechanism and the cough reflex do a remarkable job of keeping the lower airways free of these microbes—that is, the normal lower airways are essentially sterile.[12]

In mechanically ventilated critically ill patients, several factors lessen the effectiveness of these protective mechanisms. First, mechanical ventilation requires endotracheal intubation, which creates a direct channel for upper airway bacteria to access the lower airways. In addition, because the endotracheal tube is situated between the vocal cords, it thwarts cough effectiveness as the glottis cannot close to build up the airway pressure necessary for an explosive expulsion force. The endotracheal tube also injures the tracheal epithelial mucosa, impairing mucociliary function. In addition, intubation and mechanical ventilation dramatically change the bacterial flora of the oropharynx to dangerous gram-negative bacilli and *Staphylococcus aureus*;[13] in addition, the patient's immune response to bacteria is impaired. Oropharyngeal secretions contaminated with these microbes have a direct route through the vocal cords to the subglottic region of the trachea where they pool on top of the inflated endotracheal cuff. Even a properly inflated cuff cannot prevent the microaspiration of these bacteria-laden secretions past the cuff into the lower respiratory tract, where they may overwhelm the impaired defense mechanisms of a critically ill patient. Pneumonia often follows—hence the term "ventilator-associated pneumonia" (VAP). Considering the prominent causative role of the endotracheal tube, some researchers suggest that a more appropriate term for this kind of lung infection is "endotracheal tube–associated pneumonia."[13]

VAP is defined as the new occurrence of pneumonia in a patient after 48 hours of mechanical ventilation through an endotracheal tube. VAP occurs in 9% to 27% of all intubated patients, and its prevalence increases with the duration of intubation.[13] It is therefore important to limit mechanical ventilation to the shortest time possible through aggressive ventilator discontinuation or weaning protocols. The use of a specially designed endotracheal tube with a separate channel for aspiration of secretions from above the cuff and periodic swabbing of the intubated patient's oropharynx with a decontamination agent such as chlorhexidine have been shown to reduce the incidence of VAP.[14] In critically ill patients, the stomach is often colonized by bacteria, which can reflux up the esophagus into the pharynx, especially in a supine patient with a nasogastric tube in place; therefore, it is standard procedure to raise the head of the bed 30 degrees or more for mechanically ventilated patients. (A full discussion of the prevention of VAP is beyond the scope of this textbook.)

CLINICAL FOCUS 1-7

Physiological Consequences of Mucous Plugging

When airways become plugged with mucus, they no longer provide ventilation to downstream alveoli. The gas in these alveoli soon becomes absorbed by capillary blood flow, shrinking and eventually collapsing the alveoli (a condition called atelectasis). Blood flowing through (perfusing) these atelectatic alveoli can neither take up oxygen nor give up carbon dioxide; therefore, the composition of the blood remains unchanged as it passes through the lungs. This condition is called **intrapulmonary shunt**; blood is "shunted" as though it physically took a detour around the lungs. This shunted blood eventually mixes with the normally oxygenated blood from ventilated alveoli. Consequently, blood leaving the lung is low in oxygen (**hypoxemia**). The effectiveness of administering oxygen in this instance is reduced because oxygen cannot reach the blocked alveoli. Therapy is therefore focused on mobilizing and removing mucus.

Various neurohumoral and pharmacological agents regulate epithelial chloride channels. Among these agents are those that increase intracellular concentrations of cyclic adenosine monophosphate (cAMP).[10] Beta-adrenergic agonists increase intracellular cAMP levels, causing epithelial chloride channels to open and chloride secretion to increase. Increased levels of cAMP also cause smooth airway muscle relaxation and bronchodilation. Beta-adrenergic drugs, commonly administered for their bronchodilating properties, stimulate chloride secretion in normal airway cells.[10] This action may account for the enhanced mucociliary clearance observed clinically when beta-adrenergic bronchodilators are administered. (Chapter 2 discusses adrenergic receptors in more detail.)

Epithelium-Derived Relaxing Factor

Damaged or dysfunctional epithelial cells may be partly responsible for the smooth airway muscle hyperreactivity characteristic of diseases such as asthma. The normal epithelium generates

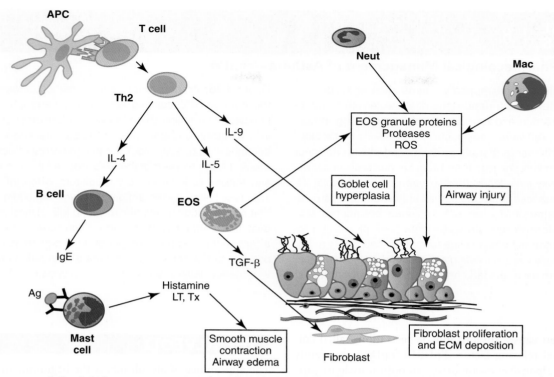

Figure 1-16 Spectrum of allergic inflammatory responses (see Clinical Focus 1-7 for discussion). *Ag,* Antigen; *APC,* antigen-presenting cell; *Th2,* T-helper 2 cell; *IL-4, IL-5, IL-9,* cytokines; *IgE,* immunoglobulin E; *EOS,* eosinophil; *LT,* leukotriene; *Tx,* thromboxane; *TGF-β,* transforming growth factor-beta; *Neut,* neutrophil; *Mac,* macrophage; *ROS,* reactive oxygen species; *ECM,* extracellular matrix. (From Jarjour NN, Kelly EA: *Med Clin North Am* 86[5]:925, 2002.)

CLINICAL FOCUS 1-8

Basis for Pharmacological Management of Asthma

Asthma is a chronic inflammatory lung disease characterized by abnormal airway responses to certain allergens and environmental irritants; the result is high resistance to airflow. Two distinct responses, a hyperreactive response and an inflammatory response, cause the patient to cough, wheeze, and experience chest tightness and shortness of breath. The hyperreactive response consists of abnormal sensitivity to inhaled allergens and irritants. The inflammatory response consists of immune reactions that injure the airway epithelium and cause it to swell and produce thick, sticky mucus. The high resistance to airflow in asthma is caused by three separate mechanisms: smooth muscle contraction (bronchospasm), mucous membrane swelling (mucosal edema), and increased mucus production. All of these mechanisms reduce airway diameter.

Ongoing airway inflammation is the major underlying defect in asthma, which can lead to permanent airway damage and structural remodeling. Remodeling occurs in response to chronic inflammation, which causes the eventual formation of fibrous tissue beneath the airway epithelium and an increase in the number (hyperplasia) of smooth muscle cells and mucous glands. In addition, chronic inflammation causes proteolytic damage

(breakdown of proteins) to the lung parenchyma, lessening its constraining tethering effect on airway narrowing.[11] Therefore, antiinflammatory drugs, such as inhaled corticosteroids, are first-line drugs for long-term maintenance and control of asthma. Quick-acting drugs that relax constricted smooth muscle (bronchodilators) are used as rescue drugs for emergency relief.

Figure 1-16 shows the spectrum of allergic inflammatory responses in asthma. Although mast cells are generally thought to be the major player in asthmatic reactions, many other cells are also involved in the inflammatory process. As Figure 1-16 shows, the allergic response begins when an inflammatory cell known as an antigen-presenting cell (APC) digests the antigen and presents it to a T-lymphocyte, one of the body's immune cells. The T-lymphocyte then produces T-helper 2 (Th2) cells, which produce inflammatory mediators known as cytokines: interleukin-4 (IL-4) stimulates plasma B cells to synthesize the antibody IgE, IL-5 causes eosinophil maturation and activation, and IL-9 promotes goblet cell hyperplasia and excessive mucus production. IgE molecules attach to the mast cell's surface, and when they are cross-linked by an antigen molecule, the mast cell membrane breaks

Continued

CLINICAL FOCUS 1-8

Basis for Pharmacological Management of Asthma—cont'd

down and releases inflammatory agents such as histamine, leukotrienes (LT), and thromboxane (Tx); the result is smooth muscle contraction and mucous membrane swelling (mucosal edema). Activated eosinophils produce inflammatory substances known as granule proteins, and along with neutrophils and macrophages, they produce protease enzymes and reactive oxygen species (toxic oxygen ions or radicals). All of these substances injure the airway epithelium and damage the lung's extracellular matrix.[11] Activated eosinophils also release transforming growth factor beta (TGF β), which promotes subepithelial fibrous tissue formation (see Figure 1-16).

Various drugs used in treating asthma work to block or inactivate one or more of the inflammatory pathways illustrated in Figure 1-16. Among other actions, corticosteroids decrease the number of circulating eosinophils, neutrophils, and lymphocytes and inhibit the synthesis of leukotrienes and other inflammatory mediators after mast cell breakdown. Leukotriene inhibitors directly block the inflammatory effects of leukotriene. Mast cell membrane stabilizers inhibit the breakdown and release of inflammatory mediators when IgE molecules are cross-linked by the antigen. Anti-IgE antibodies are drugs that reduce blood levels of circulating IgE; clinical studies suggest that therapy with this agent can have a major positive effect on the treatment of moderate to severe asthma and on patients at risk for serious asthma exacerbations that require emergency department visits or hospitalizations.[15]

---

a substance that causes smooth muscle relaxation, called epithelium-derived relaxing factor (EpDRF). EpDRF apparently modifies the responsiveness of airway smooth muscle to various stimuli. In theory, patients with damaged or dysfunctional airway epithelium do not produce EpDRF, and the response of the smooth muscle to various stimuli goes unchecked. Therefore, the airways are hyperreactive and prone to bronchospasm. EpDRF may help regulate smooth muscle tone by modifying autonomic neural impulses.[16]

CONCEPT QUESTION 1-8

Tobacco-induced release of protease enzymes may destroy elastic fibers surrounding small noncartilaginous airways; why does this affect small airway diameter?

Antiproteases in Lung Tissues and Airway Secretions

Airway secretions and lung tissues contain inhibitors of proteolytic enzymes, known as antiproteases. In people with chronic airway inflammation (patients with CF, chronic bronchitis, asthma, or **emphysema** and cigarette smokers), neutrophils invade the airways and release neutrophil elastase (NE), a powerful proteolytic enzyme.[17] NE is designed to destroy bacteria and other microorganisms that might be present in the airway; however, when it is chronically present, NE degrades elastin and collagen, which are major structural components of the healthy lung. Healthy people have natural antiproteases in the blood, lung tissues, and secretions, the major one being alpha$_1$ protease inhibitor (A1PI), also known as alpha$_1$-antitrypsin. Secretory leukoprotease inhibitor is another antiprotease found in healthy airway secretions, which, along with A1PI, protects the lung from the NE released during episodes of airway inflammation.[17] However, in chronic inflammatory lung conditions, NE overwhelms the antiproteases, and lung tissue damage occurs. Balance between the proteases and antiproteases is important for normal lung function.

THE ALVEOLI

The appearance of alveoli marks the beginning of the respiratory, or gas-exchange, zone. Alveoli first appear in the respiratory bronchioles (see Figure 1-13). The distance from the beginning to the end of the acinus is only a few millimeters, but most of the lung's volume is contained in acinar structures (about 3000 mL at rest). As mentioned, the conducting airways contain only about 150 mL of gas. The lungs of an adult contain about 300 million alveoli, representing a gas-exchange surface area of 50 to 100 m^2. Alveolar diameters range from 100 to 300 μ. Capillaries that are in contact with the alveolar membrane are only 10 to 14 μm in diameter, which is just large enough to allow the passage of red blood cells. These tiny capillaries are wrapped around the alveoli in an extremely dense network; each alveolus may be associated with up to 1000 capillary segments (Figure 1-17).

Alveolar Capillary Membrane

Alveolar epithelium has type I and type II cells (Figure 1-18). Type I cells constitute most of the alveolar surface and are extremely flat. Type II cells are compact, polygonal-shaped cells protruding into the alveolar airspace. The adjoining basement membranes of the alveolar epithelium and capillary endothelium form an extremely thin blood-air barrier, less than 0.5 μm thick in the flattest regions of the type I cell. The space between these membranes is the **interstitium**. The alveolar epithelium is highly permeable to respiratory gases, but the tight junctions between epithelial cells form an impermeable barrier to liquid solutions. Endothelial capillary cell junctions are loose and more permeable to water than alveolar epithelium (see Figure 1-18). Inhaled or circulating toxic agents may injure the alveolar capillary membrane, increasing its permeability, a major feature of **acute respiratory distress syndrome (ARDS)**.

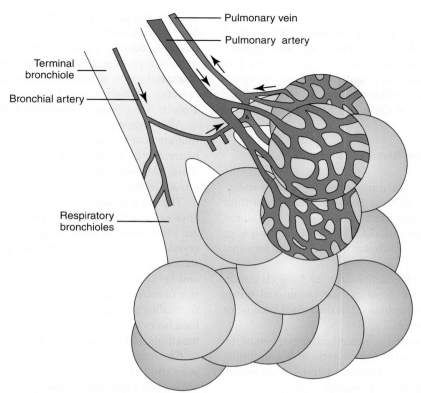

Figure 1-17 Pulmonary arteries carry deoxygenated blood (*blue*) to the capillary beds surrounding the alveoli. Oxygenated blood (*red*) flows out of these capillaries to the left atrium and ventricle, where it is pumped into the systemic circulation.

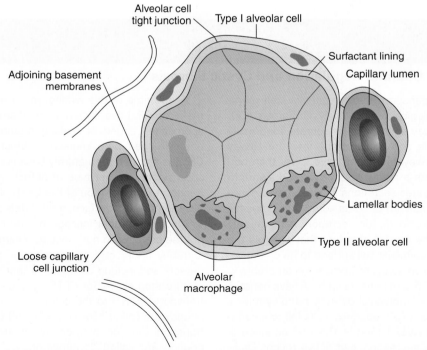

Figure 1-18 Alveolar and capillary membranes showing alveolar type I and type II cells. Lamellar bodies in type II cells are responsible for surfactant secretion.

Type II Cells and Surfactant Secretion

Type II cells have short, blunt projections (microvilli) on their alveolar surfaces and contain many internal organelles, including organelles known as lamellar bodies (see Figure 1-18). The lamellar bodies are the source of alveolar surfactant phospholipid, an agent that reduces surface tension and is essential for keeping the alveoli open. (See Chapter 3 for the properties of pulmonary surfactant.)

Alveolar Macrophages and Alveolar Clearance Mechanisms

Alveolar macrophages are large migratory phagocytes wandering freely throughout the alveolar airspaces and interstitium (see Figure 1-18). Their main function is to engulf and digest microorganisms and foreign material. The alveolar macrophage is the major lung clearance mechanism distal to the terminal bronchiole.

The acinus is the most ineffective area for lung clearance. Inorganic dusts such as coal or silica dust (from coal mines and stone quarries) tend to be retained in the acinus because of extremely slow clearance rates.

Alveolar macrophages in the acinus engulf foreign material (organic and inorganic), destroying bacteria and entrapping inorganic particles. Some phagocytized material is dissolved, and some is simply surrounded and isolated. Macrophages synthesize potent enzymes and oxidizing agents that kill bacteria, viruses, and fungi. These oxidizing agents are extremely lethal to microorganisms, even in small quantities. Enzyme systems in the macrophage chemically reduce oxygen in a stepwise fashion, generating large amounts of superoxide ions (O_2^-), hydrogen peroxide (H_2O_2), hydroxyl ions (OH^-), and ultimately water (H_2O). The mitochondria of other tissue cells produce minute quantities of these toxic oxygen radicals in the process of normal oxidative (aerobic) metabolism. However, these cells normally contain catalytic enzymes that speed up the oxygen reduction process, preventing accumulation of toxic radicals. Overproduction of these toxic oxygen radicals occurs in the presence of high inspired oxygen concentrations, leading to alveolar tissue injury, a condition known as oxygen toxicity.

After ingesting foreign matter, the macrophage may (1) migrate into the airways, where ciliary activity moves it to the pharynx; (2) migrate into the interstitial space and remain there; (3) enter the lymphatic system; or (4) simply die and remain in the alveolus.

The lung interstitium has the slowest macrophage clearance rate; particles carried to the interstitium by macrophages are most likely to cause lung tissue damage. Sharp inorganic crystals can damage and kill macrophages, releasing toxic substances, which attract cells called fibroblasts that synthesize and lay down collagen fibers over the area. Eventually, excessive fibrous tissue accumulates in the interstitium, and a condition called pulmonary interstitial fibrosis develops. The fibrous lung becomes stiff and difficult to inflate, increasing the work of breathing and impairing gas diffusion.

Cigarette smoke increases phagocytosis and the release of powerful proteases by macrophages and neutrophils (proteases are enzymes that can eventually degrade and destroy surrounding cellular protein and elastic tissue).[17] Although the lung normally contains protective antiprotease enzymes, these enzymes may be overwhelmed by the continual activation of alveolar macrophages and neutrophils caused by chronic smoking. A state of chronic inflammation and alveolar destruction develops, which is the primary feature of emphysema, an irreversible airway obstructive disease.

CLINICAL FOCUS 1-9

Defective Chloride Channel Regulation and Cystic Fibrosis

Defective chloride ion transport across epithelial cell membranes is a major pathological feature of cystic fibrosis (CF). In patients with CF, airway epithelial cells secrete abnormally low amounts of chloride and sodium ions into the airway lumen, which means airway secretions have lower than normal osmotic pressure. As a result, less water is drawn into the airway, which dehydrates secretions and impairs mucociliary clearance.[10] In patients with CF, beta-adrenergic drugs fail to bring about epithelial chloride ion secretion. A genetically mutated gene causes the protein structure that controls the chloride channel on the epithelial cell surface to be defective. In CF, this protein is known as cystic fibrosis transmembrane regulator (CFTR). About 75% of patients with CF have genetic-encoding errors that cause molecular defects in the synthesis or function of CFTR; as a result, epithelial cells fail to secrete chloride ions into the airway lumen.[18] The consequence is dehydrated, thick airway secretions; ineffective mucus clearance; mucous plugging of airways; and chronic lung infections.

At the time of this writing, major research efforts in treatment of CF have focused on pharmacological therapeutic approaches aimed at making mutant CFTR function properly.[19] In one type of molecular defect, the cell's synthesis of CFTR is stopped prematurely because of an improper genetic code signal; another type of defect causes improper folding, transport, and insertion of the CFTR protein into the epithelial cell membrane's surface; a third defect allows CFTR proteins to reach the proper location on the cell membrane surface, but the proteins do not function. Pharmacological compounds currently under clinical investigation address each of these defects and include compounds that (1) "read through" premature stop codes for CFTR synthesis, (2) properly fold and transport CFTR into the cell membrane surface (these compounds are called "correctors"), and (3) improve the chloride transport function of properly situated CFTRs (these compounds are called "potentiators").[18] Ongoing clinical trials have shown promising results.[19,20]

- The lower airways are normally well protected by the ability of the upper airways to filter, warm, and humidify inspired gas.
- Artificial heat and humidity must be supplied to artificial airways that bypass the upper airways to prevent dried, thickened secretions.
- Respiration, or gas exchange between air and blood, occurs only in alveoli; all other airspaces in the lung are known as conducting airways.
- Mucociliary clearance is a major mechanism whereby the lung is kept free of foreign material and infectious microorganisms; the lower airways are normally sterile.
- A functional larynx is essential for preventing aspiration and allowing an effective cough.
- Because of their great number and large combined cross-sectional area, small airways offer less resistance to airflow than large airways.
- Asthma is a condition in which the airway epithelium is chronically inflamed and hypersensitive to various stimuli; antiinflammatory drugs are first-line drugs in the long-term control of asthma.
- Small noncartilaginous airways are kept open by the tethering forces of the surrounding elastic lung tissue, which normally limit the extent to which bronchospasm narrows the airways.
- Rigid cartilage keeps the large airways patent.
- Surfactant, secreted by alveolar type II cells, prevents surface tension forces from collapsing the alveoli.

References

1. Clemente CD, editor: *Gray's anatomy*, ed 30, Philadelphia, 1985, Lea & Febiger.
2. Van Cauwenberge P, et al: Anatomy and physiology of the nose and paranasal sinuses, *Immunol Allergy Clin North Am* 24(1):1, 2004.
3. Dolovich M: Clinical aspects of aerosol physics, *Respir Care* 36(9):931, 1991.
4. Pien GW, Pack AI: Sleep disordered breathing. In Mason RJ, et al, editors: *Murray and Nadel's textbook of respiratory medicine*, ed 5, Philadelphia, 2010, Saunders.
5. Balkissoon RC, Baroody FM, Togias A: Disorders of the upper airways. In Mason RJ, et al, editors: *Murray and Nadel's textbook of respiratory medicine*, ed 5, Philadelphia, 2010, Saunders.
6. Amirav I, et al: Factors that affect the efficacy of inhaled corticosteroids for infants and young children, *J Allergy Clin Immunol* 125(6):1206, 2010.
7. Chen EY, Inglis AF Jr: Bilateral vocal cord paralysis in children, *Otolaryngol Clin North Am* 41(5):889, 2008.
8. McFadden ER Jr, et al: Thermal mapping of the airways in humans, *J Appl Physiol* 58(2):564, 1985.
9. Ettinger DS: Lung cancer and other pulmonary neoplasms. In Goldman L, Ausiello D, editors: *Cecil textbook of medicine*, ed 23, Philadelphia, 2007, Saunders.
10. Folkesson HG, Matthay MA: Alveolar and distal airway epithelial fluid transport. In Mason RJ, et al: *Murray and Nadel's textbook of respiratory medicine*, ed 5, Philadelphia, 2010, Saunders.
11. Schellenberg RR, Seow CY: Airway smooth muscle and related extracellular matrix in normal and asthmatic lung. In Adkinson NF, et al, editors: *Middleton's allergy: principles and practice*, ed 7, Philadelphia, 2008, Mosby.
12. Safdar N, Christopher CJ, Maki DG: The pathogenesis of ventilator-associated pneumonia: its relevance to developing effective strategies for prevention, *Respir Care* 50(6):725, 2005.
13. Pneumatikos IA, Dragoumanis CK, Bouros DE: Ventilator-associated pneumonia or endotracheal tube-associated pneumonia? *Anesthesiology* 110(3):673, 2009.
14. Deem S, Treggiari MM: New endotracheal tubes designed to prevent ventilator-associated pneumonia: do they make a difference? *Respir Care* 55(8):1046, 2010.
15. Niven R: Effectiveness of omalizumab in patients with inadequately controlled severe persistent allergic asthma: an open-label study, *Respir Med* 102:1371, 2008.
16. Barnes PJ: Pathophysiology of allergic inflammation. In Adkinson NF, et al: *Middleton's allergy: principles and practice*, ed 7, Philadelphia, 2008, Mosby.
17. Shapiro SD, Reilly JJ, Rennard SI: Chronic bronchitis and emphysema. In Mason RJ, et al: *Murray and Nadel's textbook of respiratory medicine*, ed 5, Philadelphia, 2010, Saunders.
18. Zemanick ET, et al: Measuring and improving respiratory outcomes in cystic fibrosis lung disease: opportunities and challenges to therapy, *J Cyst Fibrosis* 9(1):1, 2010.
19. Cuthbert A: New horizons in the treatment of cystic fibrosis, *Br J Pharmacol* 163(1):173, 2011.
20. Sears EH, Gartman EJ, Casserly BP: Treatment options for cystic fibrosis: state of the art and future perspectives, *Rev Recent Clin Trials* 6(2):94, 2011.

CHAPTER 2

The Lungs and Chest Wall

OBJECTIVES

After reading this chapter, you will be able to:
- Differentiate between the lobes and segments of the right and left lungs
- Explain why the pleural membranes normally have a subatmospheric pressure between them and the way in which this subatmospheric pressure is related to lung volume
- Describe why the systemic bronchial circulation in the lungs prevents alveolar gas and arterial blood oxygen pressures from being equal
- Explain why sympathetic stimulation, parasympathetic stimulation, and nonadrenergic noncholinergic nerve stimulation cause different effects in the lung

- List the neuronal effects a drug must have to elicit bronchodilation
- Describe the essential components of an effective cough and factors that impair cough effectiveness
- Identify which spinal cord levels correlate with diaphragmatic muscle function
- Discuss the assessment of abnormally high respiratory efforts by inspecting the chest
- Explain the functional difference between primary and accessory muscles of ventilation

KEY TERMS

adrenergic
anastomoses
angle of Louis
cardiac notch
C-fibers
cholinergic fibers)
costal parts
costophrenic
crura
diaphragm
dyspnea
ganglion (*pl.*, ganglia)
Hering-Breuer reflex
hilum
intercostal retractions

J-receptors
lingula
manubrium
mediastinum
nitric oxide synthase (NOS)
nonadrenergic noncholinergic (NANC) nerves
P(A-a)O_2 (alveolar-to-arterial oxygen pressure difference)
parietal pleura
pectoralis major
phrenic nerves
pleural effusion
pneumothorax
postganglionic fibers
preganglionic fibers
rapidly adapting receptors (RARs)

slowly adapting receptors (SARs)
sternomastoids
thoracentesis

thorax
visceral pleura
xiphoid process

THE LUNGS AS ORGANS

The inflated lungs are conical; the upper part is the rounded apex, and the lower concave part is the base (Figure 2-1). The costal (rib) surface of the lungs is smooth and convex and adjoins the inner chest wall. The surfaces adjoining the **mediastinum** are concave; the mediastinum is the central portion of the chest cavity containing the heart, aorta, esophagus, great veins, trachea, and mainstem bronchi.

Figure 2-1 shows that the apices of the lung extend above the clavicles into the base of the neck, with their top borders lying at the level of the first thoracic vertebra. The anterior border of the left lung forms the **cardiac notch**, which accommodates protrusion of the heart into the left half of the thoracic cavity.

CONCEPT QUESTION 2-1

The volume of the left lung is slightly less than the volume of the right lung. Explain the reason for this difference.

The lung bases rest on the **diaphragm**, the major muscle of ventilation, which consists of two distinct, separately innervated muscles—the left and right hemidiaphragms. The diaphragm separates the thoracic and abdominal cavities, bowing deeply upward into the thoracic cavity (see Figures 2-1 and 2-9, *A*). The concave lung bases fit over the domes of the diaphragm. When the body is at rest, the outer margins of the lung's bases lie at the level of the tenth thoracic vertebra; however, the highest points of their concave diaphragmatic surfaces bow up to the level of the eighth to ninth thoracic vertebra. The left hemidiaphragm surface is slightly lower than the right hemidiaphragm surface because (1) the heart rests on the left half of the diaphragm, pushing it downward, and (2) the liver, situated in the abdominal cavity directly below the right half of the diaphragm, props up this area (see Figure 2-1).

The area on the lung's mediastinal surfaces through which arteries, veins, and the main bronchus enter is called the **hilum** and can be thought of as the "root" of the lung (Figure 2-2). The pulmonary ligament just below the hilum connects the membrane that covers the lung's surface with the diaphragm below. The hilar structures and pulmonary ligament suspend and stabilize the lungs in the chest cavity. A thin anterior portion of the upper lobe of the left lung overlaps the heart and continues downward to a narrow point, forming the **lingula**, the tongue-like anatomical counterpart of the middle lobe of the right lung (see Figure 2-2).

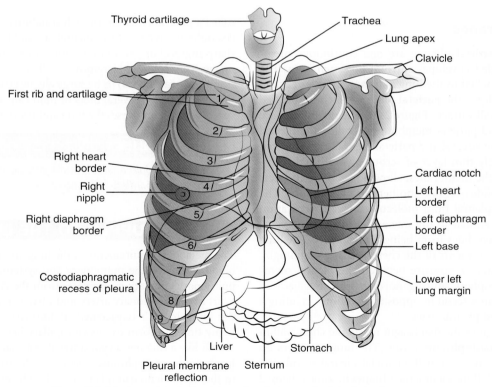

Figure 2-1 The lungs in relationship to the rib cage and other thoracic structures.

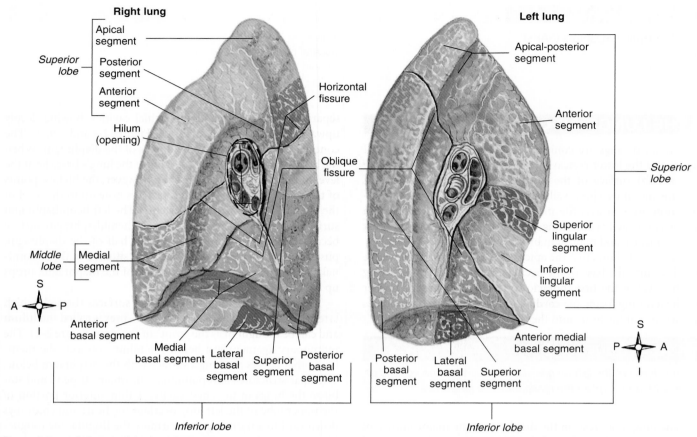

Figure 2-2 Medial view of the lungs. The hilum is the entry point for the mainstem bronchi and major blood vessels. The lingula of the left lung corresponds with the middle lobe of the right lung. (From Thibodeau GA, Patton KT: *Anatomy & physiology*, ed 3, St Louis, 1996, Mosby.)

Pleural Membranes

The visceral and parietal pleurae are one continuous membrane, forming sealed envelopes surrounding each lung. The **visceral pleura**, attached to the lung's surface, doubles back at the hilar region to form the **parietal pleura**, which is attached to the inner chest wall surface (Figure 2-3). The potential space between visceral and parietal membranes is called the pleural space. Normally, the visceral and parietal pleurae are separated only by an extremely thin layer of serous pleural fluid. Pleural fluid lubricates the membranes, allowing nearly frictionless movement as they slide over one another during breathing. The cohesive forces of pleural fluid molecules prevent separation of the membranes, similar to the way a film of water prevents two glass microscope slides from being pulled apart. The lung passively follows movements of the chest wall and diaphragm. Intrapleural pressure, or pressure between the pleural membranes, is subatmospheric during normal breathing because the chest wall and lung recoil in opposite directions, creating a vacuum in the sealed pleural space.

The lowest margin of the diaphragm meets the chest wall in an area called the **costophrenic** recess. The lung's borders do not extend into this recess, but the parietal pleural membrane does (see Figure 2-1). If the pleural membranes become inflamed by disease, fluid may form in the pleural space, creating what is called a **pleural effusion**; in such situations, fluid settles into the costophrenic recess of the pleural space, blunting the normally sharp angles of the costophrenic junctions as seen on a chest x-ray image. This fluid can be removed with a syringe and large-gauge needle (**thoracentesis**) or by surgically inserting a chest tube into the pleural cavity; several liters of fluid can collect in the pleural space, which compresses the lung and restricts its expansion.

CONCEPT QUESTION 2-2

What effect would a large pleural effusion have on the pressure required to inflate the lungs?

BLOOD SUPPLY TO THE LUNGS

The metabolic requirements of the lung are met by two separate blood supplies—the pulmonary and systemic circulations. The pulmonary circulation originates from the right ventricle of the heart as the pulmonary artery and carries oxygen-poor blood to the lungs to be reoxygenated. Pulmonary arterioles subdivide many times to form extensive capillary beds that surround the alveoli like a fine net. Beyond the alveoli, capillaries converge to form venules and pulmonary veins, which carry oxygenated blood to the heart's left atrium (Figure 2-4). The entire cardiac output flows through the pulmonary circulation and its fine capillary

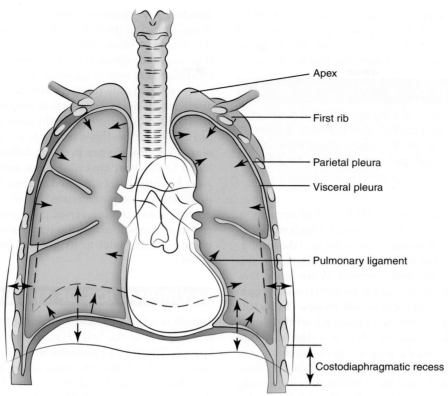

Figure 2-3 The visceral and parietal pleural membranes form a sealed envelope around each lung. *Single arrows* represent retractive lung recoil. *Double arrows* represent dimensional changes between deep inspiration and expiration. (Modified from Fishman AP: *Assessment of pulmonary function*, New York, 1980, McGraw-Hill.)

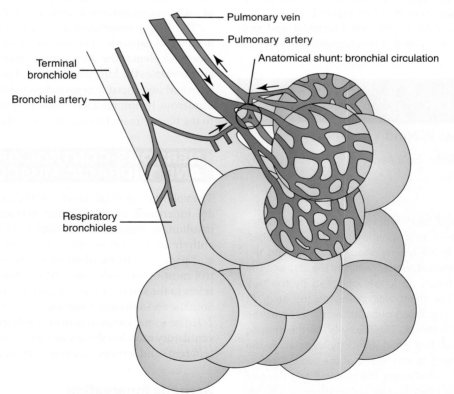

Figure 2-4 Bronchial and pulmonary circulations. Interconnections between systemic bronchial veins and pulmonary veins allow deoxygenated bronchial venous blood flow (*blue*) to merge with oxygenated pulmonary venous blood flow (*red*). This anatomical shunt causes blood entering the left atrium to have a lower oxygen pressure than alveolar gas.

network; in this way, the pulmonary capillaries act as a kind of filter through which all blood flow must pass. The main function of this circulation is to bring blood into contact with alveolar gas so that oxygen and carbon dioxide exchange (respiration) can occur.

CONCEPT QUESTION 2-3

A person with a large bruise in a leg muscle or a person who remains stationary for long periods during a transcontinental airplane journey is at risk for developing blood clots in the deep leg veins. Why are such persons also at risk for developing a pulmonary embolus?

The lung's systemic blood supply, the bronchial circulation, arises from the aorta as the bronchial arteries, which supply all of the airway walls from the major bronchi down to the respiratory bronchioles. In contrast to the pulmonary circulation, it is only a small fraction of the cardiac output. When blood flow passes through the capillary beds of the bronchial wall, oxygen diffuses out of the blood into airway wall tissues. On leaving the capillaries, this oxygen-poor blood takes at least two different courses: (1) one third to one fourth of it is channeled into the true bronchial veins into the azygos vein and then into the heart's right atrium and (2) the remaining two thirds to three fourths of it drains directly into the pulmonary veins, mixing oxygen-poor bronchial venous blood directly with the freshly oxygenated blood of the pulmonary veins. This mixing reduces the overall oxygen content of the pulmonary venous blood that enters the left atrium, which the left ventricle eventually pumps into the systemic arterial circulation (see Figure 2-4).

These vascular connections between bronchial and pulmonary circulations are called bronchopulmonary-arterial

CLINICAL FOCUS 2-1

Penetrating Chest Wound

Consider the events following a penetrating chest wall injury such as a stab wound.

Discussion

A penetrating chest wall injury breaks the pleural seal, opening the pleural space to atmospheric pressure. The subatmospheric pressure in the pleural space sucks air into the chest, creating a **pneumothorax**, or air in the thorax. The lungs' inward recoil force, no longer opposed by the outward recoil force of the chest wall, collapses the lung. At the same time, the unopposed outward recoil force of the chest wall expands the thorax. This injury is life-threatening because the individual has great difficulty ventilating the lung. Depending on the size and nature of the wound, reflex muscle spasms may partially seal the opening and prevent total lung collapse. The treatment for pneumothorax is placement of a chest tube into the pleural space and application of suction to remove the air and reexpand the lung.

anastomoses, which constitute part of the normal "anatomical shunt" found in the pulmonary circulation. Shunting refers to the mixing of unoxygenated blood with oxygenated blood. In this case, unoxygenated venous blood from the bronchial circulation mixes with oxygenated blood in the pulmonary veins, which is eventually pumped into the aorta and the systemic arteries. This normal anatomical shunting means that systemic arterial blood can never have the same partial pressure of oxygen as alveolar gas; this gives rise to the normal **P(A-a)O$_2$ (alveolar-to-arterial oxygen pressure difference)**. Vessels carrying blood to the heart are called veins, and vessels carrying blood away from the heart are called arteries. In the systemic circulation, arteries carry oxygenated blood, and veins carry deoxygenated blood; this is reversed in the pulmonary circulation. In common medical usage, the terms arterial blood and venous blood generally refer to oxygenated blood and deoxygenated blood.

LYMPHATICS OF THE LUNG

Lymph is a clear, protein-containing fluid found in the interstitial spaces of the body (i.e., extracellular and extravascular spaces). The body's capillaries filter about 30 L of fluid per day out of the blood into interstitial spaces but reabsorb only about 27 L back into the blood. If the extra 3 L of fluid remained in the interstitial spaces, fluid would accumulate and eventually flood the alveoli, causing pulmonary edema. The lymphatic system normally removes this interstitial fluid and returns it to the bloodstream. In addition, lymph nodes filter and clear the fluid of microorganisms and foreign materials.

The lung's lymphatics are organized into superficial and deep vessel networks. The superficial vessels drain the lung surfaces and pleura; the deep vessels drain the main lung tissues, also known as the lung parenchyma. The flow of lymph through deep and superficial systems is directed toward the hilum, where numerous lymph nodes are located. Lymph eventually returns to the bloodstream through the right thoracic lymph duct.

NERVOUS CONTROL OF THE LUNGS AND THORACIC MUSCULATURE

The voluntary skeletal muscles of the chest wall and diaphragm are innervated by the somatic nervous system, whereas the involuntary smooth airway muscle of the lung is innervated entirely by the autonomic nervous system. The sympathetic and parasympathetic divisions of the autonomic system control most of the body's visceral functions. (The term "viscera" refers to the soft organs of the thoracic and abdominal cavities.) Somatic and autonomic nervous systems are compared in Table 2-1. The somatic system provides only motor innervation to the ventilatory muscles; the autonomic system supplies both motor (efferent) and sensory (afferent) nerves to the lung.

Somatic Innervation

The paired **phrenic nerves** supply motor innervation to the hemidiaphragms. Phrenic nerves originate from the right and

TABLE 2-1

Comparison of Autonomic and Somatic Motor Nervous Systems

Features	Somatic Motor Nervous System	Autonomic Nervous System
Target tissues	Skeletal muscle	Smooth muscle, cardiac muscle, and glands
Regulation	Control of all conscious and unconscious movements of skeletal muscle	Unconscious regulation, although influenced by conscious mental functions
Response to stimulation	Skeletal muscle contracts	Target tissues are stimulated or inhibited
Neuron arrangement	One neuron extends from the CNS to skeletal muscle	Two neurons in series; the preganglionic neuron extends from the CNS to an autonomic ganglion, and the postganglionic neuron extends from the autonomic ganglion to the target tissue
Neuron cell body location	Neuron cell bodies are in motor nuclei of the cranial nerves and in the ventral horn of the spinal cord	Preganglionic neuron cell bodies are in autonomic nuclei of the cranial nerves and in the lateral horn of the spinal cord; postganglionic neuron cell bodies are in autonomic ganglia
Number of synapses	One synapse between the somatic motor neuron and the skeletal muscle	Two synapses—first in the autonomic ganglia, second at the target tissue
Axon sheaths	Myelinated	Preganglionic axons myelinated, postganglionic axons unmyelinated
Neurotransmitter substance	Acetylcholine	Acetylcholine released by preganglionic neurons; either acetylcholine or norepinephrine released by postganglionic neurons
Receptor molecules	Receptor molecules for acetylcholine are nicotinic	In autonomic ganglia, receptor molecules for acetylcholine are nicotinic; in target tissues, receptor molecules for acetylcholine are muscarinic, whereas receptor molecules for norepinephrine are either α- or β-adrenergic

Modified from Seeley RR, Stephens TD, Tate P: *Anatomy & physiology*, ed 3, New York, 1995, McGraw-Hill.
CNS, Central nervous system.

left cervical nerve plexuses as branches of cervical spinal nerves C3 to C5 (Figure 2-5). Phrenic nerves cross in front of the scalenus anterior muscles of the neck and enter the chest, sandwiched between subclavian arteries and veins. Thoracic surgery, neck trauma, and cancerous tumors sometimes injure or compress the phrenic nerve, causing paralysis of the diaphragm. However, breathing may still be possible even with a paralyzed diaphragm if intercostal nerves and muscles are intact.

The intercostal nerves are spinal nerves that provide motor innervation to the muscles between the ribs, the intercostal muscles. They originate from the thoracic portion of the spinal column and follow the ribs anteriorly.

Autonomic Innervation

The lung is innervated entirely by autonomic sensory and motor nerves; no voluntary motor control over airway smooth muscle exists. The general pattern of autonomic innervation for both sympathetic and parasympathetic divisions is a two-neuron system in which a nerve fiber leaves the central nervous system (brainstem or spinal cord) and forms a junction (synapse) with a second neuron. The second neuron synapses with muscle cells of the innervated organ, known as the effector organ. The synapse between two neurons outside of the spinal cord is known as a **ganglion**. The synapses between nerves and effector organs are generally known as the neuromuscular junction. Nerve impulses are transmitted across ganglionic synapses and neuromuscular junctions by chemical substances known as neurotransmitters. Neurotransmitters are stored in nerve fiber endings and are released into the synaptic region in response to electrical neural impulses. Neurotransmitter molecules travel across the synapse and stimulate the cell membrane of the next neuron or the effector organ, propagating the impulse or causing an organ to respond. The two main neurotransmitters of the autonomic system are acetylcholine and norepinephrine

Fibers between the spinal cord and ganglia are **preganglionic fibers**; the fibers between the ganglia and the innervated organ are **postganglionic fibers** (Figure 2-6). In the parasympathetic system, the ganglia are near, or even *in*, the structures they innervate; preganglionic fibers are long, and postganglionic fibers are short. The opposite is true for the sympathetic system, in which the ganglionic junctions are located a short distance from the spine, forming linked ganglia resembling a chain of beads called the sympathetic chain (Table 2-2 and see Figure 2-6). To some extent, postganglionic fibers from both systems innervate the same structures, producing a balance between excitatory and inhibitory responses (Table 2-3).

CLINICAL FOCUS 2-2

Effects of Phrenic Nerve and Spinal Cord Injuries on Ventilation

Your patient is a 25-year-old woman who was involved in a one-car rollover. She sustained fractures of the second and third cervical vertebrae and trauma to the spinal cord at the same levels.

What problems do you think your patient will have as a result of this injury? What will your role as a clinician be in caring for her?

Discussion

The diaphragm receives its motor innervation (stimulus) from the phrenic nerve, which originates from the damaged portion of the spinal cord. Phrenic nerve injury may cause partial or total loss of diaphragm stimulation. The high level of the spinal cord injury means this woman will likely require positive pressure mechanical ventilation through an endotracheal tube placed into her trachea. She may require this support temporarily or long-term, depending on the degree of diaphragm paralysis.

Spinal cord injury at C2 and C3 levels impairs respiratory muscle function because respiratory muscles receive nerve input from the spinal cord at or below these cervical vertebrae. This includes the major muscles involved in inspiration and expiration: the diaphragm, external and internal intercostals, and abdominals. At best, this patient might be able to use accessory muscles to breathe, but her inability to take deep

breaths will reduce her lung volumes, increasing the likelihood of alveolar collapse (atelectasis). Expiratory muscle impairment means she will not cough effectively and will not clear normal secretions effectively. Secretions will tend to collect in the lungs, providing a breeding ground for bacteria.

Your role is to ensure adequate ventilation and bronchial hygiene (secretion removal) for this patient. To provide adequate ventilation, you must set the mechanical ventilator to deliver appropriate breath volumes at an adequate respiratory rate. You will periodically insert a suction catheter down into the endotracheal tube to suction secretions from the airway. This suctioning helps prevent secretion retention and aids in bronchial hygiene. If she recovers enough diaphragmatic function to breathe on her own, you might take measures to improve her remaining respiratory muscle strength. You will regularly encourage her to inhale deeply and may need to use a manual ventilating device to help her take deep breaths. You can help her cough to clear secretions by placing your hands on her abdomen just below the ribs and giving a forceful thrust during exhalation. This simulated cough increases abdominal pressure and moves the diaphragm sharply upward, forcing air and secretions out of the lungs. You also may place the patient in positions that use gravity to drain secretions from the lungs (postural drainage).

Sympathetic preganglionic fibers originate in the thoracic and lumbar portions of the spinal cord—hence the term "thoracolumbar" in reference to the sympathetic division. A single preganglionic neuron may synapse with many postganglionic neurons that branch out to numerous organs. Thus, sympathetic stimulation usually elicits a widespread response involving many different organs.[1]

Parasympathetic fibers originate from the brainstem and sacral spinal cord—hence the term "craniosacral" in reference to the parasympathetic division. About three fourths[1] of all parasympathetic fibers are in the vagus nerve (see cranial nerve X in Figure 2-6), which sends out many branches to the visceral organs. Vagal stimulation is synonymous with parasympathetic stimulation. In contrast to the sympathetic division, a parasympathetic preganglionic fiber usually synapses with a single postganglionic fiber; parasympathetic stimulation often evokes the response of a single organ.[1]

Efferent (Motor) Responses

Sympathetic Responses. Sympathetic postganglionic fibers secrete the neurotransmitter norepinephrine, also known as noradrenaline, and these neurons are called **adrenergic** fibers. Sympathetic stimulation causes smooth airway muscle relaxation, which increases airway diameter (bronchodilation) and decreases resistance to airflow. Drugs that elicit sympathetic responses in the airways are called adrenergic bronchodilators; they are

commonly used to reverse bronchoconstriction in patients with asthma and chronic bronchitis. Paradoxically, there is little or no anatomical evidence for sympathetic innervation of the airways, and yet sympathetic nervous system stimulation causes bronchodilation.[2] Sympathetic bronchodilation occurs as follows: an extension of the sympathetic ganglionic chain, called the greater splanchnic nerve (see Figure 2-6), carries sympathetic impulses to the adrenal gland medulla, which secretes epinephrine directly into the bloodstream. Circulating epinephrine stimulates adrenergic receptors on smooth airway muscle cells, which are abundant in the lung despite the scarcity of sympathetic innervation. Circulating epinephrine is the only natural mechanism for sympathetic bronchodilation in humans.[2]

Parasympathetic Responses. Parasympathetic postganglionic fibers innervate lung smooth airway muscle, mucous glands, and pulmonary blood vessels. They secrete the neurotransmitter acetylcholine, and they are called **cholinergic fibers**. Parasympathetic impulses are the major neural bronchoconstrictor mechanism and the major determinant of airway diameter.[2] These cholinergic impulses normally maintain a mild degree of continuous smooth muscle contraction, providing a normal baseline smooth muscle tone. However, excessive cholinergic stimulation can cause intense airway muscle contraction or bronchospasm, greatly increasing resistance to airflow. Drugs used to block cholinergic impulses in such circumstances are called anticholinergic bronchodilators.

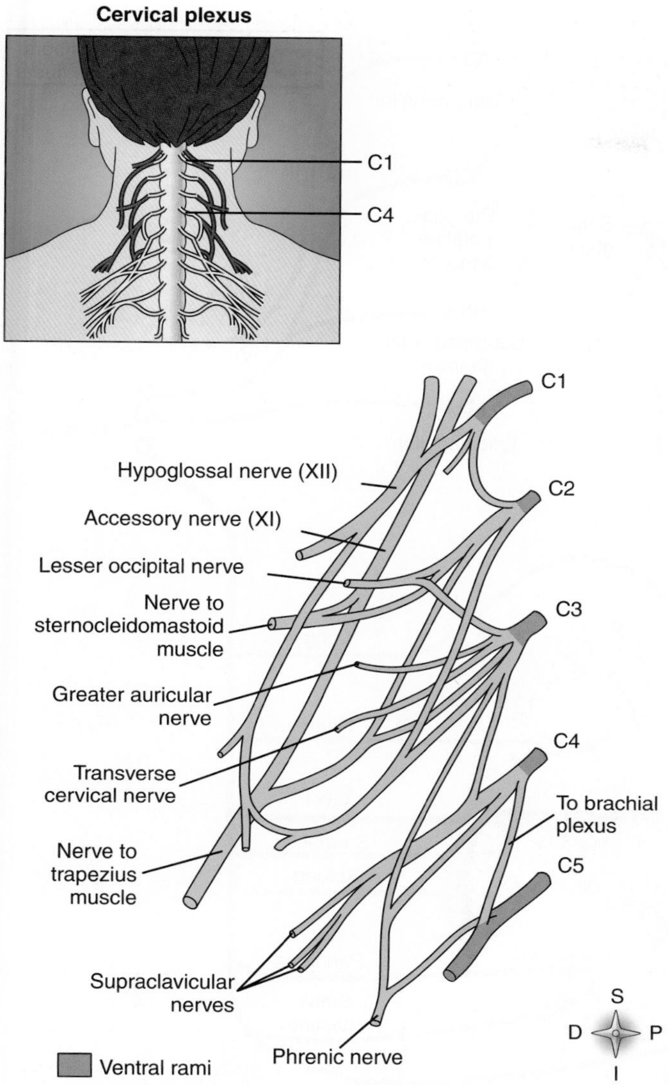

Cervical plexus

- Hypoglossal nerve (XII)
- Accessory nerve (XI)
- Lesser occipital nerve
- Nerve to sternocleidomastoid muscle
- Greater auricular nerve
- Transverse cervical nerve
- Nerve to trapezius muscle
- Supraclavicular nerves

C1
C2
C3
C4
To brachial plexus
C5
Phrenic nerve

S
D — P
I

■ Ventral rami

Figure 2-5 Cervical nerve plexus. The phrenic nerves exit this plexus from C3, C4, and C5 levels. Spinal cord transactions above the C3 level paralyze the diaphragm and all other ventilatory muscles. (From Habif TP: *Clinical dermatology*, ed 2, St Louis, 1990, Mosby.)

Parasympathetic stimulation also increases the production of mucous glycoproteins, increasing the viscosity of airway secretions. In contrast, sympathetic stimulation produces thin, watery secretions. The balance between these two autonomic divisions helps determine the viscosity of airway secretions. Neither parasympathetic nor sympathetic fibers exert control over the pulmonary circulation in an adult.

Cholinergic innervation is greatest in the large airways, diminishing peripherally as airways become smaller. This characteristic may explain why anticholinergic bronchodilator drugs are less useful than adrenergic bronchodilator drugs when bronchoconstriction involves mostly small airways. In contrast, sympathetic receptors are more uniformly distributed, and adrenergic bronchodilators are equally effective in large and small airways.[2]

Adrenergic and Cholinergic Receptors. Before a neurotransmitter can stimulate a postganglionic fiber or an effector organ

cell, it must first bind with the cell's highly specific transmembrane receptor known as a G protein–coupled receptor; the intracellular end of the receptor is linked to a G protein molecule (so named because it is part of a family of guanine nucleotide-binding proteins).[2] When a neurotransmitter molecule binds with the extracellular end of the receptor, the receptor's shape changes, activating the G protein inside the cell. G protein activation stimulates an intracellular enzyme, initiating a complex sequence of events that ultimately stimulates or inhibits the nerve fiber or effector organ, depending on the type of receptor and neurotransmitter molecule involved.

Both sympathetic and parasympathetic preganglionic fibers secrete acetylcholine at ganglionic junctions where they synapse with postganglionic fibers. At these junctions, receptors on postganglionic nerve fibers of both divisions are cholinergic; that is, they are specific for the acetylcholine. These cholinergic receptors are called nicotinic receptors because of their sensitivity to nicotine; when acetylcholine binds with nicotinic receptors, postganglionic fibers propagate the nerve impulse to the neuromuscular junction of the effector organ. At the neuromuscular junction, sympathetic (adrenergic) fibers secrete norepinephrine, and parasympathetic (cholinergic) fibers again secrete acetylcholine. The organs innervated by these fibers have adrenergic and cholinergic transmembrane receptors in their cell membranes specific for norepinephrine and acetylcholine molecules. Cholinergic receptors at the neuromuscular junction are different from receptors at the ganglionic junction and are called muscarinic receptors because of their sensitivity to muscarine, a substance derived from a mushroom. When acetylcholine molecules bind with muscarinic receptors, they produce smooth airway muscle contraction (bronchoconstriction) and increased glandular mucus secretion. In contrast, when norepinephrine molecules bind with adrenergic receptors of effector organ cells, they produce bronchodilation, which decreases airway resistance. Figure 2-7 illustrates the locations of neurotransmitters and receptors.

Parasympathetic Muscarinic Receptor Subtypes. At least five muscarinic receptor subtypes have been identified, three of which are present in the human lung. These subtypes are designated M_1, M_2, and M_3 receptors, and all are sensitive to acetylcholine.[2] M_1 receptors are present along with nicotinic receptors on the preganglionic fiber at the ganglionic junction. Although nicotinic receptors are primarily responsible for transmitting neural impulses through the parasympathetic ganglion, M_1 receptor stimulation enhances transmission. M_2 receptors are present on the postganglionic nerve ending at the neuromuscular junction. M_2 receptors have a negative feedback function; when bound by acetylcholine, they inhibit its further release from the nerve ending, limiting the effects of parasympathetic stimulation. M_3 receptors are present in airway smooth muscle and mucous glands; when bound by acetylcholine, they cause smooth muscle contraction and increased mucus production (Figure 2-8).

Adrenergic Receptor Subtypes. As with cholinergic receptors, there are different types and subtypes of adrenergic receptors; the major types are designated alpha (α) and beta (β) receptors (see Figure 2-7). Beta receptors are subdivided further into

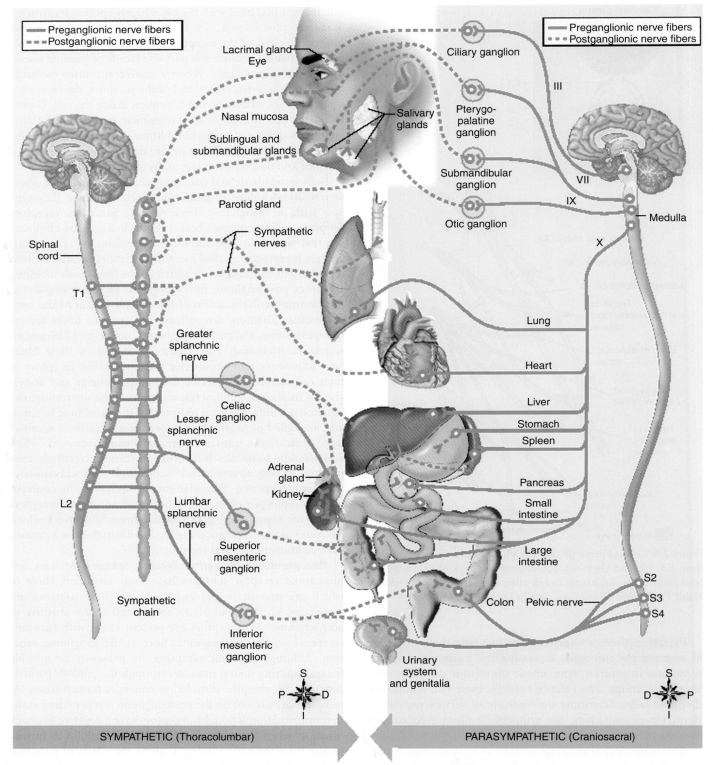

Figure 2-6 Major autonomic pathways. Parasympathetic nerves (*right*) originate from cranial and sacral segments of the spinal cord; the vagus nerve (cranial nerve X) sends branches to most visceral organs. Sympathetic nerves (*left*) originate from thoracic and lumbar segments of the spinal cord. (From Patton KT, Thibodeau GA: *Anatomy & physiology*, ed 7, St. Louis, 2010, Mosby.)

TABLE 2-2

Comparison of Sympathetic and Parasympathetic Divisions

Feature	Sympathetic Division	Parasympathetic Division
Location of preganglionic cell body	Lateral horns of spinal cord gray matter (T1-L2)	Brainstem and lateral horns of spinal cord gray matter (S2-S4)
Outflow from central nervous system	Spinal nerves, sympathetic nerves, and splanchnic nerves	Cranial nerves and pelvic nerves
Ganglia	Sympathetic chain ganglia along spinal cord for spinal and sympathetic nerves; collateral ganglia for splanchnic nerves	Terminal ganglia near or on effector organ
Number of postganglionic neurons for each preganglionic neuron	Many	Few
Relative length of neurons	Short preganglionic; long postganglionic	Short postganglionic

From Seeley RR, Stephens TD, Tate P: *Anatomy & physiology*, ed 3, New York, 1995, McGraw-Hill.

TABLE 2-3

Comparison of Sympathetic and Parasympathetic Divisions

Organ	Effect of Sympathetic Stimulation	Effect of Parasympathetic Stimulation
Heart		
Muscle	Increased rate and force (β_1)	Slowed rate (c)
Coronary arteries	Dilated (β_2), constricted (α)*	Dilated (c)
Systemic blood vessels		
Abdominal	Constricted (α)	None
Skin	Constricted (α)	None
Muscle	Dilated (β_2), constricted (α)	None
Lungs		
Bronchi	Dilated (β_2)	Constricted (c)
Liver	Glucose released into blood (β_2)	None
Skeletal muscles	Breakdown of glycogen to glucose (β_2)	None
Metabolism	Increased up to 100% (α, β)	None
Glands		
Adrenal	Release of epinephrine and norepinephrine (c)	None
Salivary	Constriction of blood vessels and slight production of a thick, viscous secretion (α)	Dilation of blood vessels and thin, copious secretion (c)
Gastric	Inhibition (α)	Stimulation (c)
Pancreas	Decreased insulin secretion (α)	Increased insulin secretion (c)
Lacrimal	None	Secretion (c)
Sweat		
Merocrine	Copious, watery secretion (c)	None
1.1 Apocrine	Thick, organic secretion (c)	None
Gut		
Wall	Decreased tone (β_2)	Increased motility (c)
Sphincter	Increased tone (α)	Decreased tone (c)
Gallbladder and bile ducts	Relaxed (β_2)	Contracted (c)
Urinary bladder		
Wall	Relaxed (β_2)	Contracted (c)
Sphincter	Contracted (α)	Relaxed (c)
Eye		
Ciliary muscle	Relaxed for far vision (β_2)	Contracted for near vision (c)
Pupil	Dilated (α)	Constricted (c)
Arrector pili muscles	Contraction (α)	None
Blood	Increased coagulation (α)	None
Sex organs	Ejaculation (α)	Erection (c)

From Seeley RR, Stephens TD, Tate P: *Anatomy & physiology*, ed 3, New York, 1995, McGraw-Hill.
α, Alpha-adrenergic receptors; β, beta-adrenergic receptors; *c*, cholinergic receptors.
*Sympathetic stimulation of the heart normally increases coronary artery blood flow because of increased cardiac muscle demand for oxygen. (Local control is discussed in Chapter 17.)

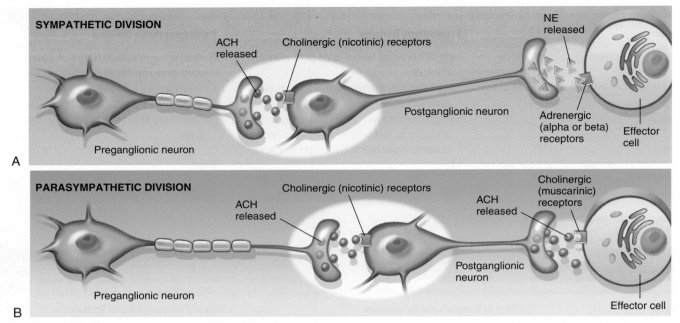

Figure 2-7 Locations of neurotransmitters and receptors of the autonomic nervous system. All preganglionic fibers are cholinergic, secreting acetylcholine (ACH), which binds with nicotinic receptors on postganglionic fibers. **A,** Sympathetic postganglionic fibers are adrenergic, secreting norepinephrine (NE), which binds with adrenergic alpha and beta receptors. **B,** Parasympathetic postganglionic fibers remain cholinergic, secreting ACH, which binds with muscarinic receptors on the effector cells. (From Thibodeau GA, Patton KT: *Anatomy & physiology*, ed 5, St Louis, 2003, Mosby.)

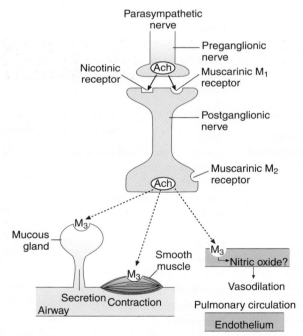

Figure 2-8 Muscarinic receptor subtypes (M$_1$ through M$_3$) of the parasympathetic nervous system in the lung. *Ach,* Acetylcholine. (From Gardenhire DS: *Rau's respiratory care pharmacology*, ed 8, St. Louis, 2008, Mosby.)

beta$_1$ (β_1) and beta$_2$ (β_2) receptors. Alpha receptors are less distinctly subdivided into alpha$_1$ and alpha$_2$ receptors.[2] Chemical substances that stimulate these receptors are called agonists, whereas substances that block their responses are called antagonists. Alpha and beta agonists generally produce opposite effects;

for example, beta$_2$ agonists cause vasodilation, whereas beta$_1$ agonists cause vasoconstriction. Similarly, some alpha-mediated functions can be excitatory, and some can be inhibitory.

Norepinephrine and epinephrine, both secreted into the bloodstream by the adrenal glands, excite alpha and beta receptors differently. Norepinephrine excites alpha receptors much more than beta receptors, whereas epinephrine excites them both about equally.[1] Table 2-3 lists some of the differences between alpha and beta receptor functions. About two thirds of the beta receptors in the lung are of the beta$_2$ type.[2] Pulmonary beta$_2$ receptors are concentrated in airway smooth muscle, airway epithelium, vascular smooth muscle, and submucosal glands, whereas the smaller number of beta$_1$ receptors are restricted to alveolar walls and submucosal glands.[2] There is no evidence of alpha receptors on airway smooth muscle, although they are present on the smooth muscle associated with blood vessels that supply the airways.[2]

From the foregoing discussion, one can see that both cholinergic blocking drugs and beta$_2$ agonist drugs cause bronchodilation. Beta$_2$ agonists and cholinergic antagonists are the two major drug types used to reverse bronchospasm in diseases such as asthma and chronic obstructive pulmonary disease (COPD). COPD includes diseases that narrow the airways for purely structural reasons (e.g., because of loss of elastic recoil or airway mucosal edema), which means that normal cholinergic smooth muscle tone decreases airway diameter more than it does in normal airways. This characteristic of COPD may explain why anticholinergic drugs are often more effective than beta$_2$ agonists as bronchodilators in patients with COPD.[2]

The preceding characterizations of neural airway control have been simplified; it is now known that the autonomic nervous system comprises more than just adrenergic and cholinergic neurons and that all neurons interact in complex ways.[2] One autonomic division can modify the function of the other. Every nerve secretes multiple transmitters, although each division is generally associated with one primary neurotransmitter.[2]

Nonadrenergic Noncholinergic Responses. Bronchodilator nerves exist in human airways that are not blocked by drugs that block adrenergic or cholinergic receptors. These nerves are called **nonadrenergic noncholinergic (NANC) nerves**; other neurotransmitters besides norepinephrine and acetylcholine bind with autonomic receptors.[2] It was previously thought that each autonomic nerve type had its own unique neurotransmitter, but a newer theory of cotransmission holds that in addition to secreting norepinephrine or acetylcholine, all postganglionic fibers release or cotransmit a host of NANC transmitters that modify autonomic receptor responses. These additional transmitters can either facilitate or antagonize the effects of the primary neurotransmitter. NANC neurotransmitters play an important role in modulating not only airway smooth muscle tone but also immune system homeostasis.

Similar to sympathetic and parasympathetic autonomic divisions, NANC neurons can be either inhibitory (i-NANC) or excitatory (e-NANC). i-NANC neurons are efferent fibers that cause bronchodilation, whereas e-NANC neurons are sensory fibers (also known as **C-fibers**) that lead to bronchoconstriction. The main i-NANC neurotransmitters in human airways are nitric oxide (NO) and vasoactive intestinal peptide (VIP); VIP is the most potent bronchodilator of the two. NO and VIP are coreleased with acetylcholine in cholinergic fibers, where they are believed to exert an important limiting effect on cholinergic bronchoconstriction.[2] (i-NANC fibers share a common ganglion with parasympathetic fibers.[2]) VIP also exists in mast cell granules where it is thought to limit the bronchoconstriction caused by mast cell histamine release (see Chapter 1). Superoxide ions generated by inflammatory cells in asthma may deplete neuronally generated NO, possibly reducing the limiting effect that NO has on cholinergic bronchoconstriction.[2]

Exhaled Nitric Oxide in Asthma. i-NANC neurons contain the enzyme **nitric oxide synthase (NOS)**, which is responsible for the synthesis of NO. In contrast to acetylcholine and norepinephrine, NO is not stored in vesicles in the neuron fiber ending but is synthesized in response to neural stimuli; it then diffuses out of the neuron into extracellular spaces and nearby smooth muscle. There are three forms of NOS: constitutive NOS (cNOS), which is constituted in the neuron; inducible NOS (iNOS), which is induced in airway epithelial cells by inflammation; and endothelial NOS (eNOS), which is another constitutive form of NOS that is generated in vascular endothelial cells.[2] Because asthma is an inflammatory disease of the airways, it stimulates the production of iNOS, which would be expected to elevate the concentration of NO in the exhaled gas of asthmatics. Asthmatics have higher concentrations of exhaled

---

CLINICAL FOCUS 2-3

Role of Bronchodilator Drugs in Asthma

Asthma is a lung disease characterized by episodes or "attacks" of bronchoconstriction, mucosal edema, and excessive secretion of thick mucus that can partially or completely obstruct the airways. Various stimuli, including dust, mold, pollens, exercise, and infections can trigger an asthma attack. The asthmatic may quickly develop symptoms of cough, wheezing, a feeling of chest tightness, excess sputum production, and shortness of breath. Respiratory therapists often administer inhaled aerosolized drugs that work rapidly to dilate the airways, reversing the sometimes life-threatening bronchoconstriction. Thus, bronchodilator drugs are often called rescue drugs in asthma treatment. As mentioned in Chapter 1, asthma is primarily an airway inflammatory disease, and anti-inflammatory drugs, such as corticosteroids, are considered first-line drugs for long-term control of asthma.

Bronchodilator drugs either mimic sympathetic nervous stimulation or block parasympathetic nervous stimulation. Sympathetic stimulation causes the adrenal glands to secrete epinephrine into the blood, which stimulates adrenergic receptors in the lung and causes smooth airway muscle relaxation (bronchodilation). Bronchodilator drugs inhaled by patients with asthma stimulate the same receptors, specifically the beta$_2$-adrenergic receptors responsible for bronchodilation. For this reason, these drugs are called beta$_2$ agonists. Beta$_2$ agonists are also known as sympathomimetic drugs because they mimic sympathetic neuronal transmission. Sympathomimetic drugs, specifically beta$_2$ agonists, are most commonly inhaled directly into the lungs to reverse the bronchoconstriction associated with asthma. A common example of such a drug is albuterol (Proventil).

Parasympathetic or cholinergic stimulation is the major cause of bronchoconstriction; drugs that block cholinergic receptors (cholinergic antagonists or, more specifically, muscarinic antagonists) cause bronchodilation. Atropine is the prototype of a cholinergic blocker, but it has widespread side effects throughout the body if used as an inhaled bronchodilator drug.[3] Ipratropium bromide (Atrovent) is a nonselective M$_1$, M$_2$, and M$_3$ antagonist with fewer side effects than atropine. The ideal anticholinergic bronchodilator drug would block only M$_1$ and M$_3$ muscarinic receptors, keeping the inhibitory effect of M$_2$ stimulation intact. An example of such a selective muscarinic blocker is tiotropium bromide (Spiriva); although tiotropium binds to all muscarinic receptors, it dissociates from M$_2$ receptors 10 times faster than from M$_3$ receptors.[3] In addition, tiotropium has a long duration of action, allowing once-daily dosing; compared with ipratropium, it dissociates from M$_1$ and M$_3$ receptors 100 times more slowly.[3] Cholinergic blockers are generally used to reduce airway resistance in COPD rather than asthma.

CLINICAL FOCUS 2-4

Alpha Agonist Drugs and Laryngeal Edema

Immediately after removing an endotracheal tube from a patient (a procedure called extubation), you notice that the patient has difficulty breathing, and inspiration creates a harsh crowing sound (called stridor). You immediately give the patient an inhaled drug, racemic epinephrine, to treat the problem.

Discussion

An endotracheal tube rests between the vocal cords of the larynx. The tube is a foreign object and creates some degree of trauma to the vocal cords as it presses against their delicate, vascular epithelium. It is common for the vocal cords to swell after extubation in response to the trauma; this is called

postextubation laryngeal edema. Edema, or swelling, occurs when vessels become engorged with blood and fluid leaks out of the capillaries into the extravascular tissues. The air passage is narrowed, creating resistance to airflow and a high-pitched crowing sound as high-velocity flow passes between the cords. An alpha-adrenergic drug, such as racemic epinephrine, causes the small arterioles that bring blood to the laryngeal epithelium to constrict; this limits blood flow and pressure that can reach the capillaries. Consequently, capillary blood volume decreases, epithelial tissues shrink, and edema subsides. For this reason, aerosolized racemic epinephrine is the drug of choice for quick relief of postextubation laryngeal edema.

NO than normal individuals, especially during exacerbations of the disease.[2] Monitoring exhaled NO is one way to identify early stages of asthma exacerbations.

CONCEPT QUESTION 2-4

Sometimes beta-blocking drugs are given to patients with heart disease to slow the heart rate and decrease the force of contraction, both of which decrease the oxygen demand of the heart. What adverse effect might beta-blocker drugs have in a patient with asthma?

Afferent (Sensory) Responses

Most sensory afferent nerves from the lung are parasympathetic (vagal) in origin. At least three kinds of afferent receptors have been identified:[2] (1) slowly adapting stretch receptors; (2) rapidly adapting irritant receptors; and (3) C-fibers, also classified as NANC excitatory nerves.[3] These nerves play a critical role in defense of the airways; their stimulation evokes powerful reflexes that limit the penetration of harmful substances into the respiratory tract that could injure the delicate alveolar gas-exchange surface.

Slowly Adapting (Stretch) Receptors. **Slowly adapting receptors (SARs)** continue to fire as long as the stimulus persists. These stretch receptors are located in the smooth muscle of conducting airways. They are stimulated by a deep inspiration, which is part of the **Hering-Breuer reflex**. A deep inspiration inhibits vagal discharge and causes smooth muscle relaxation and bronchodilation.[2]

Deep inspirations have bronchodilating and bronchoprotective effects in normal healthy people, and these effects are not present in patients with asthma; the airway smooth muscle fibers in asthmatics are not stretched by deep inspiration as much as they are in subjects without asthma.[4] In one study, subjects with and without asthma performed several deep inspirations before inhaling methacholine, a provocative substance that elicits bronchospasm. Asthmatic subjects had a much greater bronchospastic response to methacholine than subjects

without asthma. The investigators concluded that deep inspiration is a normal physiological protective mechanism that is absent in patients with asthma, even if asthma is mild.[4] Apparently, deep inspiration does not stretch asthmatic airways as much as it stretches healthy airways; in addition, asthmatic airways reconstrict more rapidly after deep inspiration compared to healthy airways.[4]

Rapidly Adapting (Irritant) Receptors. **Rapidly adapting receptors (RARs)** are activated by various irritants, including inhaled gases (e.g., cigarette smoke, ozone, sulfur dioxide), water, hypertonic solutions, acidic substances, mechanical stimulation (including distortion from bronchoconstriction), and histamine-induced bronchoconstriction.[2] RARs are widespread in the larynx, trachea, carina, and mainstem bronchi, firing vigorously on stimulation and then quickly adapting to a slower firing rate.

Stimulation of RARs causes reflex bronchoconstriction, expiratory narrowing of the larynx, cough, deep inspiration, and mucous secretion. These receptors are protective mechanisms in healthy humans because they elicit bronchospasm, limiting penetration of injurious substances into the lung. They also help expel foreign material from the lung by stimulating mucous secretion and cough.

Stimulation of irritant receptors in the larynx, trachea, carina, and major bronchi induces a strong cough reflex, and these RARs are often called cough receptors. These receptors transmit impulses via the vagus nerve to the central nervous system, where the efferent somatic system sends motor signals to appropriate ventilatory muscles. The cough is produced in the following sequence:

1. The diaphragm contracts, causing a deep inspiration.
2. A slight inspiratory pause occurs.
3. The muscles in the larynx close the glottis, sealing the upper airway.
4. The abdominal expiratory muscles contract forcefully, generating a high intrapulmonary pressure against the closed glottis (100 to 200 cm H_2O in healthy adults).
5. The glottis suddenly opens, explosively releasing compressed gas.

The sudden release of highly compressed gas produces an explosive burst of air that may achieve an instantaneous velocity greater than 100 miles per hour. The compressive narrowing of airways during the explosive expiratory burst helps generate this high velocity as air is expelled through the narrowed bronchial and tracheal slitlike openings. In this way, the cough produces shearing forces that dislodge mucus and foreign particles from the airways, expelling them from the lungs. The cough is an important lung defense mechanism against aspiration of foreign material. Artificial airways such as endotracheal and tracheostomy tubes greatly diminish cough effectiveness because they prevent glottic closure and the ability to generate high intrapulmonary pressures.

Irritant receptors in the more distal bronchi cause bronchoconstriction rather than cough.[7] Bronchoconstriction increases cough receptor sensitivity resulting from mechanical distortion, whereas bronchodilation decreases their sensitivity.[2] For this reason, persistent cough in patients with asthma can often be diminished by treatment with bronchodilator drugs.

C-Fibers. C-fibers (e-NANC fibers) are located in the lung parenchyma, conducting airways, and pulmonary blood vessels; they play an important role in defending the lower respiratory tract and respond to various chemical and physical stimuli by causing bronchoconstriction.[2] Bronchial C-fibers are apparently involved in the bronchoconstriction caused by cold air breathing in exercise-induced asthma.[5] C-fiber endings are located deep in the lung parenchyma near pulmonary capillaries and alveoli and are often called **J-receptors** (juxtacapillary receptors).[2] Stimulation of J-receptors causes rapid, shallow breathing; severe laryngeal constriction on expiration; slowed heart rate (bradycardia); and mucous secretion. J-receptors are stimulated by alveolar inflammatory processes such as pneumonia and by increased pulmonary capillary pressure and pulmonary edema as seen in patients with congestive heart failure. J-receptors probably contribute to the sensation of **dyspnea** (shortness of breath) that accompanies such conditions.[2]

THORACIC ANATOMY

The **thorax** is a cavity formed by the rib cage and its muscles (intercostal muscles), the vertebrae, sternum, and diaphragm. It can be subdivided into three cavities: the left and right pleural cavities and the mediastinum (Figure 2-9).

Thoracic Cage

The ribs are situated such that their vertebral attachments are higher than their sternal attachments, making them slant downward anteriorly (Figure 2-10). The 12 thoracic vertebrae articulate with all 12 ribs, but not all ribs connect directly with the sternum anteriorly. Ribs 1 to 7 connect directly with the sternum via cartilages and are called vertebrosternal ribs; ribs 8 to 10 are connected to the lower sternum by a common cartilage and are called vertebrochondral ribs. The last two ribs, 11 and 12, do not connect with the sternum and are called floating ribs.

The head of a typical rib articulates with the bodies of two adjacent vertebrae, and the rib tubercle articulates with the transverse process of one vertebra (Figure 2-11). A costal groove on the underside of each rib provides a protective channel for nerves, arteries, and veins; needles or tubes inserted between the ribs into the chest should be placed immediately above the

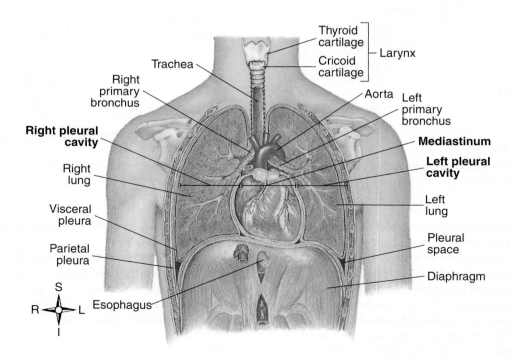

Figure 2-9 The thoracic cavity is divided into left and right pleural cavities and the central mediastinal cavity. (From Thibodeau GA, Patton KT: *Anatomy & physiology*, ed 3, St Louis, 1996, Mosby.)

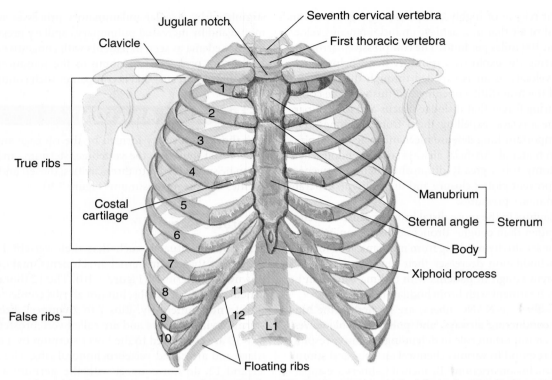

Figure 2-10 Anterior view of the thoracic cage. (From Seeley RR, Stephens TD, Tate P: *Anatomy & physiology*, ed 3, New York, 1995, McGraw-Hill.)

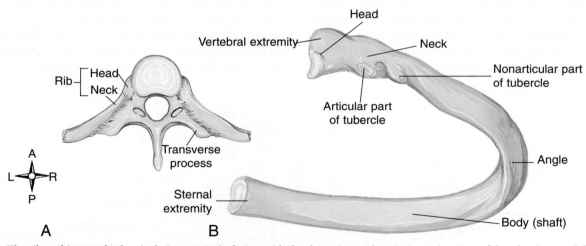

Figure 2-11 The rib and its vertebral articulation. **A,** Articulation with the thoracic vertebra. **B,** Posterior view of the rib. (From Thibodeau GA, Patton KT: *Anatomy & physiology*, ed 3, St Louis, 1996, Mosby.)

rib to prevent damage to nerves or vessels. The first two or three ribs are extremely short and have limited movement. Lower ribs are more likely to be fractured or separated from their sternal attachments in traumatic accidents. Fractured first and second ribs indicate an extremely severe blow to the thorax.

The sternum, sometimes called the breast bone, consists of the **manubrium**, body, and **xiphoid process** (see Figure 2-10). At the junction of the manubrium, the body, and the second rib is the sternal angle, also called the **angle of Louis**. The angle of Louis marks the level of the carina in the lung and is adjacent to the second rib; it is a reference point for counting ribs.

Counting ribs is necessary for locating intrathoracic structures and inserting chest tubes.

The xiphoid process at the bottom of the sternum projects downward between the ribs. During cardiopulmonary resuscitation involving cardiac compressions, care must be taken not to compress the xiphoid process because a fracture of this process may damage underlying organs.

Rib Movements

During breathing, the rib heads rotate on their vertebral articulations, but the vertebral column itself remains stationary; the

CLINICAL FOCUS 2-5

Intercostal Retractions and Expiratory Grunting in Premature Newborn Infants

Your patient, a 2-lb newborn girl, was born prematurely with immediate signs of respiratory distress. Her skin color 1 hour after delivery remains blue-purple. Her breathing rate is 75 breaths per minute, her rib cage exhibits intercostal retractions with each breath, her nostrils flare on inspiration, and she makes a grunting sound every time she exhales. Based on your patient's prematurity and symptoms, you conclude that she has respiratory distress syndrome (RDS) of the newborn.

Discussion

RDS is a disease caused by inadequate amounts of surfactant in the lungs of a premature infant. Surfactant is secreted late in fetal life by alveolar type II cells (see Chapter 3). The main reason surfactant is so important to a neonate is that it decreases alveolar surface tension; this helps prevent alveolar collapse and aids in keeping the alveoli free of fluid.

Insufficient surfactant results in high alveolar surface tension, causing widespread alveolar collapse. The newborn must generate high subatmospheric intrapleural pressures with each breath to open collapsed alveoli; this causes the observed intercostal retractions.

High subatmospheric intrapleural pressure may pull fluid out of pulmonary capillaries into the lung's interstitial spaces. J-receptors are stimulated by this process and induce the rapid, shallow breathing pattern characteristic of RDS. J-receptor stimulation also causes a reflex narrowing of the glottis, producing the grunting expiratory sound. The narrowed glottis resists airflow during expiration. This resistance increases pressure in the airways during expiration, which helps maintain a larger lung volume at the end of expiration. Expiratory grunting seems to be a natural compensatory response in newborns with RDS.

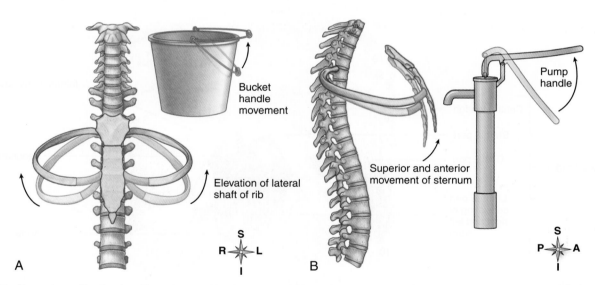

Figure 2-12 Illustration of bucket-handle and pump-handle rib movements. (From Drake R, Vogl AW, Mitchell A: *Gray's anatomy for students*, Philadelphia, 2005, Churchill Livingstone.)

sternal ends of the ribs rise and fall, whereas the vertebral ends are fixed. Muscular contraction elevates only the sternal ends of the ribs, causing a pump-handle motion that moves the sternal ends of the ribs up and away from the vertebral column. This motion increases the anterior-posterior distance between the sternum and vertebra, enlarging the thoracic cavity volume (Figure 2-12).

The so-called bucket-handle movement occurs simultaneously with the pump-handle movement. In the bucket-handle movement, the sternum and vertebral column act as fixed attachment points for the semicircular rib, which is shaped like a bucket handle. At the end of an expiration, the rib is positioned

such that its curved midpoint loops downward (similar to the handle of a pail) below its attached sternal and vertebral ends. During inspiration, an upward swing of the rib causes its midpoint to move out laterally, away from the thoracic midline, increasing the side-to-side (transverse) distance between the left and right sides of the rib cage (see Figure 2-12). Combined pump-handle and bucket-handle rib movements create a two-dimensional enlargement of the thoracic cavity as the ribs elevate during inspiration. Return of the ribs to their resting positions causes thoracic volume to decrease. This changing thoracic volume provides the basis for generating pressure gradients necessary for air movement into and out of the lungs.

Ventilatory Muscles

The muscles of ventilation are classified as primary and accessory. The major primary muscle active in quiet breathing is the diaphragm. To a much smaller extent, the parasternal intercostal and scalene muscles are involved in quiet breathing. Accessory muscles, which are used only when the work of breathing or ventilatory demand increases, include the **sternomastoids**, **pectoralis major**, and abdominals. Only the abdominals are accessory muscles of expiration.

Diaphragm

At rest, the diaphragm is bowed deeply into the thoracic cavity (Figure 2-13, *A*). It consists of two functionally distinct components: **costal parts** and crural parts. Costal diaphragm fibers originate from the lower inner rib borders (costal margins) and the lower end of the sternum. Crural fibers originate from the first three lumbar vertebrae, forming two muscle bands, the left and right **crura** (see Figure 2-13, *A*). These crural portions of the diaphragm have no direct rib cage attachments. Costal and crural fibers converge and insert into a common central tendon. The central tendon separates the diaphragm into two leaflets, the right and left hemidiaphragms. Each hemidiaphragm is innervated by its own phrenic nerve, allowing it to function independently. Normally, the hemidiaphragms function synchronously.

During inspiration, costal and crural diaphragmatic muscle fibers contract, pulling the central tendon downward. Costal

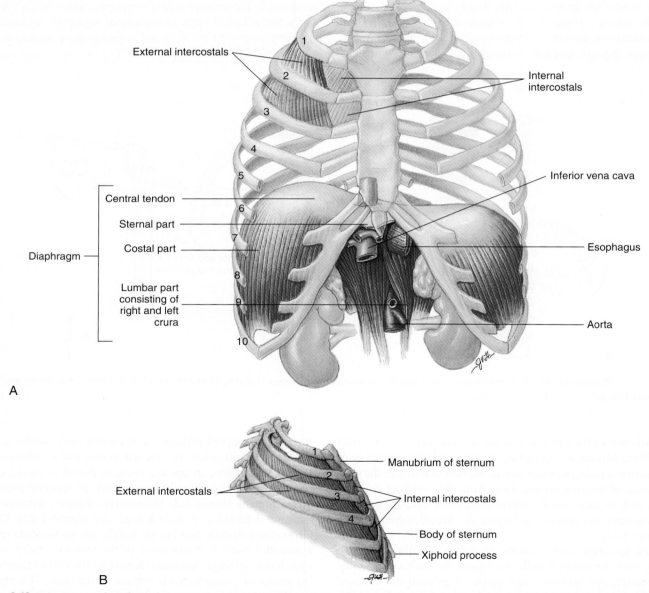

Figure 2-13 Primary muscles of ventilation. **A,** Intercostal muscles and the diaphragm. **B,** Lateral view of intercostal muscles. (From Seeley RR, Stephens TD, Tate P: *Anatomy & physiology*, ed 3, New York, 1995, McGraw-Hill.)

fiber contraction flattens the diaphragm dome, compressing the abdominal organs below. At the same time, the abdominal wall muscles relax and bulge outward as they accommodate the descending diaphragm. To the extent that compressed abdominal organs resist displacement, they form a fulcrum against which costal fibers pull and lift up the inner borders of the lower ribs. Costal diaphragmatic contraction creates a two-dimensional expansion of the thoracic cavity; it expands the lower rib cage and simultaneously increases the vertical dimensions of the thorax. Crural fibers do not have rib cage attachments, and their contraction during inspiration increases only the vertical dimensions of the thorax.

The combined rib and diaphragm movements during inspiration cause a three-dimensional increase in thoracic volume: anterior-posterior, transverse, and vertical dimensions all increase simultaneously. The downward movement of the diaphragm is the most significant cause of thoracic cavity enlargement and is most responsible for generating subatmospheric pressure in the thoracic cavity during inspiration. Only 1.5 cm of downward diaphragmatic movement (the amount of movement in a normal quiet inspiration) is responsible for a lung volume increase of more than 500 mL. Under extreme ventilatory demand, the diaphragm may move downward 6 to 10 cm.

The diaphragm is essentially inactive during quiet exhalation, although it may maintain some muscle tone in the early phase of exhalation. This delayed relaxation creates a "braking" action, making the transition between inhalation and exhalation smoother and less abrupt. The return of the diaphragm to its highly domed resting position after inhalation is passive; however, it is pulled upward by the elastic recoil of the lungs as they return to their resting end-exhalation volume.

If the lungs fail to empty normally during exhalation, because of either weakened elastic recoil forces or high resistance to airflow, the retained volume abnormally flattens the diaphragm at the end of exhalation. Then, when costal fibers contract during inspiration, they are not in a good position to lift and expand the lower rib borders. Instead, their flattened position causes their contraction to pull the lower rib cage inward, decreasing lower thoracic dimensions. An abnormally flat diaphragm at rest also reduces the volume of air that can be inhaled with each breath because the potential downward travel of the diaphragm is diminished.

Although the diaphragm is the principal muscle of inspiration, it is not essential for survival. If paralyzed, the diaphragm is passive, moving up and down only in response to changes in pressure gradients. A paralyzed diaphragm moves upward instead of downward during inspiration because the subatmospheric pressure generated by inspiration sucks the diaphragm up into the chest. This kind of diaphragmatic movement is called paradoxical because it is the opposite of what occurs during normal breathing.

CONCEPT QUESTION 2-5

How might severe obesity affect diaphragmatic movement and ventilation?

Intercostal Muscles

The intercostal muscles and the ribs form the semiflexible chest wall. The internal intercostal muscles are actually two separate muscles, the parasternal and the interosseous intercostal muscles. Both muscles are located between the ribs, but only the parasternals have an upper insertion into the sternum. Parasternal muscle contraction tends to elevate the ribs, assisting inspiration. Interosseous fibers are situated between the ribs such that their contraction depresses the ribs, causing expiration. The external intercostal muscles along with the parasternal intercostals elevate the ribs, resulting in inspiration (see Figure 2-13).

The intercostal muscles are only slightly active during quiet breathing; they mainly act to keep the ribs in a constant position rather than expand the thorax to any great extent. All intercostals become more active under heavy ventilatory demand or in cases in which the diaphragm is paralyzed. Intercostal muscle tone stabilizes the chest wall, creating a semirigid barrier in the spaces between the ribs, the intercostal spaces. However, strong inspiratory efforts may create enough subatmospheric pressure in the thoracic cavity to suck the intercostal muscles inward, clearly outlining the individual ribs. Such **intercostal retractions** are a sign of intense respiratory efforts and reflect increased work of breathing. Intercostal retractions may be observed in patients with high resistance to airflow (e.g., asthma, croup) or stiff, noncompliant lungs.

CONCEPT QUESTION 2-6

What kinds of changes in lung mechanics might cause a person to use accessory respiratory muscles at rest?

Scalene Muscles

Contraction of the scalene muscles on either side of the neck elevates and fixes the first and second ribs (Figure 2-14). Traditionally, the scalenes were considered accessory inspiratory muscles that remained inactive during quiet breathing. Clinical studies have shown evidence to the contrary. Electromyographic recordings revealed low discharge frequencies from some scalene muscle units during quiet breathing in normal subjects.[5] Extremely active scalene muscles at rest indicates an abnormally high work of breathing and implies abnormal lung mechanics. Scalene muscle activity is easily detected by observation and palpation. Assessment of scalene muscle participation in ventilation at rest is an important part of physical examination of the chest and yields important information about the severity of underlying lung disease.

Sternomastoid Muscles

The sternomastoids originate from the manubrium of the sternum and insert into the mastoid process of the skull on either side of the neck (see Figure 2-14). When the head is held in a fixed position, contraction of the sternomastoids elevates the sternum, slightly elevating the anterior ends of the ribs. If the sternomastoids actively assist each inspiration at rest, work of breathing and inspiratory effort are great. Use of these accessory muscles at rest implies abnormal lung mechanics—that is, high resistance to airflow or noncompliant lungs.

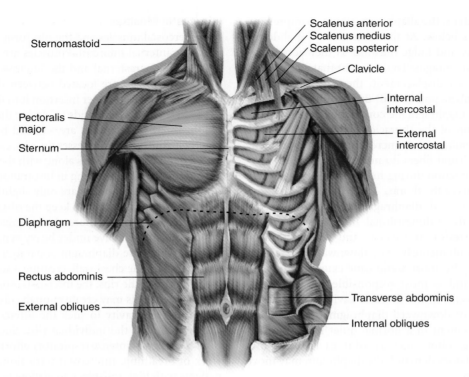

Sternomastoid

Scalenus anterior
Scalenus medius
Scalenus posterior

Clavicle

Internal intercostal

Pectoralis major

External intercostal

Sternum

Diaphragm

Rectus abdominis

External obliques

Transverse abdominis

Internal obliques

Figure 2-14 Muscles of ventilation, including accessory muscles. (From Wilkins RL, Stoller JK, Scanlan CL: *Egan's fundamentals of respiratory care*, ed 8, St Louis, 2003, Mosby.)

Pectoralis Major Muscle

The pectoralis major muscle is a fan-shaped, powerful muscle arising from the lateral borders of the sternum and inserting at the narrow end into the humerus of the arm (see Figure 2-14). If the arms and shoulders are fixed by grasping a wide stationary object, the pectoralis major can elevate the sternum and ribs. The typical posture of a person with advanced COPD is sitting, leaning forward over a table or the back of a chair, and grasping the widest portion of the object. All accessory inspiratory muscles may come into play at rest in patients with severe lung disorders characterized by high airway resistance or stiff, noncompliant lungs.

Abdominal Muscles

The abdominals are the only accessory muscles of expiration. The most important abdominal expiratory muscle is the rectus abdominis (see Figure 2-14). When contracted, it compresses the abdominal cavity, increasing pressure of the cavity.

The abdominals are normally inactive during quiet resting exhalation. They become active during heavy ventilatory demand when the passive recoil of the lung-thorax system is insufficient to provide the high expiratory flow rate needed for a rapid breathing rate. They also become active when resistance to expiratory airflow is abnormally high (e.g., severe asthma, COPD). Tensing of abdominal muscles during expiration at rest is a sign of advanced obstruction to airflow in patients with pulmonary disease. Generally, any accessory muscle use at rest is an important sign that work of breathing is greatly increased. However, during heavy exercise, all accessory muscles become active, even in normal, healthy individuals.

CONCEPT QUESTION 2-7

Why might a person with major abdominal surgery be at risk for retention of airway secretions and possible pulmonary complications?

POINTS TO REMEMBER

- The visceral and parietal pleurae, covering the lung surface (visceral pleura) and inner chest wall (parietal pleura), are one continuous membrane forming a sealed envelope surrounding the lungs.
- Oppositely directed recoil forces of the lungs and chest wall generate subatmospheric pressure in the airless space between the pleural membranes.
- Both the bronchial systemic and pulmonary circulations supply the lungs, but only the pulmonary circulation supplies the alveoli and participates in gas exchange.
- A small amount of deoxygenated bronchial systemic venous blood mixes with oxygenated blood in the pulmonary veins creating a small anatomical shunt, which is responsible for the normal difference between alveolar gas and arterial blood oxygen pressures.
- The lung receives only autonomic innervation, consisting of the sympathetic (adrenergic), parasympathetic (cholinergic), and nonadrenergic noncholinergic (NANC) systems.
- The parasympathetic system is responsible for airway smooth muscle resting tone.

- Cholinergic stimulation causes bronchoconstriction, and adrenergic stimulation causes bronchodilation.
- Beta$_2$-adrenergic agonist (stimulators) and cholinergic antagonist (blockers) drugs both elicit bronchodilation and reduced resistance to airflow.
- Sympathetic stimulation of airway smooth muscle is indirect, occurring through adrenal gland secretion of circulating epinephrine.
- Sensory afferent nerves from the lung are parasympathetic (vagal) in origin, including slowly adapting stretch receptors, rapidly adapting irritant receptors, and C-fibers; the latter two are crucial in defense of the airways because they evoke powerful reflexes that limit penetration of harmful substances into the respiratory tract.
- Movements of the thoracic ribs and diaphragm work in concert to create three-dimensional changes in thoracic volume.
- In normal quiet breathing, the diaphragm contracts and flattens to cause inspiration; it relaxes and passively returns to its resting shape during expiration because of elastic lung recoil.

- Forceful exhalation below the resting level requires the contraction of abdominal muscles.
- Accessory muscle use while at rest always signals increased ventilatory work, implying underlying lung abnormalities.

References

1. Guyton AC, Hall JE: *Textbook of medical physiology*, ed 12, Philadelphia, 2010, Saunders.
2. Barnes PJ: Pharmacologic principles. In Mason RJ, et al, editors: *Murray and Nadel's textbook of respiratory medicine*, ed 5, Philadelphia, 2010, Saunders.
3. Fryer AD, Jacoby DB: Cholinergic mechanisms and anticholinergic therapy in respiratory diseases. In Adkinson NF, et al, editors: *Middleton's allergy: principles and practice*, ed 7, Philadelphia, 2008, Mosby.
4. Crimi E, et al: Airway responsiveness to methacholine and deep inhalations in subjects with rhinitis without asthma, *J Allergy Clin Immunol* 121(2):403, 2008.
5. Gandevia SC, et al: Discharge frequencies of parasternal intercostal and scalene motor units during breathing in normal and COPD subjects, *Am J Respir Crit Care Med* 153(2):622, 1996.

CHAPTER 3

Mechanics of Ventilation

OBJECTIVES

After reading this chapter, you will be able to:
- Explain how elastic recoil forces of the lungs and chest wall interact to establish the resting lung volume
- Describe how static lung volumes and capacities are influenced by changes in the elastic recoil forces of the lungs and chest wall
- Explain which pressure gradients maintain alveolar volume and create airflow into and out of the lung
- Describe how spontaneous breathing and positive pressure mechanical ventilation are different and similar in the way they create pressure gradients throughout the respiratory cycle

- Describe how the rib cage, diaphragm, and abdomen components of the thorax move and interact differently in normal and abnormal conditions
- Interpret static and dynamic pressure-volume curves of the lungs, thorax, and lung-thorax system
- Determine whether high inflation pressure during mechanical ventilation is caused by a change in lung compliance or in airway resistance
- List factors that cause lung compliance and airway resistance to change

KEY TERMS

abdominal paradox
airway resistance (R_{aw})
asynchrony
auto-PEEP
barotrauma
body plethysmograph
closing volume
compliance
compliance curve
critical closing pressure
critical opening pressure
dipalmitoyl phosphatidylcholine (DPPC)
dynamic compliance (C_{dyn})
elasticity
equal pressure point (EPP)
exocytosis
expiratory reserve volume (ERV)
frequency dependence of compliance
frequency-to-V_T (f/V_T) ratio
functional residual capacity (FRC)
Hooke's law
hysteresis
inspiratory capacity (IC)
intrinsic PEEP
isovolume pressure-flow curve
kyphoscoliosis
Laplace's law
maximum expiratory pressure (MEP)
maximum inspiratory pressure (MIP)
peak pressure (P_{peak})

pendelluft
phosphatidylglycerol (PG)
plateau pressure (P_{plat})
Poiseuille's law
positive end-expiratory pressure (PEEP)
pressure gradients
pressure-time index (PTI)
pulmonary fibrosis
residual volume (RV)
respiratory distress syndrome (RDS)
Reynolds' number (Re)
single breath nitrogen elimination test
specific compliance
sphingomyelin
spirogram
spirometer
static compliance (C_{st})
surface tension
tension-time index of the diaphragm (TT_{di})
tension-time index of the inspiratory muscles (TT_{mus})
tidal volume (V_T)
time constant (TC)
total lung capacity (TLC)
transdiaphragmatic pressure (P_{di})
transpulmonary pressure (P_L)
transrespiratory pressure (P_{rs})
transthoracic pressure (P_w)
viscosity
viscous resistance
vital capacity (VC)

R esistance to lung inflation is categorized as (1) elastic resistance and (2) frictional resistance. Frictional resistance exists only under dynamic conditions—that is, when gas is moving through the airways. However, elastic resistance exists under both dynamic and static (no air movement) conditions. Normally, the ventilatory muscles easily overcome elastic and frictional resistances, and the work of breathing (WOB) is minimal and endlessly sustainable.

The lungs and chest wall (thorax) have equal but oppositely directed recoil forces that exactly balance each other when the respiratory muscles are relaxed and there is no airflow; the equilibrium between these forces determines the resting lung volume when ventilatory muscles are relaxed. The static and dynamic characteristics of the lung and chest wall system influence the WOB and distribution of inspired gas in the lung.

Understanding normal lung-thorax mechanics is essential in treating patients needing respiratory therapy.

STATIC LUNG AND CHEST WALL MECHANICS

Elastic Recoil of the Lungs and Thorax

Elasticity is the tendency of an object to return to its original shape after being deformed. Stretching an object that has high elasticity generates a strong recoil force. The healthy lung has a tendency to recoil inward and pull away from the chest wall. At the same time, the thorax has a tendency to recoil outward, away from the lung. These two oppositely directed recoil forces create a subatmospheric pressure between the lung and chest wall. The

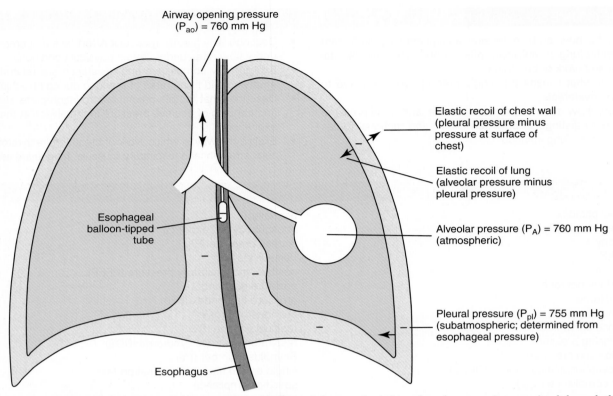

Figure 3-1 Measuring intrapleural pressure with an esophageal balloon. Subatmospheric intrapleural pressure is transmitted through the esophagus to the balloon-tipped catheter. Equal and oppositely directed recoil forces of the lungs and chest wall create this subatmospheric pressure. (From Martin L: *Pulmonary physiology in clinical practice*, St Louis, 1987, Mosby.)

lung's elastic recoil force is generated by (1) elastic and collagen fibers of the lung parenchyma and (2) surface-tension forces of the thin liquid film lining the alveoli. Of these two factors, surface tension contributes the most to the elasticity of the lung.

As the lung and chest wall recoil in opposite directions, the pressure between the pleural membranes decreases (Boyle's law). No true space exists between the visceral and parietal pleurae. However, if a small tube were placed through the chest wall between these membranes, a space would be created, and the pressure measured through the tube would be subatmospheric. This method of obtaining intrapleural pressure (P_{pl}) would be too invasive and hazardous for clinical purposes; changes in P_{pl} can be measured more safely through a balloon-tipped catheter placed in the esophagus with the tip of the catheter well inside the thoracic cavity (Figure 3-1). The thin-walled esophagus has little muscle tone and easily transmits P_{pl} changes to the balloon on the end of the catheter. Changes in intraesophageal balloon pressure reflect changes in P_{pl}. Figure 3-1 shows lung and thorax recoil forces and the resulting pressures.

CONCEPT QUESTION 3-1

The pressure in the alveoli (P_A) just before inhalation begins is 0 cm H_2O; at the end of a 500-mL inspiration, just before expiration begins, P_A is also 0 cm H_2O. Explain why P_A is 0 cm H_2O in both instances, even though the lung contains more volume at the end of the inspiration.

Pressure Gradients during Ventilation

Figure 3-2 illustrates various pressure differences or gradients involved in ventilation. Airway pressures are usually expressed using atmospheric pressure as the zero reference value. A pressure of 0 mm Hg does not refer to an absolute lack of pressure but to atmospheric pressure (760 mm Hg at sea level). In this sense, a subatmospheric pressure of 755 mm Hg is below 0 mm Hg, or "negative." Likewise, a pressure of 765 mm Hg is above 0 mm Hg, or "positive." (All pressures are positive and cannot be truly negative. However, in this book, the terms negative and positive with regard to pressure refer to subatmospheric and above atmospheric pressures.)

Pressure at the mouth or the airway opening (P_{ao}) is always equal to atmospheric pressure, or 0 mm Hg during normal spontaneous breathing. Pressure at the body surface (P_{bs}) is also by definition 0 mm Hg. Alveolar pressure (P_A), sometimes called intrapulmonary pressure, is negative during inspiration, 0 mm Hg when airflow is absent, and positive during expiration. P_{pl} is always negative during normal quiet breathing for reasons discussed previously. The more strongly the lung's recoil force tries to pull the lung away from the chest wall, the more negative the P_{pl}. When no air is moving and the lung is stationary, the inward recoil pressure of the lung is exactly balanced by the outward recoil pressure of the chest wall, creating a negative pressure between the two structures (i.e., the P_{pl} is negative); because there is no air movement, the P_A is zero. In other words, P_A is equal to the sum of chest wall and lung recoil pressures.

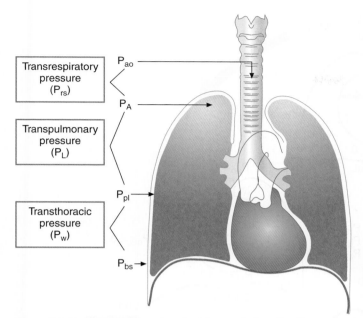

Figure 3-2 Pressure gradients involved in ventilation. P_{ao}, Pressure at the airway opening; P_A, alveolar pressure; P_{pl}, intrapleural pressure; P_{bs}, pressure at the body surface; P_{rs}, transrespiratory pressure; P_L, transpulmonary pressure; P_W, transthoracic pressure. P_{rs} is equal to either $(P_{ao} - P_A)$ or $(P_{bs} - P_A)$ in a spontaneously breathing individual and can be thought of as the pressure gradient between the mouth and alveoli or the transairway pressure.

Pressure gradients are simply pressure differences between two points that cause air to move in or out of the lungs and are responsible for keeping the lungs in an inflated state. Air always flows from a point of high pressure to a point of low pressure; a pressure gradient of 0 mm Hg means there is no pressure difference between the two points and thus no airflow. Important pressure gradients in ventilation are the **transpulmonary pressure (P_L)**, **transthoracic pressure (P_w)**, and **transrespiratory pressure (P_{rs})** (see Figure 3-2). (See Appendix I for a summary of pressure symbols in ventilatory mechanics.)

P_{rs} is the difference between alveolar and body-surface pressures ($P_{rs} = P_A - P_{bs}$) or the pressure gradient across the entire respiratory system (lungs plus chest wall). Because both P_{bs} and P_{ao} are atmospheric during normal breathing, P_{ao} can be substituted for P_{bs} in the previous equation ($P_{rs} = P_A - P_{ao}$, as shown in Figure 3-2). This equation shows that P_{rs} is also equal to the pressure gradient across the airways, between the mouth and alveoli; thus, this pressure gradient is sometimes called the transairway pressure (P_{TA}). P_{TA} is responsible for airflow in and out of the lung. No airflow exists at the end of inspiration or at the end of expiration because P_A is equal to P_{ao} under both of these conditions; P_{rs} or P_{TA} is 0 mm Hg at these two points in the breathing cycle. In normal spontaneous breathing, P_{rs} changes only when the P_A changes because P_{ao} is atmospheric and remains constant at 0 mm Hg. The magnitude of P_{rs} (i.e., the difference between mouth and alveolar pressures) reflects the airways' frictional resistance to airflow: the greater the pressure gradient needed to drive gas through the airways, the greater the airway resistance.

The transpulmonary pressure (P_L) gradient is the difference between alveolar and intrapleural pressures ($P_L = P_A - P_{pl}$); in other words, P_L is the distending pressure across the alveolar walls. P_L is equal to the elastic recoil force of the lungs when there is no airflow—that is, the lung's inward recoil creates a subatmospheric P_{pl} that exactly counterbalances the lung's recoil force and prevents it from recoiling further. P_A is always greater than P_{pl} in the intact normal lung-thorax system; thus, P_L is a pressure gradient that keeps the alveoli inflated. If P_L increases, alveolar volume increases, and vice versa; lung volume can change only if P_L changes. Breathing, whether spontaneous or mechanically induced, consists of the increase or decrease of P_L.

CONCEPT QUESTION 3-2

Refer to Figure 3-4. At the end of a spontaneous 500-mL inspiration, the P_A is 0 mm Hg; at the end of a positive pressure lung inflation to 500 mL, P_A is 10 mm Hg. Explain how it is possible for the lung to contain the same volume at these two different alveolar pressures.

Transthoracic pressure (P_w) is the difference between P_{pl} and P_{bs}, or the pressure difference across the thoracic wall ($P_w = P_{pl} - P_{bs}$). It is equal to the outward recoil force of the thorax when there is no airflow. The stronger this outward recoil force, the greater the P_w. P_w is a reflection of thoracic wall recoil force alone.

Figure 3-3 illustrates changes in pressures during the respiratory cycle (inspiration and expiration). At the end of a resting expiration when all airflow has ceased, $P_A = 0$ cm H_2O, and the elastic recoil force of the lungs (P_{el}) is equal to a pressure of about 5 cm H_2O (Figure 3-3, *A*). This means P_{pl} must be −5 cm H_2O (P_A is the sum of alveolar recoil pressure plus P_{pl}). Therefore, transpulmonary pressure (P_L) at this point is about 5 cm H_2O. The P_L is calculated as follows:

$$P_L = P_A - P_{pl}$$
$$P_L = 0 - (-5)$$
$$P_L = 5 \text{ cm } H_2O$$

By convention, P_L is expressed as a positive number because it is the pressure that distends the lung. Corresponding with a P_L of 5 cm H_2O is a counterbalancing transthoracic pressure of −5 cm H_2O, shown as follows:

$$P_w = P_{pl} - P_{bs}$$
$$P_w = (-5) - 0$$
$$P_w = -5 \text{ cm } H_2O$$

When all muscles are relaxed and no air is flowing, the inward and outward recoil forces of the lungs and thorax are in equilibrium with each another (see Figure 3-3, *A*). The P_{rs} (pressure difference between the alveoli and the body surface) is the sum of P_L plus P_w and is 0 mm Hg under the resting conditions just described. This is illustrated as follows:

$$P_{rs} = P_L + P_w$$
$$P_{rs} = 5 \text{ cm } H_2O + (-5 \text{ cm } H_2O)$$
$$P_{rs} = 0 \text{ cm } H_2O$$

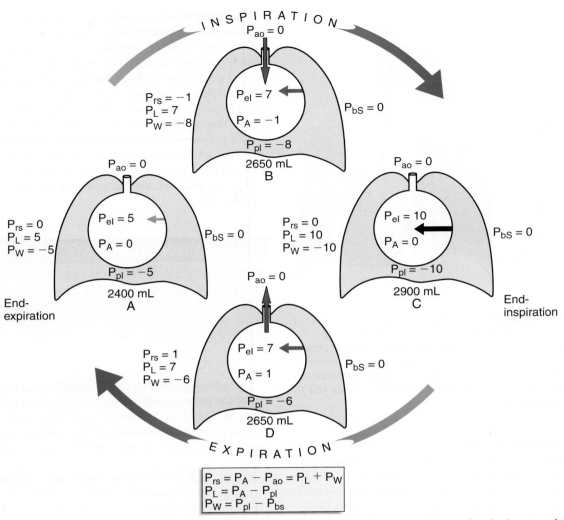

Figure 3-3 Changes in pressure and volume during a quiet 500-mL inspiration and expiration. **A,** Beginning inspiration or end-expiration. **B,** Midinspiration. **C,** End-inspiration or beginning expiration. **D,** Midexpiration. Increases and decreases in lung volume are induced by increases and decreases in P_L. P_A is always equal to $P_{el} + P_{pl}$. P_{ao}, Pressure at the airway opening; P_{el}, lung elastic recoil pressure; P_A, alveolar pressure; P_{pl}, intrapleural pressure; P_{bs}, pressure at the body surface; P_{rs}, transrespiratory pressure; P_L, transpulmonary pressure; P_W, transthoracic pressure.

The act of inspiration (see Figure 3-3, moving from *A* to *B* to *C*) disrupts the equilibrium between lung and thoracic recoil forces. The ventilatory muscles contract and increase the thoracic dimensions as explained in Chapter 2. Consequently, P_{pl} decreases (Boyle's law), which increases the P_L gradient ($P_A - P_{pl}$), "pulling" the alveoli to larger volumes. This causes P_A to fall below P_{ao}, establishing a pressure gradient for airflow into the lungs (see Figure 3-3, *B*). Air stops flowing into the lungs when P_A equalizes with P_{ao} (see Figure 3-3, *C*). At this point, P_L is at its maximum value in the respiratory cycle (i.e., the difference between P_A and P_{pl} is greatest), corresponding with an inhaled volume of 500 mL in this example.

Expiration begins when ventilatory muscles relax, allowing lung recoil forces to shrink the thoracic cavity passively (see Figure 3-3, moving from *C* to *D*). As the thoracic volume decreases, P_{pl} increases (becomes less negative), narrowing the gap between P_{pl} and P_A. This decreases P_L, reducing the lung's dimensions, which compresses the lung's air, increasing P_A

above P_{ao}. Gas flows out of the lungs, reestablishing the initial preinspiratory conditions (see Figure 3-3, from *D* to *A*).

Rib Cage and Diaphragm-Abdomen Components of the Thorax

To this point, the thorax has been considered as if it were a single unit. It is more accurate to think of the thorax as having two components: the rib cage and the diaphragm-abdomen complex.[1] The rib cage and diaphragm are coupled but can act independently during ventilation. Rib cage movements change the anterior-posterior and lateral dimensions of the thorax, and diaphragm movements displace the abdominal organs and change vertical thoracic dimensions. Normally, abdominal displacement predominates during quiet breathing, whereas rib cage displacement predominates when one breathes large volumes near maximum lung capacity.[1] If abdominal displacement by the diaphragm is hampered by obesity, pregnancy, or an otherwise distended abdomen, breathing becomes more dependent on rib cage displacement. The work of breathing increases because it is more difficult to inflate the lung when the diaphragm resists movement.

Static Lung Volumes and Capacities

The **total lung capacity** (**TLC**) is the amount of gas the lung contains after a maximal inspiratory effort. All other lung volumes are natural subdivisions of the TLC. The term "capacity" refers to the combination of two or more volumes, which are basic, nonoverlapping entities in the TLC.

Measurement of Lung Volumes—Spirometry

Spirometry is the process of measuring volumes of air moving in and out of the lungs. A **spirometer** is the device used to measure these volumes. The **spirogram** is a graphical volume versus time representation of the lung volumes made by the spirometer. A classic water-seal spirometer is shown in Figure 3-5. Knowledge of the function of the water-seal spirometer helps a

---

CLINICAL FOCUS 3-1

Pressure Gradients in Positive Pressure Ventilation and Spontaneous Breathing

During mechanical positive pressure ventilation (PPV), P_{ao} is increased above atmospheric pressure during inspiration, forcing gas into the alveoli. This is the opposite of spontaneous breathing (SB), in which P_A first decreases below P_{ao}. During PPV, the alveoli transmit some of their positive pressure into the intrapleural space. This causes P_{pl} to increase toward zero (become less negative), which is again the opposite of spontaneous inspiration, in which P_{pl} decreases and becomes even more negative. Two important points to remember are (1) both SB and PPV accomplish inspiration by increasing P_L, the pressure distending the lungs, and (2) because PPV raises the P_{pl}, it tends to compress the veins that bring blood back to the heart, ultimately impeding cardiac output. SB has the opposite effect because inspiration lowers P_{pl} further, augmenting venous blood return to the heart.

Figure 3-4 compares PPV and SB. The lung diagrams illustrate conditions at the end of an inspiration. Although the transpulmonary pressures were achieved by different means in SB and PPV, P_L is 10 cm H_2O in both instances. This means elastic lung fibers are stretched to the same extent in both instances. The PPV inspiration places no more stress on the lung than the SB inspiration, although P_A is 10 cm H_2O greater in PPV than in SB. This fact has relevance to therapeutic lung-expansion techniques used in respiratory care. Given normal inspiratory muscle function, a mechanical positive pressure inspiration is not superior to a spontaneous inspiration in expanding the lung, and a 500-mL positive pressure breath is not any more likely than a 500-mL spontaneous breath to injure the lungs. PPV may generate a greater P_L and volume than SB only in a person with weakened inspiratory muscles.

CLINICAL FOCUS 3-2

Misguided Therapy: Why High Alveolar Pressure Does Not Always Expand the Lung

In years past, respiratory therapists and nurses taught patients to use blow bottles, thinking this technique would help expand the lungs. Blow bottles consisted of two large capped jars half full of water connected by a single long tube penetrating through each bottle cap. Each end of the connecting tube was submerged below the water surface near the bottom of each jar. Each jar had an additional short tube fitted through its cap that did not reach the water's surface. By blowing forcefully through this short tube, the patient could force water up through the long connecting tube into the other jar. The high pressure generated in the lungs during the water transfer was believed to reexpand collapsed alveoli. However, a rational examination of pulmonary mechanics reveals that the high P_A created in a blow bottle exercise cannot expand the lungs.

Discussion
The P_L (i.e., the pressure difference between the alveoli and the intrapleural space) determines the lung's volume. This gradient increases during inspiration (enlarging the lung's volume) and decreases during expiration (reducing the lung's volume). Exhaling against resistance through the blow bottles' tubes increases P_A, but it increases P_{pl} even more, decreasing the transpulmonary pressure gradient. Consequently, lung volume decreases during this expiratory maneuver, even though P_A is high—the opposite of the intended therapeutic outcome. Coughing maneuvers (because they are bursts of forced expiration) also do not increase the transpulmonary pressure gradient for the same reasons. The deep breath individuals must take before a cough or before they can blow water from one bottle to the other is the only part of the procedure that can produce lung expansion. It is more rational simply to coach the patient to take deep breaths, which focuses attention on inspiration and lung expansion rather than on expiration and lung deflation—which is precisely what modern incentive spirometry techniques accomplish.

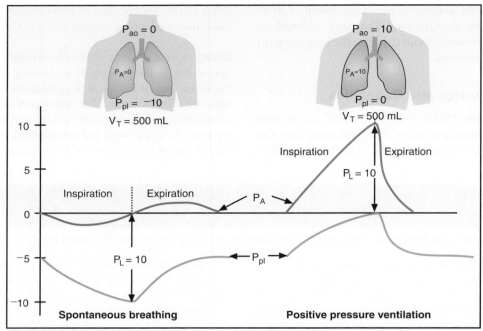

Figure 3-4 Airway and intrapleural pressure changes during spontaneous and positive pressure mechanical ventilation. Tidal volumes (V_T) are identical in both instances because the distending transpulmonary pressures (P_L) are equal. P_{ao}, Pressure at the airway opening; P_A, alveolar pressure; P_{pl}, intrapleural pressure.

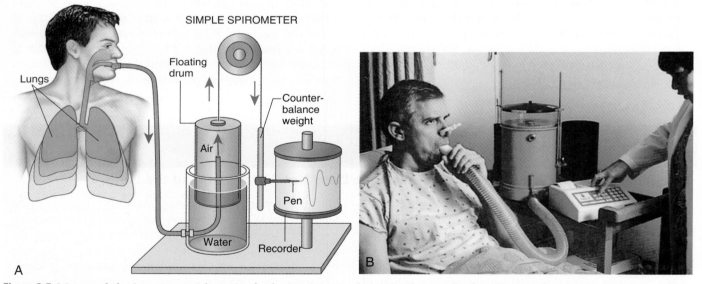

Figure 3-5 Water-sealed spirometer. **A,** Schematic of a classic spirometer design. **B,** Photograph of a pulmonary function test in progress. (From Wilson SF, Thompson JM: *Respiratory disorders*, St Louis, 1990, Mosby-Year Book.)

person understand the interrelationships between volumes and capacities. (Modern spirometers are electronic, microprocessor-controlled devices.)

While wearing nose clips to occlude the nostrils, the patient inhales and exhales through a large tube inserted snugly into the mouth (see Figure 3-5). Exhaled air enters the inverted cylinder (bell) suspended by a chain and pulley. This bell fits loosely over a smaller cylinder and floats in a water-filled sleeve. The other end of the chain is attached to a recording pen and counterweight, which exactly balance the weight of

the floating bell. The water provides a seal from atmospheric air and allows nearly frictionless movement of the bell. Bell movements cause the pen to move up and down, inscribing reciprocal tracings on recording paper wrapped around a drum rotating at a constant speed, creating a graphic representation of volume (vertical axis) versus time (horizontal axis) (Figure 3-6).

Figure 3-6 reveals that not all of the TLC is accessible to the spirometer. The **residual volume (RV)** cannot be exhaled, even with the greatest expiratory effort, because the rigid rib cage

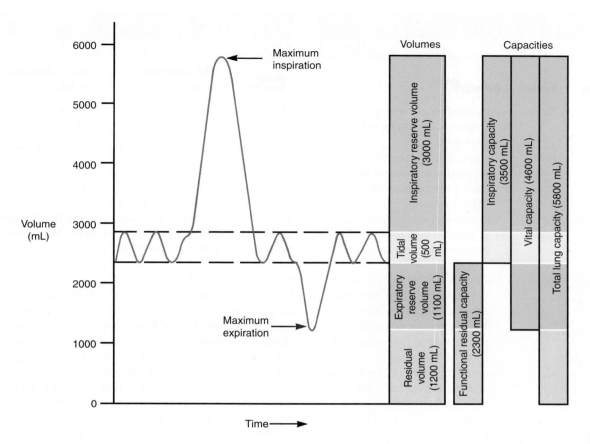

Figure 3-6 Lung volumes and capacities as displayed by a time versus volume spirogram. Values are approximate. Tidal volume is measured under resting conditions. (From Seeley RR, Stephens TD, Tate P: *Anatomy & physiology*, ed 3, New York, 1995, McGraw-Hill.)

prevents total lung deflation. RV must be measured indirectly through other techniques (see Chapter 5).

Figure 3-6 illustrates the four lung volumes and four lung capacities. The measurements for each are approximate and vary according to an individual's height, gender, and age. The descriptions and symbols for the static lung volumes and capacities are shown in Table 3-1. (See also Appendix I.)

The **tidal volume (V$_T$)** is the volume of air inhaled or exhaled with each breath. The **vital capacity (VC)** defines the maximum limits of a single breath—that is, from a maximum-effort inspiration to a maximum-effort expiration. Theoretically, the V$_T$ can increase until it equals the VC, but this never occurs, even with the most strenuous exercise. The **functional residual capacity (FRC)** is the amount of air in the lungs at the point of ventilatory muscle relaxation, also known as the resting level, or end-tidal exhalation level. Normally, about 40% of the TLC is contained in the lung at this resting FRC level. Expiratory (abdominal) muscle contraction is required to exhale any portion of the FRC, which involves the exhalation of **expiratory reserve volume (ERV)**. The balance point between inward lung recoil and outward chest wall recoil determines the FRC level. Any factor that decreases lung recoil force increases the FRC and decreases the **inspiratory capacity (IC)**. Any factor that increases lung recoil force decreases the FRC and decreases the TLC and VC. (Chapter 5 reviews these interrelationships in more detail.)

CONCEPT QUESTION 3-3

Referring to Figure 3-6 and Table 3-1, what effect does an increased RV have on other volumes or capacities, assuming TLC stays the same?

During resting V$_T$ breathing, only inspiration requires muscular (diaphragmatic) contraction. The end-tidal level is the point of total relaxation for all ventilatory muscles. Tidal exhalation is passive, a result of passive lung recoil. Tidal exhalation ends when lung and chest wall recoil forces reestablish their equilibrium point.

Maximum Static Inspiratory and Expiratory Pressures

Maximum inspiratory pressure (MIP) and **maximum expiratory pressure (MEP)** depend on ventilatory muscle strength. (Alternative symbols are PI$_{max}$ and PE$_{max}$.) These pressures are measured under static conditions while a person inhales or exhales with maximal effort against an occluded tube attached to a pressure gauge. During this measurement, the nose is blocked and the lips are sealed tightly around the tube to prevent air leaks.

The maximum pressures generated depend on the lung volumes at which they are measured. The MIP generating capacity

TABLE 3-1
Static Lung Volumes and Capacities

Volume and Capacity	Symbol	Definition
Residual volume	RV	Volume of air remaining in the lung after a maximal-effort expiration
Expiratory reserve volume	ERV	Volume of air that can be exhaled with maximal effort from a resting (tidal) end-expiratory level
Tidal volume	TV or V_T	Volume of air normally inhaled or exhaled with each breath during resting, quiet breathing
Inspiratory reserve volume	IRV	Volume of air that can be inhaled with maximal effort from the tidal end-inspiratory level
Total lung capacity	TLC	Volume of air in the lung after a maximal-effort inspiration; the sum of all volumes
Inspiratory capacity	IC	Volume of air that can be inhaled with maximal effort from a resting (tidal) end-expiratory level; sum of TV and IRV
Vital capacity	VC	Maximum volume of air that can be exhaled after a maximal-effort inspiration; sum of IRV, TV, and ERV
Functional residual capacity	FRC	Volume of gas remaining in the lung at the end of a normal tidal exhalation (relaxed ventilatory muscles); sum of ERV and RV

TABLE 3-2
Maximum Inspiratory and Expiratory Pressures

Gender	MIP—Measured at RV	MEP—Measured at TLC
Males	-126 cm H_2O	229 cm H_2O
Females	-92 cm H_2O	151 cm H_2O

MIP, Maximum inspiratory pressure; *RV*, residual volume; *MEP*, maximum expiratory pressure; *TLC*, total lung capacity.

is greatest at RV because diaphragmatic muscle fibers are maximally lengthened. The same principle is true for MEPs. At TLC, expiratory muscles are fully stretched, and a maximal expiratory effort may generate 230 cm H_2O. At RV, expiratory muscle fibers are maximally contracted, and no expiratory pressure can be generated.

Average MEP and MIP results for adults are shown in Table 3-2.[2] These pressures represent high reserve muscle strength, which may become involved during a cough or the birth process. Measurements of MIP and MEP are often used clinically to assess the ability of a patient to maintain spontaneous, unassisted ventilation; MIP is more often used in this regard. Severe compromise of ventilatory muscle strength is evident when no more than -20 cm H_2O MIP can be generated.[3]

Static Pressure-Volume Relationships

The elastic properties of the lung-thorax system are assessed by measuring the pressure required to inflate the lung under static conditions. Inflation pressures are measured many times at several volumes, and a pressure-volume (P-V) graph is constructed. Static pressures are plotted on the horizontal axis, and volumes are plotted on the vertical axis.

Hooke's Law and Elastic Recoil

Over the normal physiological range of tidal breathing, the lung's expansion in response to increasing pressures conforms to **Hooke's law**. Hooke's law states that an elastic structure changes dimensions in direct proportion to the amount of force applied. Each unit of pressure applied to the lung causes an additional unit of volume to be generated. As the lung volume increases, the recoil force increases. This linear relationship is maintained up to the elastic limit. If the elastic limit is exceeded, lung rupture is imminent.

Hooke's law oversimplifies the response of the lungs to increasing pressures. Although the P-V curve is relatively linear in the V_T range, a curve that plots the VC against the lung's distending pressure (P_L) is more S-shaped. The deflation curve follows a different path than the inflation curve, which is explained in the next section.

Static Pressure-Volume Curve

The lung's P_L (i.e., $P_A - P_{pl}$) must be measured to create a static P-V curve for the lung alone (not taking the chest wall into account). The P_{pl} can be measured with an esophageal balloon, as described previously. P_A is measured at the mouth under static conditions (i.e., when air flow is absent, mouth and alveolar pressures are equal).

An inspiratory P-V curve can be constructed (Figure 3-7) by applying pressure to the trachea, inflating the lung in volume increments in a stepwise fashion from RV to TLC. Each volume increment is held in the lung until all airflow ceases and P_L is recorded. If the lung is deflated in an identical stepwise fashion back to RV, an expiratory P-V curve is constructed. The inflation-deflation curves are traced in a counterclockwise fashion when the lung is inflated by positive pressure applied to the trachea. The curves are nonlinear, partly because the collagen and elastic fibers composing the lung parenchyma are not uniform springs. Elastic fibers are easily stretched, whereas collagen fibers are more resistant to deformation. As the lung volume approaches TLC during inspiration, collagen fibers resist stretching more, causing the slope of the P-V curve to flatten at its upper end, creating an upper inflection point (see Figure 3-7).

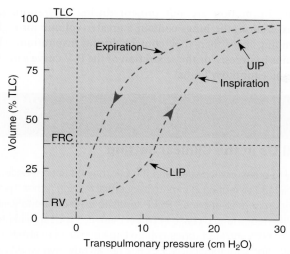

Figure 3-7 Pressure-volume curve of the lung during inspiration and expiration. The phenomenon of surface tension at the alveolar air-liquid interface creates hysteresis or different inspiration and expiration pathways. *TLC*, Total lung capacity; *FRC*, functional residual capacity; *RV*, residual volume; *UIP*, upper inflection point; *LIP*, lower inflection point. (Modified from Berne RM, Levy MN: *Physiology*, ed 3, St Louis, 1993, Mosby.)

Hysteresis and Mechanism of Lung Volume Change

The inflation and deflation limbs of the P-V curve in Figure 3-7 trace different paths, showing that for the same distending pressure, lung volume is greater during deflation than inflation. This phenomenon is called **hysteresis**, which occurs because the lungs dissipate energy during inflation.[4] In other words, part of the energy used to inflate the lungs is not recovered during deflation; this means it takes less force to keep the lungs inflated during deflation than it does during inflation. This phenomenon has been experimentally shown: at the same pressure, the lung volume fixed in inflation is lower than the volume fixed in deflation.[4]

The phenomenon of hysteresis is related to the mechanism whereby lung volume changes. The idea that lung inflation and deflation are the result of collective balloon-like changes in 300 million alveolar diameters is overly simplistic. It is now widely understood that the major mechanism of lung expansion and retraction involves the sequential opening and closing (recruitment and derecruitment) of peripheral alveoli.[4,5] At the end of a maximally forceful expiration (at RV), numerous alveoli are closed; lung volume increases during the subsequent inspiration mainly because an increasingly greater number of alveoli open up, not because individual alveolar diameters increase. The lungs dissipate energy in the alveolar recruitment process, mostly in overcoming the molecular adhesive forces of surface tension—forces not present during expiration when alveoli are already open.[4]

The lung's recruitment expansion mechanism has been confirmed by in vivo microscopy of subpleural alveoli in animal models; inflation of the lung from 20% to 80% of TLC increased the number of recruited alveoli but did not increase individual alveolar diameters.[5] A different investigation yielded similar results; when lung inflation pressure was increased from 10 cm H_2O to 20 cm H_2O and then again from 20 cm H_2O to 30 cm H_2O, alveolar size did not change, but the number of recruited alveoli changed in direct proportion to applied pressure.[4]

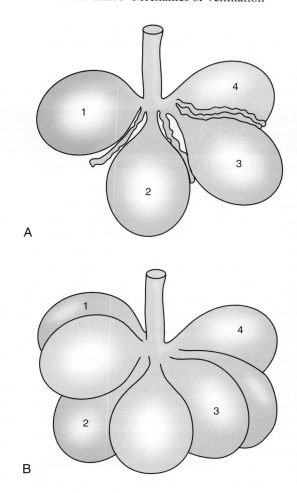

Figure 3-8 Lung inflation through alveolar recruitment. **A,** At the beginning of inspiration, some alveoli are closed, their walls stuck together. **B,** As transpulmonary pressure increases during inspiration, these alveoli are opened (recruited) with little or no change in the diameters of previously open alveoli (numbered *1-4* in **A** and **B**).

The alveolar recruitment-derecruitment mechanism is illustrated in Figure 3-8. At the beginning of inspiration (Figure 3-8, *A*), numerous alveoli are closed, their walls stuck together. As inspiration continues, these alveoli are forced open and recruited by the increasing P_L (Figure 3-8, *B*). Recruitment occurs in two phases: in the first phase, from deflation to about 50% of the TLC, lung volume increases secondary to a linear increase in the number of alveoli recruited (i.e., the number recruited is directly proportional to P_L). From 50% to 100% of TLC, the rate of recruitment accelerates, and the number of recruited alveoli increases exponentially. This accelerated recruitment rate is reflected by a steeper slope on the P-V curve, marked by a lower inflection point (LIP) on the inspiratory limb (see Figure 3-7).[4]

It was previously thought that the LIP marked the point at which alveolar recruitment was complete and that if expiratory pressure were not allowed to fall below this point in mechanically ventilated critically ill patients, alveolar closure on expiration would be prevented. It is now known that alveolar recruitment continues beyond the LIP to TLC; the entire P-V curve can be thought of as a recruitment curve.[4,6] (See Clinical Focus 3-3 for a discussion of the clinically obtained P-V curve and significance of LIP.)

When the lung deflates, all alveoli are already open; the molecular adhesive forces opposing the recruitment process during inspiration are not present during expiration. During expiration, the lungs contain a greater volume for a given distending force than they contain during inspiration, which explains hysteresis, or the separation of the P-V curve's inspiratory and expiratory limbs.

CLINICAL FOCUS 3-3

What Static and Dynamic Pressure-Volume Curves Tell Us in the Clinical Setting

Static P-V curves (no airflow conditions) are sometimes constructed in mechanically ventilated patients with acute lung injuries with the belief that these curves might be helpful in ventilator management. Beginning at the FRC level, the respiratory therapist progressively inflates the lungs in measured increments, pausing after each inflation to record its corresponding pressure. In healthy lungs, the P-V curve over the V_T range is linear, but in severe lung injury (e.g., acute respiratory distress syndrome [ARDS]), the tidal P-V curve often has a sigmoid shape with a distinct lower inflection point (LIP) and possibly an upper inflection point (UIP), as shown in the figure. Traditionally, the LIP was thought to be the critical pressure at which collapsed alveoli reopened, and the UIP was believed to mark the volume at which alveolar overstretching occurred. The conventional wisdom was to ventilate patients with airway pressures between the two inflection points; the ventilator could be set to maintain positive end-expiratory pressure (PEEP) to keep pressures above the LIP on expiration, and V_T could be limited to keep inspiratory pressure below the UIP. This strategy, sometimes called the "open-lung" approach to mechanical ventilation, was used to protect against ventilator-induced lung injury.

However, pressures measured at the endotracheal tube reflect the summation of many simultaneously occurring events in a highly complex lung composed of 300 million alveoli; alveolar P-V relationships inferred from measurements made at the endotracheal tube introduce uncertainty, limiting the helpfulness of P-V curves in ventilator management. It is now widely accepted that alveolar reopening in acute lung injury continues along the linear middle part of the static P-V curve even above the UIP and that the UIP probably indicates the end of alveolar recruitment, not necessarily the beginning of overdistention.[6] It is possible that overdistention of some alveoli occurring simultaneously with the recruitment of others might delay the appearance of the UIP, which means overdistention and alveolar injury could occur even at pressures below the UIP.[6] Regarding the use of the LIP to set PEEP at a level that prevents expiratory alveolar closure, one must keep in mind that PEEP is applied on expiration. The LIP is a feature of the inspiratory P-V curve, more related to alveolar reopening during inspiration than it is to alveolar closure, which occurs during expiration. The LIP appears to be of limited relevance to expiratory alveolar closure and optimal PEEP levels.[6]

What causes the LIP, and what does it mean? The LIP is probably due to the instantaneous reopening of many alveoli with the same threshold opening pressures, as occurs in evenly distributed (homogeneous) lung disease. In unevenly distributed (heterogeneous) lung disease, alveoli with different threshold opening pressures coexist, and the LIP may be absent because alveoli tend to reopen in a more sequential fashion rather than in large numbers all at once.[6] PEEP tends to be more beneficial in homogeneous lung disease in which there is a widespread presence of nonventilated zones, where large numbers of alveoli can be recruited simultaneously. PEEP is not as effective when lung disease is heterogeneous (characterized by interspersed ventilated and nonventilated zones), where an increase in inspiratory pressure is more likely to overdistend already open alveoli rather than recruit large numbers of alveoli en masse. The P-V curve contour may simply indicate the presence of homogeneous or heterogeneous lung disease and the potential for recruitment, not the optimal level of PEEP needed to prevent alveolar closure.[6]

The V_T P-V curve can be displayed in a breath-to-breath real-time fashion on the monitoring screens of modern mechanical ventilators. However, this dynamically traced P-V curve is affected by airflow resistance and the P-V relationships in the ventilator tubing, humidifier, and endotracheal tube; it cannot provide accurate information about the P-V relationships in the alveoli.[28] The ventilator pressure sensor measures pressure at the patient connection part of the ventilator tubing. During inflation, tubing pressure increases rapidly (depending on the ventilator's flow setting) with little initial volume change as endotracheal tube and airway resistances are overcome. Volume increases more rapidly relative to pressure as elastic resistance is overcome. This transition from frictional to elastic resistance creates an "inflection point" on the lower part of the inspiratory P-V loop, but it does not have the same meaning as the inflection point on the static P-V curve.[28]

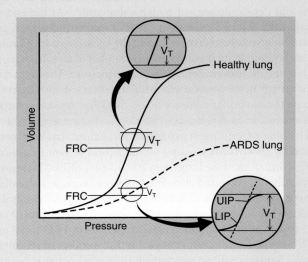

Lung Distensibility: Static Compliance

Compliance is a measure of the lung's opposition to inflation. The P-V curve (see Figure 3-7) is a **compliance curve**. Lung compliance (C_L) is defined as the change in lung volume produced by a unit of pressure change and is measured in liters per centimeter of water pressure (L/cm H_2O), shown as follows:

$$C_L = \frac{\Delta V \text{ (liters)}}{\Delta P \text{ (cm } H_2O)}$$

Compliance can be conceptualized as distensibility; if the lung is easily distended, it has high compliance. A lung with low compliance is stiff and difficult to inflate. Static C_L can be obtained from the P-V curve in Figure 3-9 by measuring the volume change (vertical axis) produced by a pressure change (horizontal axis). Normal compliance of the lung alone (C_L) is 0.2 L/cm H_2O or 200 mL/cm H_2O.

The opposite of compliance is elastance, defined as the change in pressure required to produce a unit of volume change (cm H_2O/L). Elastance is the mathematical reciprocal of compliance (elastance = 1/compliance). The more elastic the lung, the less its compliance. Elastance can be conceptualized as recoil force; highly elastic lungs are stiff and difficult to inflate and exhibit a high recoil force. By convention, in pulmonary medicine, the elastic characteristics of the lung are quantified in terms of compliance rather than elastance.

CONCEPT QUESTION 3-4

In a quiet, passive exhalation, which of the following requires the longest exhalation time: the person with high C_L or the person with high lung elastance?

Compliance and Lung Volume

The value of C_L depends on the volume at which it is measured. The compliance curve is not linear, as shown in Figure 3-9. Near TLC, lung fibers are stretched and close to their elastic limits; a 500-mL inspiration taken at a point near TLC requires more muscular effort than a 500-mL inspiration beginning at FRC. The slope of the compliance curve is steepest and C_L is greatest at FRC; this is beneficial because an individual normally inhales the V_T from the FRC level where volume changes require little effort. Even during strenuous exercise, people breathe over the lower 70% of the P-V curve, keeping the elastic WOB relatively low. The larger inspired volumes during exercise produce higher lung recoil, which helps provide the force needed to produce high expiratory flow rates during rapid breathing rates.

Compliance (L/cm H_2O) is greater in an adult than an infant because adult lungs are larger and accept more volume for a given pressure. Although the inherent elastic properties of lung tissues may be identical in adult and infant lungs, the infant's measured C_L is lower. To correct for lung size, compliance should be calculated per unit of lung volume (C_L/vol). This measurement is called **specific compliance** and is generally referenced to the individual's FRC (specific compliance = C_L/FRC). Adults and infants have about the same specific C_L.

Figure 3-10 illustrates the effects of different disease types on C_L. Emphysema is characterized by a loss of elastic lung tissue, which means the lungs can be easily distended and have an abnormally low recoil force. Small pressure changes produce large volume changes. Weakened elastic lung recoil changes

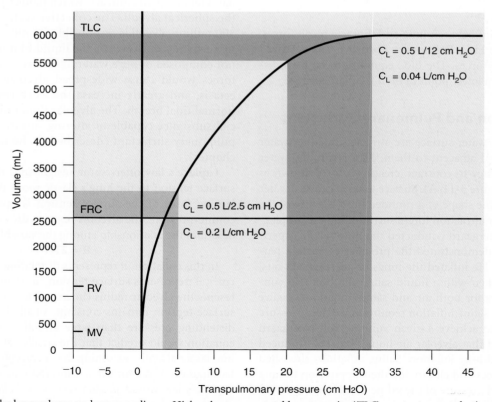

Figure 3-9 Effect of the lung volume on lung compliance. High volumes near total lung capacity (*TLC*) create stronger elastic recoil forces than lower volumes at functional residual capacity (*FRC*). Compliance is much lower at high than at low lung volumes. *RV*, Residual volume; *MV*, minimal volume.

CLINICAL FOCUS 3-4

Effect of Airway Obstruction on Functional Residual Capacity and Breathing Position on the Compliance Curve

Emphysema is a disease characterized by the destruction of elastic lung tissue. Consequently, the lung's elastic recoil force decreases (i.e., the lungs become highly compliant). The lungs do not empty completely to their normal resting volume at the end of an exhalation, which increases the FRC. Because of the increased FRC, a patient with emphysema begins each inspiration at a level closer to the TLC (see Figure 3-20, A). Patients with emphysema appear to be in a continuous inspiratory position, even when they are at the end of a normal expiration. However, breathing at this higher lung volume is actually advantageous for the highly compliant emphysematous lung because it increases lung recoil force and assists expiration (i.e., even the highly compliant lung recoils with greater force if it is stretched). In other words, the lung with emphysema has such little recoil force that it must be stretched to near its TLC to generate enough recoil to drive passive expiration. Even then, recoil force is lower than normal. This low recoil force drives expiratory flow out of the lung slowly, unduly prolonging expiratory time. For this reason, patients with emphysema often contract their abdominal expiratory muscles during normal ventilation (always an abnormal sign) to aid exhalation.

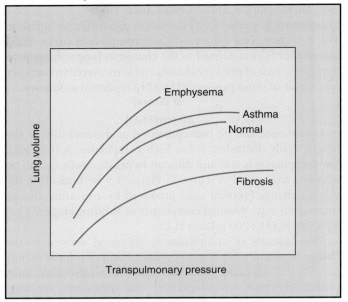

Figure 3-10 Lung compliance curves in normal, emphysematous, and fibrotic lungs. (From Berne RM, Levy MN: *Principles of physiology*, ed 2, St Louis, 1996, Mosby.)

the equilibrium point between lung and thoracic recoil forces, which increases the FRC. **Pulmonary fibrosis** is characterized by high lung recoil forces. The FRC equilibrium point is displaced, this time to a lower point in the TLC than normal.

Surface Tension and Pulmonary Surfactant

The molecules of a water surface are attracted by other water molecules below and adjacent to them. As a result, the water surface has a tendency to contract, creating a force known as **surface tension** (Figure 3-11, *A*). Surface tension causes a water droplet to take on the shape of a rounded bead because of the tight intermolecular attraction forces surrounding the droplet.

In 1929, von Neergaard conducted the now classic experiment in which he demonstrated the presence of surface tension in the alveoli. He inflated the lungs of anesthetized cats, first with air and then with a liquid saline solution. He constructed P-V curves for both air and saline inflations. Figure 3-12 illustrates that saline inflation requires much less pressure than air inflation to achieve a given volume. von Neergaard correctly concluded that alveolar air-liquid surfaces produced forces that opposed lung inflation. Saline inflations abolished the air-liquid surfaces and eliminated their opposition to lung inflation. The recoil pressure of the saline-filled lungs reflected only elastic tissue retractile forces, whereas the recoil pressure

of the air-filled lung reflected retractile forces of the elastic tissues *plus* surface tension. von Neergaard found that surface-tension forces are responsible for more than half of the lung's elastic recoil force.[7]

The film of water lining the alveoli surrounds alveolar air, similar to a soap bubble. As just described, the water surface has a tendency to contract, which tends to shrink or collapse the spherical alveoli. The collective surface tension of about 300 million alveoli is responsible for most of the lung's elastic recoil force. However, the liquid film lining the alveoli is not composed of pure water; if it were, high surface-tension forces would cause widespread alveolar collapse, or atelectasis, and greatly increase the work required to inhale a normal tidal breath. The alveolar fluid lining contains a special substance capable of altering surface tension known as pulmonary surfactant (described in the next section of this chapter).

Laplace's law offers some insight into the contribution of surface tension to the lung's elastic recoil pressure. If the collapsing force of the surface tension is opposed by an equal counterpressure, the alveolus remains distended. Laplace's law describes the relationship among the variables as follows:

$$P = 2T/r$$

In this equation, P represents distending pressure (in dynes/cm^2), T represents surface tension (in dynes/cm^2), and r represents the alveolar radius (in cm). The equation shows that if surface tension remains constant, small alveoli require higher distending pressure than large alveoli (Figure 3-13, *A*); the equation would predict that the smaller alveoli should empty into larger alveoli—assuming that all alveoli have the same surface tension. If the surface tension were the same for all alveoli, Laplace's law would predict serious alveolar instability; small alveoli would collapse into larger ones, producing coexisting

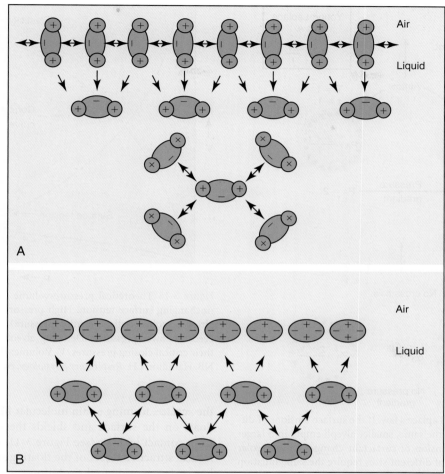

Figure 3-11 Surface tension. **A,** Water molecules at the surface are attracted to each other and to molecules below, creating a force leading to surface contraction. **B,** Water molecules repel surfactant molecules (*circles*), pushing them to the liquid's surface. Surfactant molecules repel one another when squeezed together, lowering the air-liquid surface tension.

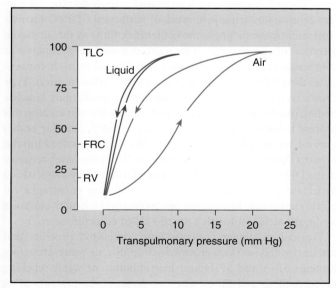

Figure 3-12 Comparison of pressure-volume curves for air-filled and saline-filled lungs. Note the absence of hysteresis in the saline-filled lung. *TLC,* total lung capacity; *FRC,* functional residual capacity; *RV,* residual volume. (From Berne RM, Levy MN: *Principles of physiology,* ed 2, St Louis, 1996, Mosby.)

areas of overdistention and complete collapse (Figure 3-13, *B*). Alveolar pressures throughout the lungs are the same, however, because they all are connected to a common airway—the trachea. How then is alveolar stability maintained, and how can the lung inflate evenly?

The explanation is that pulmonary surfactant alters alveolar surface tension in such a way that larger alveoli have a higher surface tension than smaller alveoli. Because variations in alveolar radii are associated with equivalent variations in surface tension, the same pressure can keep all alveoli inflated. As shown by Laplace's law (P = 2T/r), if r and T both double or if both are cut in half, P remains the same. Because of pulmonary surfactant, the recoil pressure for all alveoli, regardless of their size, is the same.

Figure 3-14 illustrates **critical opening pressure** and **critical closing pressure**. A relatively high pressure is required to expand a collapsed alveolus. When enough pressure is applied to produce an alveolar radius equal to that of the alveolar duct supplying it, the critical opening pressure has been reached. When the critical opening pressure is exceeded, the alveolus abruptly opens and expands easily. This phenomenon is similar to the inflation of a toy balloon. High pressure is required

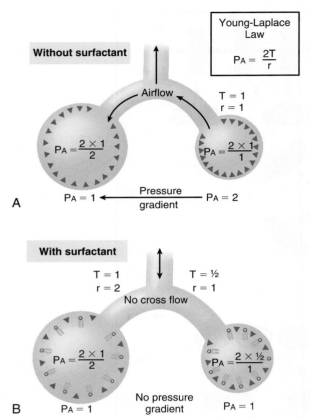

Without surfactant

Young-Laplace Law

$$P_A = \frac{2T}{r}$$

Airflow

$T = 1$
$r = 1$

$$P_A = \frac{2 \times 1}{2}$$

$$P_A = \frac{2 \times 1}{1}$$

A $P_A = 1 \longleftarrow$ Pressure gradient $\longrightarrow P_A = 2$

With surfactant

$T = 1$
$r = 2$

$T = \frac{1}{2}$
$r = 1$

No cross flow

$$P_A = \frac{2 \times 1}{2}$$

$$P_A = \frac{2 \times \frac{1}{2}}{1}$$

B $P_A = 1$ No pressure gradient $P_A = 1$

Figure 3-13 Illustration of Laplace's law. If the surface tensions of different-diameter alveoli are the same, smaller alveoli empty into larger alveoli (**A**). The surface tension of surfactant changes with alveolar diameter such that alveoli of different sizes require the same inflation pressure (**B**). (From Berne RM, Levy MN: *Principles of physiology*, St Louis, 1990, Mosby.)

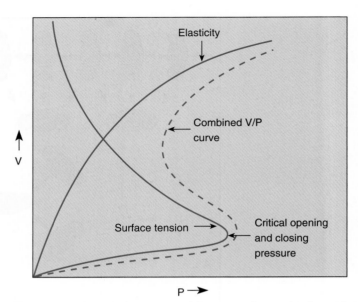

Elasticity

Combined V/P curve

V

Surface tension $\longrightarrow$ Critical opening and closing pressure

$P \longrightarrow$

Figure 3-14 Theoretical pressure-volume curve for an alveolus with unchanging surface tension. High pressure is required to inflate the airless alveolus (critical opening pressure), after which inflation proceeds at lower pressures. Deflating alveoli suddenly collapse below their critical closing pressures. *V*, Volume; *P*, pressure. (From Slonim NB, Hamilton LH: *Respiratory physiology*, ed 5, St Louis, 1987, Mosby.)

initially until the balloon abruptly expands; thereafter, the balloon inflates easily. The critical opening pressure is identical to the critical closing pressure; pressures below this measurement result in the abrupt collapse of the alveolus. The radius of the alveolar duct and the surface-tension force determine the critical opening pressure.

CONCEPT QUESTION 3-5

Why does a person with an abnormally low FRC experience a high WOB?

Adhesive molecular surface-tension forces are the major opposition to alveolar inflation when the alveolus is collapsed and below its critical opening pressure. Above the critical opening pressure, elastic tissue recoil becomes a progressively greater opposition to inflation (see Figure 3-14).

Nature and Composition of Pulmonary Surfactant

Surfactant molecules in a water medium have extremely weak attractive forces for each other and for the surrounding water molecules. Strong intermolecular attractive forces between water molecules push the neutral surfactant molecules up to

the surface, forming a thin molecular film. This surfactant film floats on the surface and shields the water molecules below from contact with air (see Figure 3-11, *B*). The weak intermolecular attractive forces of the floating surfactant film impart a low surface tension to the solution.

Pulmonary surfactant is a complex substance composed of 90% phospholipid and 10% protein. **Dipalmitoyl phosphatidylcholine (DPPC)** constitutes about 50% of surfactant's phospholipid content and is primarily responsible for the surface-tension–lowering properties of surfactant.[8] DPPC forms a tight monolayer (a single-molecule-thick film) at the air-liquid interface of the alveolus. The more this surface monolayer is compressed (as occurs in smaller alveoli), the more it concentrates the DPPC molecules and lowers the surface tension. Type II cells secrete surfactant phospholipids by discharging lamellar bodies into the liquid film that lines the inner alveolar surface; this process is known as **exocytosis**. Once secreted, lamellar bodies unravel and transform into a lattice-like structure called tubular myelin (Figure 3-15). Tubular myelin is the immediate precursor of the DPPC surface monolayer; when facilitated by a specialized surfactant protein (described in the following paragraphs), it quickly spreads to form a film one molecule thick on the alveolar air-liquid surface through a process called adsorption.

Normal surfactant contains four specialized proteins that can be divided into two groups: hydrophilic, or water-attracting proteins SP-A and SP-D and hydrophobic, or water-repelling proteins SP-B and SP-C. The two hydrophilic proteins SP-A and SP-D are not as critical for surfactant function as the two extremely hydrophobic surfactant proteins SP-B and SP-C; the presence of SP-B in particular is essential for the formation of tubular myelin and its adsorption on the monolayer film surface.[8]

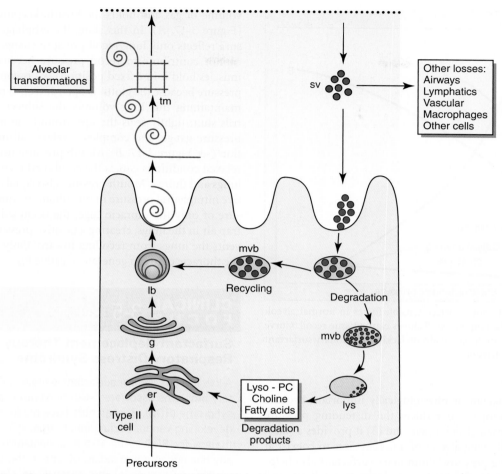

Figure 3-15 Production of pulmonary surfactant by type II cells. *tm,* Tubular myelin; *sv,* small vesicles; *mvb,* multivesicular bodies; *lys,* lysosomes; *er,* endoplasmic reticulum; *g,* Golgi; *lb,* lamellar bodies; *PC,* phosphatidylcholine.

Adequate functional surfactant must be present in the fetal lung at birth to allow a successful transition to air breathing; otherwise, high surface tension causes widespread alveolar collapse and severe respiratory distress. DPPC is first present in lamellar bodies of the human fetal lung at 24 weeks of gestation.[8] Avery and Mead[9] were the first investigators to describe low surfactant levels in premature newborns with **respiratory distress syndrome (RDS)**. It was later confirmed that deficient synthesis and secretion of pulmonary surfactant causes RDS to occur in a premature infant. Specifically, the absence of SP-B is responsible for respiratory distress and gas exchange abnormalities in a premature newborn.[8]

The concentration of DPPC, also known as lecithin, increases during the last 20% of gestation in the full-term fetus. At the same time, the concentration of another phospholipid, **sphingomyelin**, remains relatively constant.[10] The ratio of lecithin to sphingomyelin (L/S ratio) in amniotic fluid is predictive of fetal lung maturation. An L/S ratio greater than 2:1 indicates fetal lung maturity in nondiabetic pregnancies; the L/S ratio is falsely high in mothers with diabetes.[10] The L/S ratio is generally 1:1 at 31 to 32 weeks of gestation and 2:1 at 35 weeks of gestation.[10] **Phosphatidylglycerol (PG)** is another

phospholipid component of surfactant that is produced quite late in gestation. Its presence in amniotic fluid almost guarantees lung maturity; the risk of RDS is low if PG is present.[10] The L/S ratio and the presence of PG in amniotic fluid continue to be the "gold standard" for determining fetal lung maturity.[10] More recently, the lamellar body count in amniotic fluid has been shown to correlate significantly with the L/S ratio and PG levels. The advantage of the lamellar body count is that it can be performed more quickly and easily and is less costly than phospholipid analysis; in addition, it is less subject to false elevations in diabetes.[10] Maternal administration of steroids may accelerate the production of fetal DPPC.[8]

Physiological Significance of Pulmonary Surfactant

In Figure 3-16, curve *C* shows that when the alveolar diameter is small in the surfactant-deficient lung, extremely high P_L is required to offset surface-tension forces and prevent alveolar collapse. Therefore, alveoli are quite prone to collapse at low lung volumes, as Laplace's law predicts. In the presence of pulmonary surfactant, surface tension decreases dramatically as the alveolar volume decreases (curve *A*); this allows small alveoli to remain inflated at an extremely low P_L.

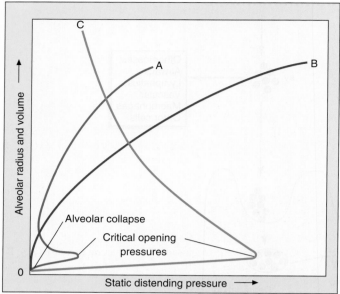

Figure 3-16 Curve *A* shows surface-tension forces in normal alveoli with pulmonary surfactant. Curve *B* shows elastic tissue recoil. Curve *C* shows surface-tension forces in alveoli lacking pulmonary surfactant (unchanging surface tension).

Pulmonary surfactant is physiologically important because (1) it reduces WOB; (2) it reduces the distending pressure required to keep small alveoli open; and (3) it provides a stabilizing influence, allowing alveoli of different sizes to coexist at the same distending pressure. Pulmonary surfactant also helps reduce the tendency for fluid to leave pulmonary capillaries and enter the interstitial space. In the absence of pulmonary surfactant, high surface-tension–retracting forces create too much negative intrapleural and interstitial pressure, which pulls fluid out of the capillaries. By decreasing alveolar surface tension, pulmonary surfactant helps prevent the development of undue negative interstitial pressure.[8]

CONCEPT QUESTION 3-6

Why might C_L decrease in conditions that block pulmonary blood flow to the alveoli, such as in pulmonary embolus?

Lung and Chest Wall Interactions

Lung, Thorax, and Total Compliance

If the lungs were removed and the empty thoracic cavity inflated with air, the measured compliance of the thoracic cage would be equal to that of the lungs (i.e., 0.2 L/cm H_2O). Thoracic compliance (C_T) can be measured directly or calculated by finding the difference between C_L and the combined lung-thorax compliance (C_{LT}).

C_L and C_{LT} can be obtained simultaneously by measuring esophageal balloon pressure and mouth pressure under static conditions, which is equivalent to measuring intrapleural and alveolar pressures (mouth pressure equals alveolar pressure under static, no-flow conditions). The subject inspires a known

volume of gas and holds the breath, keeping the glottis open (Figure 3-17, *A*). In this state, the esophageal (pleural) pressure reflects only lung recoil pressure changes (i.e., the thorax cannot contribute to recoil pressure because the ventilatory muscles hold it in a fixed position). P_A is equal to atmospheric pressure because the glottis is open and air is not moving. While maintaining this lung volume, the subject pinches the nostrils shut, tightly seals the lips around the mouthpiece of the pressure gauge, and completely relaxes all muscles of ventilation (see Figure 3-17, *B*). Mouth pressure under these no-flow relaxed conditions equals the combined recoil pressures of the lungs and thorax. Mouth pressure also equals the P_A. The negative intrapleural pressure in this situation equals the recoil pressure of only the thoracic cage; the occluded mouth and nose trap air in the lungs, creating a positive pressure splint that prevents the lungs from recoiling inward. Only outward recoil of the thoracic cage can generate negative P_{pl}.

CLINICAL FOCUS 3-5

Surfactant Replacement Therapy in Neonatal Respiratory Distress Syndrome

A low level of alveolar surfactant is the main cause of respiratory problems associated with newborn respiratory distress syndrome (RDS). Researchers have made much progress in developing various surfactants to treat RDS. Introduced as a therapy for RDS in the 1980s, surfactant replacement therapy has become a standard of care in the treatment of this condition. Because it is not naturally developed in the body, this surfactant is called exogenous surfactant.

Several kinds of exogenous surfactant, both natural and synthetic, are available; however, the essential surfactant proteins SP-B and SP-C are present only in natural surfactants derived from purified extracts of animal lungs. Attempts to formulate equally effective synthetic preparations of SP-B and SP-C have been unsuccessful, although more recent synthetic analogues of these surfactant proteins have shown promise.[11] Exogenous surfactant is instilled directly into the trachea of a premature infant through an endotracheal tube, with the infant held in several different positions. Repeat doses are sometimes given if necessary. Surfactant replacement therapy does not prevent RDS but instead reduces the severity and shortens the course of the disease. By decreasing surface tension, surfactant instillation increases lung compliance and decreases WOB, reducing the need for oxygen and positive pressure mechanical ventilation in infants with RDS.

The data needed to calculate C_L (volume inspired/[$P_A - P_{pl}$]) and C_{LT} (volume inspired/[P_A − atmospheric pressure]) are obtained from the ventilatory maneuvers just described. The compliance of the thoracic cage alone can be calculated from the following equation:

$$1/C_{LT} = 1/C_L + 1/C_T$$

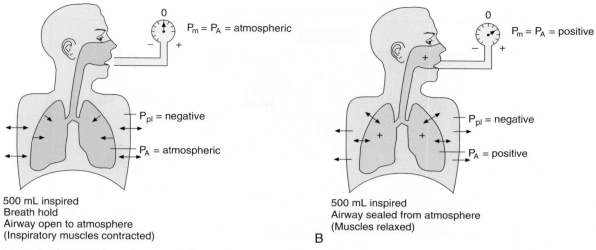

Figure 3-17 Measuring lung and lung-thorax compliance. **A,** Lung recoil force alone determines the magnitude of intrapleural pressure (P_{pl}). **B,** Combined lung-thorax recoil forces determine alveolar pressure, whereas thoracic cage recoil alone determines P_{pl}. P_{m}, Pressure at the mouth; P_A, alveolar pressure.

Another way to state this is as follows:

$$1/C_T = 1/C_{LT} - 1/C_L$$

In this equation, C_L represents lung compliance, C_T represents thoracic cage compliance, and C_{LT} represents combined lung and thoracic cage compliance. The normal value is 0.1 L/cm H_2O for C_{LT} and 0.2 L/cm H_2O for C_L. C_T is normally 0.2 L/cm H_2O, calculated as follows:

$$1/C_T = 1/0.1 - 1/0.2$$
$$1/C_T = 10 - 5$$
$$1/C_T = 5$$
$$C_T = 0.2 \text{ L/cm } H_2O$$

Thoracic cage compliance is decreased in persons with skeletal deformities of the chest wall (e.g., **kyphoscoliosis** and ankylosing spondylitis), spastic skeletal muscle diseases, and severe obesity. The reason the addition and subtraction of compliance values involves using their reciprocals becomes more apparent as the interactions between the lungs and thoracic cage are examined later in this chapter.

Relaxation Pressure-Volume Curves

At FRC, the lungs are stretched outward above their unstressed resting volume, and the thoracic cage is compressed inward, below its unstressed resting volume. The lungs and thorax are coupled by the cohesive seal of the parietal and visceral pleurae. If the pleural seal is broken, exposing the intrapleural space to atmospheric pressure, the lungs recoil inward to their resting minimal air volume, and the thoracic cage recoils outward to its unstressed resting volume (about 75% to 80% of the TLC, or 70% of the VC). The relative strengths of outward thoracic recoil and inward lung recoil determine FRC, which is the resting unstressed volume of the intact lung-thorax system.

Passive relaxation P-V curves can be constructed separately for the lungs and thoracic cage. Figure 3-18, *A*, shows the relaxation pressures for the lung alone (as if it were outside of the thorax) plotted against TLC. Pressure in the lung is 0 at collapsed resting state (see Figure 3-18, *A, 1*) and

increases to its maximum level as the lung is inflated to TLC, where elastic tissues are stretched maximally (see Figure 3-18, *A, 3*). At each lung-inflation point in the figure, the airway is sealed, airflow stops, and the positive pressure is the result of passive lung recoil. Figure 3-18, *B*, shows that if the empty thoracic cage is compressed to the RV level, it generates a strong outward recoil force. This force generates a negative intrathoracic pressure if the thoracic opening is sealed and the compression force is removed, allowing the thorax to recoil freely (see Figure 3-18, *B, 1*). When the thorax is allowed to recoil outward to the volume it would contain at 70% of the VC, the thorax is at rest, generating neither inward nor outward recoil force (see Figure 3-18, *B, 2*). Inflation beyond this point expands the thoracic cage above its resting level and generates an inward recoil force. In other words, from 70% of the VC to TLC, the thorax recoils in the same direction as the lungs (see Figure 3-18, *B, 3*).

Figure 3-19 shows relaxation P-V curves for the lungs and thorax plotted on the same graph along with the coupled lung-thorax system curve. The resting equilibrium point between inward lung recoil force and outward thoracic recoil force defines FRC and normally occurs between 40% and 50% of TLC. This FRC balance point between the two opposing recoil forces is shown in Figure 3-19 as the point where the horizontal distances between 0 pressure and the two recoil curves are identical (distance *a* is equal to distance *b* in the figure).

The lung-thorax compliance curve (see *solid line* in Figure 3-19) is the algebraic sum of the lung (*dotted line*) and thorax (*dashed line*) compliance curves. At all points along the lung-thorax curve, its slope is less than the slope of either the lung curve or the thoracic curve, which means that the combined lung-thorax system is less compliant than either of its components alone (i.e., C_{LT} is less than either C_L or C_T). Put in terms of elastance, combined lung-thorax elastance (the reciprocal of compliance) is greater than either lung or thorax elastance; this helps explain why reciprocals of C_L and C_T must be added to obtain the compliance of the total system. Compliance is a

Relaxation Pressure Curves

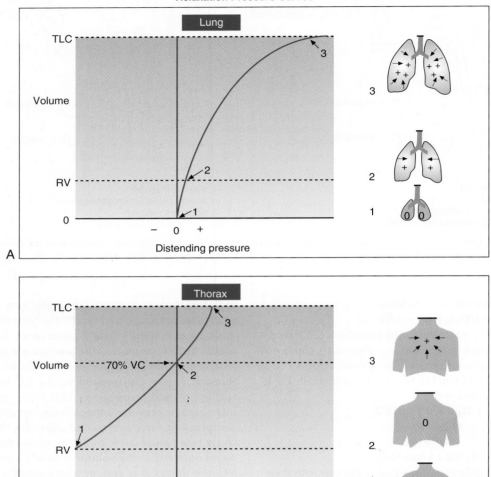

Figure 3-18 A, The lung has no recoil force when it is airless (*1*); as positive pressure inflates the lung, static relaxation pressures increase as elastic fibers stretch (*2-3*). All recoil pressures are positive. **B,** The thorax has no recoil force at about 70% of vital capacity (*VC*) (*2*). At residual volume (*RV*) (*1*), the thorax attempts to spring outward strongly, generating negative recoil pressure. Above its resting level at total lung capacity (*TLC*) (*3*), the thorax recoils inward, generating positive recoil pressure.

measure of the lung's distensibility, whereas elastance is a measure of the lung's resistance to inflation. The thorax and lungs actually represent elastances, not compliances, arranged in series with one another. As with an electrical circuit, total resistance is equal to the sum of the resistances in the series ($R_T = R_1 + R_2 + R_3 + \ldots$). In this equation, R_T represents total resistance, and R_1 through R_3 represent the individual resistances.

Likewise, lung and thorax elastances (resistance to inflation) can be summed to obtain total elastance ($E_{LT} = E_L + E_T$). In this equation, E_{LT} represents total system elastance, and E_L and E_T represent individual lung and thorax elastances. Because compliance is the reciprocal of elastance, reciprocals of compliance must be added to calculate total compliance. This is shown as follows:

1. $E_{LT} = E_L + E_T$
2. $E = 1/C$

Substituting 1/C for E in equation 1:

3. $1/C_{LT} = 1/C_L + 1/C_T$

Relaxation Pressure-Volume Curves and Disease

A change in lung elasticity alone alters the lung-thorax recoil curve because it changes the equilibrium point between lung and thorax recoil forces. Thus, FRC must change.

If the lung at FRC in Figure 3-19 develops decreased elasticity, the equilibrium between lung recoil and thoracic recoil is disrupted; outward, thoracic recoil predominates, pulling the lungs outward to a larger volume. The thorax stops expanding, and the lung stops enlarging when the stretching lung generates enough recoil force to again balance the oppositely directed thoracic recoil force. This establishes a new equilibrium point at a larger volume than before (i.e., FRC is increased, and V_T is breathed at a higher level in TLC). The lung curve and lung-thorax curve would shift leftward, showing that smaller pressures are required to inflate the lung to a given volume. Pulmonary emphysema, characterized by the destruction of elastic lung tissue, produces the changes just

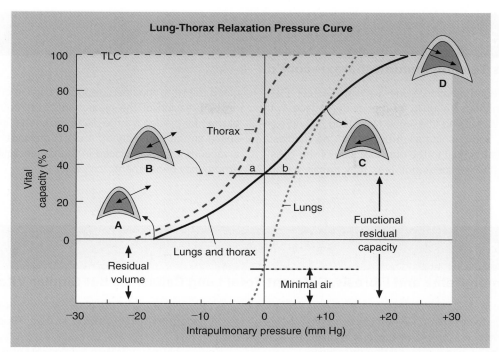

Figure 3-19 The combined lung-thorax relaxation curve is the summation of the individual lung and thorax relaxation curves. Equilibrium between lung and thoracic recoil forces determines the functional residual capacity (*FRC*) (lung model *B*). Pressure *a* equals pressure *b* at FRC, and alveolar pressure is 0. *TLC*, Total lung capacity.

CLINICAL FOCUS 3-6

Simple versus Tension Pneumothorax

You receive the following report from an emergency medical technician responding to the scene of an accident:

"A woman approximately 25 years old was thrown from a vehicle and sustained a penetrating wound to her left chest. The wound is deep and emits a sucking sound with each inspiration. The woman is complaining of severe left chest pain and has no breath sounds over the left side of the chest. Her trachea is in the midline position. We will ask her to exhale as forcefully as possible, and then we will place a sterile gauze bandage over the wound to seal it.

"The driver of the car, a man approximately 25 years old, was not thrown from the vehicle. He was found in the driver's seat complaining of severe chest pain and shortness of breath. An assessment reveals bruising over the chest area (probably caused by the impact with the steering wheel) and no breath sounds on the right side of the chest. In addition, the trachea is shifted to the left. The chest wall seems to be unstable, indicating possible broken ribs. This man's blood pressure is critically low, and he is losing consciousness. We are proceeding with immediate placement of a large-bore needle into the right upper anterior chest."

Discussion

Pressure in the pleural space is subatmospheric because of the opposing recoil forces of the lung and chest wall. Therefore, opening the pleural space to atmosphere allows air to rush into the chest cavity. The elastic recoil force of the lung, now unopposed, collapses the lung. This condition is known as a pneumothorax.

Pneumothorax can be classified as simple or tension pneumothorax. The woman in the accident sustained a simple, or open, pneumothorax. Each time she inhaled, the rib cage expanded, creating subatmospheric pressure inside her chest. Air was pulled into the chest through the wound, and the underlying lung remained collapsed. The emergency medical technician, in asking her to exhale forcefully before sealing the wound, wanted to evacuate as much air as possible from the chest. The wound was sealed to keep the pleural cavity from communicating with atmospheric pressure. When the chest wall recoiled outward, negative pressure was reestablished; this helped the underlying lung to expand. On arrival in the emergency department, a chest drainage tube attached to a vacuum source was placed into the pleural cavity to evacuate air further and aid lung reexpansion.

The driver of the car sustained a more serious tension pneumothorax. In his situation, broken ribs may have punctured the lung, creating an air leak between the lung and pleural space. In a tension pneumothorax, air is sucked from the punctured lung into the pleural space during inspiration, but it might not escape during exhalation if a torn lung tissue

Simple versus Tension Pneumothorax—cont'd

flap closes the wound creating a one-way valve effect. Positive pressure continues to build in the pleural space with each inspiration, collapsing the underlying lung, compressing large vessels, and pushing all structures in the mediastinum (including the trachea) to the opposite side of the chest. Left untreated, a tension pneumothorax may impair venous

blood return to the heart, reducing cardiac output. Immediate decompression of the pleural space is required and accomplished by placing a large-diameter needle into an intercostal space on the upper chest. A chest drainage tube attached to a vacuum source is placed in the patient later in the hospital emergency department.

Pulmonary Emphysema and Fibrosis: Different Total Lung Capacities but Similar Vital Capacities

An abnormally low TLC characterizes pulmonary fibrosis, whereas TLC in severe pulmonary emphysema is typically above normal. However, the VC of these two diseases may be similarly decreased, although for different reasons.

Discussion

The VC of people with pulmonary emphysema is typically below normal because forced expiration causes the airways to collapse prematurely and trap air. Elastic tissue that normally holds the airways open during exhalation is destroyed. Trapped gas in the lung reduces the exhaled VC. At the same time, the lung's low elastic recoil force allows the oppositely

directed recoil force of the chest wall to stretch the lungs out to an abnormally large volume at rest. Thus, TLC is greater than normal.

Conversely, patients with pulmonary fibrosis have high elastic lung recoil, making lung expansion difficult. This accounts for the low TLC and low VC in these patients. Because they cannot inhale deeply and expand their lungs normally, patients with pulmonary fibrosis have abnormally low exhaled VCs.

Diseases that restrict lung expansion and diseases that obstruct airflow cannot be separated on the basis of the VC alone. The corresponding TLC also must be observed, and the patient's medical history must be considered.

described. Diseases that increase lung recoil force, such as pulmonary fibrosis, shift lung and lung-thorax curves to the right and reduce FRC because increased lung recoil pulls the thorax down to lower volumes.

Figure 3-20 shows P-V relaxation curves for the lungs and thorax under normal conditions (see Figure 3-20, *B*) compared with pulmonary emphysema (see Figure 3-20, *A*) and pulmonary fibrosis (see Figure 3-20, *C*). The lungs of the patient with emphysema in *A* have extremely low recoil force; they must be stretched to near TLC before they generate enough recoil to counterbalance the thoracic recoil force and establish FRC. FRC is quite large, mainly because the RV is so large. Even minimal air is increased as a result of the low lung recoil; if these lungs are removed from the chest, their recoil is so weak that they are unable to expel much of their air, and they remain hyperinflated even at rest.

The fibrotic lungs in Figure 3-20, *C*, recoil quite strongly, even at low lung volumes. Not much inflation is required before their recoil is equal to chest wall recoil. The FRC equilibrium point is established at an abnormally low volume. TLC is reduced because the ventilatory muscles are not strong enough to stretch the strongly recoiling fibrotic lung to greater volumes.

DYNAMIC LUNG AND CHEST WALL MECHANICS

Elastic resistance to ventilation is normally much greater than frictional resistance. However, in certain diseases of the airways, frictional resistance may exceed elastic resistance.

Frictional (Nonelastic) Resistance

Nonelastic resistance is produced mostly by frictional resistance to gas flow or **airway resistance** (R_{aw}). To a small extent, friction between moving tissues in the thorax contributes to nonelastic resistance.

Resistance to Gas Flow

When gas flows through a tube, pressure decreases steadily along the tube from the inlet to the outlet. The pressure drop across the tube ($P_1 - P_2$) is the driving pressure of the gas flow. A driving pressure is required to overcome flow resistance. Greater frictional resistance causes a greater pressure decrease across the tube. Frictional resistance is present between gas molecules themselves (**viscosity**) and between gas flow and the tube wall. The greater the cohesive forces between gas molecules, the

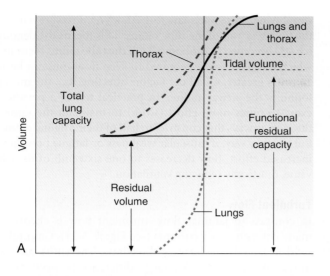

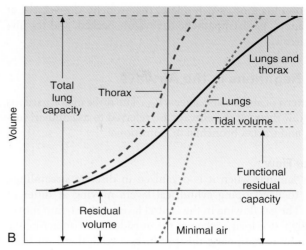

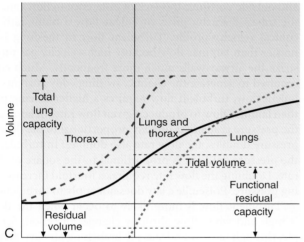

Figure 3-20 Lung-thorax relaxation curves in normal and disease states. Greatly decreased lung recoil force in emphysema (**A**) allows oppositely directed thoracic recoil to stretch the lung to a larger volume before the two forces reestablish equilibrium. This greatly increases the functional residual capacity compared with the normal lung (**B**). The high lung recoil force in pulmonary fibrosis (**C**) shrinks the lung volume, pulling the thoracic cage down to a smaller size until its outward recoil force balances that of the lungs. This decreases all lung volumes and capacities.

greater the viscosity of the gas and the greater its opposition to flow. Generally, the smaller the tube radius and the greater the gas viscosity, the greater the resistance. The greater the resistance, the greater the pressure decrease along the tube.

Resistance (R) to gas flow through a tube is expressed as the pressure decrease between the inlet and outlet divided by the flow rate ($\dot{V}$). This is shown as follows:

$$R = \frac{P_1 - P_2}{\dot{V}}$$

Airway Resistance

In the lung, R_{aw} is measured in units of cm H_2O/L/sec. For a given flow rate, a large pressure decrease across the airways indicates the presence of high resistance. Also, the higher the flow rate, the greater the pressure decrease between two points in a given airway. Normal R_{aw} in adults measured at the FRC level at a constant flow rate of 0.5 L per second is about 0.5 to 1.5 cm H_2O/L/sec; that is, to produce a flow of 1 L per second, a person must generate a pressure

difference across the airways (between mouth and alveoli) of 0.5 to 1.5 cm H_2O.

The lung volume markedly affects R_{aw}. For this reason, R_{aw} is usually measured at FRC (an easily reproducible volume at which people normally breathe). A special instrument called a **body plethysmograph** measures P_A, mouth pressure, and flow rate simultaneously to calculate R_{aw}.

R_{aw} is greater at low lung volumes than high lung volumes. High volumes near TLC create high P_L gradients and mechanically dilate the airways. Also, high elastic recoil at high lung volumes has a tethering effect on airways, pulling them to larger diameters. Both of these effects are reduced at low lung volumes. Near RV, small, noncartilaginous airways are severely narrowed, greatly increasing R_{aw}. As RV is approached, some of these small airways collapse because P_{pl} exceeds intraairway pressure.

Neurogenic factors also affect R_{aw} at different lung volumes. Stretch receptors in the lung (see Chapter 1) are stimulated at high volumes, causing a reflex decrease in parasympathetic bronchomotor tone, which dilates the bronchi. Conversely, at low volumes, parasympathetic tone is unchecked, and the airways narrow.

Flow Regimens in the Airways

The pattern of airflow also affects R_{aw}. The three major patterns of gas flow through the airways are referred to as laminar, turbulent, and tracheobronchial or transitional.

Laminar Flow

Flow is laminar when it is organized in discrete streamlines, similar to overlapping cylindrical layers moving at different speeds. The gas flowing in the central layer of the stream moves at the highest velocity, whereas the outside layer contacting the airway wall is stationary; this produces a conical stream front (Figure 3-21) or a parabolic velocity profile. The concentric cylindrical layers of gas slide over one another, creating friction between them as they travel at different velocities. This friction is determined by molecular cohesive forces (unique for each gas type) and is the source of gas viscosity. When flow is laminar, the pressure required to produce a given flow rate through the airways is influenced by gas viscosity but not by the molecular weight or density of the gas.[2]

Poiseuille's Law and Airway Resistance

Under laminar flow conditions, the pressure required to produce a given flow rate through a tube is defined by **Poiseuille's law** ($P = \dot{V}8ln/\pi r^4$). In this equation, P represents the pressure gradient across the tube, $\dot{V}$ represents the gas flow rate, l represents the tube length, n represents gas viscosity, r represents the tube radius, and 8 and π represent constants. This equation states that under laminar flow conditions, the pressure required to drive a given flow through a tube increases if the tube length or gas viscosity increase. More striking is the increased pressure needed to maintain a given flow rate when tube radius decreases. The equation shows that if an airway's radius decreases to one half of its original size (e.g., by bronchospasm or mucosal edema), 16 times more pressure is required to maintain the original flow through the airway. For practical purposes, the constants in Poiseuille's law can be lumped together to form one constant (K),

simplifying Poiseuille's law to $P = K \times \dot{V}/r^4$. Pressure varies with the fourth power of the tube radius. This means the denominator (r^4) becomes 16 times smaller if the tube radius is cut in half, which means pressure required to keep flow constant becomes 16 times greater. Of all the factors affecting R_{aw}, the most profound is the airway radius. In practical terms, a person must exert 16 times more effort (work) to maintain the same flow through airways that constrict to half of their original diameters. Put another way, if muscular weakness or fatigue prevents such increased effort, flow decreases to one sixteenth of its original value, drastically reducing ventilation.

Turbulent Flow

In contrast to laminar flow, turbulent flow is chaotic, with many churning eddy currents (see Figure 3-21). Gas molecules swirl in lateral and forward directions. The entire gas stream moves forward with no velocity difference between its center and outside portions; this lack of difference in flow rates across the tube's diameter gives turbulent flow a blunt rather than conical velocity profile. Turbulent flow in the lung is much noisier than laminar flow because high-velocity gas molecules strike the airway walls much more frequently. Much energy is required to generate the chaotic, swirling eddy currents of turbulent flow; turbulent flow requires a higher driving pressure than laminar flow to produce a given flow rate. In laminar flow, the pressure gradient is directly proportional to the flow rate; if pressure doubles, the flow rate also doubles. In turbulent flow, the pressure gradient is proportional to the square of the flow rate. Doubling the flow rate requires a fourfold increase in driving pressure. Poiseuille's law does not apply to turbulent flow.

Turbulent flow is more likely to occur when the flow rate is high and when flow abruptly changes direction, for example, through narrow and sharply branching airways. **Reynolds' number (Re)** predicts when the flow regimen will change from laminar to turbulent. Re, a dimensionless number, is derived from values for gas density, viscosity, velocity, and airway diameter. Generally, if Re is greater than 2000, flow is turbulent. In contrast to laminar flow, the pressure required to produce a given flow rate in turbulent flow is influenced by the molecular weight of the gas or its density (greater density requires greater pressure) but not by its viscosity. For this reason, helium, a gas with very low density, is sometimes used to reduce WOB in patients with abnormally turbulent airflow, as occurs in severe airway obstruction (see Clinical Focus 3-8).

Tracheobronchial or Transitional Flow

The type of flow referred to as tracheobronchial or transitional occurs where airways branch and has characteristics of laminar and turbulent flow. One or the other type of flow may predominate, depending on the airway geometry and flow velocity.

Types of Flow in the Lung and Distribution of Airway Resistance

Flow patterns in the lung are highly turbulent in the upper airways, trachea, and major bronchi but never turbulent in smaller bronchioles and distal airspaces. Normal quiet breathing

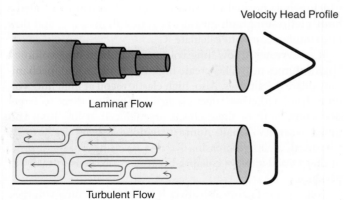

Figure 3-21 Velocity profiles of laminar and turbulent flow through a tube.

commonly produces instantaneous peak flow rates of 1 L per second, or 60 L per minute, at the mouth. Even during quiet breathing, flow is highly turbulent in the pharynx, larynx, and trachea. As the airways branch, airflow is progressively redirected into more channels until finally, at the terminal bronchiole level, flow is distributed across hundreds of millions of airways; this greatly reduces flow velocity, and flow is laminar. Even during maximal ventilation, flow in the peripheral airways remains laminar. For similar reasons, R_{aw} is normally much lower in small airways than in large airways (see Chapter 1). The increase in the number of small airways and the increase in their collective cross-sectional area far outweigh the decrease in their individual diameters.

The upper airways, including the larynx, mouth, and nose, normally account for about 50% of total R_{aw} at FRC; airways less than 3 mm in diameter account for less than 10% of the total R_{aw}.[12] However, in people who have severe emphysema, chronic bronchitis, or asthma, resistance to flow in the lower airways may exceed upper R_{aw}.

Dynamic Compliance

Lung and chest wall compliance measured while air is flowing is called **dynamic compliance (C_{dyn})**. The earlier discussions of compliance involve **static compliance (C_{st})**. Under dynamic conditions, airway pressure is a reflection of elastic plus flow-resistive opposition to lung inflation. The difference between C_{dyn} and C_{st} reflects the magnitude of R_{aw} present.

Dynamic Pressure-Volume Curves

Figure 3-22 is a plot of superimposed static and dynamic C_L curves obtained during mechanical positive pressure lung

---

CLINICAL FOCUS 3-8

Breathing Low-Density Gas (Helium-Oxygen) to Decrease the Work of Breathing

A gas mixture of 80% helium and 20% oxygen (heliox) has a lower density but higher viscosity than air. Delivering heliox to a child who has severe croup (subglottic swelling) may decrease WOB. Giving a child who has bronchiolitis (inflammation of small peripheral bronchioles) the same gas mixture would probably not decrease the child's WOB. Both children have diseases causing airway obstruction. Why does one child and not the other benefit from heliox therapy?

Discussion

The child with croup has swelling in the trachea, just below the glottis, creating increased resistance to airflow and making breathing more difficult. Because flow in the trachea and large airways is turbulent, flow rate is affected by gas density but not viscosity. Breathing a low-density gas increases the flow moving through these airways for a given effort. Laminar flow,

found in smaller airways where flow velocity is low, is influenced by gas viscosity but not gas density. The low-density but more viscous heliox does not improve flow in the smaller airways. Small airways disease is less likely to benefit from heliox therapy. Clinically, heliox is sometimes given by a special facemask in cases of severe asthma that fail to respond to medications; in this way, the clinician can "buy time," perhaps avoiding mechanical ventilation, until medications begin to have an effect.[29] Heliox is also useful in mechanically ventilated COPD patients to decompress the auto-PEEP these patients often develop and to reduce the adverse effects of positive pressure mechanical ventilation on venous blood return to the heart.[30] The low-density gas can more easily be expelled through constricted airways where flow tends to be turbulent, reducing air trapping, allowing the lung to empty to its normal FRC, and reducing mean intrapulmonary pressure.[30]

CLINICAL FOCUS 3-9

Breath Sounds and Types of Flow in the Airways

The stethoscope allows respiratory therapists and other health care personnel to listen to sounds produced in the chest; this is called chest auscultation. In the normal lung, the sounds heard on auscultation are those of air rushing through the tubelike structures of the tracheobronchial tree. Because airflow characteristics change between the trachea and alveoli (turbulent flow to laminar flow), the character and pitch of the breath sounds also change.

Over the trachea and larger bronchi, where flow is turbulent, the sound is harsh, is moderately high-pitched, and has a tubular or hollow quality. Such sounds are commonly referred to as tracheal, or bronchial, breath sounds.

Over the peripheral areas of normal lungs, where flow is laminar, the breath sounds are much softer, are lower pitched, and sound like rustling grass in the wind. These sounds are called vesicular breath sounds.

Abnormal breath sounds are called adventitious sounds. Air accelerating through constricted airways in patients with asthma often produces very high-pitched sounds called wheezes. Air pushing its way through heavy bronchial secretions produces bubbling, coarse crackling sounds, commonly called rhonchi. A measure of therapy effectiveness is the disappearance of wheezes after bronchodilator therapy, or the disappearance of rhonchi after therapy aimed at evacuating secretions.

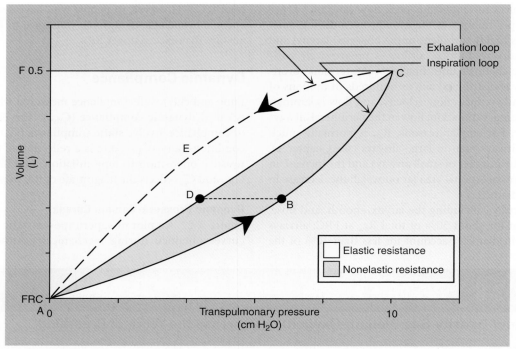

Figure 3-22 Pressure-volume curve created by a passive positive pressure lung inflation, followed by passive exhalation. Curve *ABC* is a dynamic compliance curve, and curve *ADC* is a static compliance curve. If lung inflation is stopped at midinspiration (point *B*) and exhalation is not permitted, airway pressure falls to point *D*. Elastic inspiratory resistance or work is proportional to the white triangular area, *ADCFA*; frictional inspiratory resistance or nonelastic work is proportional to the shaded area of the loop, *ABCDA*. *FRC*, Functional residual capacity. (Modified from DuPuis YG: *Ventilators: theory and clinical applications,* ed 2, St Louis, 1992, Mosby.)

inflation with the respiratory muscles completely at rest. Lung inflation begins at FRC (point *A*). The straight, solid line (*A-C*) is the C_{st} curve, which is constructed by momentarily interrupting air flow at progressively greater volumes and holding the breath (ventilatory muscles relaxed) until all airflow ceases.

The curved solid line (*ABC*) plots pressures dynamically in real time as lung volume increases during a single uninterrupted lung inflation, defining the C_{dyn} curve. The C_{dyn} curve bows away from the straight C_{st} line, reflecting the "drag" that frictional airway resistance adds to elastic resistance. If lung inflation is abruptly halted and the breath is held at point *B* on the dynamic curve, airflow stops, and its frictional resistance ceases to exist; the pressure generated by it disappears. Airway pressure falls to point *D* on the static pressure curve. Pressure at point *D* reflects only the elastic recoil forces present at that volume, whereas pressure at point *B* reflects elastic recoil forces plus flow-resistive forces. Thus, pressure *B* minus pressure *D* represents the pressure required to overcome R_{aw}. The white area in Figure 3-22 reflects static elastic resistance, and the shaded area (inspiratory portion of the loop) represents flow-dependent airway resistance. The area enclosed by the curved dashed line (*CEA* on the expiratory loop) and the straight static curve (*ADC*) reflects expiratory airway resistance. Modern positive pressure mechanical lung ventilators can graphically display breath-by-breath P-V loops (compliance curves), allowing respiratory therapists to identify and differentiate elastic and frictional resistances to ventilation.

Peak and Plateau Airway Pressure

The same positive pressure breath illustrated in Figure 3-22 can be graphically represented on a pressure versus time curve (Figure 3-23). As the ventilator inflates the lung, pressure increases to a maximum peak value (see Figure 3-23, point *B*). This **peak pressure (P_{peak})** corresponds with the pressure represented by point *B* on the C_{dyn} curve in Figure 3-22 and reflects the sum of elastic recoil force and frictional airway resistance. If the breath is held momentarily (an inspiratory pause), gas flow stops, and R_{aw} dissipates, as does the pressure that was required to overcome it; airway pressure falls to a lower level and stays there until the person is allowed to exhale. This **plateau pressure (P_{plat})** (see Figure 3-23, point *D*) reflects only the elastic recoil force of the lung-thorax system, which corresponds to point *D* on the static curve in Figure 3-22. The $P_{peak} - P_{plat}$ difference reflects only frictional R_{aw}.

CONCEPT QUESTION 3-7

In constant-volume mechanical ventilation, what effect does low C_L have on P_{peak}, P_{plat}, and the difference between peak and plateau pressures?

P_{plat} is equal to P_A because it is measured under static conditions after pressures equalize across the airways. P_{plat} is therefore more relevant than P_{peak} in assessing the potential for pressure-induced alveolar injury (**barotrauma**) during positive pressure mechanical ventilation.

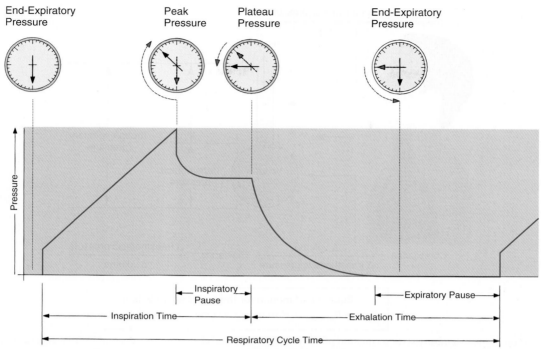

Figure 3-23 A pressure-time curve for passive positive pressure lung inflation, followed by a momentary inspiratory pause (breath hold) and passive exhalation. Peak pressure and plateau pressure correspond to points *B* and *D* in Figure 3-22. (Modified from DuPuis YG: *Ventilators: theory and clinical applications*, ed 2, St Louis, 1992, Mosby.)

Computing Lung-Thorax Compliance and Airway Resistance in Mechanical Ventilation. Respiratory system compliance (lung-thorax compliance [C_{LT}]) and R_{aw} can be easily computed on a mechanically ventilated patient. C_{LT} and R_{aw} are measures of elastic and flow-resistive opposition to ventilation. By programming the ventilator to create an inspiratory pause, as just described, the respiratory therapist can directly measure P_{peak} and P_{plat} (see Figure 3-23). The delivered V_T and the inspiratory flow rate are known values programmed into the ventilator. The C_{LT} is calculated as follows:

$$C_{LT} = V_T / (P_{plat} - \textbf{baseline pressure})$$

Baseline pressure is the airway pressure at the end of expiration, just before inspiration begins. (In critically ill patients, the ventilator is often programmed to maintain some degree of **positive end-expiratory pressure [PEEP]** in the airway to keep alveoli above their critical closing pressures.) Changes in the C_{LT} reflect changes in lung recoil forces.

A mechanically ventilated patient's R_{aw} can be computed from the ventilator's inspiratory flow rate ($\dot{V}_{insp}$) in L per second, P_{peak}, and P_{plat} as follows (assuming a constant flow rate):

$$R_{aw} = (P_{peak} - P_{plat}) / \dot{V}_{insp}$$

In this case, the computed R_{aw} includes the resistances of the ventilator tubing and the endotracheal tube, but changes in measured R_{aw} are usually a reflection of changes in the patient's airway diameter.

P_{peak} during mechanical ventilation reflects both elastic and flow-resistive opposition to lung inflation, whereas P_{plat} reflects elastic resistance only. P_{peak}, P_{plat}, C_{LT}, and R_{aw} are clinically useful in distinguishing between factors that increase lung recoil forces and factors that increase flow resistance through the airways.

Lung Inflation Pressure and Equation of Motion

We know from the previous section that the pressure required to drive gas into the airways and inflate the lungs is caused by the elastic and resistive elements that oppose ventilation. This is illustrated in Figure 3-24. Lung inflation pressure can be expressed in terms of these two resistive elements as follows:[13]

1. $P_{appl} = P_{el} + P_r$

In this equation, P_{appl} is the airway pressure applied at the mouth, P_{el} is the elastic recoil pressure (a function of lung volume), and P_r is the airway resistive pressure (a function of flow rate). The P_{appl} may be supplied totally by the respiratory muscles (P_{mus}), by a mechanical ventilator (P_{aw}), or by both ($P_{mus} + P_{aw}$). Substituting the term $P_{mus} + P_{aw}$ for P_{appl}, equation 1 can be written as follows:[14]

2. $P_{mus} + P_{aw} = P_{el} + P_r$

Breathing is spontaneous or unassisted if only the respiratory muscles supply the inflation pressure ($P_{aw} = 0$). Breathing is mechanically assisted if a mechanical ventilator helps the respiratory muscles supply the inflation pressure (P_{aw} becomes positive). Breathing is mechanically controlled if the ventilator supplies all of the inflation pressure ($P_{mus} = 0$). The inflation pressure needed to counteract the elastic recoil and airway resistance pressures can be calculated if elastance (E), resistance (R_{aw}), volume (V), and flow rate ($\dot{V}$) are known:

$$P_{el} = V \times E = L \times cm\ H_2O/L = cm\ H_2O$$
$$P_r = \dot{V} \times R_{aw} = L/sec \times cm\ H_2O/(L/sec) = cm\ H_2O$$

Substituting the term $V \times E$ for P_{el} and the term $\dot{V} \times R_{aw}$ for P_r, equation 2 can be rewritten as follows:

3. $P_{mus} + P_{aw} = (V \times E) + (\dot{V} \times R_{aw})$

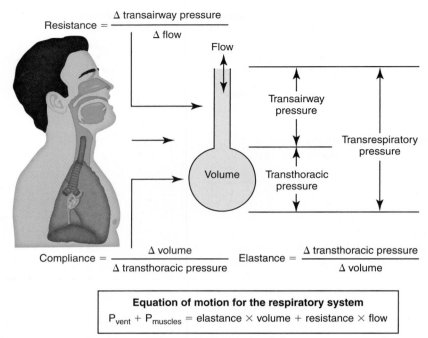

Figure 3-24 Illustration of the respiratory system equation of motion. Frictional and elastic resistances combine to create the lung inflation pressure; high inflation pressures may be the result of either increased airways resistance or decreased lung compliance, or a combination of both.

CLINICAL FOCUS 3-10

Overcoming the Resistance of the Endotracheal Tube to Breathing: Automatic Tube Compensation

The intensive care clinician must regularly evaluate the mechanically ventilated patient to determine if continued mechanical breathing assistance is necessary; the sooner the ventilator can be discontinued and the endotracheal tube (ETT) removed—a process called extubation—the fewer the complications and the shorter the patient's stay in the intensive care unit. One way clinicians can determine if patients can breathe on their own is to initiate a spontaneous breathing trial (SBT); this involves disconnecting the ventilator and allowing the patient to breathe through the ETT, while closely monitoring vital signs and other physiological data.

Because the ETT must fit inside the trachea, it has a smaller diameter than the patient's natural airway and has a greater inherent resistance to airflow. If a patient can comfortably breathe through the ETT and maintain stable cardiopulmonary function for 30 to 120 minutes, the ETT can usually be successfully withdrawn because the natural airway poses less resistance to breathing than the ETT. The ETT may impose enough airflow resistance for some patients that it causes them to fail the SBT even though they would have been able to breathe successfully without the ETT in place. As a result, these patients remain on the ventilator when they could have been extubated successfully—which means they are subjected to the hazards of mechanical ventilation longer than necessary.

The ideal SBT would allow the clinician to evaluate what the patient's response to breathing would be after extubation but without actually removing the ETT. Automatic tube compensation (ATC) is a feature of some modern ventilators that provides just enough inspiratory pressure to negate the resistance of the ETT, which simulates breathing through the natural airway while the patient remains intubated and attached to the ventilator, breathing spontaneously through the system. As stated in the text, airway resistance is measured as the pressure required to drive a given flow through the airways (R_{aw} = cm H_2O/L/sec). Airflow during a spontaneous inspiration varies continuously, which means the pressure required to drive flow through a given ETT varies in the same way. On a ventilator with ATC, the clinician enters the size of the ETT, and the ventilator's microprocessor continuously calculates the resistance of the ETT during the patient's spontaneous inspiration; based on this information, the ventilator adjusts inspiratory pressure "on the fly" to offset the resistance of the ETT precisely as the patient inhales. In this way, the patient's ability to breathe on his or her own without the added resistance of the ETT can be evaluated.

Equations 1 to 3 are consistent with Newton's third law of motion: "For every action there is an equal and opposite reaction." Each equation or a variation of each has been referred to as the respiratory system equation of motion (see Figure 3-24). In equation 3, if the patient breathes spontaneously, the airway pressure (P_{mus}) is negative during lung inflation. If the patient is attached to a mechanical ventilator and it supplies more flow than the patient demands, airway pressure becomes positive, and inspiration is assisted. If the ventilator supplies just enough flow to match the patient's inspiratory flow demand exactly, airway pressure remains at zero throughout inspiration. The respiratory system equation of motion is the theoretical basis for this kind of mechanical ventilation, known as proportional assist ventilation (PAV).[13] In PAV, the ventilator monitors volumes, pressures, and flows instantaneously as the patient breathes and uses this information to compute breath-to-breath inspiratory pressures ($P_{el} + P_r$) proportional to the patient's inspiratory demands.

Exhalation Mechanics and Cephalad Flow Bias

During expiration, P_L decreases, causing the airway diameter to decrease. The airway diameter is determined by P_L and anatomical structural support. The cartilaginous airways are better able than small, noncartilaginous airways to resist pressure-induced diameter changes. Small airways depend on elastic retractile forces of surrounding lung parenchyma for their patency (see Chapter 1). Natural airway narrowing during normal tidal exhalation causes linear flow velocity to be greater than it is during inhalation, especially in small, peripheral airways—that is, for a given flow rate, gas molecules pick up speed as they move through narrowed airways. This expiratory cephalad (toward the head) flow bias enhances the normal process of mucociliary clearance because mucus tends to move in the direction of the highest flow velocity.[16] This effect is exaggerated during a cough when small airways are narrowed further by bursts of high

intrapleural pressures; extremely high linear flow velocities provide the shearing forces necessary to propel mucus up toward the trachea and pharynx. (One must distinguish between bulk flow rate and linear flow velocity; although airway compression can reduce bulk flow rate [liters per second], it increases linear velocity [meters per second].)

Expiratory Flow Limitation

Muscular effort determines the peak flow rate that can be generated by a maximal-effort exhalation if one begins to exhale from the TLC level. However, after about 20% of the VC is exhaled (20% of the way from TLC to RV), factors other than effort limit the expiratory flow rate. At some point during exhalation from TLC to RV, the pressure inside the airways falls below the P_{pl} surrounding the airways; as a result, small airways are compressed and narrowed, limiting the maximal achievable expiratory flow rate.

At the start of a forced exhalation from the TLC level, the thorax contracts, causing the normally subatmospheric P_{pl} to become positive. As a result, P_A also increases. P_A is the sum of static elastic recoil pressure (P_{el}) and surrounding P_{pl} ($P_A = P_{el} + P_{pl}$) as shown in Figure 3-25, A. Frictional resistance to airflow causes the pressure along the airway to decrease steadily from the alveolus to the mouth, where P_{ao} is 0.

As exhalation continues and approaches RV, elastic lung recoil pressure decreases progressively as the shrinking lung approaches its resting zero recoil level. The progressively lower P_{el} associated with diminishing lung volumes means the maximum driving pressure that can be generated in the alveolus also diminishes (remember that $P_A = P_{el} + P_{pl}$). As the lungs become smaller, the driving pressure and the maximal achievable expiratory flow rate decrease. This decrease in driving pressure is the main reason why pressures inside the airways eventually drop below the surrounding P_{pl} as the lung nears RV. The point at which intraairway pressure equals the surrounding P_{pl} is called the **equal pressure point (EPP)**. Downstream from the EPP, the higher surrounding pleural pressure compresses and

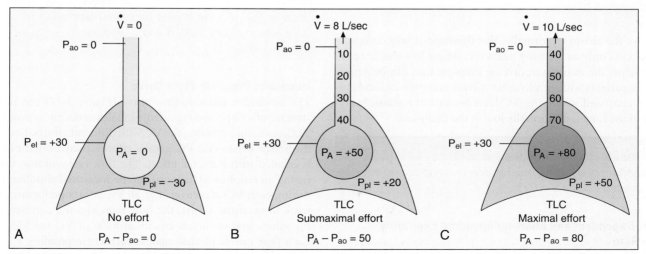

Figure 3-25 Maximum flows at high lung volume. At total lung capacity (*TLC*), expiratory flow is effort-dependent and proportional to $P_A - P_{ao}$. **A,** End-inspiration before exhalation starts. **B,** The beginning of a submaximal-effort forced exhalation. **C,** The beginning of a maximal-effort forced exhalation. *P_{ao},* Pressure at the airway opening; *P_{el},* elastic recoil pressure; *P_A,* alveolar pressure.

CLINICAL FOCUS 3-11

Detecting Causes of Increased Lung-Inflation Pressure: Increased Airway Resistance versus Increased Static Lung Recoil

You are called to the bedside of a patient who has an endo-tracheal tube in place and whose lungs are being mechanically ventilated. An alarm on the ventilator warns you of high peak inspiratory pressure (PIP).

You observe that this patient's PIP has increased significantly since your last measurement 2 hours ago. You also measure the P_{plat} and find that it has not changed. You would like to know whether the PIP increased because R_{aw} increased or because C_L decreased. How do you determine the answer?

Discussion

PIP reflects the total force required to move flow through the airways plus the force required to overcome the lung's elastic recoil. P_{plat}, measured at a time when flow is 0, reflects only the force required to overcome the lung's elastic recoil. In this situation, the unchanged P_{plat} tells you the lung's recoil force did not change. The increased peak pressure must mean your patient has increased R_{aw}; this commonly occurs in patients whose lungs are mechanically ventilated because of increased secretions. Airway mucosal edema, endotracheal tube obstruction, and bronchoconstriction may also increase R_{aw}.

Conversely, if you found that P_{plat} increased to the same extent that peak pressure increased (keeping the difference between the two constant), decreased compliance caused the increased PIP. The constant difference between PIP and P_{plat} tells you that R_{aw} remained the same.

Examples of factors that may decrease C_L include alveolar collapse (atelectasis), lung collapse (pneumothorax), overdistention of the lung, and inadvertent pushing of the endotracheal tube too far into the right mainstem bronchus.

narrows the airways. Normally, this dynamic airway compression occurs only as the lung nears RV, where low elastic recoil force limits the maximum driving pressure that can be generated. In patients with emphysema, airway compression and collapse occur well above the RV level because the elastic recoil force of the lung is abnormally low in the first place.

CONCEPT QUESTION 3-8

What effect does early dynamic airway compression have on the exhaled VC and the RV?

Effort-Dependent and Effort-Independent Expiratory Flow Rate

If forced exhalation starts from the TLC level, the initial flow rate is effort-dependent—that is, greater efforts produce greater initial flows as shown in Figure 3-25. In Figure 3-25, *A*, the subject was instructed to inhale to TLC and hold the breath, keeping the glottis open. In Figure 3-25, *B*, still at TLC, the subject was instructed to exhale with a submaximal effort. In Figure 3-25, *C*, the subject was instructed to inhale to TLC again and this time to exhale with maximal effort. The high lung volume at the beginning of these exhalations produced a high elastic recoil pressure, which made a high P_A possible. Because P_A is the sum of intrapleural and elastic recoil pressures, the higher the elastic recoil pressure, the greater the difference between P_A and the surrounding P_{pl}. Therefore, in a forced exhalation beginning from TLC, the P_A pressure head is high enough that pressures down the airway (toward the mouth) never fall below P_{pl} before gas leaves the thoracic airways. EPP and dynamic airway compression described earlier never occur at high lung volumes near TLC. In Figure 3-25, *B* and *C*, greater muscular effort produced greater $P_A - P_{ao}$ differences and greater flow rates.

In Figure 3-26, the subject was instructed exactly as in Figure 3-25 except that the exhalation maneuvers began at 60% of VC instead of from TLC. At this smaller lung volume, the beginning lung recoil is lower, and the difference between maximum achievable P_A and P_{pl} is relatively small. During even a submaximal exhalation effort (see Figure 3-26, *B*), the pressure inside the airway soon falls below P_{pl}, and EPP is reached well inside the thoracic cavity. A maximal expiratory effort (see Figure 3-26, *C*) fails to produce a greater flow rate because EPP represents a choke point between the alveolus and the mouth. In this situation, the driving pressure that produces the expiratory flow rate is not $P_A - P_{ao}$, as it is in Figure 3-25, *B* and *C*, but is instead P_A minus EPP choke point pressure, which is identical for submaximal and maximal efforts in Figure 3-26, *B* and *C*. One can think of the airway compression at EPP as a valve that controls the flow rate, similar to the way pinching the middle of a garden hose would control the outflow of water at the hose's end. Greater muscular effort in Figure 3-26, *C*, simply produced an increase in P_{pl} that exactly matched the increase in P_A. Therefore, the flow rate remained constant and was effort-independent.

CONCEPT QUESTION 3-9

Why is $P_A - P_{pl}$ the driving pressure responsible for expiratory flow in Figure 3-26, B and C, and not $P_A - P_{ao}$, as it is in Figure 3-25?

Isovolume Pressure-Flow Curve

The isovolume pressure-flow curve (Figure 3-27) can be constructed after a person repeatedly inhales as deeply as possible to TLC, each time exhaling the VC with different efforts. Each time the person exhales the VC, greater effort is used, until the last VC is exhaled with maximal effort. The flow rate, volume, and P_{pl} (using an esophageal balloon) can be measured simultaneously during each VC maneuver. For all VC efforts performed, from weak to maximal efforts, the flow rates and the corresponding P_{pl} values that occurred exactly at 60% of VC are identified. Each flow rate is plotted against each corresponding P_{pl} value obtained at 60% of each VC effort (see Figure 3-27). This curve is called an **isovolume pressure-flow curve** because all flows and pressures are measured at the same volume (60% of VC).

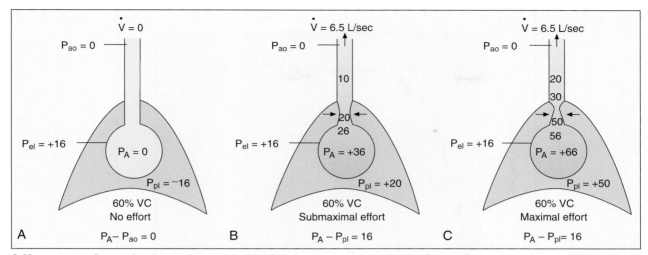

Figure 3-26 Maximum flows at low lung volumes. At 60% of vital capacity (*VC*), expiratory flow is effort-independent and proportional to $P_A - P_{pl}$. As driving pressure decreases from the alveolus to the mouth, intraluminal pressure decreases below surrounding pleural pressure; a choke point forms as the airway is compressed, establishing a gradient between the choke point and alveolus. P_{ao}, Pressure at the airway opening; P_{el}, elastic recoil pressure; P_A, alveolar pressure.

CLINICAL FOCUS 3-12

Effect of Lung Recoil on Functional Residual Capacity and Breathing Pattern in Emphysema

People with emphysema have low lung elastic recoil forces because emphysema destroys elastic tissues. Consequently, at the end of a tidal exhalation, their lungs do not recoil to normal resting volumes, and FRC is abnormally elevated. In addition, small noncartilaginous airways are prone to collapse prematurely during exhalation because few elastic fibers are available to apply retractile forces around the circumference of these airways. The result is air trapping, further enlarging the FRC. What kind of breathing pattern do you expect in people with emphysema?

Discussion

Patients with emphysema have increased WOB as a result of their high expiratory R_{aw}. To minimize this frictional work, they breathe at a low rate to reduce turbulence and increase the laminar flow characteristics of the gas stream. To keep their airways open during exhalation, they tend to purse the lips or partially close the vocal cords. This action increases pressure in the airways during exhalation, counteracting the outside collapsing force (pleural pressure) on the airway walls. At the same time, this action prolongs expiratory time. Patients with severe emphysema breathe slowly and often exhale through pursed lips or grunt through partially closed vocal cords to splint the airways open and avoid air trapping.

The points on the curve represent the flow rates and pressures produced by the different efforts, all of which are measured precisely at the moment the lung deflates through 60% of the VC. The striking feature of this curve is that flow no longer increases when expiratory efforts cause pleural pressures

to increase to greater than 10 cm H_2O. Even maximal effort (60 cm H_2O pleural pressure in Figure 3-27) fails to increase the flow rate. After the flow rate plateau is reached, the flow rate becomes effort-independent. This flow limitation is explained by the EPP phenomenon described in the previous section.

If several other pressure-flow curves are plotted at different lung volumes in exactly the same manner just described, a family of isovolume pressure-flow curves is produced, each at a different lung volume (Figure 3-28, *A*). At 90% of VC, increasing effort always produces increasing flows (i.e., a flow rate at 90% of the VC is effort-dependent). At lower lung volumes (60%, 30%, and 10% of VC), expiratory flows initially increase with greater efforts, but after a certain point, further effort fails to increase flow. Each lung volume has its own maximum achievable flow rate ($\dot{V}_{max}$). If each $\dot{V}_{max}$ is plotted against its corresponding lung volume (instead of its corresponding pleural pressure), a flow-volume curve is produced that is identical in shape to the flow-volume curve recorded instantaneously from a single exhaled, forced VC maneuver (see Figure 3-28, *B*). The FVC flow-volume curve is actually a continuous plot of all the maximum flows achievable at lung volumes ranging from TLC to RV. (The use of flow-volume curves in assessing pulmonary function is discussed in Chapter 5.)

Time Constants in Ventilation

If a constant pressure is applied to the trachea, gas flows into the lungs until the lung pressure equals the applied pressure. At this point, the lung contains a volume determined by its compliance. C_L and R_{aw} determine how *rapidly* the source pressure and lung pressure equalize. The product of C_L and R_{aw} is the **time constant (TC)**, expressed in seconds. This is shown as follows:

$$TC = C_L \times R_{aw}$$
$$TC = (L/cm\ H_2O) \times (cm\ H_2O/L/sec)$$
$$TC = seconds$$

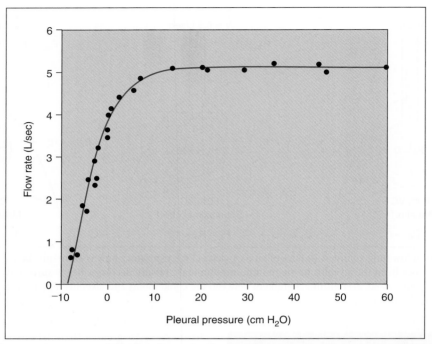

Figure 3-27 An isovolume flow-pressure curve at 60% of vital capacity obtained during a series of measurements. The points depict flow rates and intrapleural pressures at varying expiratory efforts, measured precisely as the lung deflates through 60% of vital capacity. (Redrawn from Murray JF: *The normal lung*, ed 2, Philadelphia, 1986, Saunders.)

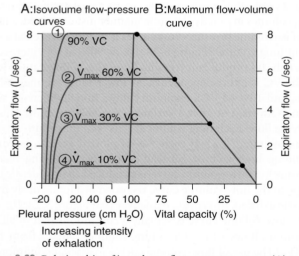

Figure 3-28 Relationship of isovolume flow-pressure curves (**A**) to the maximum flow-volume curve (**B**). (Redrawn from Murray JF: *The normal lung*, ed 2, Philadelphia, 1986, Saunders.)

When an instantaneous, constant pressure is applied to the trachea, the increase in lung pressure and increase in lung volume are exponential functions of time. After one time constant elapses, about 63% of the final equilibrium pressure or volume is achieved; 86.5% is achieved at the end of two time constants, 95% is achieved at the end of three time constants, and 99.3% is achieved at the end of four time constants. With normal values for total compliance (0.1 L/cm H_2O) and R_{aw} (1.0 cm H_2O/L/sec), TC is as follows:

TC = 0.1 L/cm H_2O × 1.0 cm H_2O/L/sec = 0.1 sec

The time required for five time constants to elapse is 5 × 0.1 = 0.5 second; this allows adequate time for normal lungs to equilibrate with an applied inflation pressure.

Effect of Compliance

Stiff lungs with low compliance achieve equilibrium with the inflation pressure quickly but at a low volume (Figure 3-29, *B*). Likewise, stiff lungs empty quickly because of their high elastic recoil. Lungs with low compliance and normal R_{aw} have short time constants. Four to five time constants are still required for complete inflation or deflation, but the absolute time required is less than for a normally compliant lung.

Effect of Airway Resistance

Figure 3-29, *C*, illustrates that high frictional resistance leads to long inflation and deflation times. If the same instantaneous inflation pressure is applied to normal lungs and lungs with high R_{aw}, more time is required for pressures to equalize across the high-resistance airways. Four or five time constants are needed for pressure equalization, but each time constant is relatively long. Given adequate time, the lung with increased R_{aw} eventually achieves the same volume as the normal lung, if inflation pressures are identical (see Figure 3-29, *C*). Equally important, lungs with high R_{aw} require long expiratory (deflation) times. Inadequate expiratory time leads to incomplete lung emptying, air trapping, and hyperinflation of the lungs.

CONCEPT QUESTION 3-10

Does a person experiencing a severe asthma attack have a short or long time constant?

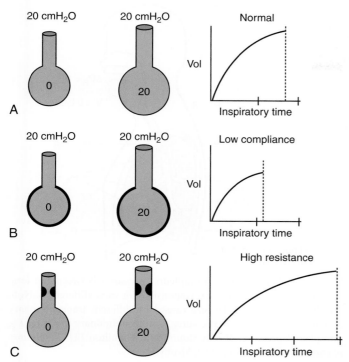

Figure 3-29 Time constants during inspiration. **A,** Normal lung filling. **B,** Low compliance, filling quickly to a low volume. **C,** High airways resistance, filling slowly; if inspiratory time is long enough, normal volume (as in **A**) is reached.

Frequency Dependence of Compliance

Because they account for less than 10% of the total R_{aw}, small airways (<2 mm in diameter) constitute a "silent zone" in which considerable disease may go undetected by conventional pulmonary function tests. One marker of increased small airway resistance is the **frequency dependence of compliance**.[15] R_{aw} is so low in people without disease that C_{dyn} and C_{st} are essentially equal at normal breathing rates. Even at 60 breaths per minute (high flow rates), C_{dyn} and C_{st} are equal in normal people. Therefore, C_{dyn} is not normally frequency-dependent, which implies that all ventilating lung units have normal and uniformly distributed resistances and time constants.

When R_{aw} is not uniformly distributed throughout the lung, different areas fill and empty at different rates. As breathing frequency increases, the difference in filling and emptying rates is exaggerated. As the breathing rate continues to increase, the high-resistance units receive less and less ventilation until eventually most of the V_T enters only normal units. High-resistance units require high driving pressures for a given V_T; measured dynamic compliance decreases. If C_{dyn} decreases by 25% or more when the breathing rate increases from 20 to 60 breaths per minute, compliance is considered to be frequency-dependent, indicating abnormally high small airway resistance. Frequency dependence of compliance may be present even if conventional R_{aw} measurements are normal.

EFFECTS OF LUNG COMPLIANCE AND AIRWAY RESISTANCE ON VENTILATION

Distribution of Inspired Air

All lung units are exposed to the same inspiratory time and are connected to the same airway. High-resistance units always lag behind the rest of the lung in filling and emptying and may continue to fill even after normal lung units start to empty. When airway resistance is high, alveoli develop differential pressures at end-inspiration because of differences in R_{aw}. After inspiration ceases, air may continue to flow within the lung from high-pressure to low-pressure areas. This intrapulmonary redistribution of gas between regions of differing R_{aw} is called **pendelluft**.

Air Trapping and Auto-PEEP

High airway resistance, as seen in patients with asthma, and weak lung recoil force, as seen in patients with emphysema, require abnormally long expiratory times. High breathing rates shorten the time available for expiration and if coupled with high airway resistance or weak lung recoil force, there may not be enough time for the lungs to empty to the normal FRC level before the next inspiration. If the lungs do not have enough time to empty, pressure in some of the slowly emptying alveoli may still be positive at the end of expiration and when the next inspiration begins. The trapped air and PEEP caused by inadequate expiratory time is called **auto-PEEP**—that is, PEEP "automatically" develops in these conditions.

CLINICAL FOCUS 3-13

Managing Auto-PEEP in the Clinical Setting

Auto-PEEP is mainly a problem of inadequate expiratory time—that is, patients with extremely high expiratory R_{aw} have such slow expiratory flows that the next inspiration occurs before their lungs have a chance to empty to the normal resting FRC level. Rapid respiratory rates exaggerate the problem. Air is trapped in the alveoli on expiration, and alveolar pressure does not fall to 0 cm H_2O at the end of expiration. Auto-PEEP can occur in spontaneously breathing or mechanically ventilated patients with high R_{aw}, such as in severe asthma attacks or severe pulmonary emphysema. In spontaneously breathing individuals, auto-PEEP increases WOB because to take a breath, the patient first must generate considerable inspiratory effort to decrease alveolar pressures below atmospheric levels before gas flow can begin to enter the lung. In mechanically ventilated patients, auto-PEEP leads to dangerously high inspiratory pressures that could injure the lungs.

Discussion

Because auto-PEEP is a problem associated with high R_{aw} and inadequate expiratory time, it stands to reason that any measure that (1) reduces R_{aw} or (2) lengthens expiratory

CLINICAL FOCUS 3-13

Managing Auto-PEEP in the Clinical Setting—cont'd

time could reduce or eliminate auto-PEEP. High R_{aw} caused by bronchospasm and mucosal edema can be treated with bronchodilator and antiinflammatory drugs. The respiratory therapist can lengthen expiratory time in spontaneously breathing patients by coaching them to exhale through pursed lips; this creates expiratory resistance that increases intraairway pressure, keeping airways splinted open while prolonging the expiratory time. If mechanically ventilated patients are controlled at a set respiratory rate and inspiratory volume, the respiratory therapist can lengthen expiratory time by (1) increasing the inspiratory flow to deliver V_T in less time, allowing more expiratory time; (2) using lower respiratory rates; and (3) using a smaller inspiratory volume, which means the patient needs less time to exhale it (which allows for a longer expiratory time.)

If a mechanical ventilator is set to sense the patient's inspiratory effort before it delivers a breath, the respiratory therapist can reduce the effort needed to trigger the machine by adjusting the ventilator to create its own PEEP, by stopping the patient's expiration before airway pressure drops to zero. Why would this kind of applied PEEP reduce the patient's inspiratory work? Consider the effects of applying a pressure to the mouth and airways equal to the pressure of the gas trapped in the alveoli at the end of expiration: the end-expiratory difference between alveolar and mouth pressures would be eliminated. If mouth and alveolar pressures are equal just before inspiration begins, the very first part of the patient's inspiratory effort decreases alveolar pressure below mouth pressure, immediately bringing gas flow into the lungs. In this way, applied PEEP can significantly reduce WOB in patients experiencing auto-PEEP. The same effect can be achieved in spontaneously breathing patients with a device that creates a continuous positive airway pressure (CPAP). CPAP in this situation is usually applied with a facemask.

Auto-PEEP increases FRC, hyperinflates the lungs, and increases WOB. WOB is increased because (1) hyperinflated lungs have decreased compliance and (2) the first part of each inspiratory effort is used to reduce the positive alveolar pressures below zero so that gas can start to flow into the lungs. For example, if at the end of expiration, P_A is +5 cm H_2O and pressure at the mouth is 0 cm H_2O, the inspiratory muscles first must work to expand the thorax and decompress P_A below 0 cm H_2O before gas can start to flow into the lung. Hyperinflation lowers the resting position of the diaphragm, shortening its muscle fibers as though it were already contracting and in a midinspiratory position. Such precontraction fiber shortening limits the diaphragm's force of contraction.

Clinicians sometimes intentionally apply PEEP to the upper airway during mechanical ventilation to prevent premature

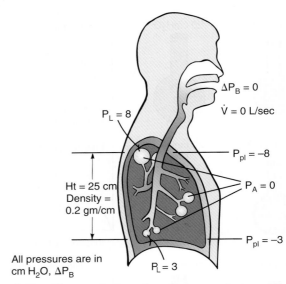

Figure 3-30 Differences in intrapleural pressures between the lung apex and lung base. Gravity is responsible for these differences. Note the differences in alveolar size caused by different transpulmonary pressures. P_B, barometric pressure; P_L, transpulmonary pressure; P_{pl}, intrapleural pressure. (From Slonim NB, Hamilton LH: *Respiratory physiology*, ed 5, St Louis, 1987, Mosby.)

collapse of alveoli during exhalation. However, auto-PEEP is an intrinsic abnormal development in patients with high airway resistance or weak lung recoil force. Other terms for auto-PEEP include **intrinsic PEEP**, inadvertent PEEP, covert PEEP, and occult PEEP. These terms allude to the fact that auto-PEEP is hidden and difficult to detect by normal means. Standard mouth pressure measurements fail to detect auto-PEEP because alveolar pressure is still positive even after mouth pressure has decreased to zero.

CONCEPT QUESTION 3-11

Which inspiratory time-to-expiratory time (I:E) ratio is most likely to cause auto-PEEP: a 1:2 ratio or a 2:1 ratio? Explain why.

Regional Pleural Pressure Gradients and Gas Distribution

P_{pl} does not have the same value throughout the pleural space from lung base to apex (Figure 3-30). In the upright position, the downward pull of lung tissue and blood creates a greater negative P_{pl} at the apex (−8 cm H_2O) than at the base (−3 cm H_2O). P_L is greater in the apex (P_L = 8 cm H_2O) than the base (P_L = 3 cm H_2O). As a result, apical alveoli are more distended and have higher recoil forces (are less compliant) than basal alveoli at the FRC level. Consequently, inspired tidal air preferentially flows to the more compliant basal lung units, ventilating them more than the apices. Although apical alveoli contain the greater volume, their decreased compliance allows less volume change per breath and less ventilation per minute.

During a VC inspiration from RV to TLC, the basal alveoli undergo a greater volume change than apical alveoli. If a person

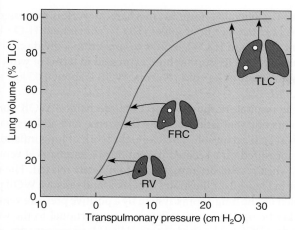

Figure 3-31 Regional distribution of lung volume. Differences in pleural pressures from the lung apex to lung base (see Figure 3-28) cause the volume to be distributed unequally between these two regions. This difference is minimal at total lung capacity (*TLC*). *RV*, Residual volume; *FRC*, functional residual capacity. (From Berne RM, Levy MN: *Physiology*, ed 3, St Louis, 1993, Mosby.)

exhales forcefully to RV, pleural pressure at the base becomes positive and small airways collapse. However, pleural pressure at the apex is still negative, and apical airways remain patent (Figure 3-31, *RV*). If the person slowly inhales to TLC, air first flows into the patent airways of apical alveoli; basal alveoli cannot receive volume until the P_{pl} is reduced below atmospheric levels and they begin to expand.

Apical alveoli at RV are small and on the steep part of the P-V curve (i.e., they are compliant and easily inflated because they are close to their resting volumes). However, at FRC (see Figure 3-31), apical alveoli are more distended and less compliant than basal alveoli. At TLC, apical and basal alveoli are nearly the same size. Although the P_L values are different, they are both on the flat part of the P-V curve, and their volumes differ only slightly. The greater portion of the inspired VC enters basal alveoli because they undergo a greater size change.

If the inspired VC described previously consists of 100% oxygen, the oxygen concentration of basal alveoli increases more than that of apical alveoli because basal alveoli receive more of the inspiratory gas. For the same reason, the nitrogen concentration of basal alveoli falls to a greater extent (i.e., nitrogen is more diluted by oxygen) than the nitrogen concentration of apical alveoli. This principle is the basis for the **single breath nitrogen elimination test**, in which the nitrogen concentration is continuously plotted against volume as a person exhales a previously inspired VC of 100% oxygen. As the exhalation approaches RV, small basal airways close and no longer contribute their nitrogen-depleted air to the exhaled gas stream. Near RV, exhaled gas originates entirely from nitrogen-rich apical alveoli. The basal airway closure point is marked by the sudden increase in exhaled nitrogen concentration. The volume in the lung at this point minus the RV is called the **closing volume**.

People with high small airway resistance have early small airway collapse, as discussed previously. Therefore, they have abnormally high closing volumes. The single breath nitrogen elimination test has been used to detect the presence of small airway obstruction.

Effect of Compliance and Resistance on Pressure Gradients in Positive Pressure Ventilation

During positive pressure ventilation (PPV), compliant lungs transmit more of the alveolar pressure into the pleural space than noncompliant lungs. Under normal conditions, when C_{LT} is about 0.1 L/cm H_2O, approximately half of the applied positive pressure in the alveoli is transmitted into the pleural space.[17] Diseased lungs with low compliance (high recoil force) may transmit only one third or one fourth of their pressures. High intrapleural pressures induced by PPV in critical care settings may compress the great veins in the mediastinum and impede the return of venous blood to the heart. This effect is more pronounced when C_L is normal but is less evident in stiff, noncompliant lungs.

R_{aw} affects the difference between P_{ao} and P_A. During PPV when R_{aw} is high, P_A may never equalize with mouth

CLINICAL FOCUS 3-14

Effects of Positive Pressure Ventilation on Cardiac Output

Your patient is a 78-year-old man admitted 5 days ago to the intensive care unit with severe bacterial pneumonia. Antibiotic therapy was started. Because of his respiratory distress, an endotracheal tube was placed, and he was connected to a positive pressure ventilator. Initially, high pressures were required to ventilate the patient's lungs because pneumonia (inflammation of the lungs) makes the lungs stiff and difficult to expand. As the pneumonia clears, his lungs require less pressure to expand them. You notice that your patient's blood pressure, which has been stable, has started to decrease. What might be responsible for change?

Discussion

When you began to ventilate your patient's lungs with positive pressure, his lungs were stiff and required high pressures to expand them. Much of this pressure was used to expand the lungs and was not transmitted to the pleural space. As the pneumonia clears, more of the inflating pressure is transmitted to the pleural space and mediastinum. These higher mediastinal pressures compress the large veins that return venous blood to the heart. This compression decreases the amount of blood flowing into the heart, decreasing cardiac output. When the cardiac output decreases, blood pressure in the body decreases, reducing blood flow to body tissues. This decrease in blood pressure is a common hazard of positive pressure ventilation, especially if the lungs are normally or highly compliant.

pressures, unless an inspiratory pause occurs at the end of inspiration. In high R_{aw}, peak inspiratory mouth pressure does not reflect P_A because much of the peak pressure is dissipated by the high resistance of the airways. For this reason, individuals with high R_{aw}, such as patients with severe asthma, can be ventilated with relatively high peak upper airway pressure without subjecting the alveoli to high pressure. The best indicator of true P_A is the pressure obtained during an inspiratory pause (P_{plat}).

Effect of Compliance and Resistance on Work of Breathing and Ventilatory Pattern

Work of Breathing

Work is required to overcome the elastic and frictional opposition to lung inflation. Expiration normally does not require muscular work under resting conditions. However, high R_{aw} may require expiratory muscular work if passive lung recoil fails to overcome frictional resistance quickly enough to accommodate normal breathing rates.

Work is performed when a force moves an object over a certain distance (work = force × distance). This equation shows that no matter how great the force, if the object does not move, no work is performed. Thus, WOB is a poor indicator of patient effort, which is one reason why it is not commonly calculated in the clinical setting. Work is measured in units of kilograms multiplied by meters (kg • m). The work equation can be modified to calculate WOB by substituting pressure for force (force equals pressure per unit of area) and lung volume for distance—WOB = P × V, which yields work units expressed in cm

H_2O • L. Generally, however, mechanical work is expressed in terms of either kg • m or joules (J). (To convert cm H_2O • L to kg • m, divide cm H_2O • L by 100; to convert to J, divide cm H_2O • L by 10.)[17] WOB is sometimes expressed in terms of work per unit of volume or kg • m/L. Normal WOB is about 0.05 kg • m/L or 0.5 J/L.[17]

The respiratory muscles affect the mechanical WOB during spontaneous ventilation because they tense and add resistance to chest wall expansion. Therefore, the work of lung inflation is best measured on a sedated patient during mechanical ventilation, when respiratory muscles are completely relaxed. The P-V curve in Figure 3-22 illustrates the elastic and resistive WOB performed on the lung-thorax system by a positive pressure ventilator. Elastic opposition to inflation is proportional to the white triangle *ADCFA*. The shaded area, *ABCDA*, represents the work required to overcome frictional resistance. The total work is represented by the sum of both areas (*ABCFA*). About 65% of the total work during quiet breathing is elastic work; the remaining 35% is frictional work. Of the frictional work, 80% is used to overcome R_{aw}, and 20% is used to overcome **viscous resistance**, or the friction between tissues as they slide over each other.

Expiratory frictional resistance, represented by the area *ADCEA* in Figure 3-22, is normally overcome by stored elastic energy of the lung. The lung deflates along the line *CEA* and inflates along the line *ABC*.

Ventilatory Pattern and Work of Breathing

Rapid breathing rates produce high flows, which increase the frictional component of work. Large tidal volumes stretch the lung, increasing its recoil force and the elastic component of

---

CLINICAL FOCUS 3-15

Mechanical Ventilation of Patients with High Airway Resistance: Why High Inspiratory Flow Rates Are Better than Low Flow Rates

A patient with status asthmaticus (an asthma attack that does not respond to treatment) is placed on a mechanical ventilator that delivers a constant volume with each breath. The lungs of this patient are difficult to ventilate because bronchoconstriction narrows the airways, creating extremely high inspiratory and expiratory R_{aw}. This condition causes high peak inspiratory pressure (PIP) and the patient needs a longer than normal time for exhalation as the lung empties to its normal resting level, or FRC. In this condition, why would setting the ventilator to deliver a high inspiratory flow rate be advantageous compared to the delivery of a low flow rate?

Discussion

A high inspiratory flow rate would seem to exaggerate the effects of high R_{aw}, making PIP even higher. Although PIP does increase, an important goal in ventilating this patient's lungs is to allow enough time for expiration. The high R_{aw} slows the expiratory flow rate of the lung so much that there is not enough time for it to empty to the normal FRC

before the next ventilator inflation occurs. This leads to dynamic hyperinflation, which is incomplete exhalation of the V_T as a result of inadequate expiratory time. Setting the ventilator to deliver a high inspiratory flow rate causes the V_T to be delivered more rapidly (shortens inspiratory time), allowing more time for exhalation. For example, assume a V_T of 600 mL is being delivered at a rate of 10 breaths per minute. The ventilatory cycle time (inspiration plus expiration) is a constant 6 seconds for each breath. Increasing the inspiratory flow rate shortens the time required to deliver the 600 mL, lengthening the time left for expiration. These longer expiratory times allow the lung to empty more completely. Although increasing the inspiratory flow increases PIP, the high R_{aw} prevents the complete transmission of this pressure to the alveoli (i.e., a large pressure decrease occurs across the airways from endotracheal tube to alveoli; thus, the alveoli are not subjected to the PIP). In extremely high R_{aw}, high PIP poses less danger to the alveoli than when R_{aw} is normal.

work. In health and disease, the body automatically chooses a breathing rate and V_T that minimize the total WOB.

A patient with chronic obstructive pulmonary disease (COPD) has a high R_{aw}, especially on expiration, and has weak elastic recoil. Therefore, patients with COPD breathe at low respiratory rates to minimize frictional work and allow more exhalation time. At the same time, these patients can afford to breathe more deeply because of the lung's weak elastic recoil force. Patients with COPD often must use a considerable amount of muscular energy to exhale through high-resistance airways and to assist the emptying force of weakly recoiling lungs.

A patient with pulmonary fibrosis chooses a rapid, shallow breathing strategy. Elastic recoil is high; therefore, work is minimized by breathing with smaller V_Ts. A normal R_{aw} allows higher breathing rates. To summarize, high R_{aw} with normal or increased C_L produces slow, moderately deep breathing, whereas normal R_{aw} with low compliance produces rapid, shallow breathing.

Muscular Weakness and Fatigue

If the respiratory muscles are already weak, increased WOB may lead to muscle fatigue. Weakness refers to the decreased force-generating capacity of the rested muscle; fatigue refers to the decreased force-generating capacity of actively working muscles, reversible by rest.[18] Respiratory muscle weakness is common in critically ill patients and predisposes them to ventilatory failure.

Clinical assessment of respiratory muscle fatigue is important in determining a patient's need for mechanical ventilation.

Overt diaphragmatic fatigue may result from excessive WOB with or without muscle weakness. Overt fatigue is defined as the inability of the diaphragm to sustain a given force of contraction throughout inspiration.[21] A measure of the diaphragm's force of contraction is the **transdiaphragmatic pressure (P_{di})**. P_{di} (pressure across the diaphragm) is measured after the subject swallows a tube with both esophageal (above the diaphragm) and gastric (below the diaphragm) balloons attached. P_{di} is the difference between esophageal and gastric balloon pressures. Any force that resists lung inflation causes the diaphragm to contract more forcefully, which increases P_{di}.

A key indicator of diaphragmatic fatigue is the ratio between quiet-breathing P_{di} and the maximal P_{di} ($P_{di}max$) a person can generate.[21] This ratio tells the clinician what percentage of the maximal force-generating capacity the patient uses for each breath. The $P_{di}/P_{di}max$ ratio increases when (1) lung recoil or R_{aw} increase or (2) muscular weakness (i.e., low $P_{di}max$) is present. The $P_{di}/P_{di}max$ ratio in normal persons breathing quietly is about 0.05. Patients with a $P_{di}/P_{di}max$ ratio of 0.4 or more eventually experience diaphragmatic fatigue.[18,19]

The "gold standard" index of diaphragmatic fatigue is the **tension-time index of the diaphragm (TT_{di})**, which relates the $P_{di}/P_{di}max$ ratio to the time spent in inspiration (T_i).[20] T_i is expressed as a fraction of the total breath cycle time, T_i/T_{tot},

CLINICAL FOCUS 3-16

Adaptive Support Ventilation: Automatic Selection of Rate and Tidal Volume That Minimize the Work of Breathing

Most modern mechanical ventilators have control panels the clinician uses to set a minimum respiratory rate and either a (1) V_T or (2) a pressure that the ventilator generates and maintains for each breath. The ventilator is sensitive to the patient's inspiratory efforts; it responds by either (1) delivering a breath at the preset volume or pressure ("mandatory" breath) or (2) allowing the patient to breathe at a volume the patient chooses ("spontaneous" breath). In either case, the patient can choose to breathe at a higher rate than the set "mandatory" rate. As explained in the text, the time it takes for the lung to exhale the V_T passively depends on the lung's time constant—which is determined by airway resistance and lung compliance. High airway resistance and high lung compliance (weak recoil force) create a long time constant, which means the lung takes a relatively long time to empty; low airway resistance and low lung compliance (high recoil force) yields a short time constant, which means the lung empties more quickly.

Patients with lungs that empty slowly (e.g., asthma) cannot breathe at high respiratory rates because expiratory time is too short to allow complete exhalation of V_T. Patients with lungs that empty quickly because of high recoil forces (low compliance, as in pulmonary fibrosis) take smaller tidal volumes to conserve energy, but they breathe at higher respiratory rates.

One can see why the clinician may have difficulty choosing the rate and volume combinations that best match lung mechanics. Adaptive support ventilation is a feature that allows the mechanical ventilator to calculate the expiratory time constant on a breath-by-breath basis; this is accomplished by the continuous calculation of airway resistance and lung compliance. Because the ventilator measures expiratory flow, pressure, and exhaled V_T, it has the necessary information to make these calculations. With adaptive support ventilation, the clinician does not set a respiratory rate or V_T; instead, the clinician enters the patient's ideal body weight, which the ventilator uses to calculate the required minute volume (MV) (i.e., respiratory rate × V_T). The clinician sets the percentage of the MV that the ventilator is to provide, ranging from 25% to 350% to account for variations in patient effort and metabolic needs. For a given % MV setting, if the patient breathes more or less, the ventilator adjusts the rate or inspiratory pressure or both to achieve the target MV. Through a complex preprogrammed formula, the ventilator calculates a rate and V_T combination that produces the least WOB. The ventilator continuously adapts to the patient's lung mechanics, increasing or decreasing V_T or rate or both to accommodate the patient's own participation in ventilation.

or the so-called duty cycle. The product of these two ratios produces the TT_{di}, shown as follows:

$$TT_{di} = P_{di}/P_{di}max \times T_i/T_{tot}$$

The greater the diaphragmatic fatigue, the greater the TT_{di}. TT_{di} takes into account (1) the percentage of maximum achievable inspiratory force the patient uses for each breath and (2) the length of time the force is applied. Clinical studies reveal that a TT_{di} of 0.15 is the fatigue threshold or critical TT_{di} above which healthy subjects cannot persistently maintain their breathing patterns.[20] It is widely accepted that TT_{di} greater than 0.15 is highly predictive of diaphragmatic fatigue.[21]

The disadvantage of TT_{di} is that it is an invasive procedure involving the swallowing of esophageal and gastric balloons, which makes it impractical for routine clinical assessment. In addition, TT_{di} focuses on diaphragmatic function alone, and does not take into account the contribution that the rib cage and accessory muscles make to vigorous inspiratory efforts. The diaphragm and rib cage muscles are uncoupled, each able to function independently. In quiet, nonstressful inspiration, only the diaphragm is active, but as inspiratory load increases (e.g., breathing through an endotracheal tube), the rib cage muscles take on an increasingly greater share of the inspiratory work.[21]

An alternative noninvasive estimate of TT_{di} is the **tension-time index of the inspiratory muscles (TT_{mus})**, which reflects the performance of all inspiratory muscles involved in respiratory effort. TT_{mus} uses easily measured mouth occlusion pressures instead of esophageal and gastric pressures. The noninvasive TT_{mus} has been validated and shown to correlate highly with the traditional invasive TT_{di}.[21,22] (TT_{mus} has also been called the **pressure-time index [PTI]**.) TT_{mus} is calculated as follows:

$$TT_{mus} = P_I/P_Imax \times T_i/T_{tot}$$

The negative inspiratory pressures, P_I and P_Imax, are measured at the mouth while the subject breathes through a tube that the clinician can abruptly occlude to make pressure measurements. P_I is the mean occlusion pressure measured during normal breathing, and P_Imax is the maximal occlusion pressure the patient can generate. T_i/T_{tot} is the fraction of the total respiratory cycle spent in inspiration. P_I is estimated from the negative airway pressure generated during normal breathing 0.1 second after the airway is abruptly occluded ($P_{0.1}$). (The greater the value of $P_{0.1}$, the greater the TT_{mus}. The reason $P_{0.1}$ increases as muscle strength decreases is that when fatiguing respiratory muscles fail to generate adequate tension, the muscle spindles become excited and stimulate the central nervous system, which increases the nervous drive to breathe.[21]) The equation for estimating P_I (the mean inspiratory occlusion pressure) is as follows:[22]

$$P_I = 5 \times P_{0.1} \times T_i$$

This method assumes that $P_{0.1}$ is the rate at which pressure increases over the inspiratory time (cm H_2O/sec). Because the pressure generated by the inspiratory muscles does not always increase linearly, this method may overestimate P_I.[21] However, a given individual's inspiratory time-pressure waveform is quite stable and repeatable; thus repeated measurements of P_I, $P_{0.1}$, and TT_{mus} for any one individual should be reliable.[23]

TT_{mus} is easily measured at the bedside or in the emergency department with the appropriate technology and correlates extremely well with TT_{di} in normal subjects, patients with COPD, and patients with restrictive lung diseases.[21-23] The fatigue threshold of the respiratory muscles above which patients fail to sustain adequate ventilation lies in a critical TT_{mus} range of 0.27 to 0.43.[24] (A normal TT_{mus} in healthy control subjects was found in one study to be about 0.05.[21]) Because TT_{mus} reflects the performance of all inspiratory muscles, it has an advantage over TT_{di} in assessing patients with high inspiratory loads, relevant especially in patients with COPD and restrictive lung disease. These patients inhale using predominantly rib cage muscles rather than the diaphragm, a pattern exaggerated by high inspiratory workloads.[21,23]

An increased use of accessory ventilatory muscles, coupled with rapid, shallow breathing, also signals impending diaphragmatic fatigue.[25] Accessory muscle use can be detected by palpating the neck and abdomen for muscle tensing. Fatiguing breathing patterns are characterized by the loss of synchronized outward inspiratory movements of the rib cage and abdomen. **Asynchrony** occurs when the outward movement of the abdomen lags behind the movement of the rib cage during inspiration. Critically ill patients exhibiting asynchrony have an increased risk of ventilatory failure. A visual sign of overt diaphragmatic fatigue is **abdominal paradox**, in which the abdomen is sucked inward during inspiration as the rib cage expands outward; this is evidence that the rib cage muscles are predominately being used.[25]

Because rapid, shallow breathing invariably accompanies respiratory muscle fatigue, the **frequency-to-VT (f/V_T) ratio** (sometimes called the rapid, shallow breathing index) is widely used in the clinical setting to assess an individual's ability to sustain adequate spontaneous ventilation. In a landmark study of patients being weaned from mechanical ventilation, patients with f/V_T ratios greater than 100 (V_T is expressed in liters and f in breaths per minute) had a 95% likelihood of developing ventilatory failure, whereas patients with f/V_T ratios less than 100 had an 80% probability of successfully sustaining spontaneous ventilation.[26] The f/V_T ratio is an attractive clinical tool for assessing WOB because it is highly predictive of ventilatory failure, is easily measured, and does not require patient effort or cooperation.

Energy Costs of Breathing

Oxygen consumed by the respiratory muscles reflects the energy costs of breathing. Oxygen consumed by the respiratory muscles alone can be assessed through a comparison of total oxygen consumption at rest with oxygen consumed at increased levels of ventilation. The oxygen cost of breathing in normal people is about 1.0 mL of oxygen consumed per liter of total ventilation; this is less than 5% of normal total body oxygen consumption. Patients with advanced COPD may have an oxygen cost of breathing as high as 10 mL of oxygen consumed per liter of ventilation.[19] The efficiency of breathing is decreased in patients with COPD because respiratory muscles consume large amounts of oxygen for each liter of ventilation they produce.

The oxygen cost of ventilation is difficult to measure directly but may be indirectly estimated from WOB measures.

However, WOB obtained from a P-V curve correlates poorly with oxygen consumed by ventilatory muscles because it does not take into account a patient effort that produces no volume change (no volume change means no work is performed, regardless of patient effort). A much more accurate indicator of oxygen consumption is TT_{di}, which takes into account the force of muscle contraction and the time over which it is applied.[27] The energy cost, and thus oxygen consumption of skeletal muscle contraction, depends on the force developed, the duration of muscular contraction, and the velocity of muscle shortening. The P-V curve reflects the mechanical work performed but does not account for the intensity of muscle contraction.

POINTS TO REMEMBER

- Both elastic and frictional forces resist ventilation; frictional forces exist only when air is flowing, whereas elastic forces are always present.
- The lung's recoil force is generated by elastic tissues and surface tension; of these two, surface tension is responsible for most of the recoil force.
- Pulmonary surfactant reduces alveolar surface tension, which prevents regional alveolar collapse and reduces WOB.
- Compliance and elastance are reciprocals of each other; low compliance implies high elastic recoil force, and high compliance implies low or weak elastic recoil force.
- The balance point between the opposing recoil forces of the lungs and thorax determine the resting level of the lung-thorax system—the FRC; low lung compliance reduces FRC, whereas high compliance increases FRC.
- Spontaneous and mechanical positive pressure breaths of equal volumes produce identical transpulmonary pressure gradients but completely different alveolar and pleural pressures.
- In mechanical positive pressure ventilation, plateau pressure is related to lung recoil force only; peak pressure is related to lung recoil force plus frictional airway resistance; peak minus plateau pressure is related to frictional airways resistance only.
- During inspiration, air preferentially goes to the high-compliance, low-resistance lung regions; during expiration, areas with the highest resistance and weakest recoil empty the slowest.
- The body chooses breathing patterns that minimize frictional and elastic work; high airways resistance requires a slow breathing rate, and low compliance requires a rapid, shallow breathing rate.
- Air trapping and auto-PEEP occur when expiratory time is too short for the lung to empty to the normal FRC level.
- High airway resistance, weak lung recoil, and rapid breathing rate predispose the lung to the development of auto-PEEP.
- At volumes less than 80% of TLC, maximal achievable expiratory flow rates are dictated by lung mechanics independent of muscular effort.
- High airway resistance enhances premature small airway collapse and expiratory flow limitation during forceful exhalation.

- Respiratory muscles may fatigue, and respiratory failure may occur if the muscles are abnormally weak or if WOB is too high.
- The best clinical indices of respiratory muscle fatigue and energy expenditure take into account both the force generated and the time over which the force is applied.

References

1. Ayas NT, et al: Respiratory system mechanics and energetics. In Mason RJ, et al, editors: *Murray and Nadel's textbook of respiratory medicine*, ed 5, Philadelphia, 2010, Saunders.
2. American Thoracic Society/European Respiratory Society: ATS/ERS Statement on Respiratory Muscle Testing, *Am J Respir Crit Care Med* 166(4):518, 2002.
3. Eskaros SM, Papadakos PJ, Lachmann B: Respiratory monitoring. In Miller RD, et al, editors: *Miller's anesthesia*, ed 7, Philadelphia, 2009, Churchill Livingstone.
4. Escolar JD, Escolar A: Lung hysteresis: a morphological review, *Histol Histopathol* 19(1):159, 2004.
5. Carney DE, et al: The mechanism of lung volume change during mechanical ventilation, *Am J Respir Crit Care Med* 160(5):1697, 1999.
6. Maggiore SM, Richard JC, Brochard L: What has been learnt from P/V curves in patients with acute lung injury/acute respiratory distress syndrome, *Eur Respir J Suppl* 42:S22, 2003.
7. Savov J: Surfactant system of the lung: historical perspective, *Semin Respir Crit Care Med* 16(1):1, 1995.
8. Mason RJ, Lewis JF: Pulmonary surfactant. In Mason RJ, et al: *Murray and Nadel's textbook of respiratory medicine*, ed 5, Philadelphia, 2010, Saunders.
9. Avery ME, Mead J: Surface properties in relation to atelectasis and hyaline membrane disease, *AMA J Dis Child* 97(5 Part I):517, 1959.
10. Druzin ML, et al: Antepartum fetal evaluation. In Gabe SG, Niebyl JR, Simpson JL, editors: *Obstetrics: normal and problem pregnancies*, ed 5, Philadelphia, 2007, Churchill Livingstone.
11. Almlen A, et al: Synthetic surfactant based on analogues of SP-B and SP-C is superior to single peptide surfactants in ventilated premature rabbits, *Neonatology* 98(1):91, 2010.
12. Albertine KH: Anatomy of the lungs. In Mason RJ, et al, editors: *Murray and Nadel's textbook of respiratory medicine*, ed 5, Philadelphia, 2010, Saunders.
13. Kacmarek RM: Proportional assist ventilation and neurally adjusted ventilatory assist, *Respir Care* 56(2):140, 2011.
14. Rubin BK: Physiology of airway mucus clearance, *Respir Care* 47(7):761, 2002.
15. Blonshine S, Goldman MD: Optimizing performance of respiratory airflow resistance measurements, *Chest* 134(6):1304, 2008.
16. Jardin F, et al: Influence of lung and chest wall compliances on transmission of airway pressure to the pleural space in critically ill patients, *Chest* 88(5):653, 1985.
17. Hess DR, Kacmarek RM: *Essentials of mechanical ventilation*, ed 2, New York, 2002, McGraw-Hill.
18. Mador MJ: Respiratory muscle fatigue and breathing pattern, *Chest* 100(5):1430, 1991.
19. Rochester DF: Respiratory muscles and ventilatory failure: 1993 perspective, *Am J Med Sci* 305(6):394, 1993.
20. Bellemare F, Grassino A: Effect of pressure and timing of contraction on human diaphragm fatigue, *J Appl Physiol* 53(5):1190, 1982.

21. Garcia-Rio F, et al: Accuracy of non-invasive estimates of respiratory muscle effort during spontaneous breathing in restrictive disease, *J Appl Physiol* 95(4):1542, 2003.

22. Ramonatxo M, Boulard P, Prefaut C: Validation of a noninvasive tension-time index of inspiratory muscles, *J Appl Physiol* 78(2):646, 1995.

23. Thompson WH, et al: Effects of expiratory resistive loading on the noninvasive tension-time index in COPD, *J Appl Physiol* 89(5):2000, 2007.

24. Capdevila X, et al: Changes in breathing pattern and respiratory muscle performance parameters during difficult weaning, *Crit Care Med* 26(1):79, 1998.

25. Tobin MJ: Breathing pattern analysis, *Intensive Care Med* 18(4):193, 1992.

26. Yang KL, Tobin MJ: A prospective study of indexes predicting outcomes of trials of weaning from mechanical ventilation, *N Engl J Med* 324(21):1445, 1991.

27. Field S, Sanci S, Grassino A: Respiratory muscle oxygen consumption estimated by the diaphragm pressure-time index, *J Appl Physiol* 57(1):44, 1984.

28. Adams AB, Çakar N, Marini JJ: Static and dynamic pressure-volume curves reflect different aspects of respiratory system mechanics in experimental acute respiratory distress syndrome, *Respir Care* 46(7):686, 2001.

29. Ho AMH, et al: Heliox vs air-oxygen mixtures for the treatment of patients with acute asthma: a systematic overview, *Chest* 123(3):882, 2003.

30. Lee DL, et al: Heliox improves hemodynamics in mechanically ventilated patients with chronic obstructive pulmonary disease with systolic pressure variations, *Crit Care Med* 33(5):968, 2005.

CHAPTER 4

Ventilation

CHAPTER OUTLINE

I. **Partial Pressures of Respiratory Gases**
II. **Classification of Ventilation**
   A. Minute or Total Ventilation
   B. Dead Space Ventilation
      1. Anatomical Dead Space
      2. Gas Composition of Anatomical Dead Space
      3. Measuring Anatomical Dead Space
      4. Alveolar and Physiological Dead Space

   C. Alveolar Ventilation
      1. Hyperventilation and Hypoventilation
      2. Alveolar Ventilation and Alveolar Partial Carbon Dioxide Pressure
   D. Partial Carbon Dioxide Pressure Equation
   E. Ratio of Dead Space to Tidal Volume
III. **Ventilatory Pattern, Dead Space, and Alveolar Ventilation**
IV. **Points to Remember**

OBJECTIVES

After reading this chapter, you will be able to:
- Calculate the partial pressures of gases under dry and 100% relative humidity conditions
- Explain how minute ventilation, alveolar ventilation, and dead space ventilation are interrelated
- Determine whether hyperventilation or hypoventilation is present by reviewing the arterial carbon dioxide pressure ($PaCO_2$)
- Explain why alveolar ventilation affects $PaCO_2$

- Explain the rationale underlying the calculation of anatomical dead space, alveolar ventilation, and physiological and anatomical dead space-to-tidal volume ratios
- Predict the effects of minute ventilation changes on alveolar ventilation, dead space ventilation, and $PaCO_2$
- Explain how ventilatory pattern affects dead space-to-tidal volume ratio and, subsequently, alveolar ventilation and $PaCO_2$
- Describe the theoretical basis for measuring and calculating dead space and alveolar ventilation

KEY TERMS

alveolar dead space (V_{DA})
alveolar ventilation ($\dot{V}_A$)
anatomical dead space (V_{Danat})
bradypnea
capnogram
capnography
capnometer
dead space ventilation ($\dot{V}_D$)
hypercapnia

hyperpnea
hyperventilation
hypocapnia
hypopnea
hypoventilation
minute ventilation ($\dot{V}_E$)
physiological dead space (V_D)
tachypnea
torr

Ventilation is the process of moving each breath, the tidal volume (V_T), in and out of the lungs. During tidal ventilation, fresh atmospheric air mixes with and replaces some of the air already in the lungs. Each exhalation removes some of the carbon dioxide (CO_2) the blood brings to the alveoli. Each inhalation replenishes the oxygen (O_2) the blood removes from the alveoli. Because not all the inspired V_T reaches the alveoli, only a portion of it participates in the gas exchange that occurs between blood and alveolar air, a process called external respiration. The depth and frequency of tidal breathing (i.e., the ventilatory pattern) greatly affects this gas exchange. Respiratory therapists and other health care clinicians must clearly understand factors affecting ventilation and respiration to assess the benefits and hazards of treatment options.

PARTIAL PRESSURES OF RESPIRATORY GASES

The measurement of respiratory gas pressures must be understood to comprehend the function of the lung as a gas-exchange organ. Air is a gas mixture of mostly nitrogen (N_2) and O_2, with traces of argon, CO_2, and other gases

(Figure 4-1, *A*). The total combined pressure exerted by these atmospheric gases, the barometric pressure (P_B), can be measured by a mercury (Hg) barometer, as shown in Figure 4-1, *B*. At sea level, atmospheric pressure exerts a force equal to the weight of a mercury column 760 mm high. By convention, standard atmospheric pressure at sea level is expressed simply as the height of the mercury column it supports, or 760 mm Hg. (The term **torr** is equivalent to mm Hg. In this book mm Hg is used.)

According to Dalton's law, the pressure of each gas that makes up air exerts a partial pressure proportional to its fractional concentration in air. The partial pressure of any gas (P_{gas}) in air is equal to its fractional concentration (F_g) multiplied by total atmospheric pressure: P_B ($P_{gas} = F_g \times P_B$).

CONCEPT QUESTION 4-1

Why is the PO₂ of tracheal gas less than the PO₂ of inspired atmospheric gas?

Because oxygen constitutes 20.93% of dry atmospheric air, its partial pressure (PO_2) at sea level is calculated as follows:

$$PO_2 = 0.2093 \times 760 \text{ mm Hg} = 159 \text{ mm Hg}$$

The partial pressure of carbon dioxide (PCO_2) is similarly calculated:

$$PCO_2 = 0.0003 \times 760 \text{ mm Hg} = 0.228 \text{ mm Hg}$$

In physiological calculations, the PCO_2 of inspired air is considered to be 0 mm Hg.

The act of inspiring heats air to body temperature (37° C) and saturates it with water vapor (100% relative humidity [RH]). The partial pressure of water vapor (P_{H2O}) is determined by only temperature and RH. Because the body maintains lung temperature and RH at 37° C and 100% RH, the P_{H2O} of gas in the lung is constant; under body temperature and humidity conditions, P_{H2O} is always 47 mm Hg. At sea level, the total pressure of all gases in the lung, including water vapor, is 760 mm Hg. Water vapor accounts for 47 mm Hg, which means the rest of the atmospheric gases account for the remaining 713 mm Hg. Therefore, 47 mm Hg first must be subtracted from P_B to calculate P_{gas} in the lung or blood. In the lung's airways, PO_2 is calculated as follows:

$$PO_2 = 0.2093 \times (760 - 47) \text{ mm Hg} = 149 \text{ mm Hg}$$

CLASSIFICATION OF VENTILATION

Minute or Total Ventilation

Minute ventilation ($\dot{V}_E$) is defined as the volume of air either entering or leaving the lung each minute; that is, the volume of air inhaled each minute must be equal to the volume exhaled each minute. In clinical practice, $\dot{V}_E$ is usually measured by adding together the exhaled tidal volumes obtained over 1 minute—hence the subscript E. Theoretically, the same result

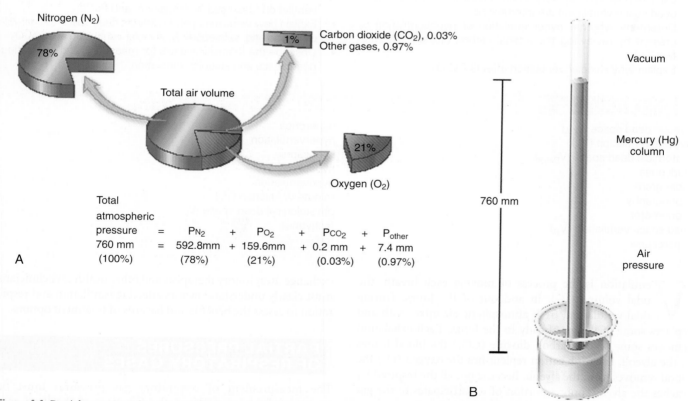

Total atmospheric pressure	=	P_{N_2}	+	P_{O_2}	+	P_{CO_2}	+	P_{other}
760 mm	=	592.8mm	+	159.6mm	+	0.2 mm	+	7.4 mm
(100%)		(78%)		(21%)		(0.03%)		(0.97%)

Figure 4-1 Partial pressures of gases in atmospheric air. **A,** Relative concentrations of atmospheric gases. **B,** Mercury barometer. Atmospheric pressure pushes mercury down in the dish and up the tube. Sea-level pressure supports a column of mercury 760 mm high in the tube. (From Patton KT, Thibodeau GA: *Anatomy & physiology,* ed 7, St Louis, 2010, Mosby.)

would be obtained by summing the inhaled tidal volumes over 1 minute, but exhaled volumes are easier to measure clinically. Regardless of the measuring method, $\dot{V}_E$ is the product of V_T and breathing frequency (f) per minute ($\dot{V}_E = V_T \times f$). If V_T is 500 mL and breathing frequency is 12 breaths per minute, $\dot{V}_E$ is calculated as follows:

$$\dot{V}_E = 500 \text{ mL} \times 12/\text{min}$$
$$\dot{V}_E = 6000 \text{ mL/min or } 6.0 \text{ L/min}$$

$\dot{V}_E$ is easy to measure but not particularly useful in evaluating the amount of ventilation that participates in gas exchange (respiration) at the alveolar level. Not all the $\dot{V}_E$ reaches the alveoli because the last part of each inspiration (about one third of the V_T) stays in the conducting airways and is eliminated with the next expiration (Figure 4-2). Likewise, the first one third of the next inspired V_T is reinspired exhaled air; it consists of the air left in the conducting airways from the last exhalation. Thus, only part of the $\dot{V}_E$ ventilates the alveoli; this part is called **alveolar ventilation** ($\dot{V}_A$). The remaining part ventilates conducting airways, which is called **anatomical dead space ventilation** ($\dot{V}_{Danat}$). $\dot{V}_E$ can be expressed in terms of its components ($\dot{V}_E = \dot{V}_{Danat} + \dot{V}_A$). This equation can be rearranged to solve for any of its components ($\dot{V}_A = \dot{V}_E - \dot{V}_{Danat}$ or $\dot{V}_{Danat} = \dot{V}_E - \dot{V}_A$). A single V_T can be similarly expressed ($V_T = V_{Danat} + V_A$), where V_{Danat} is anatomical dead space volume and V_A is alveolar volume.

Dead Space Ventilation

Anatomical Dead Space

The conducting airways from the mouth and nose down to and including terminal bronchioles constitute **anatomical dead space (V_{Danat})**. Ventilation of these airways is necessary to move gas to and from the alveoli, but no gas exchange occurs between blood and air across their walls. The fresh gas filling the conducting airways at the end of inspiration (see Figure 4-2, *left*) is exhaled and is sometimes called "wasted" ventilation because it takes no part in respiration. The term wasted ventilation is synonymous with dead space ventilation. Dead space is defined as airspaces that are ventilated but do not exchange gases with the pulmonary circulation.

The volume in the conducting airways (V_{Danat}) does not change unless surgery removes part of a lung or an artificial airway (endotracheal or tracheostomy tube) bypasses the upper airway dead space. Anatomical dead space increases slightly during a deep inspiration and with administration of drugs that relax smooth airway muscle because these factors increase the airway diameter. Diseases characterized by hyperinflation of the lungs (e.g., emphysema) increase V_{Danat} for the same reason. For clinical monitoring purposes, V_{Danat} is considered to be constant.

CONCEPT QUESTION 4-2

What effect does increasing the tidal volume have on V_{Danat} and V_A?

Gas Composition of Anatomical Dead Space

The composition of V_{Danat} gas is different at the end of expiration than at the end of inspiration (Figure 4-3). An inspired V_T of 500 mL completely flushes the normal 150 mL of V_{Danat} with atmospheric air, leaving behind a PCO_2 of 0 mm Hg and a PO_2 of 149 mm Hg (see Figure 4-3, *left*). Dead space gas is identical in composition to inspired air except that it is 100% humidified.

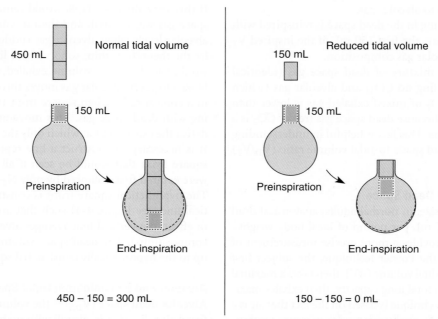

450 mL Normal tidal volume   150 mL Reduced tidal volume

150 mL   150 mL

Preinspiration   Preinspiration

End-inspiration   End-inspiration

450 − 150 = 300 mL   150 − 150 = 0 mL

Figure 4-2 Relationship among tidal volume, anatomical dead space, and alveolar volume. On the *left*, normal tidal inspiration pushes anatomical dead space volume back into the alveoli. One third of the tidal air remains in the conducting airways at end-inspiration so that alveoli receive only 300 mL of fresh gas. On the *right*, shallow tidal volume equal to anatomical dead space volume is shown. Theoretically, no fresh gas enters the alveoli. However, in reality, some gas mixing does occur. (From Forster RE, et al: *The lung: physiologic basis of pulmonary function tests,* ed 3, St Louis, 1986, Mosby.)

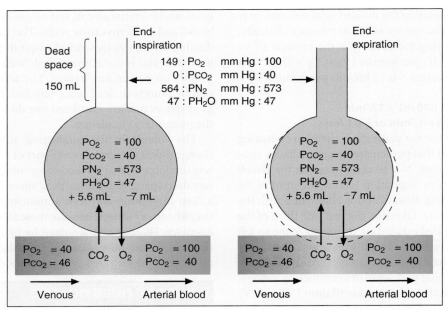

Figure 4-3 Dead space and alveolar gas compositions at end-inspiration and end-expiration. Dead space gas is identical to room air except it is saturated with water vapor (*left*). The anatomical dead space is filled with alveolar gas at end-expiration (*right*). (Redrawn from Fraser RG, Paré JA: *Organ physiology: structure and function of the lung,* ed 2, Philadelphia, 1977, Saunders.)

After the 500 mL of V_T is completely exhaled, the 150 mL of V_{Danat} (see Figure 4-3, *right*) is wholly occupied by gas that came from the alveoli. The humidified atmospheric air that occupied the dead space at end-inspiration was exhaled ahead of the alveolar gas (i.e., this gas was wasted because it did not participate in respiration). At end-tidal expiration, dead space gas is identical in composition to the average alveolar gas composition. Under normal circumstances, end-tidal expiratory gas is assumed to be identical in composition to alveolar gas.

The alveolar gas residing in the dead space is reinspired with the next breath. Therefore, the first 150 mL of the inspired V_T does not change the alveolar gas composition.

The exhaled V_T is a mixture of dead space gas (identical to inspired gas—containing no CO_2) and alveolar gas (which contains CO_2). The PCO_2 of mixed exhaled gas is lower than alveolar PCO_2 (P_ACO_2) because dead space gas free of CO_2 is a component of exhaled gas. This fact is helpful in understanding the calculation of the dead space-to-tidal volume ratio (V_D/V_T) later in this chapter.

Measuring Anatomical Dead Space

V_{Danat} is related to lung size; in normal adults, anatomical dead space is approximately 1 mL per pound of ideal body weight.[1] The Fowler technique provides a more precise measurement of V_{Danat} (Figure 4-4).[2] In the Fowler technique, the subject first exhales maximally to residual volume (RV), then takes a maximal inhalation of 100% O_2 to total lung capacity, then exhales maximally to RV again. This technique is based on the fact that air is a mixture of N_2 and O_2. An N_2 analyzer is used to measure continuously the exhaled N_2 concentration at the mouth after the single maximal inspiration of 100% O_2. N_2 concentration measured at the mouth decreases abruptly to 0 during the 100% O_2 inspiration (see Figure 4-4). At the end of inspiration, V_{Danat} contains pure O_2, which is the first gas to be exhaled. This means that N_2 concentration remains at 0% for the first part of the expiration.

As expiration proceeds, alveolar gas (which still contains some N_2) moves up into the conducting airways, and dead space N_2% gradually increases to alveolar levels—note the S-shaped curve in Figure 4-4. The increase in N_2% would be sharp and abrupt if dead space and alveolar gas were completely separated, as illustrated by the hypothetical square front in Figure 4-5, *A*. If this were the case, N_2% would remain at 0% until all dead space gas was expired, and then it would abruptly increase to alveolar levels when alveolar gas suddenly appeared, as shown by the theoretical thin, solid vertical line in Figure 4-4. V_{Danat} would simply be the volume exhaled to the sharp increase in N_2%. However, alveolar gas moves through conducting airways in a conical rather than square front (see Figure 4-5, *B*), mixing with dead space gas. This movement makes it difficult to detect the exact point at which only the V_{Danat} has been expired. It is necessary to construct a line representing the theoretical square front that would be seen if all N_2-free dead space gas were expired first, followed by only N_2-containing alveolar gas. The hypothetical square front is constructed by placing a vertical line (see Figure 4-4) such that area *A* equals area *B* (i.e., in effect, the vertical line averages alveolar and dead space gas compositions). The dead space volume is the volume expired up to the hypothetically constructed square front.

Alveolar and Physiological Dead Space

Alveolar dead space (V_{DA}) is the volume contained in nonperfused alveoli—that is, alveoli with no blood flow. The presence of V_{DA} is abnormal. Any factor decreasing pulmonary blood flow, such as extremely low cardiac output or a pulmonary embolus, increases V_{DA}. V_{DA} represents a decreased surface area for gas exchange and an increase in total wasted ventilation.

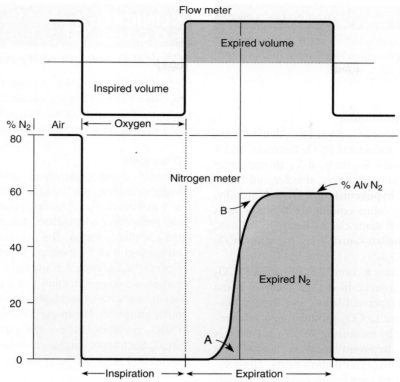

Figure 4-4 Single breath nitrogen elimination for measuring anatomical dead space. After the inhalation of a vital capacity of 100% oxygen, the nitrogen concentration of exhaled gas is continuously analyzed during the subsequent exhalation. (From Forster RE, et al: *The lung: physiologic basis of pulmonary function tests,* ed 3, St Louis, 1986, Mosby.)

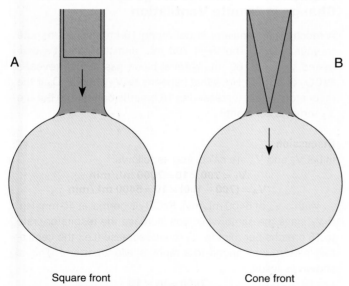

Figure 4-5 **A** and **B,** Inspired gas movement through conducting airways. Gas flow has a cone front (**B**), not a square front (**A**). (From Forster RE, et al: *The lung: physiologic basis of pulmonary function tests,* ed 3, St Louis, 1986, Mosby.)

Physiological dead space (V_D) is the sum of V_{Danat} and V_{DA} ($V_D = V_{Danat} + V_{DA}$). Similarly, physiological dead space ventilation ($\dot{V}_D$) per minute is as follows:

$$\dot{V}_D = \dot{V}_{Danat} + \dot{V}_{DA}$$

$\dot{V}_D$ is increased not only by decreased pulmonary blood flow but also by an increased breathing rate. Doubling the breathing frequency doubles the number of times the V_T moves through the V_{Danat}, doubling the $\dot{V}_{Danat}$.

Alveolar Ventilation

$\dot{V}_A$ is the amount of gas entering or leaving the alveoli per minute. It is the effective portion of the $\dot{V}_E$ in the sense that only $\dot{V}_A$ takes part in respiration. As shown previously, if $\dot{V}_D$ and $\dot{V}_E$ are known, $\dot{V}_A$ is easily calculated ($\dot{V}_A = \dot{V}_E - \dot{V}_D$).

All CO_2 in exhaled gas comes from ventilated alveoli that have blood flowing through their capillaries. The source of this CO_2 is tissue metabolism. Normal aerobic metabolism produces CO_2, which is carried by venous blood to the lungs (see Figure 4-3). The mixed venous PCO_2 ($P\bar{v}CO_2$) approaching the alveoli is several millimeters of mercury higher than P_ACO_2. Thus, CO_2 diffuses into the alveoli.

Inspiration brings fresh CO_2-free gas into the alveoli, and expiration removes a portion of the CO_2-rich alveolar gas (see Figure 4-3). The balance between metabolic CO_2 production per minute ($\dot{V}CO_2$) and its rate of elimination ($\dot{V}_A$) determines the PCO_2 of alveolar gas and the PCO_2 of the blood leaving the lung.

Hyperventilation and Hypoventilation

If $\dot{V}_A$ momentarily removes more CO_2 per minute than is metabolically produced, alveolar and blood PCO_2 decrease, and a state of **hyperventilation** exists. Similarly, if $\dot{V}_A$ momentarily removes less CO_2 than the body produces, alveolar and blood PCO_2 increase, and a state of **hypoventilation** exists. Normally, alveolar gas and blood PCO_2 values equilibrate as blood flows past alveoli and enters the left ventricle. As Figure 4-3 shows, arterial blood arising from the left ventricle has the same PCO_2 as the alveoli ($P_ACO_2 = PaCO_2$).

$\dot{V}_A$ determines $PaCO_2$ because it controls P_ACO_2. The $PaCO_2$ obtained clinically through arterial blood gas analysis is the definitive indicator of $\dot{V}_A$. Hyperventilation and hypoventilation are defined by $\dot{V}_A$ relative to CO_2 production, a relationship that can be known only by measuring $PaCO_2$. If $PaCO_2$ is above normal (**hypercapnia**), hypoventilation exists; if $PaCO_2$ is below normal (**hypocapnia**), hyperventilation exists. The presence of hyperventilation or hypoventilation cannot be reliably determined by observing only the respiratory rate or V_T depth.

Alveolar Ventilation and P$_A$CO$_2$

P_ACO_2 is inversely related to $\dot{V}_A$; if $\dot{V}_A$ is reduced by half, P_ACO_2 doubles. If $\dot{V}_A$ doubles, P_ACO_2 (and $PaCO_2$) is reduced by half. For example, if a $\dot{V}_A$ of 5 L per minute produces a P_ACO_2 of 40 mm Hg, a $\dot{V}_A$ of 10 L per minute produces a P_ACO_2 of 20 mm Hg. Similarly, a $\dot{V}_A$ of 2.5 L per minute produces a P_ACO_2 of 80 mm Hg. The $\dot{V}_A$ equation illustrates this relationship ($P_ACO_2 \times \dot{V}_A = K$).[3] In this equation, K is a constant. (See Appendix III for the derivation of this equation.) This equation is based on the assumption that during a steady state of blood flow and ventilation, CO_2 production ($\dot{V}CO_2$) is constant and equal to CO_2 elimination. Normally, P_ACO_2 and $PaCO_2$ have almost identical values; as a rule, $\dot{V}_A$ has the same relationship with $PaCO_2$ as it has with P_ACO_2. Figure 4-6 illustrates the inverse relationship between P_ACO_2 and $\dot{V}_A$.

PCO$_2$ Equation

Because dead space does not participate in gas exchange, all CO_2 in exhaled gas comes from the alveoli. The amount of CO_2 the lungs exhale each minute ($\dot{V}CO_2$) equals the $\dot{V}_A$ multiplied by the concentration of CO_2 in the alveoli. This is shown as follows:

1.　　　　　$\dot{V}CO_2 = \dot{V}_A \times F_ACO_2$

In this equation, F_ACO_2 is the fractional concentration of CO_2 in the alveoli. The P_ACO_2 can be determined by multiplying F_ACO_2 by the total alveolar gas pressure. Therefore, equation 1 can be rewritten as follows:

2.　　　　　$\dot{V}CO_2 = \dot{V}_A \times P_ACO_2 \times K$

In this equation, K is a constant that reconciles the different measurement units; $\dot{V}CO_2$ is measured in milliliters per minute,

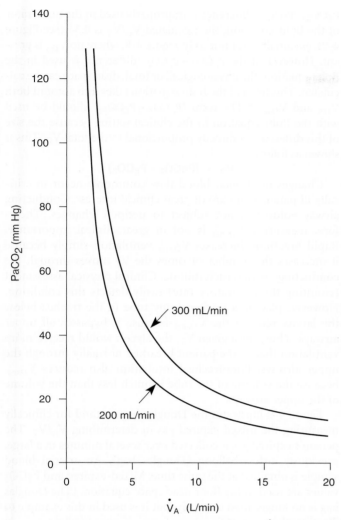

Figure 4-6 Relationship between alveolar ventilation ($\dot{V}_A$) and $PaCO_2$ at carbon dioxide production rates of 200 mL/min and 300 mL/min. (From Martin L: *Pulmonary physiology in clinical practice*, St Louis, 1987, Mosby.)

$\dot{V}_A$ is measured in liters per minute, and P_ACO_2 is measured in millimeters of mercury (see Appendix III for the derivation of K). Equation 2 can be solved for P_ACO_2 as follows:

3.
$$P_ACO_2 = \frac{\dot{V}CO_2}{\dot{V}_A \times K} = \frac{\dot{V}CO_2}{\dot{V}_A} \times \frac{1}{K}$$

In this equation, 1/K is equal to 0.863. The classic PCO_2 equation is written as follows:

4.
$$P_ACO_2 = \frac{\dot{V}CO_2 \times 0.863}{\dot{V}_A}$$

Because P_ACO_2 is usually equal to $PaCO_2$ in the absence of lung disease, $PaCO_2$ can be substituted for P_ACO_2. This is shown as follows:

5.
$$PaCO_2 = \frac{\dot{V}CO_2 \times 0.863}{\dot{V}_A}$$

Equation 5 means that the balance between the rate of CO_2 elimination ($\dot{V}_A$) and the rate of CO_2 production ($\dot{V}CO_2$) determines the $PaCO_2$. For example, under normal resting conditions, the body produces about 200 mL of CO_2 each minute, and alveolar ventilation is about 4 L per minute; using equation

5, $PaCO_2$ is calculated to be about 43 mm Hg. If $\dot{V}_A$ decreases to 3 L per minute while $\dot{V}CO_2$ stays the same, $PaCO_2$, as calculated with equation 5, would increase to about 58 mm Hg, indicating the presence of hypoventilation. If instead the metabolic rate increases, increasing CO_2 production to 300 mL per minute, but $\dot{V}_A$ stays at 4 L per minute, $PaCO_2$ increases to 65 mm Hg, again indicating hypoventilation. In the latter example, the lungs fail to increase $\dot{V}_A$ to meet the increased need for CO_2 elimination. (See Appendix III for the complete derivation of equation 5 and the 0.863 factor.) Equation 5 also can be solved for $\dot{V}_A$; if the $PaCO_2$ and $\dot{V}CO_2$ are known, $\dot{V}_A$ can be calculated as follows:

6.
$$\dot{V}_A = \frac{\dot{V}CO_2 \times 0.863}{PaCO_2}$$

Modern CO_2 measuring devices called capnometers make it feasible to measure $\dot{V}CO_2$ in the clinical setting. This information, coupled with arterial blood $PaCO_2$ analysis, allows $\dot{V}_A$ to be precisely quantified.

CONCEPT QUESTION 4-4

If V_T is 600 mL, f equals 10 breaths per minute, $PaCO_2$ equals 40 mm Hg, and $\dot{V}CO_2$ equals 200 mL per minute, what is the $\dot{V}_D$?

Ratio of Dead Space to Tidal Volume

$\dot{V}_A$ can be calculated if the fraction of V_T that is dead space (V_D/V_T) is known. Normally, about 30% to 40% of the inspired V_T remains in conducting airways, never reaching alveoli (see Figure 4-2, *left*), which means $\dot{V}_D$ constitutes about 30% to 40% of $\dot{V}_E$.[3] It follows that about 60% to 70% of the $\dot{V}_E$ is $\dot{V}_A$. Shallow tidal volumes increase V_D/V_T because conducting airway volume (V_{Danat}) remains constant (see Figure 4-2, *right*). Deep breaths decrease V_D/V_T for the same reason, causing a larger percentage of the inspired volume to reach the alveoli.

With the basic relationship ($V_T = V_D + V_A$), V_A can be expressed in terms of V_D/V_T and V_T. This is shown as follows:
$$V_A = V_T(1 - [V_D/V_T])$$
This formula is useful if V_D is unknown but V_D/V_T is known. For example, if a normal adult weighing 150 lb has a V_T of 500 mL and V_D/V_T equals 0.33, 33% of the V_T is dead space; the remaining 67% of the V_T must be V_A. This is shown as follows:
$$V_A = 500(1 - 0.33)$$
$$V_A = 500(0.67)$$
$$V_A = 335 \text{ mL}$$

The V_D/V_T can be clinically calculated if the mixed exhaled carbon dioxide ($P_{\bar{E}}CO_2$) and $PaCO_2$ partial pressures are known. The physiological dead space equation, known as the Bohr equation, allows the V_D/V_T to be calculated in the following manner:
$$V_D/V_T = \frac{PaCO_2 - P_{\bar{E}}CO_2}{PaCO_2}$$

In this equation, $P_{\bar{E}}CO_2$ is the mean carbon dioxide pressure of mixed-expired gas (dead space plus alveolar gas). (See Appendix III for the derivation of the Bohr equation.)

The Bohr equation is based on the premise that all CO_2 in mixed-expired gas originates from the alveoli and not the dead space. Figure 4-7 illustrates this point; the lightly shaded blocks represent CO_2-free inspired air, and the darkly shaded blocks represent CO_2-containing alveolar gas. The CO_2 in exhaled gas (*two dark blocks*) comes from the alveoli; dead space gas, which contains no CO_2 (*one light block*), makes up the rest of the exhaled volume.

$P_{\bar{E}}CO_2$ is always less than P_ACO_2 because the exhaled V_T consists of V_{Danat} gas, which has a PCO_2 of 0 mm Hg, mixed with alveolar gas (Figure 4-8). The degree to which V_{Danat} gas reduces the PCO_2 of mixed expired gas is reflected by the size of the difference between P_ACO_2 and $P_{\bar{E}}CO_2$. This difference is proportional ($\propto$) to V_{Danat} (see Figure 4-8), shown as follows:

$$V_{Danat} \propto (P_ACO_2 - P_{\bar{E}}CO_2)$$

In Figure 4-8, two thirds of the exhaled V_T originates from alveoli (P_ACO_2 of 40 mm Hg), and one third originates from V_{Danat} (PCO_2 of 0), yielding a mixed-expired PCO_2 of 26.7 mm Hg. The Bohr equation confirms that V_D/V_T is 0.33 (i.e., that V_{Danat} is one third of V_T). The $P_ACO_2 - P_{\bar{E}}CO_2$ difference in the numerator of the Bohr equation reflects only the presence of V_{Danat}. It does not accurately reflect the presence of V_{DA}. As illustrated in Figure 4-9, if some alveoli lose their blood flow, the PCO_2 values hypothetically decrease to 0, causing average P_ACO_2 to decrease also. (Average P_ACO_2 is measured through an analysis of the gas stream at end-expiration.) Mixed-expired gas in Figure 4-9 contains anatomical plus alveolar dead space gas, causing $P_{\bar{E}}CO_2$ to decrease to 13.3 mm Hg. (Compare Figures 4-8 and 4-9.) If alveolar dead space is present, and the

$P_ACO_2 - P_{\bar{E}}CO_2$ difference is improperly used in the numerator of the Bohr equation, the calculated V_D/V_T is 0.34 (see Figure 4-9), essentially the same as in Figure 4-8, where no V_{DA} is present. However, if the $P_ACO_2 - P_{\bar{E}}CO_2$ difference is used in the Bohr equation, the physiological, or total, dead space can be calculated. This form of the Bohr equation takes into account both V_{DA} and V_{Danat}.[4] The term ($P_ACO_2 - P_{\bar{E}}CO_2$) should be used with the Bohr equation in the clinical setting because the size of this difference is directly proportional to the total V_D. This is shown as follows:

$$V_D \propto (PaCO_2 - P_{\bar{E}}CO_2)$$

Changes in alveolar blood flow commonly occur in critically ill patients and are of great clinical interest. Conducting airway volume is not subject to periodic changes. Therefore, measuring V_{Danat} is not of great clinical importance. Rapid breathing increases V_{Danat} ventilation simply because it increases the number of times the V_T moves through the conducting airways each minute. Clinical physical assessment (counting the respiratory rate) easily detects this condition. However, placing a tracheostomy tube in the trachea below the larynx reduces the V_{Danat} because it bypasses all upper airways. Thus, for a given V_T, the alveoli would receive more ventilation than if the patient breathed normally through the upper airways. Endotracheal intubation also reduces V_{Danat} because the volume of the tube is much less than the volume of the upper airways.

Figure 4-9 illustrates the Douglas bag method for clinically measuring the mixed-expired gas in determining V_D/V_T. The person's expired gas is collected over several minutes in a large, previously airless balloon (Douglas bag). An arterial blood sample is obtained at the same time. Mixed-expired and $PaCO_2$ values are used in the Bohr dead space equation. (The Douglas bag is no longer used clinically, but it is used in this example to illustrate the concept.)

A capnometer is a device used in the clinical setting to analyze exhaled CO_2. These instruments respond instantaneously to PCO_2 changes. **Capnography** refers to the PCO_2 changes of exhaled tidal volumes graphically displayed as a waveform (capnogram). A **capnogram** allows the PCO_2 to be identified at the end of a tidal exhalation ($P_{ET}CO_2$), which corresponds to average P_ACO_2 ($P_ACO_2 = P_{ET}CO_2$). ($P_{ET}CO_2$ reflects alveolar gas composition and is not equal to mixed expired PCO_2, which reflects the composition of a mixture of dead space and alveolar gases; i.e., $P_{ET}CO_2 \neq P_{\bar{E}}CO_2$.) A microprocessor can determine the average PCO_2 over the entire exhaled V_T ($P_{\bar{E}}CO_2$).

Successive measurements over time are useful for following trends and assessing the effects of therapeutic interventions on pulmonary blood flow. V_D/V_T is a measure of ventilatory efficiency. A high V_D/V_T means much of the $\dot{V}_E$ is wasted in ventilating nonperfused alveoli, requiring high-energy expenditure to accomplish a relatively small amount of $\dot{V}_A$.

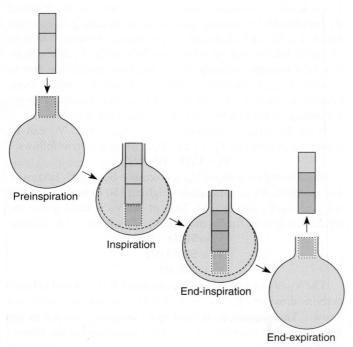

Figure 4-7 Basis for the Bohr equation. All carbon dioxide in exhaled gas originates from the alveoli (*dark-shaded blocks*). Mixed-expired gas at end-expiration consists of about two thirds alveolar gas (*dark-shaded blocks*) and one third carbon dioxide–free dead space gas (*light-shaded block*). The lower the mixed-expired PCO_2, the greater the volume of anatomical dead space. (From Forster RE, et al: *The lung: physiologic basis of pulmonary function tests,* ed 3, St Louis, 1986, Mosby.)

Labels in figure: Preinspiration, Inspiration, End-inspiration, End-expiration

---

CONCEPT QUESTION 4-5

A patient's total $\dot{V}_E$ is 18 L per minute (normal 5 to 8 L per minute), but the $PaCO_2$ is normal at 40 mm Hg. What is the physiological explanation for this situation?

CLINICAL FOCUS 4-3

Causes of and Physiological Response to Increased Dead Space-to-Tidal Volume Ratio

A 55-year-old woman is admitted to the hospital in obvious respiratory distress. Her increased rate and depth of breathing have increased her minute ventilation to 15 L per minute. Arterial blood gases show a normal $PaCO_2$ of 40 mm Hg. It seems odd that this woman, with a minute ventilation this great, has a normal $PaCO_2$. What is the explanation for this?

Discussion

A normal $PaCO_2$ associated with high minute ventilation indicates that much of this patient's ventilation is not in contact with blood flow. Dead space is the term used to describe alveoli that have normal ventilation but no blood flow (perfusion) through their capillaries. Any factor that decreases perfusion increases alveolar dead space. Increased alveolar dead space decreases alveolar ventilation if minute ventilation stays the same. Pulmonary embolism (obstruction of

pulmonary vessels by blood clots) and shock (decreased cardiac output and low perfusion) are conditions that cause increased alveolar dead space. V_D/V_T increases as a larger percentage of the V_T becomes dead space. In conditions producing dead space, the body tries to maintain a normal $PaCO_2$ by increasing the minute ventilation. This increased minute ventilation does not mean alveolar ventilation increases because much of the minute ventilation is directed toward dead space units. A physiological consequence of increased dead space is the increased work of breathing required to maintain a normal $PaCO_2$.

Patients with obstructive lung disease have impaired ventilatory capacity and may be unable to accommodate the increased demand for minute ventilation created by conditions that produce dead space. Increased dead space may precipitate ventilatory failure in these patients.

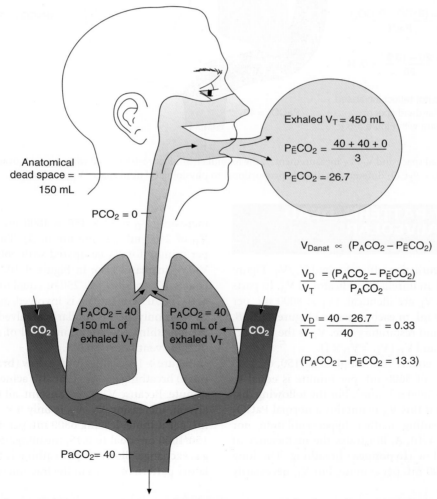

Figure 4-8 Anatomical dead space and V_D/V_T measurement. Exhaled gas is a mixture of alveolar and anatomical dead space gases. Anatomical dead space volume is directly proportional to the $P_ACO_2 - P_{\bar{E}}CO_2$ difference. The V_D/V_T of 0.33 means anatomical dead space comprises one third of the tidal volume.

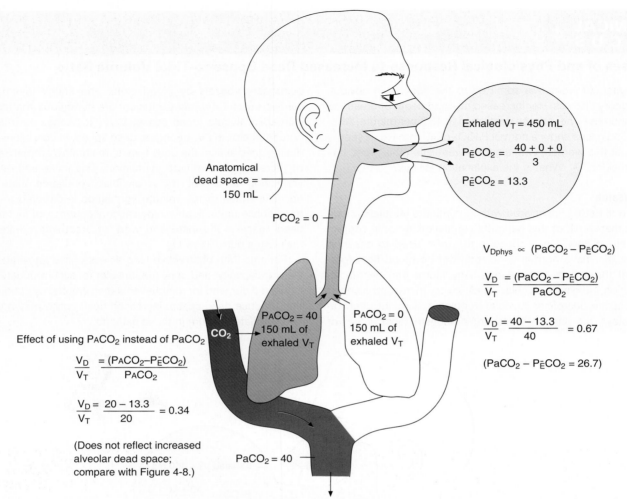

Figure 4-9 Physiological dead space and V_D/V_T measurement. If the formula from Figure 4-8 is used when alveolar dead space is present, V_D/V_T is underestimated. The $P_ACO_2 - P_{\bar{E}}CO_2$ difference is directly proportional to physiological dead space (V_{Danat} plus V_{DA}).

VENTILATORY PATTERN, DEAD SPACE, AND ALVEOLAR VENTILATION

The rate and depth of ventilation affect $\dot{V}_A$ and V_D/V_T. Figure 4-10 illustrates that $\dot{V}_E$ is an unreliable indicator of $\dot{V}_A$. In parts A, B, and C, V_{Danat} and $\dot{V}_E$ are identical. ($\dot{V}_E$ is 8000 mL per minute and V_{Danat} is 150 mL in each instance.) Figure 4-10, B, represents a normal V_T and respiratory rate. $\dot{V}_D$ is the product of respiratory frequency and V_D ($\dot{V}_D = V_D \times f$).

In Figure 4-10, B, $\dot{V}_D$ equals 16 multiplied by 150, or 2400 mL per minute. The $\dot{V}_A$ of 5600 mL per minute is equal to $\dot{V}_E - \dot{V}_D$ (8000 − 2400 = 5600 mL/min). For the following discussion, it is assumed that this $\dot{V}_A$ maintains a normal $PaCO_2$ of 40 mm Hg, representing neither hyperventilation nor hypoventilation. Figure 4-10, A, illustrates the inefficiency of rapid (**tachypnea**), shallow (**hypopnea**) breathing. The lung still achieves a $\dot{V}_E$ of 8000 mL per minute, but $\dot{V}_D$ necessarily

increases ($\dot{V}_D = 32 \times 150 = 4800$ mL/min, compared with a $\dot{V}_D$ of 2400 mL per minute in B). This leaves only 3200 mL per minute for $\dot{V}_A$ compared with 5600 mL per minute in B. V_D/V_T increases also; in Figure 4-10, B, it is 150/500, which equals 0.3, and it is 150/250 or equal to 0.6 in part A. In Figure 4-10, B, 70% of the $\dot{V}_E$ is involved in alveolar gas exchange, whereas only 40% is similarly involved in part A. Rapid, shallow breathing is a common signal of respiratory distress and possible ventilatory failure.

Figure 4-10, C, illustrates a slow (**bradypnea**), deep (**hyperpnea**) breathing pattern that also achieves a $\dot{V}_E$ of 8000 mL per minute. Because V_{Danat} is constant, all the additional V_T enters alveoli, increasing $\dot{V}_A$. $\dot{V}_D$ is only 8×150, which equals 1200 mL per minute, leaving 6800 mL per minute for $\dot{V}_A$. V_D/V_T is 150/1000 or equal to 0.15, meaning 85% of $\dot{V}_E$ participates in gas exchange. Slow, deep breathing is the most efficient ventilatory pattern in terms of the fraction of $\dot{V}_E$ received by alveoli.

CLINICAL FOCUS 4-4

Predicting the Effect of Changes in Alveolar Ventilation on Arterial Pressure of Carbon Dioxide

The lungs of a patient in the intensive care unit are mechanically ventilated with the following settings:

$$f = 12/min$$
$$V_T = 500 \text{ mL}$$

You also have the following information about your patient:

$$V_D = 150 \text{ mL}$$
$$PaCO_2 = 40 \text{ mm Hg}$$

Approximately 1 hour later, the patient seems to be agitated and is triggering the ventilator at a rate of 24/min (V_T is still 500 mL). Estimate the patient's new $PaCO_2$.

Discussion

To solve this problem, you first must determine the $\dot{V}_A$ for both situations. This is done as follows:

Initial $\dot{V}_A$

$$\dot{V}_A = \dot{V}_E - V_D$$
$$\dot{V}_A = (500 \text{ mL} \times 12) - (150 \text{ mL} \times 12)$$
$$\dot{V}_A = 6000 \text{ mL/min} - 1800 \text{ mL/min}$$
$$\dot{V}_A = 4200 \text{ mL/min}$$

New $\dot{V}_A$

$$\dot{V}_A = (500 \times 24) - (150 \times 24)$$
$$\dot{V}_A = 12,000 \text{ mL/min} - 3600 \text{ mL/min}$$
$$\dot{V}_A = 8400 \text{ mL/min}$$

Solve for $PaCO_2$ using the following equation:

$$PaCO_2 \times \dot{V}_A = K$$

This is equivalent to the following:

$$\text{Initial } (PaCO_2 \times \dot{V}_A) = \text{new } (PaCO_2 \times \dot{V}_A)$$

Solve for the new $PaCO_2$. This is done as follows:

$$PaCO_2 \text{ (initial)} \times \dot{V}_A \text{ (initial)} = PaCO_2 \text{ (new)} \times \dot{V}_A \text{ (new)}$$

$$40 \times \frac{40 \times 4200}{8400} = PaCO_2 \text{ (new)}$$

$$\frac{168,000}{8400} = 20 \text{ mm Hg}$$

The inverse relationship between $PaCO_2$ and $\dot{V}_A$ is shown. In this situation, $\dot{V}_A$ was doubled, reducing $PaCO_2$ by one half. Thus, the $PaCO_2$ of a patient whose lungs are mechanically ventilated changes if the ventilator's delivered $\dot{V}_E$ is changed (i.e., by changing V_T, respiratory rate, or both).

CLINICAL FOCUS 4-5

High-Frequency Ventilation: Tidal Volumes Smaller than Anatomical Dead Space Volume

It is possible to ventilate the lung adequately with tidal volumes smaller than the anatomical dead space volume if the respiratory rate is very high. Mechanical high-frequency ventilation (HFV) is most often used on premature newborn infants with underdeveloped lungs that do not expand properly (respiratory distress syndrome of the newborn). Less often, HFV is used on adults with severe acute lung injury. The extremely small tidal volumes place little mechanical stress on the lungs because they do not stretch the underdeveloped or injured alveoli very much. Two types of HFV are high-frequency jet ventilation (HFJV) and high-frequency oscillatory ventilation (HFOV). HFJV pulses small jets of gas very rapidly into the trachea through a small tube inside of an endotracheal tube. HFOV uses a mechanism such as a flexible diaphragm to vibrate or oscillate gas back and forth rapidly in the airways. In either type of HFV, there are no distinguishable inspiratory and expiratory phases or measurable tidal volumes. HFJV cycling rates may be 5 pulses per second (5 Hz) in adults to 7 Hz in infants (300 to 420 "breaths" per minute). HFOV uses even higher cycling frequencies, up to 15 Hz (900 cycles per minute) in infants. In HFV, the conventional relationships (discussed in this chapter) among tidal volume, frequency, dead space, and alveolar ventilation become meaningless. In HFV, alveolar ventilation and gas exchange do not occur via bulk gas flow in and out of the lungs; rather, they occur through complex gas mixing and diffusion mechanisms. As small bursts of gas are pulsed or oscillated through the airways, flow turbulence and eddy currents help mix gas and enhance diffusion. In this process, gas moves in and out of the airway at the same time. (One can appreciate this two-directional flow phenomenon by blowing air through a straw inserted halfway into a test tube.) In HFV, inspiratory gas pulses down the center of the airway, while expiratory gas streams in the opposite direction along the airway walls, a process known as coaxial flow. Whatever the physical principles involved, HFV can maintain adequate gas exchange with extremely small volumes and rapid breathing rates.

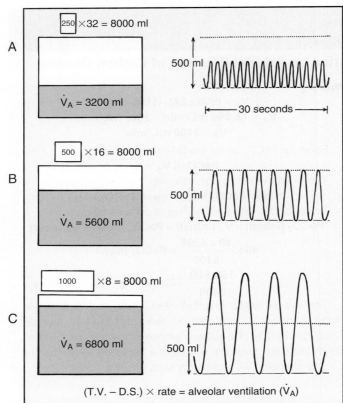

Figure 4-10 **A-C,** Effect of the ventilatory pattern on alveolar and dead space ventilation. Minute ventilation is 8000 mL per minute, or 8 L per minute, in **A, B,** and **C. B** represents normal conditions. Although minute ventilation stays the same in **A,** the anatomical dead space is ventilated more frequently. $\dot{V}_D$ increases at the expense of $\dot{V}_A$. In **C,** the tidal volume must increase because $\dot{V}_E$ remains the same. More air enters the alveoli, and $\dot{V}_A$ increases. (From Forster RE, et al: *The lung: physiologic basis of pulmonary function tests,* ed 3, St Louis, 1986, Mosby.)

POINTS TO REMEMBER

- $\dot{V}_E$ consists of V_D plus V_A; it is equal to the respiratory rate multiplied by V_T.
- V_D consists of ventilated airspaces that do not receive pulmonary blood flow; V_D does not participate in gas exchange between air and blood and contains no CO_2.

- V_{Danat} consists of conducting airway volume and it is normal; V_{DA} consists of alveoli with no blood flow and it is abnormal.
- The exhaled V_T contains a mixture of dead space and alveolar gases; therefore, the PCO_2 of the exhaled tidal gas is always lower than P_ACO_2.
- The $PaCO_2$ is determined by the balance between CO_2 production in the body and its elimination by alveolar ventilation; $PaCO_2$ is the indicator of alveolar ventilation adequacy.
- $PaCO_2$ is inversely proportional to alveolar ventilation; hyperventilation decreases $PaCO_2$, and hypoventilation increases $PaCO_2$.
- V_D/V_T, normally about one third, is the fraction of ventilation devoted to the $\dot{V}_D$ and is a measure of ventilatory efficiency with regard to gas exchange.
- A high V_D/V_T leads to a high work of breathing because too much energy is expended in ventilating airspaces that do not participate in gas exchange.
- $\dot{V}_A$ is called effective ventilation because it is responsible for gas exchange between blood and air and is the mechanism for CO_2 elimination from the body.
- $\dot{V}_A$ can be reliably assessed only through the evaluation of $PaCO_2$.
- Respiratory pattern affects V_D/V_T: identical $\dot{V}_E$ values can yield different $\dot{V}_A$ and $PaCO_2$ values depending on the rate and depth of breathing.

References

1. Wagner PD, Powell FL, West JB: Ventilation, blood flow, and gas exchange. In Mason RJ, et al, editors: *Murray and Nadel's textbook of respiratory medicine,* ed 5, Philadelphia, 2010, Saunders.
2. Anthonisen NR, Fleetham JA: Ventilation: total, alveolar, and dead space. In Fishman AP, et al, editors: *Handbook of physiology, section 3: the respiratory system, volume IV, gas exchange,* Bethesda, MD, 1987, American Physiological Society.
3. Luce JM: Respiratory monitoring in critical care. In Goldman L, Ausiello D, editors: *Cecil medicine,* ed 23, Philadelphia, 2007, Saunders.

Pulmonary Function Measurements

OBJECTIVES

After reading this chapter, you will be able to:

- Describe how the normal range of human pulmonary function values are obtained
- Explain why dilution or washout measurements of functional residual capacity (FRC) in severe obstructive airways disease generally differ from values obtained by the plethysmographic method
- Explain why both restrictive and obstructive disease mechanisms reduce the vital capacity
- Explain why restrictive and obstructive diseases affect the FRC, the residual volume, and the work of breathing differently
- Differentiate between purely obstructive and restrictive patterns of pulmonary function tests

- Explain why large and small airways resistance affects certain spirometric tests in different ways
- Explain why the results of some spirometric tests can be improved with greater effort, but the results of others are independent of effort
- Describe the theory behind the test that detects grossly uneven ventilation of the lungs
- Explain why the relationship between maximum voluntary ventilation and ventilation attained during maximal exercise is different for individuals with severe obstructive pulmonary disease compared to healthy people
- Explain the basic theory behind tests that are especially sensitive to increases in small airways resistance

KEY TERMS

ambient temperature, pressure, and saturated (ATPS) conditions
anthropometric
body temperature, pressure, and saturated (BTPS) conditions
closing capacity
closing volume test
$FEF_{25\%}$
$FEF_{25\%-75\%}$
$FEF_{75\%}$
FEV_1
FEV_1/FVC ratio
FEV_2

FEV_3
flow-volume loop (F-V loop)
forced expired flow (FEF)
forced inspiratory volume (FIV)
maximum sustainable ventilation (MSV)
maximum voluntary ventilation (MVV)
peak expiratory flow (PEF)
peak inspiratory flow (PIF)
pneumotachometer
RV/TLC ratio
volume of isoflow ($V_{iso}\dot{V}$)

ulmonary function refers to the role of the lungs in gas exchange. Pulmonary function testing is a practical application of respiratory physiology and is necessary for understanding abnormal lung function and the effects of treatment. Tests of healthy humans have identified factors that are associated with normal variations in lung function, such as age, gender, height, and body size. In clinical medicine, pulmonary function testing has helped define the natural progression of pulmonary diseases and produced a useful classification of basic functional defects. Pulmonary function tests help determine the severity of functional impairments and the extent to which treatment restores normal function. Although pulmonary function tests are diagnostic in nature, they are rarely the key factor in a definitive diagnosis. These tests reflect the combined function of the airways, alveolar-capillary membrane, respiratory muscles, and neural control mechanisms. The same pattern of abnormal pulmonary function often overlaps several diseases. The main purpose of this chapter is to provide a physiological basis for understanding pulmonary function measurements and abnormal test results. Detailed instruction on testing technique and definitive interpretation of results are beyond the scope of this chapter.

STATIC LUNG VOLUMES

Static lung volumes and their spirometric measurement are discussed in Chapter 3. Normal values and interrelationships among volumes and capacities are illustrated in Figure 5-1. **Anthropometric** differences (differences in body type and size) affect normal values, creating ranges in which normal function is presumed. Normal ranges are derived from a statistical analysis of large populations of "normal" people (i.e., people who are healthy, have no history of lung disease, and have minimal exposure to risk factors such as smoking and environmental pollution). Physical characteristics that influence pulmonary function most are age, gender, height, ethnic origin, and body size or surface area.[1] Normal values are predicted for an individual based on these physical characteristics. Function is generally classified as normal if values are within 20% of the predicted value (i.e., 80% to 120% of the predicted value). Table 5-1 displays the relationship between the percentage of the predicted normal value and the degree of functional impairment.

Theoretical Basis for Measurement

Because residual volume (RV) cannot be exhaled, it cannot be measured via direct spirometry. Therefore, no capacity containing RV can be directly measured. RV and capacities containing it are measured indirectly via one of the following methods: helium dilution, nitrogen washout, or body plethysmography. The dilution and washout techniques measure gas in the lung only if the gas communicates with unobstructed airways. These tests are started at the end of a normal expiration (i.e., the functional residual capacity [FRC] level). Washout and dilution tests measure the FRC, which is the logical starting point because it is highly reproducible and its achievement requires no patient effort—only ventilatory muscle relaxation. As shown in

Figure 5-1, after FRC is determined, spirometric measurement of the expiratory reserve volume (ERV) allows the RV to be calculated (RV = FRC − ERV). Likewise, spirometric measurement of inspiratory capacity (IC) allows total lung capacity (TLC) to be calculated (FRC + IC = TLC). Alternatively, if RV is measured, TLC can be calculated as follows: RV + vital capacity (VC) = TLC.

Helium Dilution Method

The helium dilution method requires the person to rebreathe a helium gas mixture through a closed circuit from a spirometer of known volume (Figure 5-2). Helium is a foreign gas to the lung and is inert and insoluble in the blood. Therefore, the blood does not absorb helium during the test. The lung contains no helium initially (Figure 5-2, *A*), but rebreathing causes lung and spirometric gases to mix (Figure 5-2, *B*). A helium analyzer in the circuit continuously monitors helium concentration. As rebreathing progresses, lung gases dilute the helium in the spirometer. Consequently, helium concentration decreases in the spirometer and increases in the lung until equilibrium is reached (Figure 5-2, *C*). During the rebreathing process, the spirometric volume is kept constant through the addition of oxygen to the circuit to replace oxygen taken up by the blood. Likewise, a chemical in the circuit absorbs carbon dioxide entering the lung from the blood.

The principle of the closed-circuit helium dilution method is that the amount of helium in the lung spirometric system is the same at the end of the test as at the beginning. For example, after it is charged with helium, the spirometer's volume may be 3000 mL and the helium concentration 10% (see Figure 5-2, *A*). In this example, the amount of helium present at the beginning of the test is 10% of 3000, or 300 mL ($0.10 \times 3000 = 300$ mL). Because the lung contains no helium initially, 300 mL of helium must be present in the lung spirometer system at the end of the test after helium equilibrium is achieved. Consider an example in which the helium concentration at equilibrium is 5% (see Figure 5-2, *C*). The lung volume diluting the spirometer's helium mixture is the FRC if the first inspiration of the helium mixture started from the resting FRC level. In principle, the FRC is calculated as follows:[2]

1.   **Initial helium volume = final helium volume :**
   $$(F_{in}He)(FRC) + (F_{in}He)(V_s) = (F_{fin}He)(FRC + V_s)$$

In this equation, $F_{in}He$ and $F_{fin}He$ represent the initial and final helium fractional concentrations, and V_s represents the spirometric volume.

With the values from the previous example, the following can be calculated:

2. $$0 + (0.10) \times (3000) = (0.05) \times (FRC + 3000)$$
3. $$300 = 0.05(FRC) + 0.05(3000)$$
4. $$300 = 0.05(FRC) + 150$$
5. $$150 = 0.05(FRC)$$
6. $$3000 \text{ mL} = FRC$$

This gas volume is measured under **ambient temperature, pressure, and saturated (ATPS) conditions**. Therefore, this gas volume must be converted to the volume it occupied in the lung under **body temperature, pressure, and saturated (BTPS) conditions**. (Factors for converting ATPS volumes to BTPS volumes are available in pulmonary function procedure manuals.) Modern pulmonary function machines automatically correct

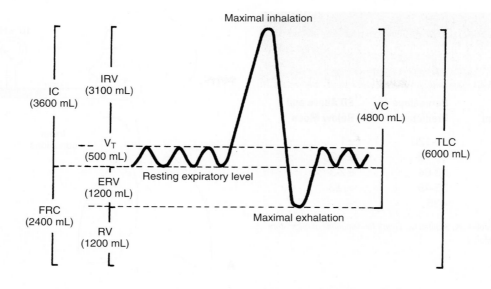

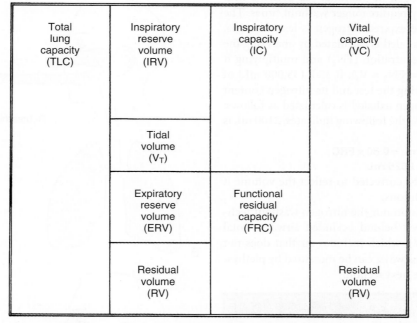

Figure 5-1 Average lung volumes and capacities in a man. (From Wilkins RL, Stoller JK, Scanlan CL: *Egan's fundamentals of respiratory care,* ed 6, St Louis, 2003, Mosby.)

measured volumes to BTPS values. If the person exhales to RV at the end of the test, the RV can be calculated by subtracting ERV from FRC.

CONCEPT QUESTION 5-1

Does a low final helium concentration in the helium dilution test mean the patient's FRC is small or large?

Nitrogen Washout Method

The nitrogen washout method requires the person to breathe a nitrogen-free gas (100% oxygen) until the nitrogen in the lung is "washed" out. The lung volume is unknown at the beginning of the test, but the nitrogen concentration in the lung is about 80% if room air is breathed. If the volume of nitrogen in the lung can be measured (in milliliters), the lung volume can be calculated as follows:

Nitrogen(mL) = 0.80(lung volume)

Nitrogen(mL)/0.80 = lung volume

In the open-circuit nitrogen washout procedure (Figure 5-3), the person breathes through a one-way valve, inspiring 100% oxygen and expiring into a large gas-collecting spirometer previously flushed with 100% oxygen. Each inspiration is nitrogen-free, and each expiration eliminates some of the nitrogen in the lung. Normally, less than 7 minutes is required to

TABLE 5-1

Severity of Pulmonary Impairments Based on the Percentage of the Predicted Normal Value or Standard Deviations of the Mean Predicted Normal Value

Degree of Impairment	Percentage of Predicted	SD Above and Below Mean
Normal	80-120	±1
Mild	65-79	±1-2
Moderate	50-64	±2-3
Severe	35-49	> ±3
Extremely severe	<35	—

Modified from Wilkins RL, Stoller JK, Scanlan CL: *Egan's fundamentals of respiratory care*, ed 8, St Louis, 2003, Mosby.
SD, Standard deviation.

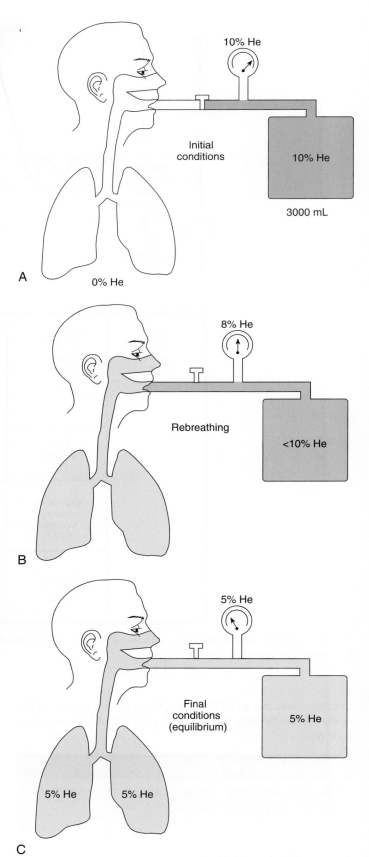

eliminate most of the nitrogen in the lung, but patients with poorly ventilated areas may require longer washout times. The test usually ends when the expired nitrogen is less than 2%. The amount of nitrogen exhaled is calculated by analyzing the spirometer's nitrogen concentration (FN_2) and multiplying it by the V_s (Nitrogen [mL] = $FN_2 \times V_s$). If 35 L (35,000 mL) of expired gas is collected during the test and its nitrogen content is 6%, the amount of nitrogen exhaled is calculated as follows: $35,000 \times 0.06 = 2100$ mL. As the following indicates, 2100 mL is 80% of the lung volume:

$$2100 \text{ mL} = 0.80 \times \text{FRC}$$
$$\text{FRC} = 2625 \text{ mL}$$

The measured FRC must be corrected to reflect the volume it occupies under BTPS conditions.

Neither the helium dilution nor the nitrogen washout techniques measure gas trapped behind occluded airways. Total thoracic gas volume (TGV), which includes air that does not communicate with patent airways, can be measured by plethysmography, described in the next section.

CONCEPT QUESTION 5-2

Does an unusually low spirometer concentration of nitrogen at the end of a nitrogen washout test mean the patient's FRC is small or large?

Body Plethysmographic Method

The plethysmographic method is based on Boyle's law. This law states that when gas volume and pressure changes occur, the initial volume (V_1) multiplied by the initial pressure (P_1) equals the final volume (V_2) multiplied by the final pressure (P_2): $P_1V_1 = P_2V_2$.

The body plethysmograph is an airtight chamber, or "body box," in which the patient sits while breathing through a mouthpiece (Figure 5-4). Sensitive pressure transducers measure mouthpiece and box pressures. Box calibration is carried out with an empty, sealed box; a known volume of gas is injected into the box with a large calibration syringe, and

Figure 5-2 A-C, Helium dilution measurement of functional residual capacity.

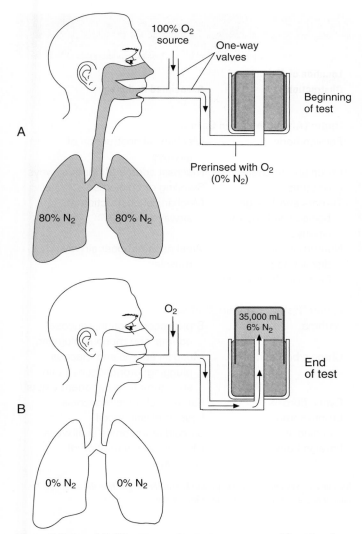

Figure 5-3 **A** and **B,** Nitrogen washout measurement of functional residual capacity.

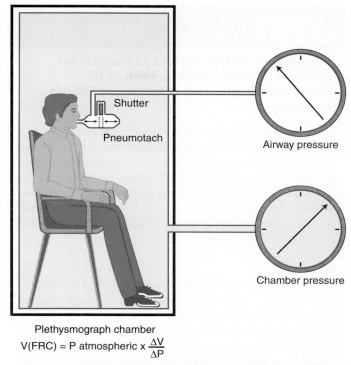

Plethysmograph chamber

$$V(FRC) = P \text{ atmospheric} \times \frac{\Delta V}{\Delta P}$$

Figure 5-4 Body plethysmographic method for measuring functional residual capacity. (From Wilkins RL, Stoller JK, Scanlan CL: *Egan's fundamentals of respiratory care,* ed 8, St Louis, 2003, Mosby.)

the change in box pressure is noted. This calibration procedure allows subsequent box pressure changes to be converted to volume changes.

At the end of expiration when gas flow ceases, mouthpiece pressure equals alveolar pressure. The lung volume at this point (the FRC) is unknown. An electrically controlled shutter occludes the mouthpiece precisely at the end expiratory point. The subsequent inspiratory effort cannot move gas. However, the respiratory muscles enlarge the thorax, decompressing the gas in the lung, decreasing its pressure (see Figure 5-4). In the absence of gas flow, intrapulmonary pressure equals mouthpiece pressure. At the same time, the enlarging thorax compresses air inside the box around the patient, increasing the box pressure. The change in box pressure is converted to the change in volume from the initial calibration procedure. The variables in Boyle's law are assigned as follows: P_1 equals initial mouth pressure (atmospheric pressure), V_1 equals FRC (unknown), P_2 equals final mouth pressure (measured during inspiratory effort through the occluded mouthpiece), and V_2 equals FRC

plus the change in lung volume (ΔV). The ΔV is known. In principle, the FRC is calculated as follows:

$$(P_1)(FRC) = (P_2)(FRC + \Delta V)$$
$$(P_1)(FRC) = (P_2)(FRC) + (P_2)(\Delta V)$$
$$(P_1)(FRC) - (P_2)(FRC) = (P_2)(\Delta V)$$
$$FRC(P_1 - P_2) = (P_2)(\Delta V)$$
$$FRC = \frac{(P_2)(\Delta V)}{(P_1 - P_2)}$$

The plethysmographic method is quite rapid; successive FRC measurements can be made as the patient pants against the occluded mouthpiece. This technique measures both the ventilated and the nonventilated air space in the thorax.

Significance of Changes in Functional Residual Capacity and Residual Volume

Physical factors that change FRC and RV are summarized in Box 5-1. Changes in lung recoil affect FRC because FRC is determined by the balance point between lung and thoracic recoil forces. An abnormally increased FRC represents hyperinflation, which may be caused by a loss of elastic recoil or partial airway obstruction. Partial airway obstruction caused by bronchospasm is generally reversed by bronchodilator drugs, and the associated increase in FRC is reversible. Increased FRC caused by a permanent loss of elastic recoil is irreversible. In severe emphysema, this loss of lung elasticity is associated with passive airway compression and collapse during expiration, causing air trapping. Bronchodilator drugs are not useful in these circumstances. (See the discussion on air trapping and auto-PEEP in Chapter 3).

CLINICAL FOCUS 5-1

Significance of Differences in Functional Residual Capacity as Determined by Plethysmography and Washout or Dilution Methods

You are asked to complete a pulmonary function study on a 68-year-old man with a suspected diagnosis of emphysema. The physician requests that both the helium dilution method and body plethysmography be performed to measure FRC.

On completing these tests, you find that the FRC obtained via body plethysmography is greater than the FRC obtained via helium dilution. What is the probable explanation for the difference in obtained FRC values?

Discussion

FRC must be measured indirectly because RV, a component of FRC, is the volume of air remaining in the lungs after the most forceful exhalation and cannot be exhaled. The helium dilution test can measure only gas that is in communication with unobstructed airways. Body plethysmography measures all gas in the chest, including gas trapped behind obstructed airways. If body plethysmography yields higher FRC values than helium dilution measurements, air trapping must be present. Air trapping is consistent with diseases such as emphysema, in which a loss of elastic lung recoil results in a loss of tethering forces that hold airways open during forceful exhalations. As a result, small noncartilaginous airways collapse prematurely, trapping air. In this patient, test results are consistent with the presence of emphysema.

TABLE 5-2

Conditions Associated with Obstruction to Airflow

Location of Airway Obstruction	Associated Pathology
Upper (Above the Main Carina)	
Foreign body	Mechanical obstruction of airways
Croup and tracheitis	Mucosal edema of upper airways
Epiglottitis	Swelling of epiglottis
Tumors and foreign bodies involving the airways	Mechanical obstruction of airways
Neuromuscular disease (e.g., Parkinson's disease)	Weakness of upper airways muscles
Lower (Below the Main Carina)	
Asthma	Bronchoconstriction, mucosal edema, and mucous plugging
Chronic bronchitis	Mucosal edema and mucous plugging; bronchoconstriction if an asthmatic component exists
Cystic fibrosis	Same as chronic bronchitis
Emphysema	Loss of elastic recoil
Sarcoidosis	Sarcoid granulomas in airways
Foreign body	Mechanical obstruction of airways

Modified from Martin L: *Pulmonary physiology in clinical practice: the essentials for patient care and evaluation*, St Louis, 1987, Mosby.

FRC and RV usually increase together, reducing the IC and VC. Regardless of the mechanism by which FRC is increased, hyperinflation flattens the diaphragm, placing it at a mechanical disadvantage. Shortened muscle fibers in flattened diaphragms have decreased contractility. In addition, flattened diaphragms cannot move downward much farther; thus, greater effort is required to inspire the tidal volume, often requiring the use of accessory muscles. Diseases increasing FRC and RV are generally classified as obstructive. An exception is neuromuscular disease in which FRC is normal but RV is increased because of weak expiratory muscles. A weak, forced exhalation reduces the ERV, increasing the RV. Table 5-2 summarizes some conditions associated with airway obstruction.

Pulmonary or extrapulmonary factors may decrease RV and FRC (Box 5-1). Fibrotic lung diseases increase lung elastic recoil, shrinking all volumes and capacities. Increased alveolar-capillary membrane permeability, characteristic of acute respiratory distress syndrome (ARDS), disrupts surfactant synthesis and increases alveolar surface tension; this decreases FRC and RV by causing widespread alveolar collapse. Extrapulmonary restriction of lung expansion by skeletal deformities also reduces all lung volumes and capacities. Regardless of the mechanisms involved, reduced FRC and high lung recoil increase the work

BOX 5-1

Factors Affecting Residual Volume and Functional Residual Capacity

Increased RV and FRC
Reduced lung recoil
  Emphysema
  Aging
Partial airway obstruction
  Active airway narrowing (e.g., asthmatic bronchospasm)
  Passive airway compression (e.g., emphysema)

Decreased RV and FRC
Increased lung recoil
  Fibrotic lung diseases (e.g., pneumoconioses)
  Surfactant abnormalities (e.g., ARDS)
Thoracic cage deformity
  Kyphoscoliosis

RV, Residual volume; *FRC*, functional residual capacity; *ARDS*, acute respiratory distress syndrome.

TABLE 5-3

Respiratory Conditions Commonly Associated with a Restrictive Breathing Pattern

Involving the Chest Bellows	Involving the Lungs
Myasthenia gravis	Atelectasis
Guillain-Barré syndrome	Pulmonary sarcoidosis
Pleural effusion and pleural disease	Pulmonary fibrosis
Flail chest (multiple broken ribs)	Pulmonary edema
Morbid obesity	Pneumonia
Diaphragm paralysis	Congestive heart failure

Modified from Martin L: *Pulmonary physiology in clinical practice: the essentials for patient care and evaluation,* St Louis, 1987, Mosby.

TABLE 5-4

Characteristics of Obstructive and Restrictive Diseases

Characteristic	Obstructive	Restrictive
Main pulmonary function characteristic	Decreased expiratory flow	Decreased volumes and capacities
Mechanism increasing work of breathing	High airway resistance	Low lung compliance

of breathing. Diseases decreasing FRC and RV are generally classified as restrictive. Table 5-3 summarizes some conditions associated with restrictive diseases.

In obstructive disease, the TLC is often normal, or it may be moderately increased in severe emphysema secondary to loss of lung recoil force. However, the major feature of obstructive disease is a reduced maximum expiratory flow rate. Obstructive diseases increase the work of breathing primarily by increasing airway resistance. In contrast, the major features of restrictive disease are reduced lung volumes and capacities. This reduction is usually accompanied by normal expiratory flow rates. Restrictive diseases generally increase the work of breathing by decreasing lung compliance, making expansion difficult. Table 5-4 summarizes the differences between obstructive and restrictive disease.

Neuromuscular diseases are unique in that they are classified as restrictive, although lung and thoracic compliance may be normal. However, they manifest as restrictive pulmonary function patterns because muscle weakness limits inspiratory and expiratory volumes.

Figure 5-5 illustrates lung volumes and capacities in normal, obstructive, and restrictive lung diseases. The normal **RV/TLC ratio** is 20% to 25% in healthy adults up to age 49 years; in people older than 50, the RV/TLC ratio may range as high as 35%, reflecting a normal loss of elastic recoil with aging. Abnormally increased RV/TLC ratios generally indicate hyperinflation, although RV/TLC may be increased in some restrictive diseases in which the VC (and the TLC) is reduced more than the RV.[1]

CONCEPT QUESTION 5-3

If the TLC stays constant, which lung volume or capacity is directly affected by an increase in the RV/TLC ratio?

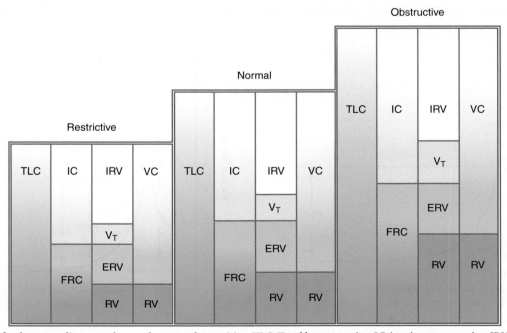

Figure 5-5 Effects of pulmonary disease on lung volumes and capacities. *TLC,* Total lung capacity; *IC,* inspiratory capacity; *IRV,* inspiratory reserve volume; *VC,* vital capacity; *V_T,* tidal volume; *FRC,* functional residual capacity; *ERV,* expiratory reserve volume; *RV,* residual volume. (From Wilkins RL, Stoller JK, Scanlan CL: *Egan's fundamentals of respiratory care,* ed 8, St Louis, 2003, Mosby.)

DYNAMIC PULMONARY MECHANICS MEASUREMENTS

Dynamic measurements reflect the ability of the lungs to move air rapidly, facilitating the detection of airway obstruction and increased airway resistance. Measuring dynamic pulmonary mechanics mainly involves measuring expiratory flows with respect to time or volume. The ability to generate high flow rates depends on muscular strength, airway patency, and neurological function. Flows are generally measured via spirometry. Modern spirometers use a compact flow-sensing device called a **pneumotachometer**. The signal from a pneumotachometer can be integrated to allow volume measurement.

Volume-Time Measurements

Forced Vital Capacity

The forced vital capacity (FVC) measurement requires the person to exhale the VC as forcefully and rapidly as possible. FVC is the most frequently performed pulmonary function test because it provides much information about large and small airways function. It is an effort-dependent test, requiring thorough patient instruction, understanding, and maximal effort. A valid test is assumed if the person can repeat three FVC maneuvers with a variation no greater than 5%.[1] FVC displayed as volume versus time is illustrated in Figure 5-6, with upward deflections denoting inspiration.

FVC and slow VC (VC performed without comparison with time) are nearly equal in individuals with normal airway resistance. Severe airway obstruction, regardless of the mechanism, often produces a smaller FVC than slow VC because of air trapping. High expiratory flows exaggerate the effect of airway resistance and may produce premature bronchiolar collapse in obstructive airways disease; exhalation of full VC is prevented, enlarging the FRC. Some people with airway obstruction may have a normal FVC, but the time required to exhale it is longer than normal. People with normal pulmonary function can exhale 100% of the FVC in 4 to 6 seconds. People who have severe airway obstruction may require more than 10 seconds.

Decreased FVC values are characteristic of restrictive diseases. Fibrotic lung tissue or thoracic cage deformities may restrict lung expansion and reduce the exhaled vital capacity. Neuromuscular disorders, severe obesity, and pregnancy also limit lung expansion. These conditions impair diaphragmatic movement, reducing FVC. The time required to exhale FVC in purely restrictive disease is normal or even less than normal because of high elastic lung recoil.

CONCEPT QUESTION 5-4

Explain the way air trapping produces both of the following abnormal test results: (1) TGV, as obtained by plethysmography is different from TLC determined by nitrogen washout; and (2) FVC is different from slow VC.

Forced Expiratory Volumes

Measuring the amount of FVC that can be exhaled within a given time interval provides additional information about airway obstruction. The time intervals often measured are 1.0 second, 2.0 seconds, and 3.0 seconds (Figure 5-7). The most commonly assessed forced expiratory volume (FEV) interval is FEV_1, the amount of FVC exhaled in 1 second. Because FEV values refer to volume measured over time, they reflect the average flow rates over their time intervals.

Patients with obstructive disease have high airway resistance and cannot exhale much of the FVC in a given time period;

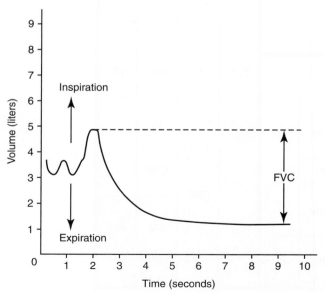

Figure 5-6 Spirographic tracing of forced vital capacity (*FVC*). (Modified from Ruppel G: *Manual of pulmonary function testing,* ed 9, St Louis, 2009, Mosby.)

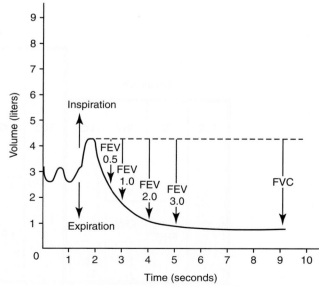

Figure 5-7 Measurement of forced expiratory volume (*FEV*) values from the forced vital capacity (*FVC*) curve. (Modified from Ruppel G: *Manual of pulmonary function testing,* ed 9, St Louis, 2009, Mosby.)

they have a reduced FEV_1. Patients with restrictive disease or neuromuscular disorders also have low FEV_1 values, but this is mainly because they have low FVC. FEV_1 expressed as a fraction of FVC—the **FEV_1/FVC ratio**—is very important in differentiating obstructive and restrictive causes of low FEV_1. The FEV_1/FVC ratio is generally expressed as a percentage (i.e., FEV_1/FVC × 100); this is not to be confused with the term FEV_1% predicted, which expresses the measured FEV_1 as a percentage of the value predicted for a given individual. A low FEV_1 and FEV_1/FVC ratio are characteristic of obstructive impairments. Restrictive impairments also have a low FEV_1 but a normal or high FEV_1/FVC ratio. Assuming good patient cooperation and maximal effort, a low FEV_1/FVC ratio indicates an obstructive (high airway resistance) abnormality.

CONCEPT QUESTION 5-5

In purely restrictive lung disease, FEV_1 is abnormally small, but the FEV_1/FVC ratio is usually normal; explain why this would be true.

FEV_1 is an index of severity in chronic obstructive pulmonary disease (COPD). The ability to work and likelihood of dying of respiratory disease are statistically correlated with the FEV_1. Healthy adults with normal pulmonary function exhale about 83% of the FVC in 1 second (FEV_1), 94% in 2 seconds (FEV_2), and 97% in 3 seconds (FEV_3). Age causes the FEV_1/FVC ratio to decrease because of reduced elastic recoil. An FEV_1/FVC ratio lower than 70% indicates that abnormal airways obstruction is present.[1]

The FVC, FEV_1, and FEV_1/FVC ratio are the three most common variables used to distinguish between obstructive and restrictive pulmonary function patterns. Table 5-5 illustrates various pulmonary function measurements in obstructive and restrictive diseases.

Forced Expired Flows: FEF$_{25\%-75\%}$ and Peak Expiratory Flow

Forced expired flow (FEF) rates are derived from the volume-versus-time FVC curve. $FEF_{25\%-75\%}$ is the average flow rate over the middle 50% of the FVC (Figure 5-8). A volume-time graph is necessary to calculate $FEF_{25\%-75\%}$ manually. The points at which 25% and 75% of the FVC have been exhaled are identified by multiplying the FVC by 0.25 and 0.75. A straight line drawn through these two points on the FVC curve is extended to intersect two vertical time lines on the graph 1 second apart. The volume between the two intersection points on the time lines is the $FEF_{25\%-75\%}$ in liters per second. As with all pulmonary function measurements, the volume must be corrected to BTPS.

The **peak expiratory flow (PEF)**, often simply called peak flow (PF) by clinicians, is the highest instantaneous flow achieved during an FVC maneuver. PEF is difficult to obtain from a volume-time graph and is usually measured via flow-sensing devices called peak flowmeters. The PEF can be precisely identified on a flow-volume graph.

PEF reflects initial expiratory flow coming from the large airways at the beginning of the FVC maneuver; because the main resistors of expiratory airflow at the beginning of the FVC are the large airways, PEF reflects function of the large airways. The PEF is an effort-dependent test; the greater the effort, the higher the test value. PEF in adults with normal pulmonary function may exceed 10 L per second. Reproducibility of PEF is a good indication of maximal patient effort. PEF is useful in assessing gross changes in airway function and evaluating the response to bronchodilator drugs. This test is very useful in managing asthma in outpatient and home settings. In asthma management

TABLE 5-5

Spirometric and Physiological Correlates of Restrictive and Obstructive Lung Disease

Clinical Example	Spirometric Measurements	Nonspirometric Lung Volumes	Lung Compliance	Airway Resistance
Restrictive				
Pulmonary fibrosis	Decreased FVC	Decreased TLC	Decreased	Decreased
	Decreased FEV_1	Decreased FRC		
	Increased FEV_1/FVC	Decreased RV		
Neuromuscular disease	Decreased FVC	Decreased TLC	Normal	Normal
	Decreased FEV_1	Normal FRC		
	Normal FEV_1/FVC	Increased RV		
Obstructive				
Asthma	Decreased FVC	Increased TLC	Normal	Increased
	Decreased FEV_1	Increased FRC		
	Decreased FEV_1/FVC			
Emphysema	Same as for asthma	Same as for asthma	Increased	Increased

Modified from Martin L: *Pulmonary physiology in clinical practice: the essentials for patient care and evaluation,* St Louis, 1987, Mosby.
FVC, Forced vital capacity; *FEV_1,* amount of FVC exhaled in 1 second; *FEV_1/FVC,* FEV compared with FVC; *TLC,* total lung capacity; *FRC,* functional residual capacity; *RV,* residual volume.

CLINICAL FOCUS 5-2

Differentiating Obstructive and Restrictive Disease Patterns

You are called to the emergency department to perform a pulmonary function test on a 52-year-old woman. She states that she had the flu approximately 2 weeks earlier and that her breathing has become more difficult since then. In addition, she has smoked two packs of cigarettes a day since age 12, and a diagnosis of pulmonary emphysema was made 7 years ago. The results of the pulmonary function test follow:

	Predicted	Actual	Percent of Predicted
FVC (L)	4.67	4.00	86
FEV_1 (L)	3.52	1.23	35
FEV_1/FVC ratio (%)	>75	31	—

Are these pulmonary function findings consistent with an obstructive or restrictive pattern? (A value ≥80% of the predicted value is considered normal.)

Discussion

Diagnoses of obstructive and restrictive patterns are traditionally based on three main variables: FVC, FEV_1, and FEV_1/FVC ratio. This woman's test shows that the FVC is normal (>80% of percent predicted), but the FEV_1 and FEV_1/FVC ratio are decreased. The normal FVC value rules out restrictive disease. These findings are consistent with an obstructive impairment because they point to expiratory airflow limitation. A person with normal pulmonary function is expected to exhale about 80% of the FVC in the first second. This woman's reduced flows are probably caused by loss of elastic support in the airways, producing premature bronchiolar collapse during forced expiration. As the obstructive disease becomes more severe, the FVC also may decrease because air trapping limits her ability to exhale as much air as normal.

What is the clinical significance of these findings? A trial of bronchodilator drugs may be administered, and follow-up pulmonary function testing may be scheduled. In this way, you can discover whether airway obstruction is reversible (i.e., whether bronchospasm contributes to airflow obstruction and whether it can be reversed by bronchodilator drugs).

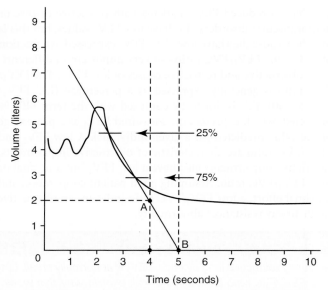

Figure 5-8 $FEF_{25\%-75\%}$ measured from the forced vital capacity curve. The vertical distance between *A* and *B* represents the average flow rate in liters per second expired during the middle 50% of the forced vital capacity maneuver. (Modified from the Ruppel G: *Manual of pulmonary function testing,* ed 9, St Louis, 2009, Mosby.)

rapidly narrowing small airways as the lung deflates. Normal $FEF_{25\%-75\%}$ for a healthy young adult is about 4 to 5 L per second. This test has more variance than other measures of flow, even in people with normal pulmonary function. $FEF_{25\%-75\%}$ equal to 65% of the predicted value may still be within statistically normal limits.[1] Because $FEF_{25\%-75\%}$ is so variable, its validity is questionable; FEV_1 is more useful and reliable in assessing the response to bronchodilators.

CONCEPT QUESTION 5-6

In which of the following tests does increased effort most likely improve measured values: PEF or $FEF_{25\%-75\%}$? Explain.

$FEF_{25\%-75\%}$ and PEF have no value in differentiating between obstructive and restrictive patterns. These flows should be considered only after the severity of obstruction has been determined from the FVC, FEV_1, and FEV_1/FVC ratio. $FEF_{25\%-75\%}$ might be valuable in further confirming or ruling out obstructive defects in asymptomatic people with a borderline low FEV_1/FVC ratio. Figure 5-9 illustrates obstructive, restrictive, and normal spirograms, including $FEF_{25\%-75\%}$, FEV_1, and FVC.

Flow-Volume Measurements

Spirometric measurements are often assessed from the perspective of flow versus volume. Figure 5-10 illustrates the FVC flow-volume curve (F-V curve). Flow is plotted vertically on the *y*-axis in liters per second; volume is plotted horizontally on the *x*-axis in liters. The expiratory (above baseline) and inspiratory (below baseline) portions of the flow-volume graph form a loop—hence the term **flow-volume loop** (**F-V loop**). The F-V

programs, respiratory therapists teach patients how to use small, inexpensive peak flowmeters to detect early onset of an asthma exacerbation before it becomes life threatening and how to use the device to assess response to bronchodilator drugs. Peak flows obtained in these settings should be periodically compared with more accurate laboratory spirometry.

PEF is not sensitive to flow coming from small airways. In early small airway obstruction, flows achieved at the beginning of the FVC are often normal because small airway collapse has not yet occurred. $FEF_{25\%-75\%}$ is more sensitive to flow coming from medium to small airways. The primary resistance to expiratory flow during the middle half of the FVC is created by the

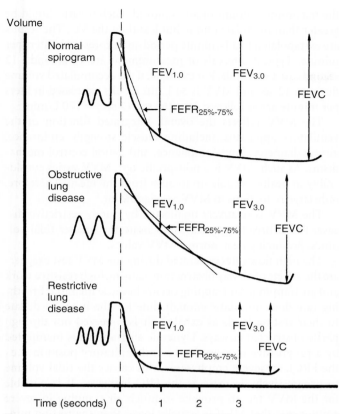

Figure 5-9 Forced vital capacity curves (*FVC*) produced by normal and diseased lungs. Reduced flow in obstructive disease and reduced volumes in restrictive disease can be noted. *FEFR$_{25\%-75\%}$*, Forced expiratory flow rate between 25% to 75% of forced vital capacity. (From Slonim NB, Hamilton LH: *Respiratory physiology*, ed 5, St Louis, 1987, Mosby.)

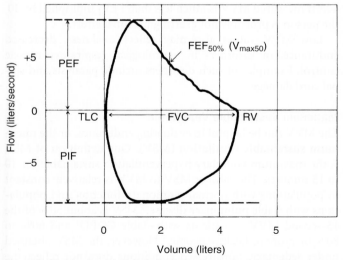

Figure 5-10 The forced (exhaled) vital capacity and forced inspiratory vital capacity displayed as a flow-volume loop. Expiration is recorded above and inspiration is recorded below the 0 L per second baseline. Instantaneous flow at any point in the forced vital capacity (*FVC*) can be observed directly. *PEF*, Peak expiratory flow; *FEF$_{50\%}$*, forced expiratory flow at 50% of forced vital capacity; *TLC*, total lung capacity; *RV*, residual volume; *PIF*, peak inspiratory flow. (From Ruppel G: *Manual of pulmonary function testing*, ed 9, St Louis, 2009, Mosby.)

loop is most commonly formed by having the person complete an FVC maneuver and then inspire forcefully back to TLC. The inspiratory maneuver is called the **forced inspiratory volume (FIV)**.

As the FVC is exhaled, the instantaneous flow at any lung volume from TLC to RV can be directly observed. For example, the maximum expiratory flow that can be generated when the lung is deflating through the 50% point of the FVC ($\dot{V}_{max50}$) can be determined directly from the graph in Figure 5-10. Likewise, PEF and **peak inspiratory flow (PIF)** are simply the highest and lowest deflections of the F-V loop. The F-V loop is actually a continuous plot of all the maximum flows achievable at an infinite number of lung volumes ranging from TLC to RV.

FEF$_{25\%-75\%}$ cannot be determined from the F-V loop. However, the display of maximum flow ($\dot{V}_{max}$) at any point during the FVC provides even more useful information. The $\dot{V}_{max}$ at a given point also may be reported as FEF, subscripted to denote the percentage of the FVC exhaled. The most frequently reported maximum flows are **FEF$_{25\%}$**, FEF$_{50\%}$, and **FEF$_{75\%}$**.

Automatic timing marks are usually superimposed on the F-V loop at 0.5 second, 1.0 second, 2.0 seconds, and 3.0 seconds, allowing these FEV values to be determined. From the F-V loop, the FVC, FEV$_1$, FEV$_1$/FVC ratio, PEF, and FEF or $\dot{V}_{max}$ can be determined at any point in the FVC. The F-V curve has advantages over the volume-time curve in that decreased flow (indicating obstruction) or volume (indicting restriction) is immediately apparent from a single curve.

Figure 5-11, *A*, compares normal (*black line*), restrictive (*red line*), and obstructive (*blue line*) F-V curves adjusted such that points of maximum inspiration coincide. This comparison does not consider the actual amount of gas in the lungs at the maximum inspiratory point. In addressing this problem, Figure 5-11, *B*, plots the same three curves with respect to the total amount of gas in the lungs at maximum inspiration (i.e., TGV). Clearly, the maximum inspiratory points are associated with different TGVs. The increases in TLC and RV are obvious in the obstructive curve (*blue line*), as are the severely reduced flows early in the FVC. Although high lung volume (normally associated with high lung recoil force) should increase expiratory flow, it is still abnormally low throughout the FVC in obstructive disease.

Severe reductions in TLC and RV are equally obvious in the restrictive curve (*red line*). Compared with the total lung volume at which they are measured, flows in the restrictive curve are above normal, even though absolute flows are reduced. For example, at a TGV of 3 L, flow is greater in the restrictive curve than the normal curve (see Figure 5-11, *B*). At the same time, flows are below normal throughout the FVC, as shown in Figure 5-11, *A* (*red curve*).

As explained in Chapter 3, the first 20% to 25% of an FVC maneuver is effort-dependent and the last 75% to 80% is effort-independent, which means that the slope of the last 80% of the F-V curve is independent of patient effort. For this reason, the expiratory F-V curve of the healthy lung descends in a linear fashion after peak flow is achieved (see Figure 5-10). PEF and FEF$_{25\%}$ occur early in the FVC, reflecting effort-dependent flow from large airways; large airways pose the major resistance to

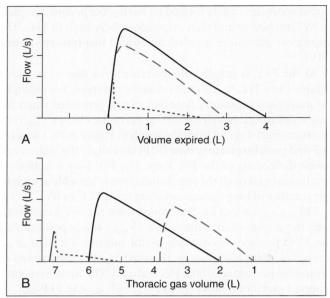

Figure 5-11 Flow rates recorded from the expiratory portion of the flow-volume loop in obstructive (*blue line*) and restrictive (*red line*) disease. **A,** Beginning points of exhaled flow-volume curves are aligned at total lung capacity. **B,** Beginning points of exhaled flow-volume curves are plotted at each patient's actual lung volume at total lung capacity. This offers more insight into the relationship between the lung volume and flow rate in disease. (Redrawn from Fishman AP: *Assessment of pulmonary function,* New York, 1980, McGraw-Hill.)

expiratory flow at high lung volumes. $FEF_{25\%-75\%}$, $FEF_{50\%}$, and $FEF_{75\%}$ occur later in the effort-independent portion of the FVC, reflecting flow from small airways; small airways pose the major resistance to expiratory flow at low lung volumes.

The decreased expiratory flow in obstructive disease is particularly evident at low lung volumes. $FEF_{50\%}$ and $FEF_{75\%}$ are most affected. When these flows are decreased, the expiratory F-V curve assumes a concave, or scooped-out, shape, as illustrated by the blue line in Figure 5-11, *A*. The sharp decrease in flow immediately after peak flow is achieved indicates severe small airway compression and collapse. The flows in restrictive disease are reduced compared with normal values because the lung volumes at which flows are measured are reduced, not because airway obstruction is present (see Figure 5-11, *A*, *red line*).

Maximum Voluntary Ventilation

The **maximum voluntary ventilation (MVV)** is the greatest amount of air a person can move in and out of the lungs with maximal effort over 10 to 15 seconds. The person is instructed to breathe as deeply and rapidly as possible in such a way that

the maximum amount of air is moved. Each breath should be greater than the tidal volume but less than the VC. The results are extrapolated to a 1-minute period and expressed in liters per minute. Typical intervals of measurement are 10 seconds, 12 seconds, or 15 seconds. For example, if the accumulated volume during a 12-second MVV is 34 L, the results expressed in liters per minute are as follows: $34 \times (60\ sec/12\ sec) = 170$ L/min.

The MVV reflects the overall integrated function of the ventilatory apparatus, including muscle strength, endurance, airway diameter, lung compliance, and neural control mechanisms. As such, MVV is a nonspecific test. MVV varies considerably in healthy people up to 30% from the mean. Therefore, only large reductions in MVV are significant.[1]

The MVV is relatively unaffected by purely restrictive disease. Faster breathing rates compensate for smaller tidal volumes, producing near-normal MVV values.

The high flow rates generated during the MVV test exaggerate the effects of airway obstruction, causing high resistive work and air trapping. Air trapping occurs because the rapid breathing rate does not allow enough time for the lungs to deflate to their resting levels as exhaled air is squeezed out through partly obstructed airways. Dynamic air trapping is manifested by a progressive increase in the end expiratory position (i.e., the FRC). In severe emphysema, this causes the tidal volume to progressively decrease as the FRC increases. It is possible for the MVV test to provoke so much air trapping in severe emphysema that MVV is actually lower than the resting minute ventilation. Even if MVV does not decrease below resting ventilation, shallow, rapid tidal volumes could possibly reduce alveolar ventilation while increasing anatomical dead space ventilation.

In COPD, the MVV is reduced proportionally with the FEV_1 and can be predicted by the following formula: $MVV = FEV_1 \times 40$.[2] If measured MVV is much less than FEV_1 multiplied by 40, the person is probably not exerting maximal effort.

Low MVV values also may reflect weakness, decreased endurance, or disorders in neurological respiratory muscle control. Examples of such disorders include paralysis and spinal cord damage.

Maximum Sustainable Ventilation

The MVV can be helpful in evaluating endurance, or the **maximum sustainable ventilation (MSV)**. One definition of MSV is the maximum voluntary hyperventilation sustainable for 10 to 15 minutes. The ratio of MSV to MVV is relatively constant in populations with normal pulmonary function and populations with stable pulmonary disease.[3] MSV is about 50% of the 15-second MVV in patients with stable COPD[4] and 60% to 80% or more in healthy people.[5] However, the MSV obtained under sedentary, nonstressed conditions does not reflect the true MSV in maximally exercising patients with severe COPD. The maximum ventilation attained during strenuous exercise in these patients can exceed 100% of the 15-second MVV[6]; this is probably because the MVV is so low in the first place. In contrast, the maximum ventilation that healthy individuals with normal pulmonary function can attain during strenuous exercise is only 55% to 65% of their MVVs.[7]

CLINICAL FOCUS 5-3

Classification of Chronic Obstructive Pulmonary Disease by Severity

COPD is the fourth leading cause of chronic illness and death in the United States and in the world; however, it is not immediately recognized by the general public and is not appropriately recognized as a major public health problem by government officials.[9] The National Heart, Lung, and Blood Institute in the United States and the World Health Organization joined resources to form the Global Initiative on Obstructive Lung Disease (GOLD); the goal was to increase awareness of COPD and to provide help for the thousands of patients with COPD throughout the world. A global workshop was held in which scientists and medical authorities around the world reviewed all that was known about COPD, its treatment, and its pathogenic mechanisms; the conference culminated in the development of a consensus document called the *Global Strategy for the Diagnosis, Management, and Prevention of Chronic Obstructive Pulmonary Disease*. One of the products of this document was a classification of COPD severity by pulmonary function test results and symptoms. The GOLD staging scheme, adopted by the American Thoracic Society, is helpful primarily as an educational tool for understanding COPD;

it is also helpful in identifying a general approach to managing COPD.[9]

GOLD Classification of COPD by Severity[9]

Stage	Characteristics
I—Mild COPD	$FEV_1/FVC < 70\%$ Sometimes but not always chronic cough and sputum production
II—Moderate COPD	$FEV_1/FVC < 70\%$ Patients with dyspnea on exertion (DOE) usually seek medical attention
III—Severe COPD	$FEV_1/FVC < 70\%$ $FEV_1 < 50\%$ but $> 30\%$ of predicted; greater DOE; repeated exacerbations; decreased quality of life
IV—Very severe COPD	$FEV_1/FVC < 70\%$ $FEV_1 < 30\%$ of predicted; life-threatening exacerbations; severe DOE

CONCEPT QUESTION 5-8

Consider the relationship between MVV and maximum exercise ventilation in people with normal pulmonary function and patients with severe COPD. What is the most likely factor that limits exercise intensity in each patient—the heart's pumping ability or the lung's ventilating capacity?

TESTS FOR SMALL AIRWAYS DISEASE

Inspiratory flow is directed into millions of small airways, greatly reducing flow velocity. (See the section in Chapter 3 on the distribution of airway resistance.) For this reason, small airways less than 2 mm in diameter account for less than 20% of total airway resistance—this means a significant amount of small airway obstruction may remain undetected by conventional spirometry. The earliest pathological changes of COPD occur in small airways. Detection of these early changes is important because they are generally reversible if appropriate therapeutic and preventive actions are taken. The more complex tests sensitive to small airway obstruction include the following: frequency dependence of compliance, closing volume, and low-density gas spirometry.

Frequency Dependence of Compliance

Frequency dependence of compliance is based on the principle that high breathing frequencies create high expiratory flows,

which exaggerate the resistive effect of small airway obstruction, decreasing dynamic compliance. In healthy people with normal pulmonary function, dynamic and static compliance are nearly equal, even at breathing frequencies of 60 breaths per minute. The dynamic compliance in people with abnormally high small airway resistance decreases as breathing frequency increases. A reduction in dynamic compliance as respiratory rates increase to 60 breaths per minute is a sensitive marker for abnormally high small airway resistance. Frequency dependence of compliance is usually expressed as the ratio of dynamic compliance to static compliance (C_{dyn}/C_{st}) for a given tidal volume at various breathing rates. In individuals with normal pulmonary function, C_{dyn}/C_{st} is greater than 0.8 in breathing rates up to 60 breaths per minute (Figure 5-12); in patients with small airway disease, this ratio is markedly decreased, even at lower breathing rates.[8]

Frequency dependence of compliance is an extremely sensitive test for early detection of abnormal small airways resistance and is the standard against which other tests are compared. However, frequency dependence of compliance tests are cumbersome and technically difficult to perform. The patient must have an esophageal balloon in place to measure pleural pressure. Simultaneous changes in tidal volume and pleural pressures are displayed on an oscilloscope at various breathing frequencies. The importance of the test is its sensitivity to early obstructive changes when routinely measured lung volumes and flow rates are still normal.

Closing Volume

The **closing volume test** is mentioned in Chapter 3 in the section on the distribution of inspired air. It is exactly the same test

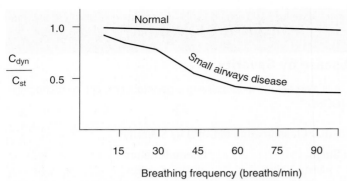

Figure 5-12 Frequency dependence of dynamic compliance. Normally, the relationship between dynamic and static compliance (C_{dyn}/C_{st}) remains constant as breathing frequency increases. In small airways obstructive disease, dynamic compliance decreases as breathing frequency increases; higher breathing rates create higher flow rates, exaggerating the effects of high airway resistance. (From Martin L: *Pulmonary physiology in clinical practice*, St Louis, 1987, Mosby.)

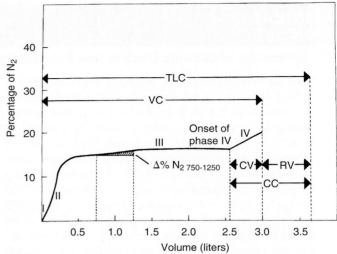

Figure 5-13 Single breath nitrogen elimination curve. First, a vital capacity of 100% oxygen is inspired; the graph shows nitrogen concentration plotted against exhaled volume during the subsequent exhaled vital capacity. (See the text for an explanation of phases I through IV and $\Delta\% N_{2\,750-1250}$.) *TLC*, Total lung capacity; *VC*, vital capacity; *CV*, closing volume; *CC*, closing capacity; *RV*, residual volume. (From Ruppel G: *Manual of pulmonary function testing*, ed 9, St Louis, 2009, Mosby.)

as the single breath nitrogen elimination test (the Fowler technique) for measuring anatomical dead space (see Chapter 4). This test is based on the principle that as a person inspires from RV to TLC, basal alveoli undergo greater volume changes than apical alveoli. In the closing volume test, a VC of 100% oxygen is inspired (i.e., from RV to TLC). When TLC is reached, basal nitrogen concentration is less than apical nitrogen concentration because basal units receive a greater share of the inspired 100% oxygen VC. Continuous nitrogen concentration analysis of the subsequent expiration from TLC to RV is the basis for the single breath nitrogen elimination or closing volume curve (Figure 5-13). The curve plots the percentage of nitrogen against the VC and is separated into four distinct phases: I, exhalation of nitrogen-free dead space gas; II, transition from dead space gas to alveolar gas; III, exhalation of alveolar gas; and IV, exhalation of only apical alveolar gas because of basal airway closure.

The alveolar phase is relatively flat (plateau phase) in healthy people because all alveoli empty synchronously. Even if some alveoli empty faster than others, they do so at a relatively constant ratio so that the nitrogen percentage of the exhaled alveolar gas mixture remains constant. To the extent that the emptying rates of different portions of the lung change, the slope of alveolar phase III increases. In other words, if emptying rates of basal alveoli steadily decrease while emptying rates of apical alveoli steadily increase, progressively greater portions of the exhaled gas stream become nitrogen because exhaled gas comes increasingly from the less diluted, nitrogen-rich apical alveoli. The increase in nitrogen percentage in the liter of gas expired after the first 750 mL has been exhaled ($\Delta\% N_{2\,750-1250}$) is a measure of nonuniform alveolar emptying; it is less than 1.5% in healthy adults.[1]

Phase IV is a dramatic illustration of nonuniform alveolar emptying. Basal alveoli abruptly cease to contribute to the expired gas stream as RV is neared because their airways suddenly close. (See the section on dynamic airway compression in Chapter 3.) The sharp increase in nitrogen percentage

is evidence that all gas now originates from apical alveoli. The onset of phase IV marks the point of basal small airways closure; the volume from this point to RV is the closing volume (see Figure 5-13). The volume of gas in the lung at the onset of phase IV is the **closing capacity**.

People with small airways obstruction experience basal airway closure earlier in the exhaled VC, which increases the closing volume. The closing volume in healthy adults is about 10% to 20% of the VC, increasing with age. This test is sensitive to small airways disease, especially in smokers with otherwise normal spirometry.[1] The closing volume cannot be determined in people who have severe obstructive disease and nonuniform distribution of ventilation. The gross variation in alveolar emptying rates creates such a steep phase III slope that it is indistinguishable from phase IV.

Low-Density Gas Spirometry (Helium-Oxygen Flow-Volume Curve)

Low-density gas spirometry involves comparing FVC flow-volume curves produced while the patient breathes room air with curves produced while breathing a mixture of 80% helium and 20% oxygen. The two curves are superimposed, as shown in Figure 5-14. The test is based on the principle that breathing a low-density gas mixture improves the flow rate for a given effort when the flow pattern is turbulent. This improvement does not occur when the flow pattern is laminar. The high flow early in the FVC is turbulent, and breathing helium and oxygen increases the flow rate for a given effort compared with air breathing (see Figure 5-14). Small airway compression greatly decreases expiratory flow velocity during the latter portion of

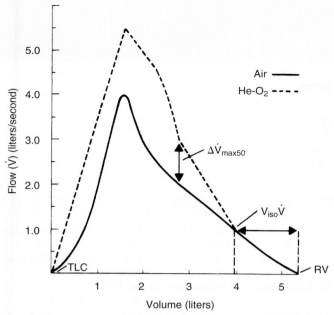

Figure 5-14 Superimposed expiratory flow-volume curves performed with air and a helium-oxygen mixture (*He-O₂*). The He-O₂ mixture offers a flow advantage throughout the forced vital capacity only when the flow pattern is turbulent. Convergence of the curves marks the point at which the expiratory flow pattern becomes laminar ($V_{iso}\dot{V}$) owing to small airways compression and low flow rates. *TLC,* Total lung capacity; *RV,* residual volume. (From Ruppel G: *Manual of pulmonary function testing,* ed 9, St Louis, 2009, Mosby.)

the FVC, creating a laminar flow pattern. Because laminar flow is density independent, the helium-oxygen mixture offers no flow advantage over air breathing. The convergence of air and helium-oxygen curves marks the point at which flow changes from a turbulent to laminar pattern (see Figure 5-14). This point coincides with dynamic airway compression in small, noncartilaginous bronchioles.

To perform the test, an F-V curve is first produced with room air (see Figure 5-14, *solid line*). Then a mixture of 80% helium and 20% oxygen is breathed over several minutes, after which a second F-V curve is produced (*dotted line*) and superimposed on the first. The **volume of isoflow ($V_{iso}\dot{V}$)** is the volume between the curves' convergence point and the RV. In adults with normal pulmonary function, the $V_{iso}\dot{V}$ ranges from 10% to 20% of the FVC. If dynamic airway compression occurs earlier in the FVC, laminar flow develops earlier, increasing the $V_{iso}\dot{V}$; this indicates increased small airway resistance and premature airway collapse. The $V_{iso}\dot{V}$ test is more sensitive to small airway obstruction than the $FEF_{25\%-75\%}$ or FEV_1.

The difference between flows in the two curves at 50% of the FVC ($\Delta\dot{V}_{max50}$) decreases in small airway obstructive disease (see Figure 5-14). In small airways obstruction, dynamic airway compression occurs earlier in the FVC, causing earlier development of laminar flow and less difference between $\dot{V}_{max50}$ values. The $\Delta\dot{V}_{max50}$ is particularly sensitive to changes in small airways resistance.

The three tests mentioned in this section require expensive equipment, are difficult to administer accurately, and require considerable patient cooperation. For this reason, these tests are not used in routine screening for pulmonary disease.

POINTS TO REMEMBER

- Pulmonary function measurements are important diagnostic tools but are insufficient in themselves to arrive at a diagnosis.
- Normal pulmonary function test values are based on the patient's age, gender, height, ethnicity, and body surface area.
- Helium dilution and nitrogen washout techniques measure only gas in communication with patent airways, whereas plethysmography measures the total TGV, whether or not it communicates with airways.
- The difference between dilution or washout techniques and plethysmography is a measure of air trapping.
- FRC and RV are increased in obstructive disease because of air trapping, low elastic lung recoil, or both.
- The major spirometric screening tests for differentiating obstructive and restrictive pulmonary function defects are FVC, FEV_1, and FEV_1/FVC ratio.
- The FEV_1/FVC ratio is an indicator of expiratory flow rate and is the major criterion for determining the presence of an obstructive defect.
- Obstructive disease primarily reduces expiratory flow rates, whereas restrictive disease primarily reduces lung volumes and capacities.
- Vital capacity is often reduced in obstructive disease because of air trapping, whereas it is reduced in restrictive disease because of low lung compliance.
- Obstructive disease increases work by increasing airway resistance and placing the diaphragm at a mechanical disadvantage; restrictive disease increases work by decreasing lung compliance.

References

1. Ruppel G: *Manual of pulmonary function testing,* ed 9, St Louis, 2009, Mosby.
2. Wasserman K, Hansen JE, Sue DY: *Principles of exercise testing and interpretation including pathophysiology and clinical applications,* ed 4, Philadelphia, 2005, Lippincott Williams & Wilkins.
3. Aldrich TK, Arora NS, Rochester DF: The influence of airway obstruction and respiratory muscle strength on maximal voluntary ventilation in lung disease, *Am Rev Respir Dis* 126(2):195, 1982.
4. Rochester DF, et al: The respiratory muscles in chronic obstructive pulmonary disease (COPD), *Bull Eur Physiopathol Respir* 15(5):951, 1979.
5. American Thoracic Society/European Respiratory Society: ATS/ERS statement on respiratory muscle testing, *Am J Respir Crit Care Med* 166(4):518, 2002.
6. Clark TJH, et al: The ventilatory capacity of patients with chronic airways obstruction, *Clin Sci* 36(2):307, 1969.
7. Pierce AK, et al: Exercise ventilatory patterns in normal subjects and patients with airway obstruction, *J Appl Physiol* 25(3):249, 1968.
8. Levitzky MG: *Pulmonary physiology,* ed 7, New York, 2007, McGraw-Hill.
9. GOLD Executive Committee: *Global initiative for chronic obstructive lung disease: pocket guide to COPD diagnosis, management, and prevention,* Gig Harbor, WA, 2009, Medical Communication Resources, Inc.

CHAPTER 6

Pulmonary Blood Flow

OBJECTIVES

After reading this chapter, you will be able to:
- Describe how the pulmonary and systemic circulations differ anatomically and functionally
- Explain how blood flow, pressure, and vascular resistance in the pulmonary circulation can be assessed through pulmonary artery catheterization
- Distinguish among causes of high pulmonary artery pressure through data obtained from the pulmonary artery catheter
- Explain how right and left ventricular pumping function can be assessed through pulmonary artery catheterization
- Calculate pulmonary vascular resistance
- Differentiate between passive and active factors that affect pulmonary vascular resistance
- Explain how the pulmonary vasculature can accommodate great increases in blood flow during exercise without significantly increasing blood pressure
- Explain why hypoxemia affects the right ventricle differently than the left ventricle

- Explain how hypoxic pulmonary vasoconstriction can be both beneficial and harmful
- Explain why the hypoxic pulmonary vasoconstriction response is diminished in certain pulmonary diseases
- Explain why inhaled vasodilators can bring about beneficial physiological changes that are not possible through systemic administration routes
- Explain why gravity creates three distinct physiological blood flow zones in the lung, and how they differ physiologically from one another
- Describe how mechanical and physiological changes can convert a blood flow zone in the lung to a different type of zone
- Explain why the match between blood flow and ventilation in an upright individual is different in the lung base than in the lung apex
- Describe the kinds of circulatory abnormalities cause pulmonary edema

KEY TERMS

acidemia
alkalemia
central venous pressure (CVP)
cyclic guanosine monophosphate (cGMP)
endothelium-derived relaxing factor (EDRF)
endotoxins
extraalveolar vessels
hydrostatic
hypervolemia
hypoxia
hypoxic pulmonary vasoconstriction (HPV)
oncotic pressure
osmotic

persistent pulmonary hypertension of the newborn (PPHN)
preload
proteinuria
pulmonary artery pressure (PAP)
pulmonary capillary wedge pressure (PCWP)
pulmonary edema
pulmonary vascular resistance (PVR)
right atrial pressure (RAP)
septicemia
shunt
systemic vascular resistance (SVR)
Valsalva maneuver
ventilation-perfusion ratio ($\dot{V}/\dot{Q}$)

PULMONARY VASCULATURE

The vascular system of the body consists of separate pulmonary and systemic circulations operating in series (Figure 6-1). Each circulation receives its blood from the other; each has its own reservoir, pump, and set of vessels. The right ventricle receives mixed venous blood through the tricuspid valve from its reservoir, the right atrium, and pumps it through the pulmonic valve, which marks the beginning of the pulmonary circulation.[1] This relatively deoxygenated blood flows through pulmonary arteries and arterioles to an immense alveolar capillary bed where it is reoxygenated. The capillary bed consists of extremely short, interconnected segments spreading 75 to 100 mL of blood over a 70-m^2 area, or about half the size of a tennis court.[1] Comroe[2] described the capillary bed as two sheets of endothelium held apart in places by posts, similar to an underground parking garage. Rather than flowing through numerous individual tubes (as in systemic capillaries), pulmonary blood flows more like a sheet over the alveoli, maximizing its exposure to alveolar gases. This structural arrangement shortens the distance for oxygen and carbon dioxide diffusion between air and blood to one tenth of the diffusion distance that exists between systemic capillaries and tissue cells.[1]

After leaving the alveoli, the capillaries converge to form venules and veins. The newly oxygenated blood flows through four major pulmonary veins (two from each lung) into the left atrium, the reservoir for the left ventricle. The pulmonary vein orifices in the left atrial wall mark the end of the pulmonary circulation.[1] Blood continues to flow out of the left atrium through the mitral valve into the left ventricle, which pumps the blood through the aortic valve into the aorta. The aortic valve marks the beginning of the systemic circulation. The aorta distributes the oxygenated blood through its many branches to systemic arteries, arterioles, and capillary beds throughout the body, supplying oxygen to tissue cells and removing the carbon dioxide they produce. Beyond the capillary beds, systemic venules and veins converge to return the oxygen-poor blood to the right atrium via the vena cavae, which mark the end of the systemic circulation.

The total cardiac output ($\dot{Q}_t$) is simultaneously pumped through both circulations each minute. Right and left ventricular outputs must be essentially equal over time; otherwise, blood would accumulate in one of the circulations. Small differences in outputs may occur briefly for a few heartbeats, but over time, individual ventricular outputs are equal in healthy hearts. Figure 6-1 illustrates pulmonary and systemic circulations with their associated pressures.

The pulmonary arteries and arterioles have much thinner walls and less smooth muscle than systemic arteries and arterioles. Therefore, pulmonary arterioles cannot constrict as effectively as systemic arterioles. Pulmonary veins and venules also have sparse smooth muscle, differing little in structure from pulmonary arteries and arterioles. Pulmonary arteries generally follow a course parallel with bronchi, whereas pulmonary veins leave the lung through different routes. Without this anatomical difference, distinguishing pulmonary arteries from veins on a chest x-ray image would be difficult because of their structural similarities.[2]

Pulmonary capillaries also differ significantly from systemic capillaries; as noted previously, pulmonary capillary blood flows in thin sheets, as opposed to the distinctly tubular flow in systemic capillaries. The thin walls of pulmonary vessels and vast area of the capillary bed make the pulmonary vasculature highly distensible compared with the systemic vasculature.

BRONCHIAL VASCULATURE

The supporting tissues of the tracheobronchial tree, including airways down through the terminal bronchioles, are supplied with oxygenated blood through the systemic bronchial arteries. (See the section on blood supply to the lungs in Chapter 1.) Bronchial systemic venous blood drains directly into the pulmonary veins, mixing oxygen-poor blood with freshly oxygenated pulmonary venous blood on its way to the left ventricle.[3] Bronchial blood flow is only 1% to 2% of the cardiac output, which means that the anatomical shunt from this source is usually less than 2%; this also means that left ventricular output is about 1% to 2% greater than right ventricular output.[3]

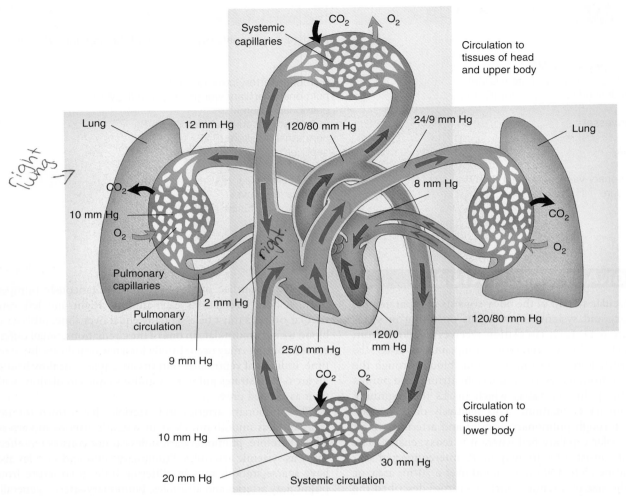

Figure 6-1 Comparison of pulmonary and systemic blood flows and pressures. (Adapted from Thibodeau GA, Patton KT: *Anatomy & physiology,* ed 5, St Louis, 2003, Mosby.)

CONCEPT QUESTION 6-1

Explain the way anatomical shunt through the bronchial circulation causes an oxygen pressure (PO_2) difference between alveolar gas and arterial blood.

PULMONARY AND SYSTEMIC PRESSURES

Figure 6-1 shows that the pulmonary circulation is a low-pressure, low-resistance system compared with the systemic circulation. The lower resistance in the pulmonary circulation is manifested by the fact that its pressures are lower even though it receives the same cardiac output as the systemic circulation receives. The resistance to blood flow in the pulmonary circulation is about one tenth as great as it is in the systemic circulation.[1]

Blood flow through the pulmonary circulation is highly pulsatile rather than continuous as in systemic capillaries. The total volume of blood in the pulmonary circulation is about 450 mL, which is only 9% of the total circulating blood volume. About 70 mL of this blood is in the capillaries at any given moment;

the rest is distributed equally between pulmonary arterial and venous vessels.[3] The capillary blood volume of 70 mL is about equal to the volume ejected by the right ventricle with each contraction (the right ventricular stroke volume). Pulmonary capillary blood is thus almost completely replaced with each heartbeat, which means a red blood cell travels through the capillaries in about 0.75 second. Pulmonary blood flow almost stops between each ventricular beat, which explains its pulsatile nature.[1,3]

The highly expandable pulmonary vascular bed serves as a backup reservoir that shields the left atrium from sudden changes in right ventricular output. If venous return to the right ventricle increases suddenly, as would occur during sudden strenuous exercise, left ventricular filling pressure increases gradually over two or three cardiac cycles rather than increasing abruptly.

Clinical Measurement of Pulmonary Blood Pressures and Flows

Measurement of Pulmonary Blood Pressures

Systemic blood pressure is easily measured by simple non-invasive means. However, measurement of pressures in the

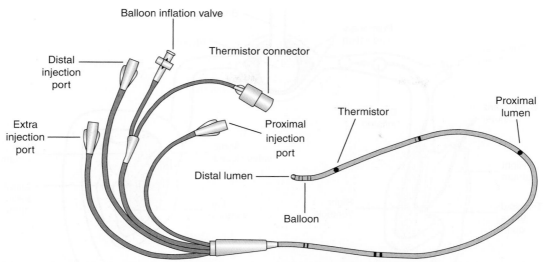

Figure 6-2 Typical quadruple channel pulmonary artery catheter. After insertion, the distal lumen rests in the pulmonary artery, and the proximal lumen rests in the right atrium. Both communicate with their respective injection ports. (From Wilkins RL, Stoller JK, Kacmarek RM: *Egan's fundamentals of respiratory care*, ed 9, St Louis, 2009, Mosby.)

pulmonary circulation requires an invasive procedure called pulmonary artery catheterization. The special catheter used for this purpose was the subject of a study published in 1970 by Swan, Ganz, and others. Since then, the catheter has been marketed under the brand name Swan-Ganz, and the term Swan-Ganz catheter has become synonymous with pulmonary artery catheter. This catheter is a very thin, multilumen flexible tube with a balloon located at its distal end. The balloon can be inflated through a separate channel inside the catheter. The catheter contains at least two additional internal channels: the distal channel, leading to an opening at the tip of the catheter, and the proximal channel, leading to an opening located several centimeters back from the tip. Pressures can be measured or blood can be withdrawn through these channels via the proximal and distal ports of the catheter (Figure 6-2).

A physician inserts the catheter under surgically sterile conditions, sometimes at the bedside of a critically ill patient in a hospital intensive care unit. Proximal and distal channels are first filled with sterile fluid to remove all air; the catheter is then inserted into a large systemic vein, usually the right internal jugular or subclavian vein, and advanced until the tip enters the right atrium. At this point the balloon is inflated, allowing the bloodstream to direct the catheter tip across the tricuspid valve into the right ventricle—hence, the term flow-directed, balloon-tipped catheter. The physician advances the catheter until the bloodstream carries it through the pulmonic valve and into the pulmonary artery (Figure 6-3). During insertion, pressures at the catheter tip are continuously recorded by an electronic pressure transducer connected to the distal port. The stationary fluid column inside the distal channel reflects these pressures precisely because it is in direct contact with the blood at the catheter's tip. The pressure waveforms are continuously displayed on the bedside monitor as the catheter is advanced; this helps the physician identify the position of the catheter tip because each cardiovascular structure produces unique pressure waveforms (Figure 6-4, *A* and *B*).

When the catheter is advanced far enough to wedge in a small branch of the pulmonary artery, the inflated balloon completely blocks blood flow to the downstream vessels supplied by that artery (see Figure 6-3, *dotted circle*). The pressure measured from the catheter tip in this wedged position is called the **pulmonary capillary wedge pressure (PCWP)**. (When the balloon is deflated, flow resumes, and the catheter tip simply measures the **pulmonary artery pressure [PAP]**.) The vessels extending beyond the artery blocked by the inflated balloon are in direct communication with the pulmonary capillaries and the pulmonary veins. Pulmonary venous pressure is nearly equal to left atrial pressure (LAP), which is essentially equal to left ventricular end-diastolic pressure (LVEDP), the pressure inside the filled ventricle just before it contracts (see Figure 6-3). This so-called filling pressure is also known as **preload** of the left ventricle. The PCWP is only slightly greater than the filling pressure of the left ventricle.[3] The PCWP accurately reflects changes in LAP (or ventricular filling pressure) because the stationary fluid column inside the catheter is functionally extended from the catheter tip to the left atrium. For this reason, the PCWP is commonly used to assess the pumping function of the left ventricle. For example, if the left ventricle fails to contract with normal force, blood flowing into it dams up in the left atrium, pulmonary veins, and capillaries; consequently, the PCWP increases. In certain rare circumstances, the PCWP might not accurately reflect left atrial pressure: (1) if the pulmonary veins constrict and downstream resistance beyond the catheter tip increases or (2) if the catheter tip is in an area in the lung where alveolar pressure exceeds pulmonary venous pressure, as might occur in positive pressure mechanical ventilation. In the latter instance, high alveolar pressure compresses capillaries distal to the catheter tip, blocking its communication with the left atrium.

CONCEPT QUESTION 6-2

Why would a narrowed (stenotic) mitral valve affect the PCWP? (See Figure 6-3.)

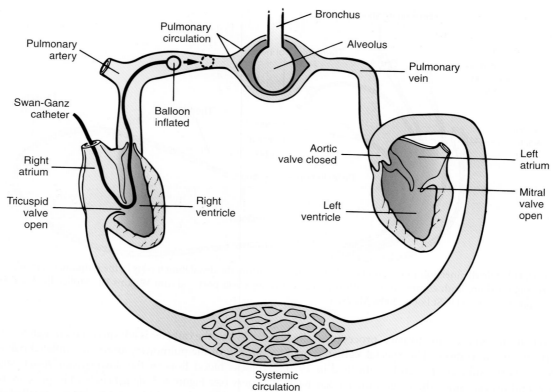

Figure 6-3 Pulmonary artery catheter in place. The *dotted circle* represents the wedge position. The heart is in diastole in this schematic. (From Martin L: *Pulmonary physiology in clinical practice*, St Louis, 1987, Mosby.)

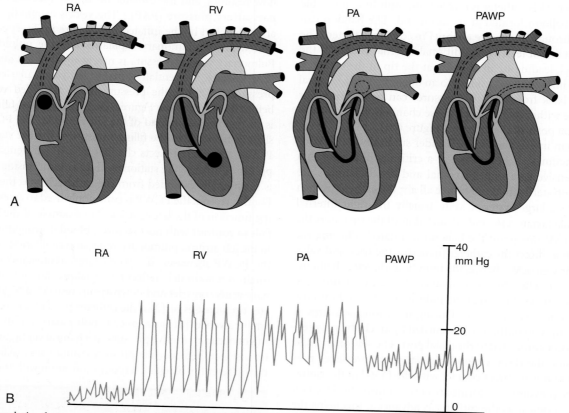

Figure 6-4 Correlation between pulmonary artery catheter positions (**A**) and pressure waveforms (**B**). *RA,* Right atrium; *RV,* right ventricle; *PA,* pulmonary artery; *PAWP,* pulmonary artery wedge pressure. (From Wilkins RL, Stoller JK, Kacmarek RM: *Egan's fundamentals of respiratory care,* ed 9, St Louis, 2009, Mosby.)

Causes of Pulmonary Artery Catheter Pressure Waveform Shapes

Proper positioning of the pulmonary artery catheter is confirmed by waveform patterns produced as the catheter is advanced into the pulmonary artery (see Figure 6-4). The first waveform appears on the monitor when the tip of the catheter reaches the great vessels. This is known as the central venous pressure (CVP) and reflects pressure in the vena cava and right atrium. A normal value for CVP is about 2 mm Hg; this produces the low-amplitude waveform in Figure 6-4, B. In the right atrium, the balloon is inflated for two reasons: (1) to decrease the risk of cardiac arrhythmias induced by the catheter tip hitting the ventricular walls and (2) to allow blood flow to catch the balloon and carry the catheter forward.

The catheter passes through the tricuspid valve into the right ventricle. The pressure waveform increases in height as the ventricle contracts (systole) and decreases sharply to near 0 as the ventricle relaxes (diastole) (see Figure 6-4, B). During diastole, the pressure waveform slowly rises as blood flows into the right ventricle through the tricuspid valve. Normal right ventricular pressure is about 25/0 mm Hg (systolic/diastolic).

The striking difference between pulmonary artery pressure (PAP) tracings and tracings created by the right ventricle is the diastolic pressure in the pulmonary artery. Closure of the pulmonic valve prevents PAP from decreasing as much as it does in the right ventricle (see Figure 6-4). The ejection of blood from the right ventricle creates a steep rise in the systolic portion of the curve. After systole, PAP decreases sharply until the pulmonic valve closes. Closure of this valve abruptly stops blood backflow, creating a shock wave responsible for the dicrotic notch on the downslope of the waveform. Normal PAPs are about 25/10 mm Hg.

As the catheter floats into a small branch of the pulmonary artery, the inflated balloon blocks blood flow. The pressure tracing is similar to right atrial waveforms but is of even lower amplitude; this is known as pulmonary capillary wedge pressure (PCWP). Normal PCWP is 4 to 12 mm Hg and is about the same as pressure in the left atrium. If pulmonary vascular resistance (PVR) is normal, the pulmonary artery diastolic pressure is about equal to the PCWP.

The pulmonary artery catheter also can be used to assess right ventricular preload and pumping function because the proximal channel (see Figure 6-2) communicates with the right atrium. The pressure measured at the catheter's proximal port reflects **right atrial pressure (RAP)**, sometimes called **central venous pressure (CVP)**.

Blood drawn from the proximal channel is a mixture of superior and inferior vena cava venous blood. Because oxygen contents of these two sources may differ considerably, proximal channel blood is not a clinically acceptable mixed venous blood

sample for purposes of measuring the average venous oxygen content of the body. A thoroughly mixed venous blood sample reflecting the true average venous oxygen content of the body must be obtained from the pulmonary artery, through the distal channel of the catheter (see Figure 6-2). By comparing the oxygen content of mixed venous blood with the oxygen content of systemic arterial blood, the oxygen consumption of the body can be assessed. (This is discussed in Chapters 8 and 12.)

By measuring and comparing pressures obtained from the pulmonary artery catheter (RAP, PAP, and PCWP), the

Differentiating Causes of High Pulmonary Artery Pressure

You have two patients with the following cardiac pressure values.

Patient A
Pulmonary artery (PA) systolic	38 mm Hg
PA diastolic	25 mm Hg
Pulmonary capillary wedge pressure (PCWP)	21 mm Hg

Patient B
PA systolic	40 mm Hg
PA diastolic	25 mm Hg
PCWP	10 mm Hg

Although both patients have elevated pulmonary artery pressures (PAPs), the reasons for this are quite different. The PCWP helps differentiate origins of high PAPs.

Discussion

In the following discussion, PCWP is used as a substitute for the left atrial pressure (LAP). PCWP (i.e., LAP) is elevated in Patient A and normal in Patient B. Pulmonary artery end-diastolic pressure (PAEDP) in Patient A is only 4 mm Hg higher than PCWP, whereas PAEDP in Patient B is 15 mm Hg higher than PCWP. In healthy people, the PAEDP is almost equal to the PCWP (PCWP = LAP) because pressures across the pulmonary capillary bed have enough time to equalize during diastole. High pulmonary vascular resistance (PVR) creates an increased PAEDP-PCWP difference because the resistance is located between the pulmonary artery and left atrium. In Patient B, PVR must be high, as shown by the high PAEDP-PCWP difference. The normal PCWP in Patient B suggests normal left ventricular pumping action. In Patient A, PVR must be normal because the difference between PAEDP and PCWP is small. The elevated PCWP (i.e., LAP) is transmitted back across the pulmonary capillaries, creating a proportionately high PAEDP, preserving the PAEDP-PCWP difference. Causes of increased PAP in Patient A may be left ventricular pumping failure or mitral valve narrowing. Causes of increased PVR in Patient B may be a pulmonary embolus or vasoconstriction induced by hypoxemia.

clinician can evaluate right and left ventricular function, differentiate the causes of increased PAP, and assess the risk of pulmonary edema. PAP might be increased because of excessive blood volume (**hypervolemia**) or because of left ventricular pumping failure in which blood dams up in the entire pulmonary circulation. The PAP might also be increased as a result of increased **pulmonary vascular resistance (PVR)**. Increased pressures in either ventricle at the end of diastole, coupled with a low cardiac output, signal a loss of ventricular pumping ability, or a loss of contractility. Increased PCWP, regardless of the cause, means that the pulmonary capillaries are engorged with blood, increasing the likelihood that fluid will be forced into interstitial lung spaces and cause pulmonary edema. Understanding these relationships is essential for taking appropriate therapeutic actions.

Measurement of Pulmonary Blood Flow or Cardiac Output

The amount of blood the heart pumps each minute can be clinically measured with a pulmonary artery catheter via a thermodilution technique. In this method, a known volume of room temperature fluid (e.g., saline) is rapidly injected into the right atrium through the proximal injection port (see Figure 6-2). This volume of cool fluid rapidly flows into the right ventricle where it is pumped into the pulmonary artery. A temperature-sensing thermistor near the end of the catheter (see Figure 6-2) in the pulmonary artery records a sudden decrease in temperature as the bolus of cool saline passes by. If cardiac output is increased, blood temperature rapidly returns to its original value; if it is decreased, the temperature increases more slowly to the original value. A microprocessor receives information from the thermistor and computes the area under the temperature-time curve. The area under the curve is small for rapid blood flow and large for slow blood flow. The microprocessor uses the area under the curve and the volume of the injected fluid to compute the blood flow rate, or the cardiac output ($\dot{Q}_t$). Several determinations of cardiac output can be made within minutes in this fashion.

PULMONARY VASCULAR RESISTANCE

PVR is measured in millimeters of mercury per liter per minute (mm Hg/[L/min]). PVR is the resistance that the vessels pose to blood flowing through the pulmonary circulation—it is the resistance against which the right ventricle pumps. Any factor that increases PVR increases right ventricular work. An increased PVR does not affect left ventricular work because this ventricle is situated on the downstream side of the pulmonary vessels.

Calculation of Pulmonary Vascular Resistance

PVR is calculated by dividing the mean pressure difference between beginning and ending points of the pulmonary circulation by the pulmonary blood flow. This is shown as follows:

$$PVR(mm\ Hg/[L/min]) = \frac{mean\ PAP - LAP}{\dot{Q}_t}$$

Clinically, values for calculating PVR are obtained from pulmonary artery catheter measurements. Cardiac output is obtained via the thermodilution technique, and PCWP is substituted for LAP. A microprocessor computes the mean PAP from the PAP waveform. The clinical equation is as follows:

$$PVR = \frac{mean\ PAP - PCWP}{\dot{Q}_t}$$

For example, at a $\dot{Q}_t$ of 5 L per minute, a mean PAP of 14 mm Hg, and a PCWP of 8 mm Hg, PVR is calculated as follows:

$$\frac{14\ mm\ Hg - 8\ mm\ Hg}{5\ L/min} = 1.2\ mm\ Hg/(L/min)$$

A pressure of 1.2 mm Hg is needed to produce a flow of 1 L per minute through the pulmonary circulation. In classic physics, pressure is measured in dynes per square centimeter (force per unit of area), and blood flow is measured in milliliters per second (cubic centimeters per second). Using these measurement units, PVR is calculated as follows:[2]

$$\frac{dynes/cm^2}{cm^3/sec} = \frac{dynes}{cm^2} \times \frac{sec}{cm^3} = \frac{dynes \times sec}{cm^5} = dynes \bullet sec \bullet cm^{-5}$$

The resistance term dynes $\bullet$ sec $\bullet$ cm^{-5} is traditionally used in clinical hemodynamic measurements. To convert mm Hg/(L/min) to its equivalent units in dynes $\bullet$ sec $\bullet$ cm^{-5}, one multiplies mm Hg/(L/min) by 80. Thus, the PVR of 1.2 mm Hg/(L/min) calculated previously is equivalent to 96 dynes $\bullet$ sec $\bullet$ cm^{-5}.

The pressure difference between beginning and ending points of the systemic circulation is the difference between mean arterial pressure (MAP) and RAP (or CVP). **Systemic vascular resistance (SVR)** is calculated as follows (using values from Figure 6-1):

$$SVR = \frac{MAP - RAP}{\dot{Q}_t}$$

$$SVR = \frac{93^* - 2}{5} = 18.2\ mm\ Hg/(L/min)$$

A pressure gradient of 18.2 mm Hg is needed to drive 1 L per minute of blood through the systemic circulation (compared with 1.2 mm Hg in the pulmonary circulation). This pressure converts to about 1456 dynes $\bullet$ sec $\bullet$ cm^{-5}. PVR is normally less than one tenth of SVR.[1] Thus, right ventricular work is about one tenth of left ventricular work, which explains why the left ventricular muscle mass is normally much greater than the right ventricular mass.

CONCEPT QUESTION 6-3

Which of the following does an increased PVR influence more: PAP or PCWP? Explain.

Distribution of Pulmonary Vascular Resistance

Figure 6-1 shows that the pressure decreases from the pulmonary arterioles to the pulmonary capillaries to the pulmonary veins are similar—that is, from 12 mm Hg to 10 mm Hg to

---

*MAP is estimated by doubling diastolic pressure, adding this value to systolic pressure and dividing by 3. (Normal diastolic time is approximately double the systolic time.) In this example, the approximate MAP is calculated as follows: [120 + 2(80)]/3 = 93.3 mm Hg.

9 mm Hg as shown in the right lung of the diagram in Figure 6-1. This means the individual resistances of these three components are nearly equal; at rest, each accounts for about one third of the total PVR. In contrast to the more muscular systemic arterioles, pulmonary arterioles do not normally function to regulate and redistribute blood flow.[4] In contrast to the pulmonary vasculature, systemic arterioles account for about two thirds of the total SVR.

FACTORS AFFECTING PULMONARY VASCULAR RESISTANCE

Passive or active factors may change pulmonary vessel diameters and vascular resistance. Passive changes occur in response to pressure differences across vessel walls. Because pulmonary vessels are thin and distensible, they are especially susceptible to pressure-induced diameter changes. Active changes in the vessel diameter and resistance occur when vascular smooth muscle contracts or relaxes.

Passive Factors

Lung Volume: Effects on Alveolar and Extraalveolar Vessels

Pulmonary vessels can be classified into two groups: vessels in direct contact with alveoli, exposed to alveolar pressure (alveolar vessels), and vessels not in contact with alveoli, exposed to intrapleural pressure (**extraalveolar vessels**). Alveolar vessels are pulmonary capillaries in intimate contact with alveolar walls. The state of alveolar inflation determines the diameters of alveolar vessels. As the lung inflates, alveolar vessels are compressed, and their resistances increase (Figure 6-5, *A* and *B*).[1,3]

Extraalveolar vessels include all pulmonary arteries, arterioles, venules, and veins not in direct contact with alveoli. The lung's elastic fibers have a tethering effect on these vessels (similar to their effect on small airways), stretching them to larger diameters as the lung inflates. In addition, during lung inflation, subatmospheric intrapleural pressure increasingly dilates these vessels, decreasing their resistance.[1,3] Extraalveolar vessels also include certain capillaries between alveoli in corners formed by the junctions of adjacent alveoli (see Figure 6-5, *A* and *B*). As the lung inflates, these corner spaces enlarge, stretching and dilating the "corner vessels" (see Figure 6-5, *B*).

To visualize this phenomenon, think of a basket of small half-inflated balloons. Similar to the balloons, the spherical alveoli touch each other, but spaces exist between them. Extraalveolar corner vessels occupy these spaces. During inspiration, the balloons (alveoli) enlarge, increasing the amount of space between them. Alveolar recoil forces attempt to increase this space further. The pressure in these spaces decreases, dilating the corner vessels and reducing their resistance.

Because alveolar and extraalveolar vessel resistances are in series with each other, their effects are additive.[1] Thus, total PVR is the composite of alveolar and extraalveolar vessel resistances, creating a U-shaped curve (Figure 6-6). Overall, PVR is lowest at functional residual capacity (FRC). At volumes less than FRC, elastic retractile forces and subatmospheric intrapleural

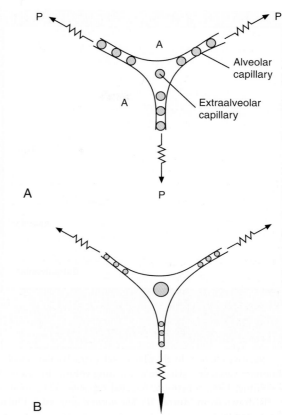

Figure 6-5 Schematic drawing of alveolar and extraalveolar (corner) vessels during normal, quiet inspiration (**A**) and deep inspiration (**B**). High lung volumes (**B**) compress alveolar vessels and dilate extraalveolar vessels. *A,* Alveoli; *P,* pleural pressure. (Redrawn from Fishman AP: *Assessment of pulmonary function,* New York, 1980, McGraw-Hill.)

pressures are weak, allowing extraalveolar vessels to narrow, shorten, and kink. The resulting increase in extraalveolar vessel resistance predominates, increasing total PVR. At volumes greater than FRC, increased alveolar vessel resistance caused by capillary compression becomes the predominant factor, again increasing total PVR (see Figure 6-6).

Vascular Pressure: Recruitment and Distention

An increase in either PAP or LAP decreases PVR. One reason is that both PAP and LAP cause an increase in distending pressure across vessel walls (transmural pressure), which dilates them.[1,4] This dilating effect is amplified if PAP and LAP increase together (Figure 6-7).[1,3] For example, consider an increasing LAP caused by inadequate left ventricular pumping action; the elevated LAP is reflected back throughout the pulmonary veins, capillaries, and arteries, dilating them and decreasing their vascular resistance.

The second mechanism responsible for the decrease in PVR when vascular pressures increase is recruitment.[1,4] Under normal resting conditions, some pulmonary capillaries in the upper regions of the lungs are completely collapsed.[1,4] As intravascular pressure increases, these collapsed capillaries are forced open (recruited), increasing the total cross-sectional area of the pulmonary capillary bed. As vascular pressures increase further,

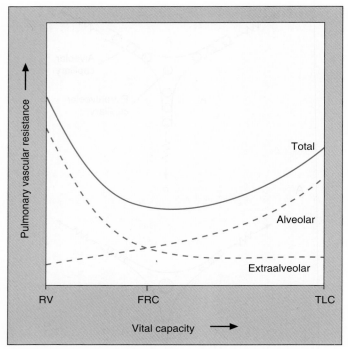

Figure 6-6 Relative changes in alveolar vessel, extraalveolar vessel, and total pulmonary vascular resistance as the lung volume increases. *RV,* Residual volume; *FRC,* functional residual capacity; *TLC,* total lung capacity. (Redrawn from Murray JF: *The normal lung,* ed 2, Philadelphia, 1986, Saunders.)

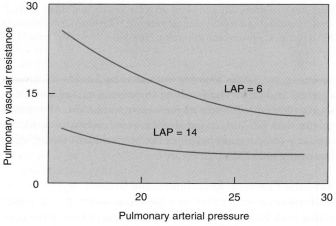

Figure 6-7 Effects of pulmonary artery pressure changes on pulmonary vascular resistance. High left atrial pressure (*LAP*) exaggerates the effect. (From Berne RM, Levy MN: *Physiology, international edition,* ed 2, St Louis, 1988, Mosby.)

individual capillaries widen or distend, decreasing PVR even more. If vascular pressure increases from an initially low level, recruitment is the chief mechanism whereby PVR decreases; conversely, if vascular pressure increases further from an initially high level when all vessels are already open, distention is the main reason why PVR decreases.[4] Recruitment and distention help explain why PAP changes little during exercise. As cardiac output increases, recruitment and distention dramatically decrease PVR, allowing PAP to increase only a few millimeters

of mercury. The opposite effect is equally important; decreased cardiac output and vascular pressures cause derecruitment, or collapse, of pulmonary capillaries.

CONCEPT QUESTION 6-4

In what circumstance may a decreased cardiac output be associated with increased pulmonary vascular pressures and pulmonary capillary distention?

Blood Volume

Pulmonary blood volume is generally constant, but it may change under certain circumstances. For example, a sustained **Valsalva maneuver** (forced expiration against a closed glottis) can squeeze 250 mL of blood into the systemic circulation.[3] Systemic blood loss can also decrease pulmonary blood volume. Left ventricular failure causes blood to dam up in pulmonary vessels, potentially increasing pulmonary blood volume by 100%.[3] Regardless of the mechanism, increased blood volume distends and recruits capillaries, decreasing the PVR.

Active Factors

Neurogenic Stimuli

There is little evidence to suggest that neurogenic stimuli play a role in controlling pulmonary blood flow in healthy adults.[1,4] Although sympathetic and parasympathetic nerves innervate the pulmonary vasculature (mostly larger arteries), their functional significance is marginally important and not well understood.[1] Some investigators have shown that sympathetic stimulation causes a slight increase in PVR, but others have shown only a stiffening of the arteries with no change in calculated resistance.[4] Parasympathetic (vagal) stimulation causes a slight decrease in vascular resistance, but its physiological significance is unknown. Overall, the effects of autonomic stimulation on the pulmonary circulation are controversial and not well understood; autonomic stimulation produces only minor changes in the smooth muscle tone of vessels in the adult lung.[1]

Humoral Agents and Nitric Oxide

The most important substance that regulates pulmonary vascular tone is nitric oxide (NO), derived from the endothelial cells lining the blood vessels.[5] Naturally occurring (endogenous) humoral substances in the body produce vasodilation by stimulating the production of NO, previously called **endothelium-derived relaxing factor (EDRF).** Endogenous substances include acetylcholine, bradykinin, histamine, thrombin, serotonin, adenosine diphosphate (ADP), and some prostaglandins.[6] In 1987, Furchgott[6] noted that acetylcholine did not cause smooth muscle relaxation in vessels stripped of their endothelium; he postulated that endothelial cells produce a smooth muscle relaxing factor. Palmer et al.[7] and Ignarro et al.[8] later identified EDRF as NO. The 1998 Nobel Prize in physiology or medicine was awarded to Furchgott, Ignarro, and Murad for their discovery of the role of NO in the human body.[9]

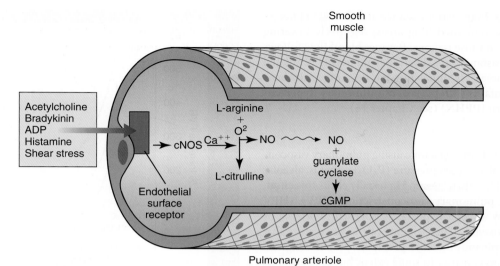

Figure 6-8 Endothelial production of nitric oxide (*NO*) in the pulmonary arteriole. Various stimuli may activate endothelial surface receptors, initiating a chain of biochemical events that produce NO and subsequent vascular smooth muscle relaxation. *ADP*, Adenosine diphosphate; *cNOS*, constitutive nitric oxide synthase; *cGMP*, cyclic guanosine monophosphate.

Nitric oxide is a potent vasodilator in the human circulation, and it plays an important role in regulating pulmonary vascular smooth muscle tone.[5] The endogenous substances previously listed are considered to be endothelial-dependent vasodilators because they depend on the endothelial release of NO for their effects. The elaboration of NO accounts for the vasodilating mechanism of nitrate drugs such as nitroglycerin (used to improve coronary blood flow) and nitroprusside (used to treat dangerously high blood pressure).[10]

NO is produced in vascular endothelial cells (Figure 6-8) by oxidation of an amino acid, L-arginine, catalyzed by an enzyme, nitric oxide synthase (NOS).[11-13] As stated in Chapter 1, there are three forms of NOS: neuronal NOS (nNOS), which is constituted in nonadrenergic noncholinergic neurons (a form of constitutive NOS [cNOS]); inducible NOS (iNOS), which is induced in airway epithelial cells by inflammation; and endothelial NOS (eNOS), another constitutive form of NOS that is generated in vascular endothelial cells (referred to as cNOS in Figure 6-8).[5,13] Production of eNOS is controlled by endothelial cell surface receptors that are stimulated by the various humoral substances previously listed. Besides these substances, mechanical factors such as stretching and shear stress stimulate cell surface receptors.[11] Whether the stress is humoral or mechanical, receptor stimulation activates eNOS but only in the presence of calcium ions (Ca++). Calcium-activated cNOS catalyzes the oxidation of L-arginine, producing small bursts of NO.

NO is highly soluble in cell membranes and diffuses instantly into vascular smooth muscle cells. In vascular smooth muscle cells, NO activates another enzyme, guanylate cyclase, which catalyzes the production of **cyclic guanosine monophosphate (cGMP)**, as shown in Figure 6-8. cGMP causes vascular smooth muscle relaxation. Physical exercise induces cNOS production, presumably by increasing vascular pressure, and may be a factor, along with recruitment and distention, in preventing significant increases in PVR during exercise.[11]

CONCEPT QUESTION 6-5

Predict the physiological effect of a drug that inhibits the action of NOS.

Endothelial cells synthesize NO in small amounts on demand, exerting a regulatory vasodilating influence on pulmonary arterioles under normal resting conditions.[11,12] A calcium-independent form of NOS (inducible NOS [iNOS]) can be induced in endothelial and inflammatory cells by **endotoxins** associated with bacterial blood infections (**septicemia**) and by various other inflammatory mediators in the body.[5] In contrast to eNOS, which is released in small pulses as needed, iNOS is always "turned on," releasing large, continuous amounts of NO not controlled by cell receptor–dependent mechanisms. Excessive induced NO production is linked to the massive vasodilation and hypotension of septic shock syndrome.[14,15] Sepsis-induced vasodilation does not respond well to vasoconstrictor drugs. If an effective iNOS-inhibiting drug could be given to patients with septic shock, it would seem that the vasodilation and associated hypotension might be reversed, increasing the blood pressure.

This hypothesis was studied in a large multicenter clinical trial in which humans with septic shock were given a drug known to inhibit NOS activity. The NOS inhibitor reduced blood nitrate levels, increased pulmonary and systemic vascular tone, maintained systemic blood pressure in an acceptable range, and reduced the need for conventional vasoconstrictor drugs, such as norepinephrine.[14] However, overall patient outcome was not improved. Although general inhibition of NOS is not ultimately beneficial in septic shock, selective inhibition of the inducible form (iNOS) was found to be more beneficial than norepinephrine in an animal study.[16]

Inhaled NO gas in extremely low concentrations has been used therapeutically to treat severe pulmonary hypertension and to selectively dilate pulmonary vessels in well-ventilated regions of the lungs. In the latter instance, inhaled NO of necessity enters the best-ventilated lung areas, selectively lowering vascular resistance in those regions. Because blood flow follows the path of least resistance, it is diverted from poorly ventilated to well-ventilated areas. NO inhalation has been especially beneficial in treating infants with **persistent pulmonary hypertension of the newborn (PPHN)** (see Chapter 16).

Chemical Factors

The most important chemical factor causing pulmonary vasoconstriction is low alveolar oxygen pressure ($P_{A}O_{2}$)—that is, alveolar **hypoxia**. A $P_{A}O_{2}$ of less than 70 mm Hg usually elicits this effect, known as **hypoxic pulmonary vasoconstriction (HPV)**.[1] HPV is brought about by alveolar hypoxia, as opposed to arterial or mixed venous hypoxemia. The elements of the vasculature that constrict are predominantly the small precapillary arterioles; small pulmonary veins also constrict to some extent but produce only 20% or less of the HPV-induced increase in PVR.[17] This constrictive venous response might explain the acute pulmonary edema sometimes seen in individuals who travel to high altitudes in the mountains where atmospheric oxygen pressure is low; hypoxia-induced venous constriction could increase pulmonary capillary pressure, which is a feature of high-altitude pulmonary edema.[17]

The constrictive response to hypoxia is unique to the pulmonary circulation; hypoxia evokes vasodilation in the systemic circulation. High $P_{A}O_{2}$ (hyperoxia) has little effect on normal pulmonary circulation, probably because pulmonary vessels in normal lungs have little muscle tone, and their vasodilating ability is minimal.[18] However, in hypoxic individuals, improved oxygenation markedly dilates pulmonary vessels and dramatically decreases PVR.

HPV is enhanced by low arterial blood pH (**acidemia**); HPV becomes progressively greater for a given $P_{A}O_{2}$ as pH decreases. At a normal arterial pH of 7.40, the maximal vasoconstrictive response occurs at a $P_{A}O_{2}$ of 60 to 70 mm Hg[18]; this corresponds with a PaO_{2} of about 50 to 60 mm Hg when the normal alveolar-to-arterial PO_{2} gradient is taken into account. A classic animal experiment showed that at arterial pH less than 7.30, a PaO_{2} less than 50 mm Hg causes a sudden, sharp increase in PVR (Figure 6-9).[19] At a normal PaO_{2}, arterial pH must decrease to less than 7.25 to cause a significant increase in PVR.[18] High $PaCO_{2}$ increases PVR indirectly by generating carbonic acid, which causes acidemia. HPV is also enhanced by NOS-inhibiting agents, suggesting that reduced endothelial NO release may be an underlying mechanism in HPV.[17]

HPV is inhibited by various mediators present in the blood that cause vasodilation, such as the endothelial-derived substances NO and prostacyclin.[17] HPV is also inhibited by drugs that block alpha-adrenergic or stimulate beta-adrenergic receptors. In addition, it is inhibited by increased LAP (a vascular distending effect), high alveolar pressure, and high blood pH (**alkalemia**).[17]

Physiological Function of Hypoxic Pulmonary Vasoconstriction

The physiological function of HPV is to match blood flow with ventilation better (i.e., to divert pulmonary arterial blood

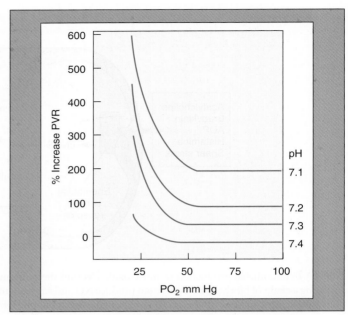

Figure 6-9 Effects of low arterial pH and hypoxemia on pulmonary vascular resistance (*PVR*) in newborn calves. The greater the acidemia, the greater the vascular resistance at any PO_{2} value. Note the abrupt increase in PVR at PO_{2} less than 50 mm Hg, especially at pH less than 7.40. (Redrawn from Rudolph AM, Yaun S: *J Clin Invest* 45[3]:407, 1966.)

away from poorly ventilated, hypoxic regions to the better ventilated areas. If HPV or a similar mechanism did not exist, pulmonary arterial blood would remain poorly oxygenated as it flows unchecked past underventilated alveoli. This blood would mix with and decrease the PO_{2} of blood leaving well-ventilated alveoli, causing systemic arterial hypoxia. Thus, HPV has a beneficial effect, even though it increases the PVR. If the entire lung is uniformly hypoxic (e.g., at high altitudes), HPV is widespread throughout the lung, increasing vascular resistance and pressures. HPV still may be physiologically helpful because elevated pressures recruit previously nonperfused pulmonary capillaries, increasing the surface area for gas exchange.

CONCEPT QUESTION 6-6

Scintiphotography, a special imaging technique, allows ventilation or blood flow distribution to be seen in the lungs (ventilation or perfusion scans). Why does regional alveolar hypoxia caused by mucous plugging produce a perfusion scan similar to one produced by a pulmonary embolus that blocks blood pulmonary flow, and how might one distinguish between these two conditions?

Mechanism of Hypoxic Pulmonary Vasoconstriction

The exact mechanism of HPV is poorly understood.[1] The response is localized, occurring only in areas of alveolar hypoxia. HPV does not depend on nervous or humoral control because it occurs in surgically removed, mechanically perfused lungs ventilated with hypoxic gas mixtures[17]; this explains why HPV occurs even in patients who receive heart-lung transplants.

CLINICAL FOCUS 6-3

Chronic Hypoxia and Right Ventricular Failure

You are called to assess a patient admitted with chronic obstructive pulmonary disease (COPD). A physician has just examined the patient and tells you that physical findings include obvious pulmonary disease, distended neck veins, ankle edema, and hepatomegaly (enlarged liver). Arterial blood gas values indicate chronic hypoxia, and the chest radiograph shows hyperinflation of the lungs with right ventricular enlargement (hypertrophy). The admitting diagnosis is COPD with right ventricular hypertrophy. What is the relationship between this patient's lung disease and cardiac function?

Discussion

Chronic hypoxia characterizes COPD. COPD is often associated with anatomical destruction of alveoli and associated capillaries, decreasing the functional surface area for gas exchange. The resulting hypoxia induces pulmonary vasoconstriction, increasing pulmonary artery pressure (PAP). The destruction of the alveolar-capillary membrane area contributes further to increased PAP by reducing the cross-sectional area of the pulmonary vasculature. High PAP poses an increased opposition to blood flow coming from the right ventricle. The muscle mass of the right ventricle increases in response to the increased workload, but it may ultimately fail to pump blood effectively into the high-resistance pulmonary vascular system. A failing right ventricle causes blood to back up into the right atrium, vena cava, jugular veins, liver, and veins in the legs and ankles; this accounts for liver enlargement (hepatomegaly) and ankle edema (pedal edema). Right heart failure induced by pulmonary disease is called cor pulmonale. This condition often improves with continuous oxygen therapy, which relieves hypoxic vasoconstriction and decreases pulmonary vascular resistance.

Animal and human studies strongly suggest that lack of normal NO release by the endothelium plays a role in the HPV mechanism. Decreased PO_2 in vascular endothelial cells diminishes NO synthesis, suggesting that reduced NO formation is a mechanism underlying HPV.[1, 20] HPV is abolished by breathing NO gas mixtures or by drugs that stimulate endothelial NO production.[1, 20] Conversely, blocking NO synthesis enhances HPV, which means that NO must have a regulating effect on HPV, holding its severity in check.[17] Even in persons without hypoxia, drugs inhibiting NO synthesis induce pulmonary vasoconstriction, confirming that the normally oxygenated pulmonary vasculature is in a continuous state of NO-mediated dilation.[20]

Whatever the cause of HPV, Ca^{++} entry into the vascular smooth muscle cell must be involved to cause muscle contraction.[1] A mechanism has been proposed whereby hypoxia directly affects vascular smooth muscle; it has been shown that hypoxia depolarizes smooth muscle cell membranes, probably by inhibiting potassium ion (K^+) channels, which is accompanied by the opening of Ca^{++} channels and Ca^{++} entry into the cell.[1,17] Ca^{++} are essential in the smooth muscle contraction process. Consistent with this proposed mechanism is the fact that Ca^{++} channel blocking drugs inhibit HPV, whereas Ca^{++} agonists enhance it.[1]

Loss of Hypoxic Pulmonary Vasoconstriction

The HPV response is often diminished in patients with acute lung injuries, such as burn and smoke inhalation, sepsis, and acute respiratory distress syndrome (ARDS).[13,14,17,21,22] This diminished response may account for the severe systemic hypoxemia these diseases cause. Acute lung injury causes the release of inflammatory mediators that induce formation of iNOS and subsequent NO release; this prevents the normal vasoconstrictive response of vessels in hypoxic lung regions. When the HPV response is lost, poorly oxygenated mixed venous blood flows unchecked through underventilated and nonventilated lung regions, creating severe shunting and systemic arterial hypoxemia. This type of intrapulmonary shunting responds poorly to oxygen inhalation because the supplemental oxygen cannot enter nonventilated alveoli.

Inflammatory mediators are also released in response to overinflation of the alveoli, which has implications for patients who are dependent on mechanical ventilatory assistance. Patients with acute lung injuries often require positive pressure mechanical ventilation. High pressures during mechanical ventilation can overstretch and injure the alveoli. This type of stretch injury is known to release inflammatory cytokines that induce iNOS and subsequent NO release, which counteracts HPV.[23-25]

A purely mechanical explanation for why acute lung injury might diminish the effect of HPV also has been proposed.[21] Injury to the alveolar-capillary membrane increases its permeability, allowing fluid to enter the alveolus and deactivate surfactant. The resulting high surface tension causes alveoli to shrink and collapse. Animal studies using an in vivo microscope revealed that as alveoli shrink, they place a tethering force on the extraalveolar vessels, causing them to dilate. In this way, portions of the pulmonary vasculature are mechanically dilated in injured, poorly ventilated lung regions, possibly negating or minimizing the effects HPV might have.[21]

Inhaled Vasodilators in Acute Respiratory Distress Syndrome

Despite the reduction of the effectiveness of HPV in acute lung injury, the overall PVR is nevertheless often elevated in ARDS.[17] For this reason, inhaled NO and other pulmonary vasodilators have been used clinically to decrease PVR. Besides decreasing PVR, an added benefit of inhaled vasodilators (as a gas or an aerosol mist) is that they selectively dilate pulmonary vessels only in well-ventilated lung regions, diverting mixed venous blood to these areas. The effect is to match blood flow with ventilation better, reducing intrapulmonary shunt and improving arterial oxygenation—in effect, enhancing the benefits of HPV. Selective dilation occurs because inhaled vasodilators can enter only ventilated portions of the lung.

Alternatives to inhaled NO have been sought because of the complex technology associated with NO administration, high NO costs, potential NO toxicity, and the failure of NO to decrease overall mortality in patients with ARDS.[26] Some of these alternative vasodilators, which are inhaled as aerosols,

include prostacyclin (PGI_2), sildenafil (Viagra), nitroprusside, and nitroglycerin.[26-28] Similar to NO, prostacyclin is synthesized in the pulmonary vascular endothelial cells; it exerts its effects by activating specialized endothelial receptors. Sildenafil exerts its effects by inhibiting phosphodiesterase, an enzyme that deactivates cyclic adenosine monophosphate (cAMP); cAMP is the intracellular substance responsible for smooth muscle relaxation. Nitroprusside and nitroglycerin induce the enzymatic release of NO. All of these NO alternatives reduce both pulmonary and systemic blood pressures if given intravenously or orally. Intravenous or oral administration of these agents not only could dangerously lower the systemic blood pressure but also indiscriminately dilate all pulmonary vessels; this would hinder HPV and worsen intrapulmonary shunt and hypoxemia. However, when administered by inhalation, these vasodilators affect only the pulmonary circulation and only in well-ventilated lung regions; this tends to preserve HPV in poorly ventilated areas.[26]

CLINICAL FOCUS 6-4

Different Therapy for Different Causes of Increased Pulmonary Artery Pressure

Increased pulmonary artery pressures (PAPs) occur for different reasons. What are the different reasons, and how does therapy differ?

Discussion

When PAP is elevated as a result of high pulmonary vascular resistance (PVR), therapy is aimed at reducing the PVR. For example, if hypoxic pulmonary vasoconstriction (HPV) in chronic hypoxemia causes high PVR and right ventricular strain, continuous oxygen therapy might be appropriate. Oxygen therapy relieves the hypoxia, removing the stimulus for pulmonary vasoconstriction.

An elevated PAP caused by left heart failure (i.e., loss of left ventricular pumping action) may be treated with inotropic drugs, which increase the heart's contractility and pumping effectiveness. Diuretics decrease the blood volume by enhancing urine production and reducing venous return to the heart. Vasodilators decrease the resistance against which the left ventricle must pump, allowing it to pump blood more effectively.

Understanding the origins of elevated PAP is important because treatment approaches are completely different for different circumstances.

DISTRIBUTION OF PULMONARY BLOOD FLOW

Gravitational and Pressure Effects: Zones of Blood Flow

Because pressures in the thin, distensible pulmonary blood vessels are low, gravity and pressures surrounding the vessels greatly affect blood flow distribution in the lung. The effects of gravity create three distinct zones of blood flow, as described in the classic model by West[4] (shown in Figure 6-10). Blood enters the lung at the hilum through the pulmonary artery. The same average PAP of about 15 mm Hg is applied to arterial vessels in all zones. Arteries in zone III (lung base) are about 12 cm below the hilum. Thus, the weight of a column of blood 12 cm high is added to the pressure in zone III vessels. A column of blood 12 cm high exerts a pressure of about 9 mm Hg, causing arterial

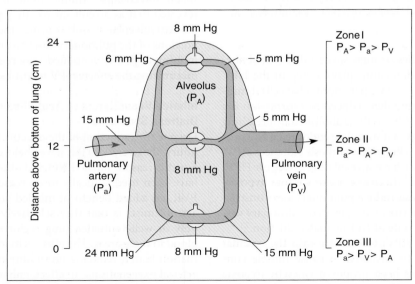

Figure 6-10 Gravitational effects create three zones of blood flow patterns in the pulmonary circulation. Zone I has no flow, zone II has intermittent flow, and zone III has continuous flow. (From Berne RM, Levy MN: *Principles of physiology*, ed 2, St Louis, 1996, Mosby.)

pressure in zone III to be 9 mm Hg higher than arterial pressure in zone II (see Figure 6-10). Blood flows down into zone III with the aid of gravity.

In contrast, blood is pumped up into zone I (lung apex) against gravitational forces. Zone I arteries are about 12 cm above the main pulmonary artery, causing the arterial pressures to be 9 mm Hg less than the arterial pressure in the main pulmonary artery. Figure 6-10 shows an upright lung (i.e., the person is standing). If the person is supine, zones I to III are redistributed from anterior to posterior lung regions, rather than from the lung apex to the lung base.[4]

Zone I Blood Flow

To illustrate zone I conditions, which are not normally present in spontaneously breathing individuals, the lung model in Figure 6-10 is receiving positive pressure mechanical ventilation such that the average alveolar pressure is about 8 mm Hg in all alveoli. In the lung apex or zone I, gravitational effects cause both arterial and venous pressures to be lower than alveolar pressure. Consequently, alveolar pressure compresses the surrounding capillaries, totally occluding them and stopping blood flow. Only extraalveolar corner vessels may still have some blood flow in this zone. In zone I, alveoli are ventilated but have no blood flow, which constitutes alveolar dead space ventilation. In spontaneously breathing healthy individuals with normal cardiac outputs and blood pressures, arterial pressures always exceed alveolar pressures, even in the uppermost apical lung regions, and zone I does not exist. However, a severe decrease in blood pressure can lower PAP so much that zone I conditions are created in the lung.

Zone II Blood Flow

Figure 6-10 shows that arterial pressure in zone II considerably exceeds alveolar pressure, but alveolar pressure still exceeds venous pressure; this produces intermittent flow through alveolar capillaries. Blood flows into a capillary at its arterial end because its pressure exceeds the surrounding alveolar pressure. As blood flows down the length of the capillary, approaching the venous end, capillary pressure progressively decreases until it falls below alveolar pressure. At this point, alveolar pressure collapses the capillary, stopping blood flow. (This is similar to the situation described in Chapter 3 in which forced expiration causes dynamic airway compression after an equal pressure point is formed.) The pressure of the stationary column of blood in the capillary quickly equalizes with its source, the arterial pressure, which is greater than alveolar pressure. This action momentarily forces the capillary open, allowing blood flow to resume. As blood flows through the opened capillary, pressure again decreases down its length, falling below alveolar pressure, recollapsing the capillary near its venous end. The cycle repeats, causing capillaries to flutter rapidly between open and closed states, producing intermittent flow.

The pressure gradient for blood flow in zone II is the difference between arterial and alveolar pressure, not arterial and venous pressure (as it is for most other vessels). As long as venous pressure is below alveolar pressure, pulmonary veins are blocked, and venous pressures cannot influence flow. This zone

---

CLINICAL FOCUS 6-5

Most Likely Location of the Pulmonary Artery Catheter Tip: Zone I, II, or III?

Blood flow must be continuous between the tip of the Swan-Ganz catheter and left atrium to reflect left heart pressure accurately. Uninterrupted blood flow is found only in zone III of the lung, where arterial and venous pressures exceed alveolar pressures. Because the Swan-Ganz catheter is flow directed (i.e., carried into place via continuous blood flow), it is most likely to migrate into zone III. Pulmonary capillary wedge pressure (PCWP) measured when the Swan-Ganz catheter is located in zone I or II does not accurately reflect left atrial pressure (LAP) because alveolar pressure momentarily or continuously stops blood flow in these zones. PCWP measured from zone I or II reflects alveolar pressures instead of LAPs.

II flow characteristic is sometimes called the waterfall effect. In this analogy, the rate of flow over the waterfall's edge is proportional to the pressure difference between a point upstream (arterial pressure) and a point at the waterfall's edge (alveolar pressure). Neither the pressure in the stream below the waterfall's edge (venous pressure) nor the height of the waterfall influences the rate of flow over the edge.

Zone III Blood Flow

The arterial and venous pressures exceed alveolar pressure in zone III because of the effects of gravity. Blood flow is continuous and proportional to the difference between arterial and venous pressures. As long as alveolar pressure is below vascular pressures, it cannot influence blood flow. Gravity causes zone III, the lung bases in the upright person, to have the greatest blood flow.

Factors Affecting Zones of Blood Flow

Blood flow zones are not fixed, anatomical boundaries; rather, they are dependent on physiological conditions. Certain respiratory maneuvers, such as exhaling against a closed glottis, blowing through a wind instrument, or coughing, can momentarily increase alveolar pressures above arterial pressure, creating zone I conditions in gravity-independent (uppermost) lung regions. Positive-pressure mechanical ventilation may increase alveolar pressure enough to convert some zone II regions to zone I. This is one mechanism whereby positive pressure ventilation increases alveolar dead space. Likewise, a loss of blood volume or massive vasodilation, as in septic shock, may decrease PAP enough to create zone I conditions. Conversely, exercise increases cardiac output and PAP, recruiting any zone I to zone II or zone II to zone III. The lung volume also affects regional distribution of blood flow, as implied in the earlier discussion regarding the effect of lung volume on PVR (see Figure 6-7). At total lung capacity when alveoli are maximally expanded, apical regions are more likely to produce zone I conditions.

Normal Matching of Ventilation and Blood Flow

As discussed in Chapter 3, tidal inspiration is preferentially distributed to basal alveoli. This distribution occurs because at FRC, the beginning point for a tidal inspiration, apical

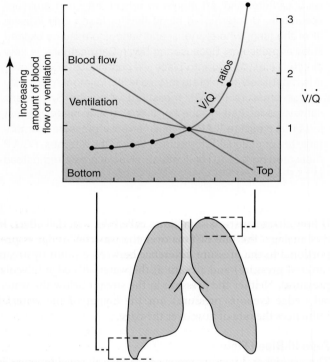

Figure 6-11 Changes in blood flow, ventilation, and $\dot{V}/\dot{Q}$ ratio in the upright lung. From the lung base to the lung apex, blood flow decreases more rapidly than ventilation. Consequently, the $\dot{V}/\dot{Q}$ ratio increases from the lung base to the lung apex. (Modified from West JB: *Ventilation, blood flow and gas exchange*, Oxford, 1965, Blackwell Science; and Martin L: *Pulmonary physiology in clinical practice*, St Louis, 1987, Mosby.)

alveoli are more distended and less compliant than basal alveoli. Although apical alveoli contain more volume at FRC, their decreased compliance allows less volume change per breath and less ventilation per minute. Similar to blood flow, ventilation is least in the lung apex and greatest in the lung base. However, the decrease in blood flow from base to apex is greater than the corresponding decrease in ventilation, which means that the lung apex has relatively more ventilation than blood flow. Likewise, the lung base has relatively more blood flow than ventilation. As a result, the **ventilation-perfusion ratio** ($\dot{V}/\dot{Q}$) *increases* from the lung base to the lung apex (Figure 6-11).

Dead Space and Shunt Effects in the Normal Lung

Shunt refers to deoxygenated blood flowing through the capillaries of unventilated alveoli; dead space refers to the ventilation of alveoli that have no capillary blood flow. Between these two extremes are shuntlike and dead space–like effects, corresponding with low and high $\dot{V}/\dot{Q}$ ratios. Because the lung apices have relatively more ventilation than blood flow (high $\dot{V}/\dot{Q}$), a dead space–like effect is produced. Likewise, because lung bases have relatively less ventilation with respect to blood flow (low $\dot{V}/\dot{Q}$), a shuntlike effect is produced. The overall average $\dot{V}/\dot{Q}$ ratio in the normal resting lung is about 0.8, which means ventilation on average is slightly less than blood flow (Figure 6-12). During exercise, the tremendous increase in ventilation causes the $\dot{V}/\dot{Q}$ ratio to increase. (Ventilation-perfusion relationships and their effects on blood gases are discussed in Chapter 12.)

LIQUID MOVEMENT ACROSS THE ALVEOLAR CAPILLARY MEMBRANE

Capillary Fluid Dynamics

Figure 6-13 illustrates **hydrostatic** and **osmotic** forces governing fluid movement across pulmonary capillary walls. The pulmonary capillary acts as a semipermeable membrane, freely permeable to water molecules but much less permeable to larger

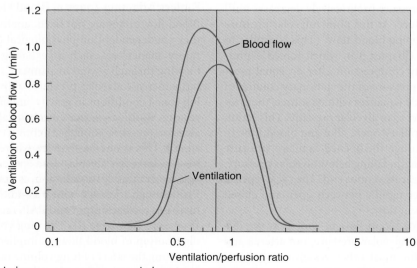

Figure 6-12 Normal human $\dot{V}/\dot{Q}$ curves. Overall average $\dot{V}/\dot{Q}$ for the lung is slightly greater than 0.8, as shown by the *thin vertical line*. On average, blood flow slightly exceeds ventilation. (From Berne RM, Levy MN: *Physiology*, ed 3, St Louis, 1993, Mosby.)

molecules. The capillary endothelial membrane is relatively impermeable to large high-molecular-weight proteins, although the membrane's leakiness allows some proteins to enter the interstitial space. Large protein molecules create osmotic pressure in solution. The influence of proteins on the osmotic pressure of blood plasma is called **oncotic pressure**. The greater the protein concentration in blood plasma, the greater the oncotic pressure. One can think of oncotic pressure as a force that "pulls" water molecules from areas of low oncotic pressure into areas of high oncotic pressure. This is the opposite of hydrostatic pressure, a force that "pushes" fluid from high to low pressures.

As shown in Figure 6-13, pulmonary capillary hydrostatic blood pressure is about 7 mm Hg, and interstitial hydrostatic fluid pressure is about 8 mm Hg. Interstitial fluid pressure is "negative" because inward alveolar recoil and lymphatic removal of fluid from this area create subatmospheric pressure. The combined effect of interstitial and capillary hydrostatic pressures is a force of 15 mm Hg, which tends to move fluid out of the capillary. Adding to this force is an interstitial oncotic pressure of about 14 mm Hg, which tends to pull fluid out of the capillary into the interstitial space. Hydrostatic and oncotic forces combine for a total of 29 mm Hg, favoring fluid movement out of the capillary into the interstitial space. The only force that moves fluid into the capillary is the blood's oncotic pressure of about 28 mm Hg. The total force favoring fluid movement out of the capillary is 29 mm Hg, whereas the total force favoring inward movement is 28 mm Hg. This yields a net mean filtration pressure of 1 mm Hg.[3]

The following Starling equation describes fluid movement across the capillary endothelium:[4]

$$\dot{Q}_f = K_f[(P_c - P_{is}) - \alpha(\pi_{pl} - \pi_{is})]$$

In this equation, $\dot{Q}_f$ represents the net flow of fluid (mL/min) out of the capillary; K_f represents the capillary filtration coefficient, describing capillary fluid permeability characteristics; P_c represents capillary hydrostatic pressure; P_{is} represents interstitial hydrostatic pressure; σ represents the reflection coefficient, describing how easily the capillary endothelium prevents passage of solute particles (when σ equals 1.0, the membrane is impermeable to solutes); π_{pl} represents plasma oncotic pressure; and π_{is} represents interstitial fluid oncotic pressure.

This filtration pressure causes a slight amount of fluid to flow continuously from capillaries into interstitial spaces. The lymphatic system, a natural sump for draining interstitial fluid, immediately removes this fluid. Lymphatic action is extremely important for preventing fluid leakage into alveoli; the alveolar epithelium is so thin and weak that positive interstitial pressure can rupture it, allowing fluid to flow into alveoli.[3]

Pulmonary Edema

Pulmonary edema is the accumulation of fluid in the interstitial spaces between capillaries and alveoli. Causes of pulmonary edema include (1) increased hydrostatic pressure, (2) increased capillary permeability, (3) decreased plasma oncotic pressure, and (4) insufficient lymphatic drainage.[3]

Increased Hydrostatic Pressure

If hydrostatic pressure in the pulmonary capillary increases enough, fluid filtration into the interstitial space may exceed lymphatic drainage, flooding the interstitial spaces. The interstitial fluid volume cannot increase by much more than 100 mL before alveolar membranes rupture, causing alveolar

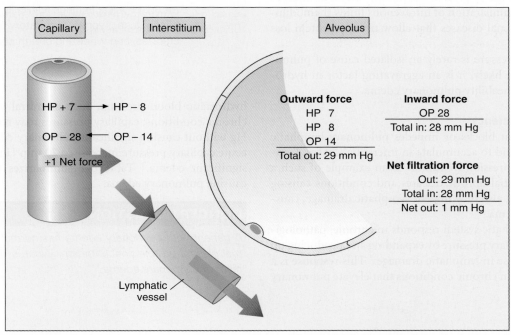

Figure 6-13 Fluid movement in pulmonary capillaries. Lymphatic vessels normally prevent fluid accumulation in the interstitium. *Outward force* and *inward force* refer to forces moving fluid out of or into the pulmonary capillary. *HP*, Hydrostatic pressure; *OP*, oncotic pressure. (Modified from Guyton AC: *Textbook of medical physiology*, ed 8, Philadelphia, 1991, Saunders.)

edema.[3] Some fluid enters alveoli even in mild pulmonary edema.

A common cause of hydrostatic pulmonary edema is left ventricular failure. Coronary artery disease may reduce blood flow to the left ventricular muscle, reducing the effectiveness of its pumping action. Blood dams up in the left atrium and pulmonary veins, increasing pulmonary capillary pressures. This type of edema is associated with a high PCWP and is called cardiogenic pulmonary edema.

Mitral valve stenosis, or narrowing of the mitral valve orifice, also may cause blood to dam up in the pulmonary capillaries and cause pulmonary edema. Overadministration of intravenous fluids may create hypervolemia, or fluid overload, with similar results.

Increased Capillary Permeability

Acute lung injuries that damage the alveolar capillary membrane may increase its permeability to fluids and cause pulmonary edema. This kind of edema is often called high-permeability pulmonary edema or noncardiac pulmonary edema. Causes of alveolar capillary membrane injury include severe infections such as pneumonia, endotoxins of sepsis, oxygen toxicity, ARDS (regardless of the cause), and inhaled noxious substances. Typically, patients with this kind of pulmonary edema have normal pulmonary capillary pressure and left atrial pressures (i.e., PCWP is generally normal).

Decreased Plasma Oncotic Pressure

Capillary blood oncotic pressure is the only force favoring fluid retention inside the capillary. If it is abnormally low, fluid easily moves out of the capillary, overwhelming the removal capacity of the lymphatic system (see Figure 6-13). Oncotic pulmonary edema may be caused by protein starvation,* blood dilution as a result of overadministration of intravenous fluids (hemodilution), or certain renal diseases that allow urinary protein loss (**proteinuria**).

Low oncotic pressure is rarely an isolated cause of pulmonary edema. More likely, it is an aggravating factor in hydrostatic or high-permeability pulmonary edema.

Lymphatic Insufficiency

Any condition that blocks or impedes pulmonary lymphatic flow may cause fluid to accumulate in interstitial spaces. Lymphatic vessel compression by tumors is an example of such a condition. Interstitial fibrotic diseases and conditions causing interstitial scarring also may impede lymphatic drainage, causing pulmonary edema.

A normal lymphatic system responds to chronic, pathologically elevated capillary pressure by expanding and producing up to a 10-fold increase in lymphatic drainage.[3] This response is a large safety factor in chronic conditions that elevate pulmonary

---

CLINICAL FOCUS 6-6

Correlation of Pulmonary Capillary Wedge Pressure with Hydrostatic Pulmonary Edema

Hydrostatic pulmonary edema is also known as cardiogenic pulmonary edema (i.e., arising from left heart failure). The inefficient left ventricle causes blood to back up in the pulmonary circulation, increasing hydrostatic pressure in the pulmonary capillaries, increasing the pulmonary capillary wedge pressure (PCWP). High capillary pressure forces fluid into the interstitium and alveoli. Differentiating between cardiogenic and noncardiogenic pulmonary edema may be difficult because the clinical presentation is similar in both. Clinical signs and symptoms of pulmonary edema (cardiogenic and noncardiogenic) include dyspnea, wheezing, fine crackling breath sounds, and hypoxemia. In cardiogenic pulmonary edema, the PCWP is usually greater than 20 mm Hg. In contrast, PCWP is usually normal in noncardiogenic pulmonary edema. The cause of pulmonary edema in this situation is often hyperpermeability, or leakiness, of the alveolar capillary membrane. A general correlation between PCWP and clinical evidence of pulmonary edema with normal capillary permeability follows.

PCWP (mm Hg)	Clinical Evidence of Hydrostatic Pulmonary Edema
16-18	No physical or x-ray findings evident
18-25	Some x-ray evidence of pulmonary edema (engorged pulmonary vessels and appearance of infiltrates); physical findings evident, including some fine crackling breath sounds
>25	Obvious x-ray evidence of pulmonary edema (greatly increased infiltrates and vascular engorgement); physical findings (clinically significant hypoxemia, tachypnea, respiratory distress, diffuse crackles, and wheezing breath sounds)

---

hydrostatic blood pressure, such as mitral valve stenosis. In chronic conditions, capillary pressures may reach 35 to 45 mm Hg without causing significant pulmonary edema, whereas an acute capillary pressure increase to 20 mm Hg normally causes significant edema.[3] Table 6-1 summarizes the mechanisms causing pulmonary edema.

CONCEPT QUESTION 6-7

A patient with pulmonary edema has normal PCWP and normal plasma protein concentration. What is the likely mechanism of pulmonary edema?

---

*Proteins are the main source of blood oncotic pressure.

Clinical Consequences and Treatment of Cardiogenic Pulmonary Edema

Cardiogenic pulmonary edema engorges pulmonary capillaries, forcing fluid into the interstitial spaces. Eventually, this fluid may enter the alveoli, disrupting the alveolar surfactant system and causing alveolar collapse. Ventilation is unevenly distributed throughout the lung because pulmonary edema does not affect all alveolar units equally. Lung compliance decreases because engorged capillaries surround the alveoli, restricting their expansion. Alveolar collapse also reduces lung compliance. As a result, the patient develops hypoxemia and dyspnea. In life-threatening situations, fluid moves into the alveoli and airways, blocking ventilation of alveoli.

The severity of pulmonary edema may vary. With evidence of respiratory failure, intubation and mechanical ventilation are required. In all situations, treatment is focused on improving cardiac pumping effectiveness and maintaining adequate oxygenation. Pharmacological agents commonly used to treat cardiogenic pulmonary edema generally have one or more of the following actions: (1) reduce blood volume, (2) increase myocardial contractility, and (3) decrease cardiac workload. Diuretics decrease the circulating blood volume by increasing urine output. Reducing the blood volume tends to decrease venous return, which decreases pulmonary vascular pressures. Vasodilators redistribute the blood volume by increasing vessel diameters. This also reduces the venous return and the pulmonary capillary wedge pressure (PCWP). In addition, vasodilators decrease the resistance against which the left ventricle must pump, making it a more effective pump. Inotropic agents increase myocardial contractility and the heart rate, improving left ventricular function. More blood is pumped out of the left atrium, decreasing the PCWP.

The goals in treating cardiogenic pulmonary edema are to reverse pulmonary capillary congestion, increase cardiac pumping effectiveness, and improve oxygenation. In addition to drugs, oxygen therapy plays an essential role in treating pulmonary edema.

TABLE 6-1
Mechanisms of Pulmonary Edema

Factor	Value	Type	Clinical Problem
Hydrostatic pressure	Increased	Cardiac	Left ventricular failure Fluid overload Mitral stenosis
Capillary permeability	Increased	Noncardiac	Sepsis Oxygen toxicity Acute lung injury
Oncotic pressure	Decreased	Noncardiac	Protein starvation Hemodilution Renal loss of proteins
Lymphatic drainage	Decreased	Noncardiac	Pulmonary interstitial fibrosis

POINTS TO REMEMBER

- The pulmonary circulation is a low-pressure, low-resistance system; the systemic circulation is a high-pressure, high-resistance system.
- The pulmonary vasculature is highly distensible; arteries and veins are structurally similar and contain little smooth muscle compared with their systemic counterparts.
- Some bronchial venous blood drains directly into pulmonary veins, introducing deoxygenated blood directly into the oxygenated blood entering the left atrium, which causes PaO_2 normally to be lower than P_AO_2.
- The balloon-tipped, flow-directed pulmonary artery catheter measures right atrial, pulmonary artery, and pulmonary capillary pressures; LAP is estimated from the PCWP.
- PCWP obtained through the pulmonary artery catheter is high in left ventricular pumping failure because blood dams up back to the capillaries behind the failing ventricle.
- Factors affecting PVR are active or passive; passive factors include alveolar pressure, vascular pressure, and vascular volume, and active factors involve smooth vascular muscle contraction or relaxation.
- NO is a potent pulmonary vasodilator and is naturally synthesized by the vascular endothelial cells to help regulate PVR.
- HPV works to match blood flow with ventilation better, which helps moderate the severity of intrapulmonary shunting.
- Acute lung injury causes release of inflammatory substances that induce NO synthesis; this tends to defeat HPV, worsening intrapulmonary shunt and decreasing the blood pressure.
- Inhaled vasodilators target well-ventilated lung regions, lowering their vascular resistance and diverting blood flow to these regions; this reduces shunting and arterial hypoxemia.
- Gravity causes pulmonary blood flow to be categorized into three distinct zones of blood flow: zone I, no blood flow; zone II, intermittent blood flow; and zone III, continuous blood flow.
- Hypotension and high alveolar pressures can convert zone II regions to zone I.
- Ventilation and blood flow increase from the lung apex to the lung base.
- The ventilation-to-blood flow ratio increases from lung base to lung apex.

- Pulmonary edema occurs when fluid filtration from capillaries into the interstitial space overwhelms the removal capacity of the lymphatic system.
- Pulmonary edema may be caused by high pressures, low plasma oncotic pressures, lymphatic insufficiency, or hyperpermeability of the alveolar-capillary membrane.

References

1. Jacobson JR, Garcia JGN: Pulmonary circulation and regulation of fluid balance. In Mason RJ, et al: *Murray and Nadel's textbook of respiratory medicine*, ed 5, Philadelphia, 2010, Saunders.
2. Comroe JH: *Physiology of respiration*, ed 2, Chicago, 1974, Year Book Medical Publishers.
3. Hall JE: *Guyton and Hall textbook of medical physiology*, ed 12, Philadelphia, 2011, Saunders.
4. West JB: *Respiratory physiology: the essentials*, ed 8, Baltimore, 2008, Lippincott Williams & Wilkins.
5. Steendijk P: Going on and on with NO? (Editorial), *Crit Care Med* 33(5):1157, 2005.
6. Furchgott RF: Endothelium-derived relaxing factor: discovery, early studies, and identification as nitric oxide, *Biosci Rep* 19(4):235, 1999.
7. Palmer RM, Ferrige AG, Moncada S: Nitric oxide release accounts for the biological activity of endothelium-derived relaxing factor, *Nature* 327(6122):524, 1987.
8. Ignarro LJ, et al: Endothelium-derived relaxing factor produced and released from artery and vein is nitric oxide, *Proc Natl Acad Sci U S A* 84(24):9265, 1987.
9. Altman LK: Three Americans awarded Nobel for discoveries of how a gas affects the body, *The New York Times* 309:A14, October 13, 1998.
10. Reeves JT, Kinsella JP, Abman SH: Nitric oxide in treatment of persistent pulmonary hypertension of the newborn, *Semin Resp Crit Care Med* 15(6):495, 1994.
11. Anggard E: Nitric oxide: mediator, murderer, and medicine, *Lancet* 343(8907):1199, 1994.
12. Lorente JA, et al: L-Arginine pathway in the sepsis syndrome, *Crit Care Med* 21(9):1287, 1993.
13. Enkhbaatar P, Traber DL: Pathophysiology of acute lung injury in combined burn and smoke inhalation injury, *Clin Sci* 107(2):137, 2004.
14. Watson D, et al: Cardiovascular effects of the nitric oxide synthase inhibitor NG-methyl-L-arginine hydrochloride (546C88) in patients with septic shock: results of a randomized, double-blind, placebo-controlled multicenter study (study no. 144-002), *Crit Care Med* 32:282, 2004.
15. Nduka OO, Parrillo JE: The pathophysiology of septic shock, *Crit Care Clin* 25:677, 2009.
16. Su F, et al: Effects of a selective iNOS inhibitor versus norepinephrine in the treatment of septic shock, *Shock* 34:243, 2010.
17. Naeije R, Brimioulle S: Physiology in medicine: importance of hypoxic pulmonary vasoconstriction in maintaining arterial oxygenation during acute respiratory failure, *Crit Care* 5(2):67, 2001.
18. Fishman AP: Pulmonary circulation. In Fishman AP, editor: *Handbook of physiology, section 3: the respiratory system, volume I, circulation and nonrespiratory functions*, Bethesda, MD, 1985, American Physiological Society.
19. Rudolph AM, Yuan S: Response of the pulmonary vasculature to hypoxia and H^+ ion concentration changes, *J Clin Invest* 45(3):399, 1966.
20. Wagner PD, Powell FL, West JB: Ventilation, blood flow and gas exchange. In Mason RJ, et al: *Murray and Nadel's textbook of respiratory medicine*, ed 5, Philadelphia, 2010, Saunders.
21. McCann UG, et al: Alveolar mechanics alter hypoxic pulmonary vasoconstriction, *Crit Care Med* 30(6):1315, 2002.
22. Ogasawara H, et al: Effects of selective nitric oxide synthase inhibitor on endotoxin-induced alteration in hypoxic pulmonary vasoconstriction in sheep, *J Cardiovasc Pharmacol* 42(4):521, 2003.
23. Carney D, DiRocco J, Nieman G: Dynamic alveolar mechanics and ventilator-induced lung injury, *Crit Care Med* 33(Suppl 3):S122, 2005.
24. Broccard AF, et al: Effects of L-NAME and inhaled nitric oxide on ventilator-induced lung injury in isolated, perfused rabbit lungs, *Crit Care Med* 32(9):2004, 1872.
25. Ricard JD, Dreyfuss D, Saumon G: Ventilator-induced lung injury, *Curr Opin Crit Care* 8(1):12, 2002.
26. Lowson SM: Inhaled alternatives to nitric oxide, *Crit Care Med* 33(3 Suppl):S188, 2005.
27. Fattouch K, et al: Inhaled prostacyclin, nitric oxide, and nitroprusside in pulmonary hypertension after mitral valve replacement, *J Card Surg* 20(2):171, 2005.
28. Lee AJ, Chiao TB, Tsang MP: Sildenafil for pulmonary hypertension, *Ann Pharmacother* 39(5):869, 2005.

Gas Diffusion

CHAPTER OUTLINE

OBJECTIVES

After reading this chapter, you will be able to:
- Differentiate between diffusion and bulk gas flow
- Use the alveolar gas equation
- Explain why the respiratory exchange ratio affects the calculation of alveolar oxygen pressure (P_AO_2)
- Identify the factors that affect diffusion, as illustrated by Fick's law
- Use Graham's law and Henry's law to explain the differences in oxygen (O_2) and carbon dioxide (CO_2) diffusion rates in the lung
- Explain why O_2 transfer from lung to blood is perfusion limited, whereas carbon monoxide (CO) transfer is diffusion limited

- Explain why CO and not O_2 is the test gas normally used for measuring the diffusion capacity of the lung
- Explain how diffusion capacity is measured in a pulmonary function laboratory
- Correlate disease entities with the abnormal processes that decrease diffusion rate
- Explain why the diffusion capacity of the lung for carbon monoxide (D_LCO) test detects oxygenation problems in the natural progression of disease before abnormalities in arterial blood oxygen pressure (PaO_2) are evident

KEY TERMS

diffusion
diffusion capacity of the lung for carbon monoxide (D_LCO)
Fick's law
Graham's law

Henry's law
polycythemia
respiratory exchange ratio (R)
single breath carbon monoxide diffusion test

WHAT IS DIFFUSION?

Diffusion is the result of high-speed random motion of gas or liquid molecules. For example, if the number of molecules present in area *A* is greater than in area

B, mathematical probability dictates that more molecules will move from *A* to *B* than from *B* to *A*. This net movement of molecules from high to low concentrations is called diffusion. **Diffusion** in the above-mentioned example continues until the molecules are evenly distributed such that the number of

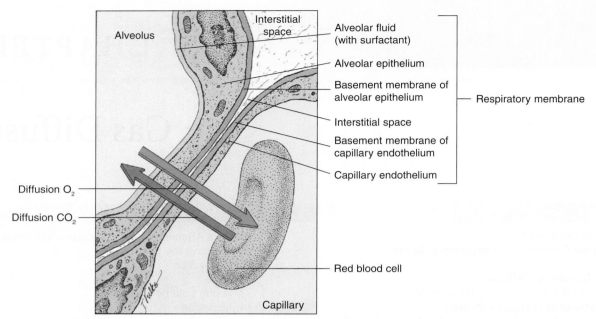

Figure 7-1 Alveolar capillary gas-exchange membrane. (From Seeley RR, Stephens TD, Tate P: *Anatomy & physiology*, ed 3, New York, 1995, McGraw-Hill.)

molecules moving from *A* to *B* and from *B* to *A* is the same. This state is called equilibrium.

The high-speed random impacts of atmospheric air molecules on solid surfaces create the atmosphere's pressure. Air is a gas mixture; the contribution that each gas makes to the atmospheric pressure is proportional to the number of its molecules present (i.e., each gas exerts its own partial pressure, as explained in Chapter 4). A gas diffuses from one point to another when there are differences in its partial pressures within the mixture; the direction of diffusion is always from high to low partial pressure. When no partial pressure difference exists for any gas throughout the mixture, equilibrium is present. Individual gas partial pressure differences are called diffusion gradients. During diffusion, each gas in a mixture moves according to its own diffusion gradient. That is, two different gases may simultaneously diffuse in opposite directions because of oppositely oriented partial pressure gradients. This occurs for oxygen (O_2) and carbon dioxide (CO_2) across the alveolar capillary membrane (Figure 7-1).

Diffusion is not the same as bulk gas flow, in which a large pressure gradient causes all molecules of all gases to move together in one direction. An example of bulk gas flow is ventilation, in which mouth and alveolar pressure differences cause gas to move in and out of the lungs. In terminal airways and alveoli, random molecular diffusion is the main mechanism whereby gas molecules reach the alveolar surface.

CONCEPT QUESTION 7-1

Which of the following problems—both of which cause hypoxemia—can be attributed to a diffusion defect: partially obstructed airways that reduce ventilation in certain lung regions or destruction of alveolar tissues and associated capillaries?

DIFFUSION GRADIENTS OF RESPIRATORY GASES

Figure 7-2 illustrates diffusion gradients between alveolar gas and blood and between blood and body tissues. Inspired air contains about 21% O_2 and essentially no CO_2. Inspired oxygen partial pressure (P_IO_2) is about 160 mm Hg, as the following calculation shows:

1. $P_IO_2 = 0.2095 \times 760 \text{ mm Hg} = 159 \text{ mm Hg}$

Conducting airway PO_2 is lower than the air's PO_2 because gas in the lung is 100% saturated with water vapor. At body temperature, the partial pressure of water vapor in the lung (P_{H2O}) is 47 mm Hg. PO_2 in conducting airways is about 150 mm Hg, as the following calculation shows:

2. $P_IO_2(\text{humidified}) = 0.2093 \times (760 - 47) = 149 \text{ mm Hg}$

Alveolar PO_2 (P_AO_2) is lower still because CO_2 diffuses into the alveoli, diluting incoming O_2 and lowering P_AO_2 to about 100 mm Hg. (Calculation of P_AO_2 is discussed in the next section.)

The diffusion gradient between alveolar gas and mixed venous blood is much larger for O_2 than it is for CO_2 (60 mm Hg vs. 6 mm Hg), as shown in Figure 7-2. At rest, these diffusion gradients transfer about 250 mL of O_2 into the blood and 200 mL of CO_2 into the alveoli each minute. By the time blood leaves the alveolar capillary, the PO_2 and PCO_2 of the blood have reached equilibrium with alveolar gases, even during exercise when blood flows very rapidly through the capillary. PO_2 of blood entering the left atrium is never as high as PO_2 of blood leaving the pulmonary capillaries (see Figure 7-2) because a small amount of deoxygenated bronchial venous blood mixes with capillary blood; this constitutes a normal anatomical shunt. Anatomical shunt is mostly responsible for the normal $P(A-a)O_2$ (alveolar-to-arterial oxygen pressure difference). Left atrial blood normally flows unaltered into the systemic arteries.

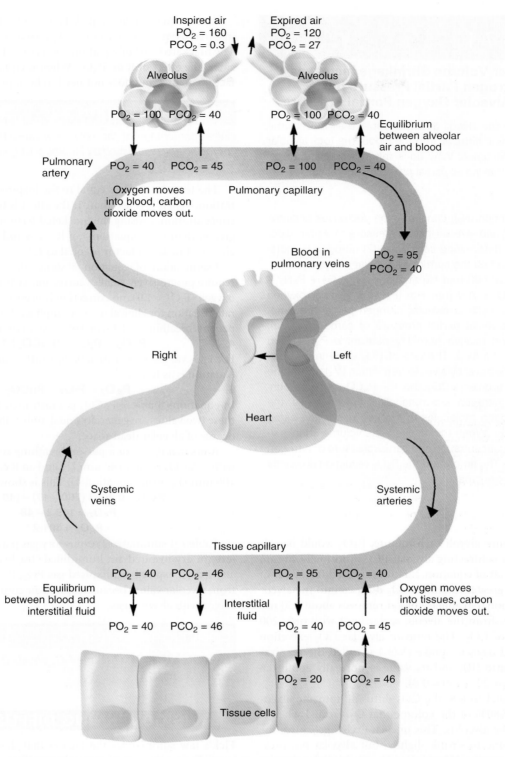

Figure 7-2 Partial pressure diffusion gradients for oxygen and carbon dioxide (CO_2) at the alveolar and systemic tissue levels. (From Seeley RR, Stephens TD, Tate P: *Anatomy & physiology,* ed 3, New York, 1995, McGraw-Hill.)

Alveolar Air Equation

The sum of all gas pressures at any point in the lung must equal 760 mm Hg at sea level. When air—which is CO_2-free—is inspired and enters the alveoli, its PCO_2 immediately increases

to 40 mm Hg as it mixes with the CO_2 present in the alveoli; because the sum of all alveolar gas pressures is constant (760 mm Hg), the inspired air PO_2 decreases by about 40 mm Hg. If the amount of O_2 diffusing out of alveoli into the blood each minute were exactly equal to the amount of CO_2 diffusing

CLINICAL FOCUS 7-1

Why Alveolar Volume Shrinkage Increases Alveolar Nitrogen Partial Pressure but Decreases Alveolar Oxygen Partial Pressure

If CO_2 entering the alveoli does not replace all the volume vacated by O_2 as it diffuses into the blood, the total alveolar volume must decrease. Why does this not concentrate all alveolar gases, making all partial pressures increase?

Discussion

O_2 (but not nitrogen [N_2]) concentration decreases because (1) alveolar CO_2 and alveolar partial pressure of water vapor (P_AH_2O) are predetermined constants, (2) nitrogen is metabolically inert, and (3) the sum of all alveolar gas partial pressures must equal 760 mm Hg at sea level ($P_AO_2 + P_AN_2 + P_ACO_2 + P_AH_2O = 760$ mm Hg) (P_AO_2 is alveolar oxygen partial pressure, P_AN_2 is alveolar nitrogen partial pressure, and P_ACO_2 is alveolar partial pressure of carbon dioxide). Temperature and relative humidity determine P_AH_2O and are constant in the lung. The rate of CO_2 entry into alveoli ($\dot{V}CO_2$) and its removal by alveolar ventilation ($\dot{V}_A$) determine the P_ACO_2; for a given $\dot{V}CO_2$ and $\dot{V}_A$, P_ACO_2 remains constant. Because nitrogen is a metabolically inactive gas, the number of nitrogen molecules in inspired gas is the same as in expired gas. When the inspired gas volume shrinks in the alveoli, the concentration and partial pressure of nitrogen (P_AN_2) increase. The amount of the P_AO_2 reduction is exactly equal to the P_AN_2 increase.

from the blood into alveoli each minute, P_AO_2 would be calculated by simply subtracting alveolar PCO_2 (normally 40 mm Hg) from the result of equation 2. However, O_2 diffuses out of the alveolus at a greater rate than CO_2 diffuses into the alveolus. At rest, pulmonary capillary blood removes about 250 mL per minute of O_2 from the alveoli, replacing it with only 200 mL per minute of CO_2. The ratio of alveolar CO_2 excretion ($\dot{V}CO_2$) to blood oxygen uptake ($\dot{V}O_2$) is called the **respiratory exchange ratio (R)**, and its value is normally about 0.8 ($R = \dot{V}CO_2 / \dot{V}O_2 = 200 / 250 = 0.8$).

When R is equal to 0.8, the CO_2 diffusing into the alveolus replaces only 80% of the volume that O_2 vacated when it diffused out of the alveolus. This uneven exchange causes the alveolar gas volume to shrink slightly, but alveolar gas pressure remains constant at 760 mm Hg. The shrinkage in alveolar volume concentrates the alveolar nitrogen molecules, which the alveolar air equation takes into account. This equation is known as the ideal alveolar air equation because it assumes the ventilation-to-blood flow ratios of each alveolus in the lung are identical, as the following calculation shows:

3. $$P_AO_2 = P_IO_2 - P_ACO_2 \left[F_IO_2 + \frac{1 - F_IO_2}{R} \right]$$

In this equation P_IO_2 equals F_IO_2 (760 − 47). F_IO_2 represents inspired oxygen concentration expressed as a decimal fraction. The bracketed part of equation 3 is a correcting factor that considers the effect of R on P_AO_2. When R equals 1, the correction factor equals 1 and does not need to be applied.

CONCEPT QUESTION 7-2

What percentage of the volume vacated by O_2 diffusing out of the alveoli is replaced by incoming CO_2 when R equals 1.0?

The term $1 - F_IO_2$ is equal to the inspired nitrogen concentration. When R is less than 1, the effect is to increase nitrogen concentration, causing the bracketed term to increase to values greater than 1. In equation 3, if R = 0.8 and F_IO_2 = 0.21 (room air), the bracketed factor is equal to 1.2.

Examination of equation 3 shows that higher F_IO_2 values require progressively smaller correction factors; at 100% inspired oxygen (F_IO_2 = 1.0), no correction is needed. A sufficiently accurate equation for clinical use is a simplified form of equation 3 for patients breathing an F_IO_2 of 0.60 or less. This is shown as follows:[1]

4. $$P_AO_2 = P_IO_2 - (PaCO_2)\, 1.2$$

For F_IO_2 values greater than 0.60, a sufficiently accurate clinical equation is as follows:[1]

5. $$P_AO_2 = P_IO_2 - PaCO_2$$

In equations 4 and 5, $PaCO_2$ is substituted for P_ACO_2 because these two values are generally equal, unless the lungs have a high degree of alveolar dead space.

A normal P_AO_2 for a person breathing room air at sea level, with a $PaCO_2$ equal to 40 mm Hg and an R equal to 0.8, is about 100 mm Hg (using equation 4). This is shown as follows:

$$P_AO_2 = 0.2093\,(760 - 47) - (40 \times 1.2)$$
$$P_AO_2 = 149.2 - 48$$
$$P_AO_2 = 101.2$$

Table 7-1 summarizes respiratory gas partial pressures at sea level in dry inspired air, humidified (tracheal) air, alveolar air, and mixed expired air. Expired gas PO_2, PCO_2, and PN_2 differ from alveolar values because expired air contains dead space gas mixed with alveolar gas.

CONCEPT QUESTION 7-3

Calculate the P_AO_2 when the F_IO_2 equals 0.40 and the $PaCO_2$ equals 35 mm Hg.

LAWS GOVERNING DIFFUSION

Fick's law summarizes the factors that determine the rate of gas diffusion through the alveolar capillary membrane. This is shown as follows:

$$\dot{V}_{gas} = \frac{A \times D \times (P_1 - P_2)}{T}$$

In this equation the following are represented:

$\dot{V}_{gas}$ represents the volume of gas diffusing through the membrane per minute (mL per minute).

A represents the surface area of the membrane available for diffusion (cm^2).

TABLE 7-1

Partial Pressures of Gases at Sea Level

Gases	Dry Air		Humidified Air		Alveolar Air		Expired Air	
	mm Hg	%	mm Hg	%	mm Hg	%	mm Hg	%
Nitrogen	600.2	78.98	563.4	74.09	569.0	74.9	566.0	74.5
Oxygen	159.5	20.98	149.3	19.67	104.0	13.6	120.0	15.7
Carbon dioxide	0.3	0.04	0.3	0.04	40.0	5.3	27.0	3.6
Water vapor	0.0	0.0	47.0	6.20	47.0	6.2	47.0	6.2

Modified from Seeley RR, Stephens TD, Tate P: *Anatomy & physiology*, ed 3, New York, 1995, McGraw-Hill.

CLINICAL FOCUS 7-2

Using the Alveolar Air Equation: Effect of Hypoventilation on Alveolar Partial Pressure of Oxygen When Room Air is Breathed

A healthy 60-year-old woman was brought to the emergency department in a comatose state, breathing very shallowly. The family stated that she had taken an excess number of sleeping pills. Arterial blood gases obtained while she was breathing room air (fractional concentration of oxygen in inspired gas [F_IO_2] = 0.21) revealed arterial oxygen partial pressure (PaO_2) of 55 mm Hg, partial pressure of carbon dioxide in arterial blood ($PaCO_2$) of 70 mm Hg, and pH of 7.15. Normal $PaCO_2$ is equal to 40 mm Hg. Her elevated $PaCO_2$ is explained by her hypoventilation; she cannot remove CO_2 from her lungs as rapidly as it diffuses in from the capillary blood. But why is her PaO_2 reduced?

Discussion

The high partial pressure of carbon dioxide in alveolar gas (P_ACO_2) of hypoventilation reduces the alveolar oxygen partial pressure (P_AO_2) and the PaO_2. This can be shown by calculating the P_AO_2 during hypoventilation ($PaCO_2$ = 70 mm Hg) and comparing it with P_AO_2 when ventilation is normal ($PaCO_2$ = 40 mm Hg), using the following alveolar air equation:

$$P_AO_2 = F_IO_2(PB - 47) - (PaCO_2 \times 1.2)$$

P_B represents barometric pressure.

Situation 1: Hypoventilation on Room Air, $PaCO_2$ = 70 mm Hg

$$0.21(760 - 47) - (70 \times 1.2)$$
$$= 0.21(713) - 84$$
$$= 149.73 - 84$$
$$P_AO_2 = 65.73 \text{ mm Hg}$$

Situation 2: Normal Ventilation on Room Air, $PaCO_2$ = 40 mm Hg

$$0.21(760 - 47) - (40 \times 1.2)$$
$$= 0.21(713) - 48$$
$$= 149.73 - 48$$
$$P_AO_2 = 101.73 \text{ mm Hg}$$

In situation 1, hypoventilation caused high $PaCO_2$, and low PaO_2 is a secondary consequence. Hypoventilation is the major abnormality present, not O_2 transfer across the lung. Correction of oxygenation in this situation involves improving the patient's ventilation, not administering O_2. Although administering O_2 might eliminate hypoxemia, it would not address the underlying defect (hypoventilation) that causes the hypoxemia.

D represents the diffusion coefficient (D), or diffusivity, of a particular gas. It is directly proportional to the gas solubility (sol) but inversely proportional to the square root of the gas molecular weight (mw):

$$D \propto \frac{sol}{\sqrt{mw}}$$

$P_1 - P_2$ represents the partial pressure difference across the membrane (i.e., diffusion pressure gradient [mm Hg]).

T represents the membrane thickness, or diffusion path distance (cm).

This equation states that $\dot{V}_{gas}$ increases if there are increases in the membrane surface area, gas diffusivity, or diffusion pressure gradient. The diffusion rate decreases if membrane thickness increases. Doubling the membrane surface area or diffusion pressure gradient doubles the overall diffusion rate; doubling the membrane thickness reduces the diffusion rate by half. Figure 7-3 illustrates the factors involved in Fick's law.

CONCEPT QUESTION 7-4

Why does exercise increase the diffusion rate of O_2?

Physical Gas Characteristics and Diffusion

O_2 and CO_2 diffuse through gaseous and liquid phases in the lung; the alveolar capillary membrane (see Figure 7-1) is a liquid barrier. Light gases diffuse more rapidly than heavier gases, and highly soluble gases diffuse through liquids more rapidly than less soluble gases. The rate of gas diffusion in the lung is inversely proportional to its molecular weight and directly

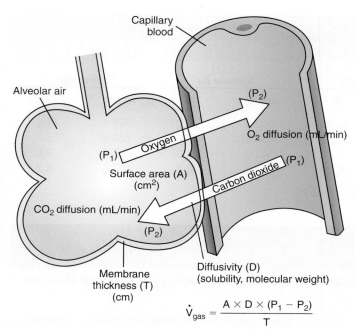

$$\dot{V}_{gas} = \frac{A \times D \times (P_1 - P_2)}{T}$$

Figure 7-3 Fick's law of diffusion states that oxygen and carbon dioxide diffuse from high (P_1) to low (P_2) pressures across the alveolar capillary membrane.

proportional to its solubility; the diffusion coefficient in Fick's law is derived from these two factors. Specifically, the gas diffusion rate is inversely proportional to the square root of its gram molecular weight (gmw) (**Graham's law**). Relative rates of diffusion for O_2 (molecular weight = 32) and CO_2 (molecular weight = 44) in a gaseous medium are as follows:

$$\frac{O_2 \text{ rate}}{CO_2 \text{ rate}} = \frac{\sqrt{gmwCO_2}}{\sqrt{gmwO_2}} = \frac{\sqrt{44}}{\sqrt{32}} = \frac{6.63}{5.66} = \frac{1.17}{1.0}$$

Because O_2 is a lighter molecule, it diffuses through a gas medium 1.17 times faster than CO_2.

Conversely, CO_2 is much more soluble in water than O_2. **Henry's law** states that the amount of gas dissolving in a liquid is directly proportional to the gas partial pressure. At body temperature (37° C) and 760 mm Hg pressure, 0.592 mL of CO_2 and 0.0244 mL of O_2 dissolve in 1 mL of water. CO_2 is about 24 times more soluble than O_2, as the following equation shows:

$$\frac{CO_2 \text{ sol}}{O_2 \text{ sol}} = \frac{0.592}{0.0244} = \frac{24.3}{1.0}$$

Combining Graham's law and Henry's law, CO_2 diffuses across the alveolar capillary membrane about 20 times faster than O_2. This is shown as follows:

$$\frac{CO_2 \text{ rate}}{O_2 \text{ rate}} = \frac{\sqrt{32}}{\sqrt{44}} \times \frac{0.592}{0.0244} = \frac{3.35}{0.16} = 20.7$$

For this reason, alveolar capillary membrane defects limit O_2 diffusion long before they limit CO_2 diffusion. In a practical clinical sense, the alveolar capillary membrane never limits outward diffusion of CO_2 from blood to alveoli. Discussion of diffusion in this chapter is therefore primarily focused on O_2 diffusion.

LIMITATIONS OF OXYGEN DIFFUSION

Factors influencing the rate of O_2 transfer across the alveolar capillary membrane include (1) the partial pressure gradient across the membrane, (2) the diffusion path length, and (3) the membrane surface area. (All factors are included in Fick's law of diffusion.)

Effects of the Partial Pressure Gradient and Capillary Blood Transit Time on Gas Equilibrium

At a resting cardiac output, a red blood cell spends about 0.75 second traveling through the pulmonary capillary. Normally, the equilibrium between alveolar gas and capillary blood PO_2 occurs within 0.25 second, or about one third of the distance through the capillary (Figure 7-4, *dark curved line*). The time to reach equilibrium may be prolonged if alveolar capillary membranes are thickened (*light curved line* in Figure 7-4). Even so, equilibrium is virtually always achieved at rest. The rate of diffusion is rapid at first when the partial pressure gradient across the alveolar capillary membrane is greatest. The diffusion rate continuously slows as the partial pressure gradient diminishes (notice the shape of the PO_2 curve [*dark line*] in Figure 7-4) until diffusion completely ceases at equilibrium. Thus, during the last two thirds of travel through the pulmonary capillary, no diffusion normally occurs.

Even when capillary transit time is shortened to 0.25 second by a high blood flow rate during exercise, complete O_2 equilibrium normally occurs between alveolar gas and end-capillary blood; it simply occurs at some point farther along the capillary path. In such a situation, the number of O_2 molecules transferred into the blood each minute is greatly increased because the greater rate of blood flow takes up more O_2 molecules from the alveoli each minute. Another reason exercise increases the number of O_2 molecules transferred each minute is that previously nonperfused capillaries are recruited, which increases the surface area for diffusion.

If a healthy person exercises vigorously at a high altitude, where atmospheric PO_2 is very low, the O_2 diffusion gradient may be so low that O_2 cannot diffuse across the alveolar capillary membrane fast enough to establish equilibrium during the shortened capillary transit time. Alternatively, if disease thickens the alveolar capillary membrane, the diffusion rate across the membrane may be slowed enough to prevent complete O_2 equilibrium by the time blood leaves the capillary. In the clinical setting, this situation rarely occurs at rest, even in severe lung disease.[2] However, exercise immediately exposes the diffusion abnormality problem because it shortens the blood's transit time through the capillary, making it likely that alveolar and capillary O_2 equilibrium never occurs (Figure 7-5). Patients with thickened alveolar capillary membranes are most likely to show evidence of O_2 diffusion impairment during exercise.[3]

Perfusion and Diffusion Limitations to Oxygen Transfer

Figure 7-4 shows that diffusion normally stops when O_2 equilibrium is reached between the alveolus and capillary, which occurs

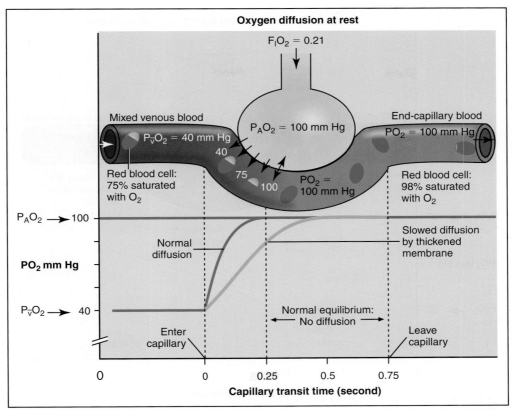

Figure 7-4 Resting capillary transit time and gas pressure equilibrium time for pulmonary blood flow. Oxygen diffusion normally ceases after blood traverses one third of the capillary distance (within 0.25 second) because alveolar and capillary partial pressures of oxygen (PO_2) equilibrate. PO_2 equilibrium usually occurs even across alveolar capillary membranes thickened by disease. Oxygen diffusion is normally perfusion limited.

long before the blood travels the length of the capillary. If blood flow (perfusion) increases, more O_2 leaves the lung each minute because the O_2-saturated blood moves out of the capillary more quickly, which means deoxygenated blood enters more quickly to take up more O_2. Therefore the O_2 diffusion rate through the alveolar-capillary membrane is normally perfusion limited (see Figure 7-4); that is, a change in blood flow rate alters the number of O_2 molecules that cross the alveolar-capillary membrane each minute. If O_2 equilibrium between the alveolus and capillary never occurs because of thickened membranes, O_2 transfer is truly diffusion limited. In such an instance, it is the alveolar capillary membrane, not blood flow rate, that influences the O_2 transfer rate (see Figure 7-5).

CONCEPT QUESTION 7-5

In what way would changes in pulmonary blood flow interfere with the measurement of diffusion capacity of the lung for O_2 (as opposed to carbon monoxide)?

If one wishes to evaluate the extent to which the alveolar capillary membrane itself impedes the diffusion rate (milliliters per minute of O_2 transfer per millimeters of mercury pressure gradient), one should not measure the O_2 diffusion rate because it is affected by blood flow rate. Instead, one should measure the diffusion rate of a gas that never reaches equilibrium between

alveolar gas and capillary blood, even in resting conditions. In other words, the blood's capacity for this gas should be so great that the gas cannot diffuse across the membrane fast enough to saturate the blood to capacity before it leaves the capillary. For such a gas, the only factor that limits diffusion is the resistance of the alveolar capillary membrane itself. Carbon monoxide (CO) is the ideal gas for this kind of measurement because blood can absorb it at a greater rate than CO can diffuse across the alveolar capillary membrane, even under resting conditions. For this reason, CO is always diffusion limited. Figure 7-6 illustrates the diffusion-limited characteristics of CO. All events that are illustrated in Figure 7-6 occur at rest; increased blood flow cannot result in greater CO uptake because CO is already diffusing through the alveolar-capillary membrane at its maximum rate. For this reason, CO is commonly used in pulmonary function laboratories to evaluate the lung's true diffusion capacity.

CONCEPT QUESTION 7-6

What is the main reason CO_2 diffuses across the alveolar capillary membrane so much more rapidly than O_2?

Hemoglobin in the blood makes O_2 and CO much more soluble in whole blood than they are in the alveolar-capillary membrane fluid or the blood plasma. In contrast, a gas such as nitrous oxide (N_2O), highly soluble in the alveolar-capillary membrane

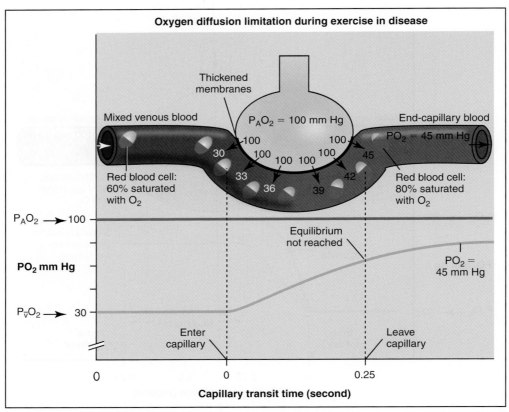

Figure 7-5 Exercise increases blood flow velocity, shortening capillary transit time. In this situation, diseased, thickened alveolar capillary membranes slow the diffusion rate enough to prevent oxygen equilibrium by the time blood leaves the capillary. Exercise unmasks diffusion defects not apparent at rest (compare with Figure 7-4).

and plasma, does not chemically bind with hemoglobin; its solubility in whole blood is much less than that of CO or O_2. If N_2O is inhaled, the pulmonary capillary blood reaches its maximum capacity for N_2O almost instantly (Figure 7-7). N_2O partial pressures across the alveolar capillary membrane reach equilibrium in the first one twentieth of the distance along the capillary.

Increased blood flow causes N_2O-saturated blood to exit the capillary sooner, allowing more mixed venous blood to enter and take up alveolar N_2O. Thus, diffusion of N_2O in the lung is strictly perfusion limited. This characteristic makes N_2O an ideal test gas to measure pulmonary blood flow.

O_2 diffusion is normally perfusion limited because it equilibrates across the alveolar capillary membrane long before blood leaves the capillary; increased blood flow increases the amount of O_2 taken up from the alveolus. Exercise increases blood flow and may cause O_2 to become diffusion limited if the alveolar capillary membrane is thickened.

Diffusion Path Length

The distance for diffusion includes the entire path length from alveolar gas to the hemoglobin in the red blood cell. It was originally thought that the alveolar capillary membrane was the only important rate-limiting barrier to diffusion; it is now known that the red blood cell membrane and rate of O_2 combined with hemoglobin limit the lung's O_2 uptake to the same extent

as the alveolar-capillary membrane.[4] The total diffusion path distance is normally less than 0.1 μ and includes the following (see Figure 7-1): (1) surfactant layer that is lining the alveolar surface, (2) alveolar epithelium, (3) basement membrane of the alveolar epithelium, (4) extremely thin interstitial space, (5) basement membrane of the capillary endothelium, (6) capillary endothelium, (7) plasma, (8) red blood cell membrane, and (9) intracellular fluid bathing the hemoglobin molecule.

Various abnormal conditions can increase the diffusion path length, including the following: (1) fibrotic thickening of alveolar and capillary walls; (2) interstitial edema fluid, separating alveolar and capillary membranes; (3) fluid in the alveoli; (4) interstitial fibrotic processes that thicken the interstitial space; and (5) dilated, engorged capillaries, which allow red blood cells to flow side by side. Abnormalities that increase the distance for diffusion are rarely the cause of decreased end-capillary or arterial PO_2 at rest. The major cause of resting hypoxemia in these patients is a mismatch between ventilation and blood flow.[2] That is, the processes that increase diffusion distance generally decrease lung compliance, which decreases ventilation in these areas. Blood perfusing these underventilated areas tends to be inadequately oxygenated.

Diffusion Surface Area

Diffusion surface area is the total area of contact between ventilated alveoli and perfused capillaries. A decrease in the

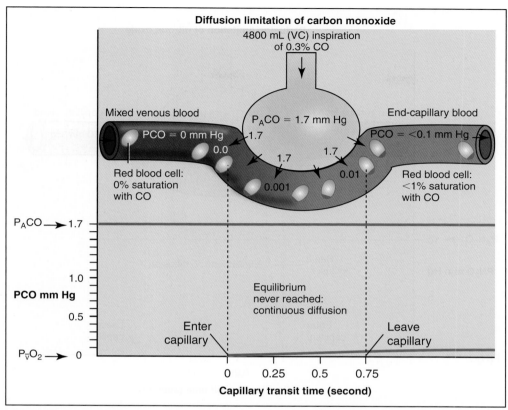

Figure 7-6 Hemoglobin removes carbon monoxide (CO) so rapidly from the plasma that it maintains the diffusion gradient of CO all along the capillary. This makes CO the ideal test gas for evaluating diffusion defects. Hemoglobin removes CO from the plasma faster than it can diffuse across the alveolar capillary membrane. The only factor limiting CO diffusion is the membrane itself.

number of open, perfused capillaries or in the number of open, ventilated alveoli decreases the diffusion surface area and the lung's diffusion capacity. In such instances, diffusion capacity is decreased, although the diffusion path length may be normal at all points. For example, emphysema destroys alveolar walls and their associated capillaries, which decreases the diffusion surface area. Although the diffusion path length is not thickened at any point, overall diffusion rate is decreased because much of the functional gas-exchange surface area is lost.

CONCEPT QUESTION 7-7

Pulmonary embolism blocks blood flow to alveolar capillaries; completely obstructed airways block ventilation to alveoli. What category of diffusion limitation do these two defects represent?

MEASURING DIFFUSION CAPACITY

General Principles

A diffusion-limited test gas such as CO is used to measure the diffusion capacity of the lung. As clinically performed, the **single breath CO diffusion test** measures the amount (in milliliters) of CO that diffuses out of the lung into the pulmonary capillaries during a 10-second breath-holding period after first inhaling a known concentration of CO. The average diffusion

pressure gradient also must be calculated during the breath-holding period, that is, mean P_ACO − mean capillary PCO. (Partial pressure of CO in the capillary blood is denoted by the symbol PćCO). The theoretical formula for the **diffusion capacity of the lung for CO (D_LCO)** is as follows:

$$D_LCO = \frac{\text{milliliters of CO transferred to the blood per minute}}{\text{mean } P_ACO - \text{mean capillary PćCO}}$$

Normal Values

Normal D_LCO values in healthy individuals vary considerably depending on age, body size, and body position as explained in subsequent sections. A large cross-sectional study of healthy, never-smoking adult men and women in the United States yielded a mean D_LCO of 26.4 mL/min/mm Hg (single breath testing method).[5] The mean D_LCO was about 33 mL/min/mm Hg in men and about 24 mL/min/mm Hg in women. The diffusion capacity of the lung for oxygen (D_LO_2) is obtained by multiplying D_LCO by 1.23. A mean D_LCO of 26 mL/min/mm Hg yields a normal D_LO_2 of about 32 mL/min/mm Hg. It may seem odd that D_LO_2 is greater than D_LCO, considering the much greater affinity of hemoglobin for CO than O_2. This peculiarity is explained by the fact that O_2 is more soluble than CO in the alveolar capillary membrane and the plasma and diffuses more rapidly. The fact that hemoglobin has 210 times greater affinity

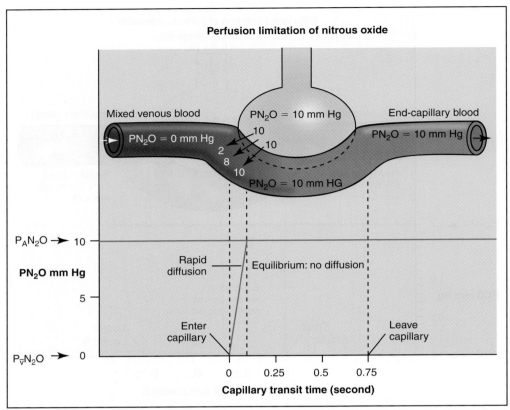

Figure 7-7 Nitrous oxide (N_2O) is extremely soluble in the alveolar capillary membrane and plasma but does not combine with hemoglobin (no red blood cells are shown). Plasma N_2O pressure reaches equilibrium with alveolar N_2O almost instantly. The rate of N_2O uptake by the blood depends strictly on the blood flow rate.

for CO than O_2 simply means that at a given partial pressure (PCO or PO_2), the hemoglobin carries more CO than O_2. This fact is unrelated to O_2 and CO diffusion rate across the alveolar capillary membrane, which is determined by molecular weight and solubility coefficients.

Factors Affecting Measured Carbon Monoxide Diffusion in the Lung

Body Size

D_LCO increases with body size. Larger lungs have a greater absolute D_LCO than smaller lungs because they have a greater gas-exchange surface area.

Age

D_LCO increases as the lungs develop from infancy to adulthood. In people older than 20 years, D_LCO decreases gradually as the lung ages and structural changes reduce the functional gas-exchange surface area. A 10-year age increase is associated with a decline of about 1.32 mL/min/mm Hg in D_LCO.

Lung Volume

D_LCO is significantly greater at high lung volumes than low volumes. This may reflect increased pulmonary blood volume at high lung volumes (greater subatmospheric pressure near total

lung capacity [TLC] draws more blood into the pulmonary circulation) or an increased functional surface area for diffusion. Dividing D_LCO by the lung volume at which it was measured (D_LCO per unit of lung volume [D_L/V_L]) eliminates the effect of volume on D_LCO. For example, the abnormally large lung volume of a patient with emphysema may have a total D_LCO in the normal range, obscuring the true decrease in surface area per unit of lung volume. Calculating the D_L/V_L in this instance yields an abnormally low value, revealing the loss of diffusion capacity.

Exercise

D_LCO increases markedly with exercise as previously unperfused capillaries are recruited; this greatly increases the surface area for diffusion. Increased cardiac output means capillary transit time decreases, and more O_2 can be transferred into the blood each minute. During exercise (in contrast to rest), blood stays in the capillary only long enough to reach equilibrium with alveolar gas. Increased cardiac output dilates capillaries, exposing more hemoglobin to alveolar gas and allowing greater O_2 uptake per minute.

Body Position

D_LCO is 15% to 20% greater in supine than in standing positions.[4] This is probably because gravitational effects decrease pulmonary blood volume in the standing position.

CLINICAL FOCUS 7-3

Technique for Measuring Carbon Monoxide Diffusion in the Lung

When measuring the carbon monoxide diffusion in the lung (D_LCO), a volume of gas equal to vital capacity containing about 0.3% CO is inhaled through a tube attached to a spirometer. This means the patient first exhales forcefully to the residual volume (RV), then inhales the CO gas mixture maximally to total lung capacity (TLC). This breath is held at TLC for 10 seconds, after which the vital capacity is forcefully exhaled back to the RV level. As the exhalation approaches RV, a gas sample from the exhaled stream is collected in a small balloon by opening a valve in the apparatus. This gas represents the composition of alveolar gas. The amount of CO that diffused into the blood is calculated by analyzing the alveolar gas sample for CO and comparing it with the calculated initial alveolar CO concentration. (The amount diffusing in 10 seconds is multiplied by 6 to obtain the amount diffusing in 1 minute.) The spirometer's microprocessor performs a complicated calculation of the average CO diffusion gradient over the 10-second breath-holding interval. The calculation is complicated because it is not simply the average of beginning and final PCO diffusion gradients but the average of an infinite number of continuously changing pressure gradients occurring over 10 seconds. The pressure gradient driving CO diffusion changes continuously as pressures between alveolus and capillary approach equilibrium. This means the CO diffusion rate changes continuously over the 10-second breath-hold period as well. (Note the changing pressure gradient examples in Figure 7-6.) The microprocessor calculates the average diffusion rate in units of milliliters per minute per millimeter of mercury (mL/min/mm Hg).

CLINICAL FOCUS 7-4

Abnormally High and Abnormally Low Lung Volumes: Mechanisms of Reduced Carbon Monoxide Diffusion in the Lung

A person with advanced pulmonary emphysema and a total lung capacity (TLC) 150% of the predicted value has an abnormally low carbon monoxide diffusion capacity (D_LCO). Another person with advanced pulmonary fibrosis and a TLC 60% of the predicted value also has a low D_LCO. What are the mechanisms producing the low D_LCO in these two people?

Discussion

Emphysema, an obstructive lung disease, destroys alveolar walls and their capillaries, reducing elastic recoil and functional tissue for gas exchange. D_LCO is decreased because less gas can diffuse into the blood per unit of lung tissue. A loss of elastic lung tissue increases lung compliance, which eventually leads to increased TLC.

Pulmonary fibrosis is characterized by inflammation and scar tissue in the alveolar capillary area. This scar tissue stiffens the lungs, creating high elastic recoil, low lung compliance, and a reduced TLC. Alveolar capillary membranes are thickened, and some are destroyed. These defects slow the diffusion rate and reduce the gas-exchange surface area, decreasing D_LCO. Diffusing capacity is decreased when there is loss of functional alveolar capillary membranes, regardless of the lung volume.

Alveolar Partial Pressure of Oxygen and Partial Pressure of Carbon Dioxide

Increased P_AO_2 is associated with decreased D_LCO because in the blood O_2 competes with CO for binding sites on the hemoglobin molecule. In other words, the rate of CO uptake by hemoglobin is hindered by increased arterial PO_2 values but is enhanced by decreased arterial PO_2 values. People with severe hypoxia have higher D_LCO values because of this phenomenon and because hypoxia increases cardiac output, pulmonary blood flow, and capillary recruitment and distention.[4] This phenomenon also explains why elevated P_ACO_2 increases D_LCO; an elevated P_ACO_2 means hypoventilation is present, which means P_AO_2 is of necessity also low.

Alveolar Partial Pressure of Carbon Monoxide

Heavy smokers already have CO in their mixed venous blood. The presence of CO in mixed venous blood lowers the diffusion pressure gradient across the alveolar-capillary membrane and slows the diffusion rate.

Hemoglobin Concentration

The blood of patients with anemia has abnormally low hemoglobin content and low CO-carrying capacity. Less CO can be taken up per minute during the D_LCO test. The opposite is true for **polycythemia** (increased red blood cells and hemoglobin concentration).

Pulmonary Diseases

Box 7-1 lists conditions that decrease diffusion capacity. D_LCO is useful in differentiating emphysema from other obstructive diseases not associated with destroyed alveolar architecture, such as chronic bronchitis and asthma. Asthma is often associated with an increased D_LCO. An explanation may be that high inspiratory resistance created by narrowed airways increases negative intrathoracic pressure during maximal inspiration of the test gas, which increases the gas diffusion pressure gradient and the blood flow in lung apices.[6]

Clinical Use of Carbon Monoxide Diffusion in the Lung

The D_LCO test assesses the extent to which the alveolar capillary membrane is a barrier to gas diffusion. Because O_2 equilibrium normally occurs before blood traverses one third of the

BOX 7-1
Conditions That Decrease Diffusion Capacity

Increased Diffusion Path Distance
Interstitial or alveolar edema
Interstitial or alveolar fibrosis
Dilated, engorged capillaries (congestive heart failure)

Decreased Diffusion Surface Area
Destruction of alveolar capillary bed (emphysema)
Reduced capillary blood flow
Pulmonary embolus
Low cardiac output (heart failure and blood loss)
Tumors

Decreased Uptake by Red Blood Cells
Anemia
Low pulmonary capillary blood volume
High carbon monoxide blood levels (smokers)

Ventilation-Perfusion Mismatch (Low $\dot{V}/\dot{Q}$)
Obstructive lung diseases (reduced regional ventilation)
Atelectasis (small airway and alveolar collapse)
Pneumonia (fluid-filled alveoli)

CLINICAL FOCUS 7-5
Using Carbon Monoxide Diffusion in the Lung to Differentiate Emphysema from Chronic Bronchitis

You are asked to perform a complete pulmonary function study on a 53-year-old woman who has chronic obstructive pulmonary disease (COPD). Results show markedly reduced expiratory flow rates, increased residual volume (RV), and a normal carbon monoxide diffusing capacity (D_LCO). Later that day, you perform a pulmonary function study on a 55-year-old woman who also has COPD. Her results show markedly reduced expiratory flow rates, increased RV, and an abnormally low D_LCO. Why is D_LCO reduced in only one of these women, even though they both have COPD?

Discussion
Emphysema and chronic bronchitis both cause chronic airflow obstruction but in different ways. Emphysema destroys alveolar structures, including the gas-exchange surface area. This destruction decreases the D_LCO. Chronic bronchitis refers to chronic airway inflammation and overproduction of abnormally thick mucus, which may partially obstruct the airways. The alveolar surface area for gas exchange remains intact, maintaining a normal D_LCO.

The first woman had a bronchitic component of COPD. The second woman had a predominantly emphysematous component of COPD.

pulmonary capillary distance, a 50% reduction in D_LCO can exist without affecting end-capillary and arterial PO_2. In this sense, the D_LCO test is more sensitive than the PaO_2 to potential O_2 transfer problems (i.e., as disease progresses, D_LCO becomes abnormal before PaO_2). Impairment of diffusion across the alveolar capillary membrane is only one mechanism that can cause arterial hypoxemia. Many factors decrease PaO_2 without affecting the diffusion path length or membrane surface area, such as ventilation–blood flow mismatches. The D_LCO test can help clarify the mechanism of arterial hypoxemia; if D_LCO is normal, diffusion impairment cannot be a contributing factor.

CONCEPT QUESTION 7-8

As alveolar capillary membranes gradually thicken in the course of disease, the O_2 diffusion rate gradually decreases. Which test reveals this problem first: the D_LCO test or the blood gas analysis that measures arterial blood PO_2? Explain.

POINTS TO REMEMBER

- Gas always diffuses from an area of high partial pressure to an area of low partial pressure.
- Diffusion ceases when partial pressure equilibrium across the alveolar capillary membrane occurs; this normally occurs for O_2 long before blood flows through the length of the capillary.
- Gas transfer from alveolus to blood is diffusion limited if blood is able to take up the gas faster than the gas can diffuse through the alveolar capillary membrane.
- Gas transfer from alveolus to blood is perfusion limited if its pressures in the alveolus and blood equalize so quickly that diffusion ceases before blood leaves the capillary.
- Diffusion impairments rarely cause hypoxemia at rest because gas equilibrium between alveolus and blood virtually always occurs; exercise unmasks the impairment because blood flows so fast that there is not enough time for equilibrium to occur.
- Diffusion rate is affected by membrane functional surface area, physical gas characteristics, partial pressure gradient for diffusion, and membrane thickness (diffusion path length).
- Light and soluble gases diffuse faster than heavy insoluble gases; because of its much greater solubility, CO_2 diffuses across the lung 20 times faster than O_2.
- Diseases affect diffusion capacity chiefly by increasing the membrane thickness or decreasing the functional surface area.
- D_LCO can be significantly reduced before any decrease in arterial PO_2 occurs.

References

1. Martin L: Abbreviating the alveolar gas equation: an argument for simplicity, *Respir Care* 31:40, 1986.
2. Hegewald MJ, Crapo RO: Pulmonary function testing. In Mason RJ, et al, editor: *Murray and Nadel's textbook of respiratory medicine*, ed 5, Philadelphia, 2010, Saunders.

3. West JB: *Respiratory physiology: the essentials*, ed 8, Baltimore, 2008, Lippincott Williams & Wilkins.

4. Hughes JM, Bates DV: Historical review: the carbon monoxide diffusing capacity (DLCO) and its membrane (DM) and red cell (Theta. Vc) components, *Respir Physiol Neurobiol* 138(2-3):115, 2003.

5. Neas LM, Schwartz J: The determinants of pulmonary diffusing capacity in a national sample of U.S. adults, *Am J Respir Crit Care Med* 153(2):656, 1996.

6. Saydain G, et al: Clinical significance of elevated diffusing capacity, *Chest* 125(2):446, 2004.

CHAPTER 8

Oxygen Equilibrium and Transport

OBJECTIVES

After reading this chapter, you will be able to:

- Describe how the blood takes up, transports, and releases oxygen
- Explain the difference between arterial and venous oxygen contents, and how they are related to oxygen consumption and cardiac output
- Show how oxygen content, oxygen saturation, oxygen partial pressure (PO_2), and hemoglobin concentration are related to each other
- Explain why the hemoglobin-oxygen binding process produces a sigmoid-shaped rather than linear PO_2-hemoglobin equilibrium curve
- Explain why the sigmoid-shaped oxyhemoglobin equilibrium curve is physiologically advantageous
- Describe how various factors affect the release and binding of oxygen by changing affinity of hemoglobin for oxygen
- Explain why a change in the value of P_{50} means hemoglobin's affinity for oxygen has changed
- Explain why changes in cardiac output affect mixed venous PO_2, the difference between arterial and mixed venous oxygen content, and the amount of oxygen the tissues extract from the arterial blood each minute

- Calculate oxygen delivery rate, oxygen consumption, and tissue oxygen-extraction percentage
- Explain why arterial oxygen partial pressure (PaO_2) and arterial oxygen saturation (SaO_2) are insufficient indicators of tissue oxygenation
- Explain why PaO_2 is a more sensitive indicator than SaO_2 of changes in the lung's ability to oxygenate the blood
- Define critical oxygen delivery threshold
- Explain why cyanosis may be absent in people who have high percentages of desaturated hemoglobin and why cyanosis may be present in people who have normal arterial oxygen contents
- Describe how anemia caused by low hemoglobin content differs physiologically from anemia produced by carbon monoxide poisoning
- Explain how fetal hemoglobin, methemoglobin, and sickle cell hemoglobin differ physiologically from normal hemoglobin

anemia
arterial oxygen content (CaO_2)
arterial oxygen saturation (SaO_2)
arterial-venous oxygen content difference ($C(a-\bar{v})O_2$)
Bohr effect
carbaminohemoglobin
cyanosis
deoxyhemoglobin (Hb)
HbO_2 equilibrium curve
hypothermia

ischemia
methemoglobin (metHb)
mixed venous oxygen saturation ($S_{\bar{v}}O_2$)
mL/dL
oxygen-extraction ratio (O_2 ER)
oxyhemoglobin (HbO_2)
thromboemboli

HOW DOES BLOOD CARRY OXYGEN?

Mixed venous blood enters the pulmonary capillary with a partial pressure of oxygen (PO_2) of about 40 mm Hg and is exposed to an alveolar partial pressure of oxygen (P_AO_2) of about 100 mm Hg. Oxygen (O_2) diffuses down this pressure gradient into the blood until equilibrium is established. Both liquid (plasma) and cellular (erythrocytes) components of blood carry O_2. O_2 is dissolved in plasma and bound to hemoglobin in the erythrocyte.

Oxygen Dissolved in Plasma

The amount (in milliliters) of O_2 that dissolves in plasma is determined by the P_AO_2 to which the plasma is exposed (Henry's law). The relationship between PO_2 and dissolved O_2 is linear (i.e., doubling or tripling PO_2 doubles or triples the amount of dissolved O_2) (Figure 8-1). Chapter 7 explained that the solubility coefficient of O_2 is 0.0244 mL O_2/mL plasma/atmosphere of pressure (atm). This means a PO_2 of 760 mm Hg causes 0.0244 mL of O_2 to dissolve in 1 mL of plasma at a body

temperature of 37° C (Figure 8-2, *A*). It also means that a PO_2 of only 1 mm Hg causes 0.00003 mL of O_2 to dissolve in 1 mL of plasma, as shown in Figure 8-2, *B* (0.0244/760 = 0.00003). By convention, blood O_2 content units are expressed in milliliters of O_2 per 100 mL of blood, or **mL/dL**. (The unit mL/dL has replaced the outdated term vol%.) To express O_2 content in its proper units, the amount of O_2 that dissolves in 100 mL of plasma for each millimeter of mercury (mm Hg) of PO_2 is 0.003 mL/dL (0.00003 mL O_2/mL plasma/mm Hg × 100 mL plasma = 0.003 mL/dL/mm Hg, as shown in Figure 8-2, *C*). At a normal arterial partial pressure of oxygen (PaO_2) of 100 mm Hg, 0.3 mL of O_2 dissolves in 100 mL of plasma, or 0.3 mL/dL (PO_2 of 100 mm Hg × 0.003 mL/dL/mm Hg = 0.3 mL/dL dissolved O_2, as Figure 8-2, *D*, shows). The 0.003 factor can be used to calculate dissolved plasma O_2 content at any PO_2 as follows:

$$PO_2 \times 0.003 = \text{mL/dL dissolved } O_2$$

PO_2 in the blood plasma is sometimes called the blood's O_2 tension, which comes from the concept that dissolved gases have an "escaping tendency." That is, if the PO_2 of a gas to which the plasma is exposed suddenly decreased, dissolved O_2 would immediately diffuse out of the plasma into the gaseous phase. Although it is correct to think of PO_2 as a force that dissolves O_2 in the plasma, it is also correct to think of dissolved O_2 as creating a force as it tries to escape to the gaseous phase—a force responsible for the plasma PO_2. The plasma PO_2 is extremely important in determining the adequacy of blood and tissue oxygenation because it determines the direction and rate of O_2 diffusion in the lungs and body tissues. Plasma PO_2 is intimately related to how O_2 binds with hemoglobin, as described later in this chapter.

CONCEPT QUESTION 8-1

What is the PO_2 of normal plasma with a dissolved O_2 content of 1.8 mL/dL?

Oxygen Combined with Hemoglobin

Most O_2 in the blood is bound to hemoglobin inside the erythrocyte. Without hemoglobin, blood could not carry enough O_2 to meet minimal tissue oxygenation requirements.

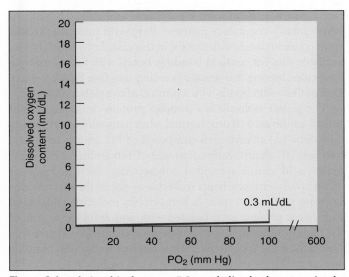

Figure 8-1 Relationship between PO_2 and dissolved oxygen in the blood plasma (dissolved O_2 in mL/dL = PO_2 × 0.003).

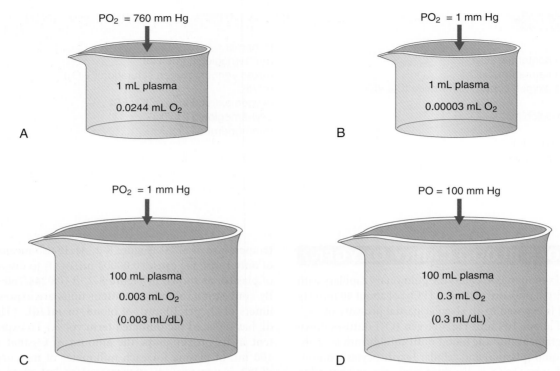

Figure 8-2 Solubility coefficient of oxygen in blood plasma at 37° C. **A,** At 1 atm (760 mm Hg) of oxygen pressure, 0.0244 mL of oxygen dissolves in 1 mL of plasma. **B,** 1 / 760 of this amount dissolves in 1 mL of plasma at a PO_2 of 1 mm Hg. **C,** 100 times the amount in **B** dissolves in 100 mL of plasma. **D,** At a normal arterial PO_2 of 100 mm Hg, 100 times the amount of oxygen dissolved in **C** dissolves in 100 mL of plasma; normal dissolved oxygen content in arterial blood is about 0.3 mL/dL.

Hemoglobin allows whole blood (plasma plus cellular components) to carry about 20 mL of O_2 per 100 mL of blood at a normal PaO_2 of 100 mm Hg. This is about 67 times more than the capacity of plasma alone when PaO_2 is 100 mm Hg ([20 mL/ dL]/[0.3 mL/dL] = 66.6). A normal cardiac output ($\dot{Q}$) of 5 L per minute delivers about 1000 mL of O_2 to the body's tissues each minute. This is more than enough O_2 to meet the resting requirement of tissues, which is only 250 mL per minute. This is shown as follows:

1. **mL O_2/L blood = 20 mL O_2/100 mL blood × 10 dL/L = 200 mL O_2/L**
2. **O_2 DEL = 5 L/min blood flow × 200 mL O_2/L = 1000 mL O_2/min**

Oxygen delivery (O_2 DEL) rate is normally about four times the resting requirement of the body tissues. From another perspective, the tissues normally extract only one fourth of the O_2 present in the blood they receive. The remaining three fourths (750 mL per minute) is an available reserve for increased metabolic demands.

Hemoglobin Molecule

Hemoglobin is a large, complex protein molecule found inside the erythrocyte. It has a molecular weight of about 64,500 and accounts for about one third of the red blood cell volume. Because hemoglobin exists inside the red blood cell, high concentrations can be carried without affecting the blood's oncotic pressure.

As its name suggests, hemoglobin consists of heme (an iron-containing pigment) and globin (a protein). Heme is an organic molecule consisting of four symmetrically linked pyrrole rings, with a ferrous iron ion (Fe^{++}) at its center (Figure 8-3, A-C). A pyrrole is an organic molecule organized in a ringlike structure. In addition to carbon atoms, a nitrogen atom helps form the ring. Pyrroles are building blocks for respiratory pigments that take up O_2. The four pyrrole rings are linked with methylene bridges (see Figure 8-3, B) to form a porphyrin molecule, the basis for hemoglobin's respiratory pigment. Porphyrin molecules readily form covalent bonds with metals. In this case, Fe^{++}, which has six available sites for covalent bonding, bonds with four porphyrin molecules, leaving two unused bonding sites (see Figure 8-3, C). One of these sites bonds with a portion of the globin molecule.

The globin molecule is a complex protein consisting of four linked amino acid chains; normal adult hemoglobin (HbA) has two alpha (α) chains, each composed of 141 amino acids, and two beta (β) chains, each composed of 146 amino acids. These amino acid chains are called polypeptides. Each polypeptide chain bonds with one heme molecule at one of the two remaining sites of the Fe^{++} ion. A hemoglobin molecule consists of four heme groups, each bonded with and enfolded in one of the globin molecule's four polypeptide chains (see Figure 8-3, D). Each of the four heme groups has one remaining bonding site on the Fe^{++} ion. This sixth site binds rapidly and reversibly with an O_2 molecule, but iron remains in the nonoxidized, ferrous state (Fe^{++}). Because each of the four polypeptide-heme

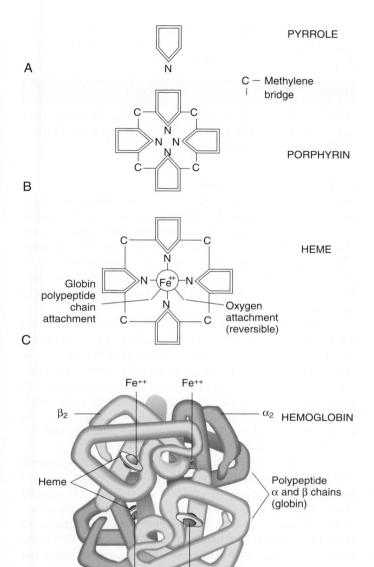

Figure 8-3 Hemoglobin molecule. Pyrrole rings (**A**) linked by methylene bridges form porphyrin molecules (**B**), which form covalent bonds with iron to form heme (**C**). The two remaining bonding sites on the Fe^{++} ion bond with a globin polypeptide chain and an oxygen molecule. Each of the four polypeptide chains of the globin molecule bind with a heme group to form the hemoglobin molecule (**D**).

combinations can bind one molecule of O_2, a single hemoglobin molecule can bind four O_2 molecules. The hemoglobin molecule is called a tetramer because it contains four polypeptide subunits.

By themselves, heme, iron, and globin cannot take up O_2; all three must be combined chemically with ferrous iron in a precise spatial arrangement before O_2 can be taken up from the plasma. The precise amino acid sequence of each polypeptide chain is important for normal O_2 uptake. A variation in this sequence changes how readily hemoglobin binds O_2 (i.e., it changes the affinity of hemoglobin for O_2). Variations of HbA are discussed later in this chapter.

Hemoglobin Combined with Oxygen

Combined with O_2, hemoglobin is called **oxyhemoglobin** (**HbO_2**). O_2 does not normally oxidize hemoglobin; rather, it oxygenates hemoglobin. Unoxygenated hemoglobin is called **deoxyhemoglobin (Hb)**. The term "reduced" hemoglobin, which is sometimes used, is chemically incorrect because iron remains in the ferrous (Fe^{++}) state.

The four heme groups of the hemoglobin molecule take up and release their O_2 molecules in succession in a process known as cooperative O_2 binding.[1] The binding of an O_2 molecule to one heme group induces a structural change in the shape of the hemoglobin molecule, which increases the affinity of the next heme subunit for O_2. Binding of each O_2 molecule makes the remaining bonds occur with successively greater speed and ease. Similarly, the release of the first O_2 molecule facilitates the release of each remaining molecule. This cooperative binding mechanism is an efficient way to take up O_2 when PO_2 is increased (in the alveoli) and to release O_2 when PO_2 is decreased (in the body's tissues). Cooperative binding means that a hemoglobin molecule either is bound to four O_2 molecules or is bound to none. In other words, the hemoglobin molecule either is fully oxygenated or is fully deoxygenated.

The change in shape of the hemoglobin molecule that occurs as it binds and releases O_2 causes it to reflect and absorb light differently when it is oxygenated than when it is deoxygenated. This phenomenon is responsible for the bright red color of oxygenated hemoglobin and the deep purple color of deoxyhemoglobin. This difference in light absorption and reflection makes it possible to measure the amount of oxygenated hemoglobin present in a blood sample through a process known as spectrophotometry or, as it is clinically known, oximetry.

Hemoglobin Saturation and Oxygen Partial Pressure

Hemoglobin is 100% saturated with O_2 if every hemoglobin molecule is combined with four O_2 molecules. Saturation is expressed as the percentage of hemoglobin molecules in the blood that are oxygenated. Normally, at sea level about 97.5% of the hemoglobin molecules in arterial blood are oxygenated; the remaining 2.5% are unoxygenated. This means that **arterial oxygen saturation (SaO_2)** is about 97.5% at a normal PaO_2 of 100 mm Hg. Only 75% of the hemoglobin molecules in mixed venous blood are oxygenated. That is, **mixed venous oxygen saturation ($S\bar{v}O_2$)** is normally 75%, which corresponds to a partial pressure of oxygen in mixed venous blood ($P\bar{v}O_2$) of about 40 mm Hg.

Saturation can be thought of as a percentage of hemoglobin's capacity for O_2. An SaO_2 of 90% means the hemoglobin in the blood is carrying 90% of its O_2 capacity. Mixed venous blood hemoglobin normally carries only 75% of its O_2 capacity. It is important to understand that hemoglobin's O_2 saturation percentage is not a measure of blood O_2 content, nor is it relevant to the concentration of hemoglobin in the blood. In other words, 100% saturation does not automatically imply that blood O_2 content is normal or that hemoglobin concentration is normal. If hemoglobin concentration is low (as it is in **anemia**), blood O_2 content is low even if the hemoglobin present is 100% saturated with O_2. Likewise, low saturation does not automatically mean that blood O_2 content is below normal, although this is generally the meaning. For example, hemoglobin concentration may be abnormally high (polycythemia) in individuals who have chronic hypoxia, which makes it possible for blood O_2 content to be normal even though hemoglobin saturation percentage is below normal.

Hemoglobin Capacity for Oxygen

When hemoglobin is 100% saturated with O_2, each gram (g) of hemoglobin carries 1.34 mL of O_2. The normal concentration of hemoglobin in the blood ranges from 12 to 15 g per 100 mL blood (12 to 15 g/dL). Assuming a hemoglobin concentration of 15 g/dL, hemoglobin's O_2-carrying capacity (100% saturation) is as follows: $15 \times 1.34 = 20.1$ mL/dL. Mixed venous blood

CLINICAL FOCUS 8-1

Clinical Measurement of Blood Oxygen Saturation

The measurement of the oxygen saturation of hemoglobin in the clinical setting involves a process called spectrophotometry. Spectrophotometry measures light wavelengths. All substances absorb and emit a unique spectrum of light wavelengths, known as an absorption spectrum. Each form of hemoglobin (e.g., HbO_2, Hb, and carboxyhemoglobin [HbCO]) has its own absorption spectrum. A spectrophotometer specifically designed to measure the absorption spectra of various hemoglobin forms is called an oximeter.

An oximeter passes the light of specific wavelengths through a blood sample to a photodetector on the opposite side. The photodetector senses the light's intensity and converts it to a proportional electrical current. When light enters the blood sample, certain wavelengths may be absorbed, transmitted, or reflected. The greater the optical density or opaqueness of the blood sample, the less light can be transmitted through it. The oximeter differentiates between HbO_2 and deoxyhemoglobin based on their different absorption spectra and quantifies their concentrations. Oximeters that use only two light wavelengths can detect only Hb and HbO_2; they cannot detect other forms of hemoglobin such as HbCO. An instrument called a CO-oximeter distinguishes among all forms of hemoglobin and displays their relative percentages. CO-oximeters are used in blood gas laboratories with blood gas analyzers, allowing SaO_2 to be included in the blood gas report. Pulse oximeters are compact portable devices that pass two wavelengths of light through an extremity such as a finger or toe, sensing the absorption spectrum of arterial blood during the systolic pulse. These oximeters are convenient because they do not require blood sampling, but their accuracy is limited in the presence of abnormal hemoglobin forms.

(75% saturated) carries 15.1 mL/dL of O_2 (0.75×20.1), whereas arterial blood (97.5% saturated at PO_2 of 100 mm Hg) carries about 19.7 mL/dL of O_2 (0.975×20.1).

CONCEPT QUESTION 8-2

What is the O_2 content (mL/dL) of an anemic person's blood while breathing 100% O_2 (hemoglobin concentration 10 g/dL, PaO_2 550 mm Hg, and SaO_2 100%)?

Oxyhemoglobin Equilibrium Curve

The blood plasma PO_2 determines hemoglobin's saturation with O_2. The **HbO_2 equilibrium curve** (Figure 8-4), also known as the HbO_2 dissociation curve, shows the relationship between plasma PO_2 (horizontal axis) and the percentage of hemoglobin saturated with oxygen (SO_2) (vertical axis). Because SO_2 and O_2 content are directly related (as described in the foregoing section), either one can be plotted on the vertical axis of the curve (see Figure 8-4).

The HbO_2 equilibrium curve can be constructed by exposing whole blood (which in Figure 8-4 contains 15 g Hb per 100 mL blood) to gas mixtures with successively higher PO_2 values. The blood pH, PCO_2, and temperature are held constant throughout the process. When hemoglobin is 100% saturated, each gram carries 1.34 mL of O_2. Thus, 100% saturation corresponds to a hemoglobin O_2 content of 20.1 mL/dL (15 g/dL $\times$ 1.34 mL O_2/g = 20.1 mL/dL); 50% saturation corresponds to half this content, or 10.05 mL/dL.

In contrast to the relationship between dissolved O_2 content and PO_2 (see Figure 8-1), the relationship between PO_2 and hemoglobin saturation or O_2 content is nonlinear. The sigmoid shape of the HbO_2 curve (see Figure 8-4) is caused by the hemoglobin molecule's change in O_2 affinity as each O_2 molecule binds in succession with heme. The middle steep portion of the curve reflects the rapid loading or unloading of O_2 molecules after hemoglobin's binding or release of the first O_2 molecule. Small PO_2 changes cause large blood O_2 content changes in the middle steep portion of the curve (20 to 60 mm Hg). In contrast, large PO_2 changes cause small to minimal changes in O_2 content at the extreme flatter ends of the curve, especially the flat, right end (60 to 100 mm Hg).

CONCEPT QUESTION 8-3

Is the gain in blood O_2 content when PO_2 increases from 40 mm Hg to 60 mm Hg greater than, equal to, or less than the O_2 content gain when PO_2 increases from 100 mm Hg to 600 mm Hg?

Physiological Advantages of the Oxyhemoglobin Equilibrium Curve Shape

The shape of the HbO_2 equilibrium curve has important physiological consequences. As shown in Figure 8-5, the upper flat section between PO_2 values of 60 mm Hg and 100 mm Hg can be thought of as the association part of the curve because O_2 uptake in the lung normally occurs in this PO_2 range. The lower part of the curve (PO_2 <60 mm Hg) can be thought of as the

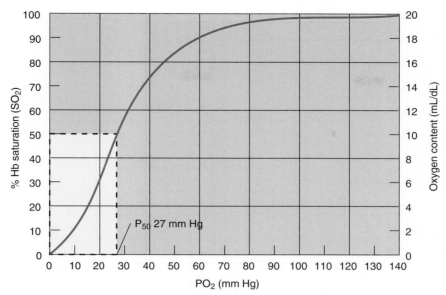

Figure 8-4 Oxyhemoglobin (HbO$_2$) equilibrium curve. P$_{50}$ is the PO$_2$ at which 50% of the hemoglobin is saturated with oxygen.

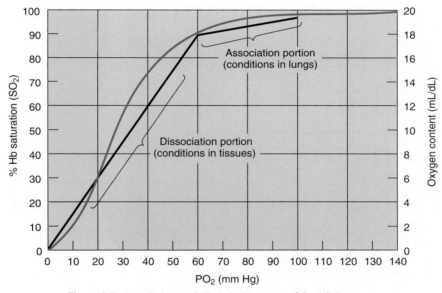

Figure 8-5 Association and dissociation parts of the HbO$_2$ curve.

dissociation part of the curve because O$_2$ release to the tissues occurs at these lower PO$_2$ values.

The flat association part of the HbO$_2$ curve provides a considerable safety margin in that blood PO$_2$ can decrease from 100 mm Hg to 60 mm Hg (Figure 8-6) and cause only a small reduction in blood O$_2$ content; SO$_2$ decreases only 7.5% (97.5% to 90%), corresponding to a reduction in **arterial oxygen content (CaO$_2$)** of only 1.5 mL/dL (19.6 mL/dL to 18.1 mL/dL). PaO$_2$ can decrease considerably without reducing the blood O$_2$ content significantly, as long as this occurs on the flat part of the HbO$_2$ curve; this is diagnostically important because a change in PaO$_2$ reflects oxygenation problems much sooner than a change in SaO$_2$. If the HbO$_2$ curve were linear rather than sigmoid, a reduction in PO$_2$ from 100 mm Hg to 60 mm Hg would greatly decrease SO$_2$ and O$_2$ content (Figure 8-7).

Increases in PO$_2$ above 60 mm Hg do not add much oxygen to the blood; this is especially true for PO$_2$ values greater than 100 mm Hg, where the HbO$_2$ curve is virtually flat. Likewise, maximal hyperventilation is ineffective in increasing SO$_2$ and O$_2$ content in healthy individuals; for example, extreme hyperventilation with room air at best might lower alveolar pressure of carbon dioxide (P$_A$CO$_2$) to about 15 mm Hg. According to the alveolar gas equation (see Chapter 7), this would produce a maximally attainable PO$_2$ in the alveolus of about 130 mm Hg and a slightly lower PO$_2$ in the arterial blood because of normal shunt. Even at a normal PaO$_2$ of 100 mm Hg when breathing room air, hemoglobin is already 97.5% saturated with O$_2$; technically, it is fully saturated at a PO$_2$ of about 250 mm Hg[2], although for all practical purposes, one can consider hemoglobin to be 100% saturated at a PO$_2$ of 130 mm Hg. Even increasing the PaO$_2$ to

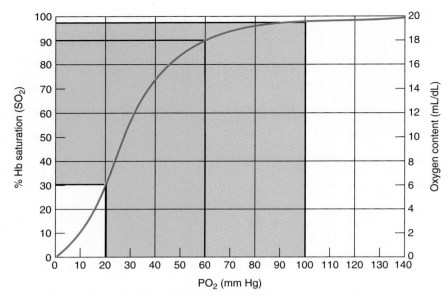

Figure 8-6 Significance of the HbO$_2$ curve shape. A 40-mm Hg decrease in PO$_2$ from 100 mm Hg to 60 mm Hg causes a 7.5% reduction in hemoglobin saturation (*pink area*). The same 40-mm Hg decrease in PO$_2$ from 60 mm Hg to 20 mm Hg causes a 60% reduction in hemoglobin saturation (*green area*).

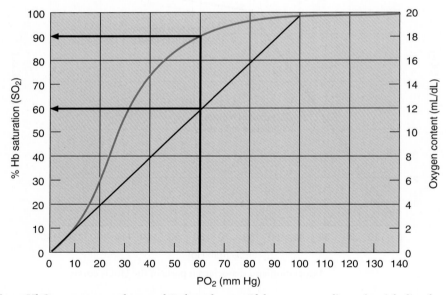

Figure 8-7 Hypothetical linear HbO$_2$ curve versus the actual S-shaped curve. If the curve were linear (straight line from 0 to 100 mm Hg), a PO$_2$ of 60 mm Hg would produce a HbO$_2$ saturation of 60 mm Hg and an oxygen content of 12 mL/dL instead of the actual saturation of 90% and oxygen content of 18 mL/dL.

600 mm Hg by breathing 100% O$_2$ increases SaO$_2$ by only 2.5%, from 97.5% to 100%. This increase adds only 0.5 mL/dL of O$_2$ to the blood (from 19.6 mL/dL to 20.1 mL/dL). The steep dissociation part of the HbO$_2$ curve is especially suited for releasing O$_2$ to the tissues, where the PO$_2$ is between 10 mm Hg and 40 mm Hg. A reduction in PO$_2$ from 60 mm Hg to 20 mm Hg causes SO$_2$ to decrease from 90% to about 32% (see Figure 8-6), corresponding to a reduction in CaO$_2$ of about 11.7 mL/dL (from 18.1 mL/dL to 6.4 mL/dL). Thus, hemoglobin releases about 11.7 mL/dL of O$_2$ into the plasma; this increases the plasma PO$_2$, which provides the pressure gradient for O$_2$ to diffuse into the tissues.

P$\bar{v}$O$_2$ reflects the average PO$_2$ of all body tissues and is normally about 40 mm Hg. A PO$_2$ of 40 mm Hg corresponds with about 75% Hb saturation with O$_2$. The body's tissues extract about 25% of the arterial O$_2$ content (about 5 mL/dL) under resting conditions. During heavy exercise, average tissue PO$_2$ may decrease to 20 mm Hg or less, and the tissues may extract 70% or more of the CaO$_2$ (Figure 8-8). Coupled with this greater O$_2$ extraction rate, cardiac output increases considerably—six or seven times the resting level in trained athletes—which can increase O$_2$ delivery to the tissues 20-fold.[1]

CLINICAL FOCUS 8-2

Sensitivity of Arterial Oxygen Saturation and Arterial Oxygen Partial Pressure to Decreased Blood Oxygen Content

You are called to the emergency department to draw arterial blood for blood gas analysis on a young teenager experiencing a severe asthma attack. Emergency department personnel assure you that the oxygen saturation, as obtained by a pulse oximeter, is "fine" at 90%. You are further informed that in the past 45 minutes the saturation decreased only "slightly" from 95% to 90%. The patient appears to be in significant respiratory distress. Before you draw the blood gas sample, what is your interpretation of the recent decrease in saturation from 95% to 90%?

Discussion

A health care provider's perspective suddenly changes when it is realized that a "slight" reduction in SaO_2 from 95% to 90% means that the PaO_2 decreased about 25 mm Hg, from 85 mm Hg to 60 mm Hg (see Figure 8-6). Health care personnel tend to be a bit more alarmed by a decrease in PaO_2 of this magnitude. The arterial oxygen content decreased only 5%. However, the PaO_2 of 60 mm Hg is on the "shoulder" of the curve. As the PO_2 falls below this point, sharp decreases in oxygen saturation and content occur for relatively small changes in PO_2. The important clinical point is that as a previously healthy person develops hypoxemia, changes in PaO_2 reflect oxygenation defects much sooner than changes in SaO_2. A decrease in a young person's PaO_2 from 85 mm Hg to 60 mm Hg indicates a significant change in the lung's oxygenation ability. The nature of hemoglobin's combination with oxygen during this decrease provides a protective margin of safety because blood oxygen content does not quickly decrease on the "flat" portion of the O_2-Hb equilibrium curve. At the same time, this protective mechanism masks the severity of the oxygenation defect. Changes in SaO_2 must be interpreted in light of the corresponding PaO_2 values to gain a true appreciation for changes in the lung's oxygenating ability.

Affinity of Hemoglobin for Oxygen

The O_2 pressure at which hemoglobin is half-saturated (P_{50}) is a measure of hemoglobin's affinity for O_2. Normally, a PO_2 of 27 mm Hg produces an SO_2 of 50% when the blood temperature is 37° C, pH is 7.40, and PCO_2 is 40 mm Hg (see Figure 8-4). An increased P_{50} means more than 27 mm Hg of PO_2 is required to saturate 50% of the hemoglobin. In this instance, one can think of Hb as being more "reluctant" to bind O_2, and greater pressure is required to make it do so. An increased P_{50} means hemoglobin's affinity for O_2 is decreased. Similarly, a decreased P_{50} means hemoglobin's affinity for O_2 is increased, causing it to bind O_2 molecules more aggressively (i.e., in this situation, hemoglobin saturation is >50% at a PO_2 of 27 mm Hg).

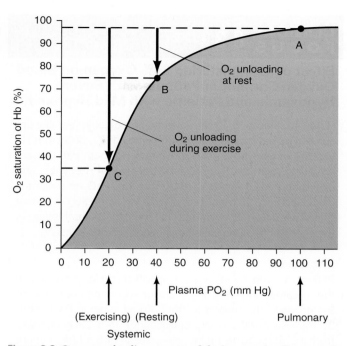

Figure 8-8 Oxygen unloading at rest and during exercise. Decreases in tissue PO_2 values occur on the steep part of the curve and cause greater oxygen unloading. (From Thibodeau GA, Patton KT: *Anatomy & physiology*, ed 3, St Louis, 1996, Mosby. Network Graphics.)

TABLE 8-1

Indicators of Hemoglobin Affinity for Oxygen

Increased Affinity	Decreased Affinity
Left HbO_2 curve shift	Right HbO_2 curve shift
Decreased P_{50} (<27 mm Hg)	Increased P_{50} (>27 mm Hg)
Greater SO_2 for given PO_2	Decreased SO_2 for given PO_2

HbO_2, Oxyhemoglobin; P_{50}, oxygen pressure producing 50% oxyhemoglobin; SO_2, oxygen saturation; PO_2, oxygen partial pressure.

In the alveoli where O_2 loading takes place, blood with a decreased P_{50} (high O_2 affinity) is advantageous. Conversely, high hemoglobin affinity for O_2 is detrimental at the tissue level where O_2 release is required. Ideally, hemoglobin affinity for O_2 changes depending on whether loading or unloading is required.

Oxyhemoglobin Curve Shifts

Factors that change Hb affinity for O_2 shift the HbO_2 curve to the left or to the right. Factors that increase Hb affinity for O_2 cause a leftward curve shift, or a decreased P_{50}; factors that decrease Hb affinity cause a rightward curve shift, or an increased P_{50} (Table 8-1). Figure 8-9 shows HbO_2 curves for blood passing through pulmonary capillaries (*left, blue curve*) and through systemic tissue capillaries of heavily exercising muscle (*right, red curve*). As blood from the lungs travels through the systemic tissue capillaries, the HbO_2 curve shifts rightward from the blue curve position in Figure 8-9 to the red curve position. This right shift reflects hemoglobin's

CLINICAL FOCUS 8-3

Effect of Administering 24% Oxygen on Blood Oxygen Content in Patients with Severe Hypoxemia and Patients with Mild Hypoxemia

Refer to Figure 8-4, the oxygen-hemoglobin equilibrium curve. You have two patients, one with a PaO_2 of 30 mm Hg and the other with a PaO_2 of 60 mm Hg; both patients are breathing room air. Both patients receive 24% oxygen, and each has a PaO_2 increase of 30 mm Hg; PaO_2 in patient A increased from 30 mm Hg to 60 mm Hg, and PaO_2 in patient B increased from 60 mm Hg to 90 mm Hg. Did both patients experience the same increase in blood oxygen content?

Discussion

Patient A, with an initial PaO_2 of 30 mm Hg, experienced the greatest increase in arterial oxygen content. Figure 8-4 provides the reason for this. An increase in PaO_2 from 30 mm Hg to 60 mm Hg corresponds to a CaO_2 increase from 12 mL/dL to 18 mL/dL, an increase of 6 mL/dL. Patient B had an equal increase in PaO_2, from 60 mm Hg to 90 mm Hg, which corresponds to a CaO_2 increase from 18 mL/dL to 19 mL/dL, an increase of 1 mL/dL. The reason is obvious on examining the oxygen-hemoglobin equilibrium curve; the curve is nearly flat beyond 60 mm Hg and quite steep from 30 mm Hg to 60 mm Hg. Equal PaO_2 increases do not produce equal CaO_2 increases; this explains why relatively low inspired oxygen concentrations are so effective in certain individuals who have severe hypoxemia. (This example is for illustration of the concept only; one would not give 24% oxygen to a patient with a life-threatening PaO_2 of 30 mm Hg.)

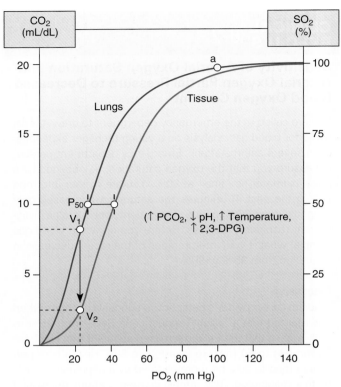

Figure 8-9 HbO_2 curve as blood passes through pulmonary (*blue curve*) and systemic (*red curve*) capillaries. These curve shifts facilitate oxygen uptake in the lung and oxygen release in the tissues. (From Berne RM, Levy MN: *Principles of physiology*, St Louis, 1990, Mosby.)

decreasing affinity for O_2 as blood enters systemic capillaries; this is shown by the increased P_{50}. Hemoglobin's decreased affinity for O_2 promotes the release of O_2 into the plasma, which increases plasma PO_2 and creates a gradient for O_2 to diffuse into the tissues. Listed to the right of the curves are factors that cause a decrease in hemoglobin affinity (increased blood PCO_2, decreased blood pH, increased blood temperature, and increased blood levels of the organic phosphate 2,3-diphosphoglycerate [2,3-DPG]).

Active tissue metabolism produces heat and carbon dioxide. Carbon dioxide combines with water to form carbonic acid (H_2CO_3), which produces hydrogen ions and decreases the pH. These factors shift the HbO_2 curve to the right, enhancing O_2 release to the tissues.

One can also examine the blue curve in Figure 8-9 to see what would happen if hemoglobin's affinity for O_2 did not change as blood passed through the systemic tissue capillaries. For example, if O_2 consumption of vigorously exercising muscle decreased tissue PO_2 to 22 mm Hg, as shown in Figure 8-9, and if hemoglobin's O_2 affinity did not change, the blood would release about 12 mL/dL of O_2 to the tissues (from point *a* [20 mL/dL] to point V_1 [8 mL/dL]). Instead, what actually

happens is that hemoglobin's affinity for O_2 decreases at the tissue level, and it gives up much more O_2 than it would otherwise release (from point *a* on the *blue curve* to point V_2 on the *red curve* in Figure 8-9). The difference in O_2 content between V_1 and V_2 (about 6 mL/dL) is the additional amount of O_2 that hemoglobin molecules released when their affinity for O_2 decreased. In other words, if hemoglobin's affinity for O_2 had not decreased, the 6 mL/dL of O_2 would have remained in the blood, bound to hemoglobin molecules.

Effects of Partial Pressure of Carbon Dioxide, pH, Temperature, and 2,3-Diphosphoglycerate on Hemoglobin Affinity for Oxygen

Figure 8-10 summarizes the effects of PCO_2, pH, temperature, and 2,3-DPG on P_{50} and hemoglobin's affinity for O_2, as manifested by the position of the HbO_2 curve. Curve shifts affect the dissociation (steep) portion of the curve much more than the association (flat) portion (i.e., curve shifts influence O_2 release to the tissues much more than they influence O_2 uptake in the lungs). The decreased affinity of hemoglobin for O_2, or the rightward curve shift caused by high PCO_2, is known as the **Bohr effect.** In normal resting conditions, changes in PCO_2, [H^+], temperature, and 2,3-DPG between arterial and venous blood are small. Figure 8-11 compares the HbO_2 equilibrium curves for arterial and venous blood. The venous blood curve is shifted slightly to the right, causing P_{50} to be about 29 mm Hg compared with 27 mm Hg for arterial blood. At an average

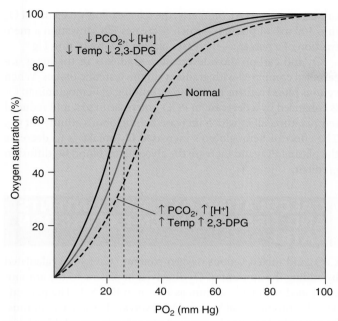

Figure 8-10 Effect of hydrogen ion concentration (pH), PCO_2, temperature, and 2,3-DPG concentration on hemoglobin's oxygen affinity. Decreased affinity shifts the curve to the right, increasing P_{50}. Increased affinity shifts the curve to the left, decreasing P_{50}. (From Berne RM, Levy MN: *Physiology*, ed 3, St Louis, 1993, Mosby.)

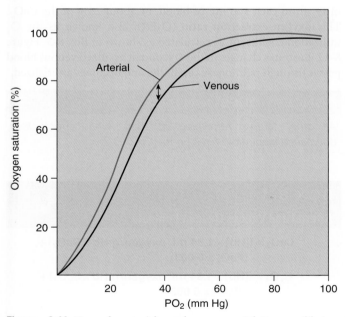

Figure 8-11 Normal arterial and venous HbO_2 equilibrium curves. (From Berne RM, Levy MN: *Physiology*, ed 3, St Louis, 1993, Mosby.)

resting tissue PO_2 of 40 mm Hg, the shift of the curve from the arterial position to the venous position increases the amount of O_2 released to the tissues.

The effect of PCO_2 on the HbO_2 equilibrium curve is mediated mostly through its formation of H^+; carbon dioxide reacts with water to produce H_2CO_3, which dissociates to produce H^+. Hydrogen ions bind directly with the hemoglobin

molecule, especially deoxygenated Hb, causing its affinity for O_2 to decrease. Carbon dioxide also directly combines with the hemoglobin molecule, forming **carbaminohemoglobin** (see Chapter 9). Increased carbaminohemoglobin decreases hemoglobin's O_2 affinity, shifting the HbO_2 curve to the right.

Temperature affects equilibrium between O_2 and Hb in the same way it affects all chemical equilibriums. Increased temperature disrupts equilibrium, causing more dissociation; decreased temperature favors association. For example, increased metabolic activity of exercising muscles generates heat, which makes hemoglobin affinity for O_2 decrease, enhancing O_2 release to tissues.

Because blood PO_2 and saturation are clinically measured under standard 37° C conditions, these values are sometimes corrected to the patient's actual temperature. Sometimes the temperature of a patient in surgery is deliberately reduced to decrease tissue O_2 requirements; this condition is called **hypothermia**. In such instances, the HbO_2 curve shifts to the left, and more O_2 remains attached to hemoglobin. If the body temperature is reduced to 20° C, Hb is 100% saturated at a PO_2 of 60 mm Hg. Although this greatly reduces O_2 release to the tissues, hypothermic tissues require less O_2 because they have a reduced metabolic rate.

CONCEPT QUESTION 8-4

Which of the following carries more O_2 at a PO_2 of 40 mm Hg: acidotic blood or alkalotic blood?

Mature red blood cells synthesize 2,3-DPG. This organic phosphate decreases Hb affinity for O_2 by binding directly to deoxygenated hemoglobin. In the absence of 2,3-DPG, the affinity for O_2 is so great that normal O_2 release to the tissues is seriously impaired. Increased 2,3-DPG synthesis is an important adaptive mechanism in people with a need for more tissue O_2; 2,3-DPG concentration in the erythrocyte is increased in anemia, vigorous exercise, high-altitude living, and diseases that cause hypoxemia, such as chronic obstructive pulmonary disease (COPD). Changes in 2,3-DPG concentration may occur rapidly (within minutes during vigorous exercise) or more slowly (1 to 2 days after high-altitude air breathing).

Changes in blood pH cause counteracting 2,3-DPG changes. Increased blood pH, or alkalemia, increases production of 2,3-DPG by red blood cells.[3] The increase in 2,3-DPG lessens the left HbO_2 curve shift caused by the increased pH. Conversely, decreased blood pH, or acidemia, decreases 2,3-DPG production. The decreased 2,3-DPG counteracts the right shift in the HbO_2 curve caused by the decreased pH.

Other factors besides acidemia that decrease 2,3-DPG concentration include septic shock (bacterial blood infection) and the storage of blood for transfusions. Banked blood stored with an acid-citrate dextrose anticoagulant loses a considerable amount of 2,3-DPG over time.[4] This loss increases hemoglobin affinity for O_2, decreasing O_2 availability to the tissues. Large transfusions of banked blood stored over several days can theoretically impair O_2 release to the tissues. In terms of O_2 delivery

Increased Hemoglobin Affinity for Oxygen When pH, PCO_2, and Temperature Are Normal

You are asked to interpret the findings of the following blood sample:

PaO_2 = 85 mm Hg
$PaCO_2$ = 40 mm Hg
pH = 7.40
Temperature = 37° C
Oxygen saturation = 99%

Normally, an oxygen saturation of 99% is associated with a PO_2 greater than 100 mm Hg. What conclusions can be drawn from these blood gas values?

Discussion

Referring to Figure 8-10, a PaO_2 of 85 mm Hg associated with an oxygen saturation of 99% can be explained only by an increased hemoglobin affinity for oxygen, a leftward shift in the HbO_2 equilibrium curve. The high SaO_2 associated with PaO_2 means that hemoglobin has increased affinity for oxygen and releases less oxygen to the tissues. If you measure P_{50}, you will find that it is low (<27 mm Hg), which is conclusive evidence of hemoglobin's increased affinity to oxygen. What could have caused the left shift in this scenario?

The pH, PCO_2, and temperature are normal and cannot be responsible for hemoglobin's increased oxygen affinity. A likely cause of hemoglobin's increased affinity is a decreased level of 2,3-DPG in the blood. Banked blood stored for transfusion has decreased levels of 2,3-DPG; this patient may have recently received a transfusion.

rate to the body's tissues, the transfusion of 2,3-DPG–depleted blood is probably physiologically insignificant.[4,5]

Clinical Significance of Changes in Hemoglobin Affinity for Oxygen

The normal changes that occur in hemoglobin's O_2 affinity enhance O_2 uptake and release in pulmonary and systemic capillaries. As blood enters the systemic capillaries, O_2 diffuses out of the plasma into the tissue cells. Plasma PO_2 decreases, causing hemoglobin to release O_2 in accordance with the HbO_2 dissociation curve (see Figure 8-8). At the same time, hemoglobin's affinity for O_2 decreases (for reasons discussed in the previous section), and hemoglobin releases even more O_2. The major physiological effect of the right shift of the HbO_2 curve is that hemoglobin releases additional O_2 into the plasma, which increases the pressure gradient for O_2 diffusion into the tissues.

The decrease in hemoglobin's O_2 affinity at the tissue level increases the blood PO_2 much more than it decreases the hemoglobin saturation. For example, when hemoglobin molecules release only 0.003 mL of O_2 into 100 mL of plasma, the plasma PO_2 increases by a comparatively large 1 mm Hg ($PO_2 \times 0.003 =$

mL/dL dissolved O_2). Similarly, the release of only 0.03 mL of O_2 into 100 mL of plasma—which decreases Hb saturation a mere fraction of a percent—increases plasma PO_2 by 10 mm Hg.

O_2 and carbon dioxide pressure gradients in the lungs are reversed compared with gradients in the systemic tissues. When venous blood returns to the lungs, binding of hemoglobin to O_2 is enhanced by a decrease in PCO_2, increase in pH, and reduced temperature, all of which increase hemoglobin's affinity for O_2. The effect of hemoglobin's increased O_2 uptake is to decrease the plasma PO_2 and increase the alveolus-to-blood O_2 diffusion gradient.

CALCULATING OXYGEN CONTENTS AND TISSUE OXYGEN-EXTRACTION RATIO

CaO_2 and mixed venous oxygen content ($C_{\bar{v}}O_2$) are calculated by adding the amount of O_2 dissolved in plasma to the amount combined with hemoglobin, as shown in Box 8-1. The percentage of saturation (SaO_2 or $S_{\bar{v}}O_2$), expressed as a decimal, must be multiplied by the O_2-carrying capacity of hemoglobin (Hb × 1.34) to arrive at the actual amount of combined O_2 present. As shown, the approximate normal values for CaO_2 and $C_{\bar{v}}O_2$ are 20 mL/dL and 15 mL/dL (Boxes 8-2 and 8-3). The **arterial-venous oxygen content difference $C(a-\bar{v})O_2$** is about 5 mL/dL (Box 8-4). This means the systemic tissues at rest extract about 5 mL of O_2 from each 100 mL of blood, or about 25% of the CaO_2. This **oxygen-extraction ratio (O_2ER)**, also known as the O_2 utilization coefficient, is calculated as shown in Box 8-5. Figure 8-12 illustrates changes in the O_2 content as mixed venous blood passes through pulmonary capillaries and becomes arterialized.

CONCEPT QUESTION 8-5

All other factors remaining constant, what effect does decreased blood flow have on the $C(a-\bar{v})O_2$?

BOX 8-1

Arterial and Venous Oxygen Contents

$$CaO_2 = ([Hb] \times 1.34 \text{ mL oxygen/g Hb} \times SaO_2) + (PaO_2 \times 0.003)$$

$$C_{\bar{v}}O_2 = ([Hb] \times 1.34 \text{ mL oxygen/g Hb} \times S_{\bar{v}}O_2) + (P_{\bar{v}}O_2 \times 0.003)$$

BOX 8-2

Normal Arterial Oxygen Content

Given the following:
Hb = 15 g/dL blood, SaO_2 = 97.5 %, PaO_2 = 100 mm Hg

$$CaO_2 = (15 \times 1.34 \times 0.975) + (100 \times 0.003)$$
$$CaO_2 = (19.9 \text{ mL/dL}) + (0.3 \text{ mL/dL})$$
$$\text{combined} \qquad \text{dissolved}$$
$$CaO_2 = \text{approximately } 20 \text{ mL / dL}$$

OXYGEN DELIVERY (TRANSPORT) TO TISSUES

Factors Affecting Oxygen Delivery and Tissue Oxygenation

Biomedical technology has made the clinical measurement of a patient's PaO_2 and SaO_2 extremely easy. Automated blood gas analyzers and pulse oximeters provide the clinician with almost instant results. However, PaO_2 and SaO_2 alone do not provide an adequate assessment of the patient's oxygenation. PaO_2 can be 100 mm Hg, and SaO_2 can be 98%, and yet an anemic patient with 5 g/dL of hemoglobin may experience serious tissue hypoxia.

Even with normal hemoglobin, PaO_2, and SaO_2 values, a person can still have inadequate O_2 DEL if the blood flow (i.e., $\dot{Q}$) is inadequate. The tendency to evaluate the oxygenation status as normal because PaO_2 and SaO_2 are normal must be resisted. Factors that affect O_2 DEL to the tissues include the following: (1) hemoglobin concentration, (2) arterial hemoglobin saturation with O_2 (this automatically takes PaO_2 into account), and (3) cardiac output $\dot{Q}$. Because hemoglobin concentration, saturation, and PaO_2 determine CaO_2, O_2 DEL depends on CaO_2 and $\dot{Q}$.

Normal Oxygen Delivery Rate

O_2 DEL in milliliters per minute is the product of CaO_2 (mL O_2/100 mL blood) and $\dot{Q}$ (L per minute). Because CaO_2 is expressed as the milliliters of O_2 contained in 100 mL (i.e., one tenth of a liter) of blood, the amount of O_2 carried in 1000 mL (1 L) of blood is calculated as follows:

$$(CaO_2 \times 10 \text{ dL/L}) = \text{mL } O_2/\text{L blood}$$

The cardiopulmonary system normally delivers about 1000 mL of O_2 to the tissues each minute at rest, as shown in Box 8-6. During exercise, $\dot{Q}$ may easily quadruple, increasing O_2 DEL to about 4000 mL per minute. The only significant way the body can increase O_2 DEL to the tissues is to increase $\dot{Q}$, because the blood is normally almost 100% saturated with O_2 at rest.

Oxygen Delivery versus Oxygen Consumption

Is the delivery of 1000 mL of O_2 per minute to the tissues adequate? Systemic tissues normally extract about 5 mL of O_2 from every 100 mL of blood perfusing them (i.e., $C[a-\bar{v}]O_2$ is about 5 mL/dL). Similarly, the tissues extract 50 mL of O_2 from every 1000 mL of blood perfusing them. Consequently, if the tissues receive 5 L of blood flow per minute, they remove a total of 250 mL of O_2 from the blood each minute (total extraction = 50 mL O_2/L $\times$ 5 L/min = 250 mL/min). Normal tissue O_2

BOX 8-3

Normal Mixed Venous Oxygen Content

Given the following:
$Hb = 15$ g/dL blood, $S_{\bar{v}}O_2 = 75\%$, $P_{\bar{v}}O_2 = 40$ mm Hg

$$C_{\bar{v}}O_2 = (15 \times 1.34 \times 0.75) + (40 \times 0.003)$$
$$C_{\bar{v}}O_2 = (15.08 \text{ mL/dL}) + (0.12 \text{ mL/dL})$$
$$\qquad\qquad\text{combined}\qquad\qquad\text{dissolved}$$
$$C_{\bar{v}}O_2 = \text{approximately 15 mL/dL}$$

BOX 8-4

Arterial-Venous Oxygen Content Difference

$$C(a - \bar{v})O_2 = CaO_2 - C_{\bar{v}}O_2$$
$$C(a - \bar{v})O_2 = 20 \text{ mL/dL} - 15 \text{ mL/dL}$$
$$C(a - \bar{v})O_2 = 5 \text{ mL/dL}$$

Tissues extract about 5 mL of oxygen from each 1 dL of arterial blood.

BOX 8-5

Oxygen-Extraction Ratio

$$O_2 \text{ ER} = C(a - \bar{v})O_2/CaO_2$$
$$O_2 \text{ ER} = [5 \text{ mL/dL}] / [20 \text{ mL/dL}]$$
$$O_2 \text{ ER} = 0.25 \text{ or } 25\%$$

Tissues extract about 25% of CaO_2.

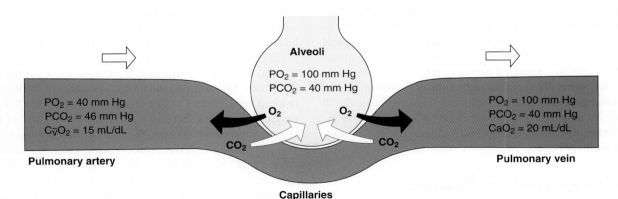

Figure 8-12 Changes in oxygen content and PO_2 as mixed venous blood passes through pulmonary capillaries and becomes arterialized. (From Berne RM, Levy MN: *Principles of physiology,* ed 2, St Louis, 1996, Mosby.)

consumption ($\dot{V}O_2$) is about 250 mL/min when the body is at rest; this is only one fourth of the amount of O_2 delivered to the tissues each minute. This fraction is consistent with earlier observations that the tissues extract and consume about 25% of the O_2 delivered to them by arterial blood. The foregoing is the basis of Fick's equation, which relates $\dot{Q}$, O_2 consumption, and $C(a-\bar{v})O_2$ (Box 8-7).

Cardiac Output and Mixed Venous Oxygen Content

As illustrated in Box 8-7, Fick's equation can be solved for $\dot{Q}$. If O_2 consumption is constant (as it usually is over relatively short time periods), an increased extraction of O_2 (i.e., an increased difference between arterial and venous O_2 contents) implies that a decrease in $\dot{Q}$ has occurred. This implication makes sense when one considers the consequences of blood moving more slowly through tissues that continue to consume O_2 at a constant rate. That is, slow moving blood gives up more O_2 to the tissues because it spends more time in contact with them; this causes the blood leaving the capillaries (now venous blood) to have a relatively low O_2 content. The result is a low $C_{\bar{v}}O_2$ and an increased difference between arterial and venous O_2 contents [$C(a-\bar{v})O_2$]. For this reason, a decrease in $C_{\bar{v}}O_2$ or an increase in $C(a-\bar{v})O_2$ generally signals a reduction in $\dot{Q}$, assuming the O_2 consumption rate remains constant. In some critically ill patients, this relationship between $C(a-\bar{v})O_2$ and $\dot{Q}$ may be unreliable because of abnormalities in blood flow distribution through capillary beds.

Critical Oxygen Delivery Threshold

Normally, O_2 DEL far exceeds tissue O_2 requirements. Variations in the O_2 DEL rate do not affect tissue O_2 uptake.[6]

However, in critically ill patients, O_2 DEL may fail to meet tissue O_2 demands. Abnormally increased tissue O_2 consumption aggravates this situation further. The point below which O_2 DEL fails to satisfy the tissue demands for O_2 is called the critical oxygen delivery threshold (DO_2crit).[6] Below DO_2crit, tissue hypoxia and lactic acid accumulation occur, marking a transition from aerobic to anaerobic metabolism at the whole-body level. In addition to increased blood lactate levels, a decrease in plasma bicarbonate (a major blood buffer) is a marker for DO_2crit.[5] The precise DO_2crit value in healthy humans is unknown and is difficult to measure experimentally.[5,7] One study of healthy human volunteers did not find blood lactate evidence that DO_2crit was reached even when O_2 DEL decreased to 7.3 mL O_2/kg body weight/min, a value that corresponds with an O_2 DEL of 511 mL O_2/min in an adult weighing 70 kg.[7] The investigators concluded that DO_2crit is below this level. Nevertheless, it is reasonable to assume that DO_2crit is higher in critically ill patients, who often have increased O_2 demands, and that an O_2 DEL rate of 500 mL per minute would likely produce tissue hypoxia. Clinicians must take measures to ensure that a critically ill patient has an adequate $\dot{Q}$ to maintain O_2 DEL above the critical delivery threshold.

CLINICAL FOCUS 8-6

Is the Patient Adequately Oxygenated?

A patient's $\dot{Q}$ in the intensive care unit (ICU) is 2.5 L/min (normal = 4 to 8 L/min). The patient has normal arterial blood gas values (PaO$_2$ 90 mm Hg, SaO$_2$ 95%, and Hb 15 g/dL). Calculate the oxygen delivery (O$_2$ DEL) for this patient. Based on your answer, decide whether this patient is adequately oxygenated.

Discussion

$$O_2 \text{ DEL } (mL/min) = CaO_2(mL/100 \text{ mL})$$
$$\times 10 \text{ dL/L} \times \dot{Q}(L/min)$$

First, calculate the CaO$_2$ as follows:

$$CaO_2 = (Hb \times 1.34 \text{ mL oxygen/g Hb} \times SaO_2)$$
$$+ (PaO_2 \times 0.003)$$
$$CaO_2 = (15 \text{ g/dL} \times 1.34 \times 0.95) + (90 \text{ mm Hg} \times 0.003)$$
$$CaO_2 = 19.4 \text{ mL/dL}$$

The next step is as follows:

$$O_2 \text{ DEL} = (19.4 \text{ mL/dL} \times 10 \text{ dL/L}) \times 2.5 \text{ L/min}$$
$$O_2 \text{ DEL} = 485 \text{ mL/min}$$

Is this patient adequately oxygenated? The normal O$_2$ DEL rate to the tissues is about 1000 mL/min. This patient's O$_2$ DEL is less than half of normal. The oxygen consumption of a healthy person at rest averages about 250 mL/min. Critically ill patients in the ICU generally have much higher oxygen requirements because of their disease. An O$_2$ DEL of 485 mL/min may not meet the oxygen requirements of this patient. Organs with high metabolic rates (e.g., heart, brain, kidneys, liver) would almost certainly be hypoxic with an O$_2$ DEL less than half of normal. Although this patient has normal values for PaO$_2$, SaO$_2$, and hemoglobin, these common measurements are not enough to assess oxygenation. The patient's O$_2$ DEL to the tissues is impaired by reduced $\dot{Q}$, not by reduced CaO$_2$.

Blood Transfusion to Improve Oxygen Delivery

It is intuitively logical to transfuse red blood cells in critically ill anemic patients to improve O$_2$ DEL to the tissues. Paradoxically, various clinical studies have shown that blood transfusions in these patients do not increase O$_2$ availability to the tissues and are associated with increased mortality, independent of disease severity.[4,6,8] Although anemia in critically ill patients is associated with increased mortality, correction with red blood cell transfusion does not decrease mortality.[4] Transfusions may increase O$_2$ DEL but are generally not associated with increased tissue O$_2$ consumption and are even linked to tissue hypoxia.[4,6] The latter may be the result of capillary bed occlusion by stored blood erythrocytes, which are less capable of being deformed than normal erythrocytes as they squeeze through capillaries.[4,6] Healthy adults can tolerate an anemia of 3.5 to 5 g/dL without organ failure, mainly by increasing cardiac output and tissue O$_2$

extraction.[4] However, blood transfusion is important in anemic patients with coronary artery disease because (1) the heart muscle has little ability to increase its O$_2$ extraction because it already extracts up to 90% of the O$_2$ from the blood it receives, and (2) obstructed or narrowed coronary arteries do not permit much increase in blood flow.[4]

A landmark Canadian study in 1999 revealed that critically ill patients in the intensive care unit who were transfused only after hemoglobin decreased to less than 7 g/dL had significantly lower mortality rates than patients with equal disease severity who were transfused after hemoglobin decreased to less than 10 g/dL.[8] Another, more recent study in the United States, the CRIT study,[9] confirmed that the number of blood transfusions a patient receives is independently associated with increased risk of death—even in patients with equal disease severity, more transfusions were associated with higher mortality. Some proposed reasons for increased mortality rates include (1) the release of proinflammatory mediators by white blood cells of stored blood; (2) transfusion-related changes in the ability to mount an immune response, which predisposes the recipient to infections; and (3) decreased erythrocyte deformability.[4]

Anemia is so common in critically ill patients that it is almost an expected problem; it is thought to be due in large part to overhydration of patients commonly seen in intensive care units.[8] The general consensus seems to be that in patients with hemoglobin levels greater than 7 g/dL who are not actively losing blood and are not hypovolemic, blood transfusions are of little or no benefit and expose patients to a potentially toxic substance.[8]

CYANOSIS

When the hemoglobin molecule releases O$_2$ and becomes deoxyhemoglobin (desaturated Hb), it changes its shape and turns deep purple in color. Severely hypoxic patients may have enough desaturated Hb in their blood that the skin, nail beds, lips, and mucous membranes appear blue or blue-gray. This condition, called **cyanosis**, is a long-recognized clinical sign associated with severe hypoxia.

Most observers do not perceive cyanosis until the average desaturated Hb concentration in the capillaries is at least 5 g/100 mL of blood (5 g/dL). The percentage of desaturated Hb in the blood is the difference between 100% O$_2$ saturation and the actual percentage of oxygenated hemoglobin present. For example, normal arterial blood contains 97.5% oxygenated hemoglobin; the remaining 2.5% is desaturated Hb. Similarly, mixed venous blood ($S_{\bar{v}}O_2 = 75\%$) contains 25% desaturated Hb. The average amount of desaturated Hb present in capillary blood is calculated by averaging the amounts of desaturated Hb present in arterial and venous blood (i.e., blood entering and leaving the capillary). Under normal conditions, hemoglobin concentration is 15 g/dL, SaO$_2$ is 97.5%, and $S_{\bar{v}}O_2$ is 75%. Normal arterial desaturation is 2.5%, and venous desaturation is 25%. The amount of desaturated arterial Hb is $0.025 \times 15 = 0.375$ g/dL, and the amount of desaturated venous Hb is $0.25 \times 15 = 3.75$ g/dL; the average of these desaturations is $(0.375 + 3.75)/2 = 2.06$ g/dL, or about 2 g/dL. Because 5 g/dL of desaturated Hb is necessary to produce observable cyanosis, normal capillary blood does not appear cyanotic.

CONCEPT QUESTION 8-6

If $\dot{Q}$ is so low that $S_{\bar{v}}O_2$ is 0.50 (hemoglobin concentration is 15 g/dL) and if SaO_2 is normal at 0.975, is cyanosis likely to be present?

Cyanosis can be classified as peripheral or central cyanosis. Peripheral cyanosis is caused by low venous O_2 saturation; arterial saturation might still be normal. This condition may occur in low blood flow states, when tissues extract more than normal amounts of O_2 from the blood. Peripheral cyanosis causes blue discoloration of the skin and nail beds and is generally limited to the extremities. Central cyanosis is caused by excessively low SaO_2, which is caused by inadequate oxygenation of the blood in the lungs. Central cyanosis involves blue discoloration of not only the skin and nail beds but also the lips, tongue, and mucous membranes in the mouth. Peripheral cyanosis involves mostly the extremities, whereas central cyanosis may be noticeable in any visible capillary bed. An arterial hemoglobin O_2 saturation of about 83% (assuming a normal Hb concentration and $C(a-\bar{v})O_2$) produces about 5 g/dL of desaturated Hb, which should produce cyanosis. Central cyanosis signals a more profound hypoxemia than peripheral cyanosis.

Cyanosis does not always accompany severe hypoxemia, and cyanosis is sometimes present even in the absence of hypoxemia. If anemia is severe enough, total hemoglobin concentration may be so low that even severe hypoxemia does not produce the 5 g/dL of desaturated Hb necessary to cause cyanosis. Conversely, people with abnormally high hemoglobin concentrations (polycythemia) may appear to be cyanotic because their capillary blood contains 5 g/dL of desaturated Hb, and yet the remaining quantity of saturated hemoglobin is high enough that the O_2 content is normal. Carbon monoxide (CO) inhalation is another example of hypoxemia without cyanosis. CO creates hypoxemia by aggressively binding to the hemoglobin molecule, blocking binding sites of O_2. Hemoglobin combined with CO is bright red; although the blood's O_2 content is very low, it is not cyanotic.

The presence or absence of cyanosis is an unreliable indicator of the blood's oxygenation status; cyanosis should always be interpreted in conjunction with the patient's actual hemoglobin concentration. Although the presence of central cyanosis often indicates hypoxia, the absence of central cyanosis does not automatically indicate normal oxygenation. However, the disappearance of cyanosis usually means oxygenation has improved.

HEMOGLOBIN ABNORMALITIES

Carboxyhemoglobin

The hemoglobin molecule's affinity for CO is 210 times greater than its affinity for O_2. This means if a person breathes a gas mixture containing 21% O_2 and 0.1% CO, O_2 and CO

molecules are on equal footing in competing for Hb binding sites. A mixture of air and 0.1% CO eventually produces 50% carboxyhemoglobin (HbCO). Because HbCO cannot carry O_2, CO decreases the concentration of functional hemoglobin available for O_2 binding. In this sense, CO poisoning has an effect similar to that of anemia in which hemoglobin concentration is physically reduced.

CO not only decreases the amount of hemoglobin available for O_2 transport, but it also hampers the ability of hemoglobin to release O_2 to the tissues. CO increases hemoglobin's affinity for O_2, shifting the HbO_2 equilibrium curve to the left, as shown in Figure 8-13. The *solid curve* in Figure 8-13 represents normal arterial blood with normal O_2 content. The *dashed curve* represents anemic blood with normal arterial saturation but half-normal O_2 content because hemoglobin concentration is half-normal. The *dotted curve* represents blood with normal hemoglobin concentration but with half of it blocked by CO. As in the anemic curve, half of the normal amount of hemoglobin is available for combination with O_2. However, CO also increases hemoglobin's affinity for O_2, as indicated by the left shift of the *dotted curve*, which means tissue PO_2 must decrease to a very low level before hemoglobin releases O_2 to the plasma. This lower tissue PO_2 is especially dangerous to heart muscle because, in contrast to other tissues, heart muscle extracts 70% to 90% of the O_2 present in the blood. Especially in people with decreased coronary blood flow, the impaired release of O_2 caused by the effect of CO on the HbO_2 curve may cause severe hypoxia of heart muscle.

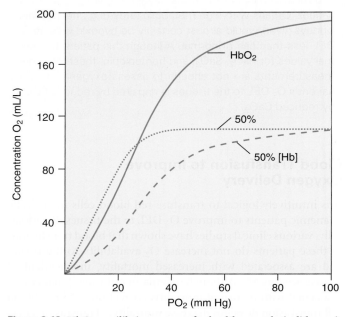

Figure 8-13 HbO_2 equilibrium curves for healthy people (*solid curve*), anemic people (*dashed curve*), and people with carbon monoxide (CO) poisoning (*dotted curve*). Anemia and CO poisoning both decrease the blood oxygen content, although SO_2 and PO_2 may be normal. However, CO also increases hemoglobin's affinity for oxygen, shifting the curve to the left and impairing oxygen release at the tissues further. (From Berne RM, Levy MN: *Principles of physiology,* ed 2, St Louis, 1996, Mosby.)

CO is produced by the combustion of organic materials. Heavy cigarette smokers may have HbCO levels of 10%. Lethal levels of HbCO most commonly occur in the smoke of house fires or automobile exhaust. In acute CO poisoning, inhalation of 100% O_2 is extremely important in displacing CO from the hemoglobin molecule. A fractional inspired oxygen concentration (F_IO_2) of 1.0 greatly decreases the half-life of HbCO (the time required to cut HbCO blood levels in half). Hyperbaric oxygen therapy (administration of O_2 at pressures greater than atmospheric) is even more effective in quickly eliminating CO from the blood.

Hemoglobin Variants

The hemoglobin discussed to this point has been normal adult hemoglobin (HbA). Researchers have identified 120 variations of HbA. As mentioned previously, slight variations in the polypeptide amino acid sequence of the hemoglobin molecule may change hemoglobin's affinity for O_2. Hemoglobin variants were originally named according to letters of the alphabet (e.g., A for normal adult hemoglobin, F for fetal hemoglobin, S for sickle cell hemoglobin). Because of the large number of variants identified, hemoglobin variants discovered later were named for geographical regions where they were first described (e.g., Hb Kansas, Hb Seattle, Hb Rainier). The most clinically significant hemoglobin variants are fetal hemoglobin (HbF), methemoglobin (metHb), and sickle cell hemoglobin (HbS).

Fetal Hemoglobin

Hemoglobin present in the fetus has a high affinity for O_2, apparently because 2,3-DPG does not bind with HbF.[2] HbF and HbA without 2,3-DPG have similar left-shifted HbO_2 equilibrium curves.[2] HbF of normal-term infants has a P_{50} of about 22 mm Hg. A cyanotic newborn infant has a much lower arterial PO_2 than an equally cyanotic adult. It is fortunate that HbF has a high affinity for O_2 because the maximum PO_2 of fetal blood is less than 40 mm Hg. Despite the low PO_2, HbF allows fetal blood to carry adequate amounts of O_2. Because of its high affinity for O_2, HbF vigorously takes up O_2 from the plasma at the placenta. This lowers fetal plasma PO_2, promoting O_2 transport across the placenta by maintaining an O_2 diffusion gradient. By 6 months after birth, most HbF has been replaced with HbA.

Methemoglobin

Methemoglobin (metHb) is formed when the ferrous ion (Fe^{++}) of normal HbA is oxidized to the ferric form (Fe^{+++}). metHb cannot carry O_2; in addition, its presence in the blood increases the remaining normal hemoglobin's affinity for O_2, hindering its ability to release O_2 to the tissues. Some methemoglobin is normally formed in the blood through spontaneous autooxidation, which is kept in check by antioxidant proteins in the erythrocyte.[2] Methemoglobinemia (high blood levels of metHb) can be caused by nitrate poisoning or toxic reactions to oxidant drugs. Normally, the antioxidant protein in the erythrocyte instantly reverses any Fe^{++} oxidation that occurs, maintaining a metHb content less than 1%. However, this protein is only 50% to 60% as active in newborn infants as in adults, making newborns, especially premature infants, more susceptible to developing methemoglobinemia.[2] Well water, which commonly contains nitrates, is a cause of methemoglobinemia in infants in rural areas. Methemoglobinemia produces a slate-gray cyanotic appearance and arterial blood that is chocolate brown in color. Generally, acquired methemoglobinemia resolves spontaneously with the removal of the offending agent; symptomatic cases can be treated with an infusion of methylene blue, a methemoglobin reduction agent.[2]

Sickle Cell Hemoglobin

Sickle cell hemoglobin (HbS) is much less soluble than HbA in the deoxygenated state. HbS tends to crystallize in the red blood cell on deoxygenation, changing the red blood cell from a biconcave to a curved, sickle shape. The sickle-shaped cell is fragile and subject to rupture. Its shape causes it to tangle with other sickle cells clumping and forming **thromboemboli** (blood clots); this may block blood flow through small vessels, creating painful areas of **ischemia** (tissue hypoxia). The fragility and ease of rupture of the sickle cell also predisposes the patient to develop anemia. Sickle cell anemia is an inherited blood disorder. The sickling phenomenon is not always present in people with sickle cell disease, but it may be precipitated by prolonged episodes of hypoxia.

POINTS TO REMEMBER

- O_2 is carried in the blood in two forms—dissolved and combined with hemoglobin—more than 98% of the O_2 carried in the blood is bound to hemoglobin.
- Although dissolved O_2 content is small compared with O_2 bound to hemoglobin, dissolved O_2 gives rise to the blood PO_2 and determines the direction and rate of O_2 diffusion.
- PO_2 determines the extent to which O_2 combines with hemoglobin, but the relationship between hemoglobin saturation and PO_2 is not linear.
- At PO_2 values less than 60 mm Hg, small changes in PO_2 produce large changes in the blood O_2 content and hemoglobin saturation; at PO_2 values greater than 60 mm Hg, large increases in PO_2 produce minimal increases in O_2 content and hemoglobin saturation.
- Except for instances of CO poisoning, little clinical rationale exists for increasing a patient's PaO_2 greater than 100 mm Hg.
- Decreased pH and increased PCO_2, temperature, and 2,3-DPG decrease hemoglobin's O_2 affinity, causing a right HbO_2 curve shift; opposite changes increase hemoglobin's affinity for O_2, causing left HbO_2 curve shifts.
- The main clinical consequence of decreased hemoglobin affinity at the tissue level is an increase in plasma PO_2, which creates a pressure gradient for O_2 diffusion into the tissues.
- O_2 transport to the tissues is the product of CaO_2 and $\dot{Q}$; PaO_2 and SaO_2 do not provide a sufficient basis for assessing oxygenation.
- The whole-body tissues normally extract 25% of the O_2 delivered to them; in exercise, low blood flow, and anemic states, the O_2 ER increases.

- Evaluating oxygenation adequacy involves evaluating CaO_2 (hemoglobin and saturation percentage) and blood flow ($\dot{Q}$).
- Cyanosis is caused by the presence of 5 g/dL of deoxygenated Hb in capillary blood.
- Cyanosis may not appear in hypoxic individuals with severe anemia or CO poisoning but may be present in patients with polycythemia who have adequate blood O_2 content.
- In anemic critically ill patients with hemoglobin concentrations greater than 7 g/dL who are not bleeding or hypovolemic, blood transfusions are generally not beneficial and are associated with increased mortality.
- CO poisoning decreases the Hb available for O_2 transport, and it decreases O_2 release at the tissues by increasing hemoglobin affinity for O_2.
- HbF has high affinity for O_2, making it possible for the fetus to carry adequate amounts of O_2 even though PO_2 is quite low.
- In methemoglobinemia, the iron in the hemoglobin molecule binds irreversibly with O_2, and hemoglobin is unable to transport or release O_2.
- In sickle cell hemoglobin, deoxygenation changes the shape of the red blood cell, causing it to clump with other sickle-shaped cells to form vascular occlusions.

References

1. Firth PG: Anesthesia and hemoglobinopathies, *Anesthesiol Clin* 27(2):321, 2009.
2. Gregg XT, Prchal JT: Red blood cell enzymopathies. In Hoffman R, et al, editors: *Hoffman: hematology: basic principles and practice*, ed 5, Philadelphia, 2008, Churchill Livingstone.
3. Gauthier PM, Szerlip HM: Metabolic acidosis in the intensive care unit, *Crit Care Clin* 18(2):289, 2002.
4. Ho J, Sibbald WJ, Chin-Yee IH: Effects of storage on efficacy of red cell transfusion: when is it not safe? *Crit Care Med* 31(Suppl 12):S687, 2003.
5. Torres Filho IP, et al: Experimental analysis of critical oxygen delivery, *Am J Physiol Heart Circ Physiol* 288(3):H1071, 2005.
6. Hameed SM, Aird WC, Cohn SM: Oxygen delivery, *Crit Care Med* 31(Suppl 12):S658, 2003.
7. Lieberman JA, et al: Critical oxygen delivery in conscious humans is less than 7.3 ml $O_2 \times kg(-1) \times min(-1)$, *Anesthesiology* 92(2):407, 2000.
8. Ward NS, Levy MM: Blood transfusion practice today, *Crit Care Clin* 20(2):179, 2004.
9. Corwin HL, et al: The CRIT study: anemia and blood transfusion in the critically ill—current clinical practice in the United States, *Crit Care Med* 32(1):39, 2004.

Carbon Dioxide Equilibrium and Transport

OBJECTIVES

After reading this chapter, you will be able to:

- Explain how blood levels of carbon dioxide partial pressure (PCO_2), dissolved carbon dioxide (CO_2), carbonic acid, and alveolar ventilation are interrelated
- Describe the way in which blood levels of CO_2 play a role in the body's acid-base balance
- Use the CO_2 hydration reaction to explain how changes in alveolar ventilation affect blood levels of CO_2 and hydrogen ions

- Explain why equal CO_2 production and elimination rates can coexist with normal ventilation, hypoventilation, or hyperventilation
- Describe how CO_2 is transported in different ways in the blood plasma and erythrocytes
- Explain how hemoglobin in the erythrocyte helps generate plasma bicarbonate ions (HCO_3^-)
- Explain how the Bohr and Haldane effects are mutually enhancing with regard to oxygen and CO_2 transport

KEY TERMS

carbonic acid
carbonic anhydrase
chemical equilibrium
chloride shift

CO_2 hydration reaction
Haldane effect
law of mass action
volatile acid

CARBON DIOXIDE, CARBONIC ACID, AND HYDROGEN ION EQUILIBRIUM

In an individual breathing room air at sea level, arterial blood enters the systemic capillary with a carbon dioxide partial pressure (PCO_2) of about 40 mm Hg. At rest, the body's tissues produce about 200 mL of carbon dioxide (CO_2)

each minute; CO_2 is a by-product of oxidative (aerobic) metabolism. Each millimole (mmol) of oxygen metabolized by the body produces about 0.7 to 1 mmol of CO_2; healthy adults produce about 13,000 mmol of CO_2 per day. Blood flow carries CO_2 from the body's tissues to the lungs where CO_2 is eliminated in exhaled gas; this is necessary to prevent CO_2 buildup in the tissues.

Inspired atmospheric gas contains a negligible amount of CO_2; the presence of CO_2 in the blood is evidence of the blood's exposure to metabolically active tissues. Normally, a steady state exists in which blood flow removes CO_2 at the same rate that the tissues produce it, maintaining an average tissue PCO_2 of about 46 mm Hg. This creates an average CO_2 diffusion gradient between tissues and arterial blood of about 6 mm Hg, causing CO_2 to diffuse into the capillary (tissue PCO_2 = 46 mm Hg and arterial PCO_2 = 40 mm Hg). The PCO_2 of blood perfusing the systemic capillaries equilibrates with tissue PCO_2, creating a venous PCO_2 of about 46 mm Hg. Venous blood returns to the lungs, where it is exposed to an average alveolar PCO_2 of about 40 mm Hg. Normal alveolar ventilation ($\dot{V}_A$), which eliminates CO_2 at the same rate that it is brought to the lungs, maintains the P_ACO_2 at about 40 mm Hg. An average CO_2 diffusion gradient of about 6 mm Hg between capillary blood and alveoli causes CO_2 to diffuse into the alveoli.

Carbon Dioxide Hydration Reaction

The presence of CO_2 in the blood creates a special problem because CO_2 reacts with water (i.e., CO_2 is hydrated) to form **carbonic acid** (H_2CO_3). The blood must possess effective buffering mechanisms to prevent harmful increases in acidity as it transports CO_2. As the following reaction shows, when CO_2 diffuses from tissues into capillary blood, the **CO_2 hydration reaction** occurs:[1]

1. $$H_2O + CO_2 \rightarrow H_2CO_3 \rightarrow HCO_3^- + H^+$$

Hydrolysis is a chemical reaction in which H_2O splits another molecule; the term is incorrect in reference to the reaction between H_2O and CO_2. Reaction 1 shows that CO_2 in the blood is associated with the formation of H_2CO_3 and the production of hydrogen ions (H^+). A fundamental characteristic of an acid is the release of H^+ into solution. Although CO_2 is technically not an acid, its immediate formation of H_2CO_3 in physiological fluids allows it to be treated as though it were an acid.

Hydration Reaction: Chemical Equilibrium (Le Chatelier's Principle)

The CO_2 hydration reaction (reaction 1) can proceed in either direction (i.e., it is reversible). **Chemical equilibrium** exists when the reaction velocities to the left and right are equal. A state of equilibrium does not mean the concentrations of substances on both sides of the equation are equal, and it does not imply a static state of affairs. At equilibrium, the reaction continues to move in both directions at equal rates but in such a way that no net change occurs in the concentrations of constituents on either side of the reaction. This state is called *dynamic equilibrium*. The reaction between CO_2 and H_2O in plasma occurs only to a slight extent; in this state of the chemical equilibrium, CO_2 and H_2O molecules far outnumber H_2CO_3 molecules. Therefore, at equilibrium, the CO_2 hydration reaction is shifted to the left, as the following reaction shows:

2. $$H_2O + CO_2 \underset{\longrightarrow}{\longleftarrow} H_2CO_3 \underset{\longrightarrow}{\longleftarrow} HCO_3^- + H^+$$
   (400) (400)   (1)

The short arrows pointing to the right and the long arrows pointing to the left indicate that at equilibrium the reaction is left shifted. The numbers in parentheses indicate relative concentrations of the constituents.[2] At equilibrium, concentrations to the left of the arrows are greater than concentrations to the right of the arrows. Despite these concentration differences, the velocities of right-directed and left-directed reactions are identical at equilibrium.

According to Le Chatelier's principle, if a system at equilibrium is placed under stress, it will react in such a way that counteracts the stress and creates a new equilibrium at a different point.[3] For example, in reaction 2, if we add a certain amount of CO_2 molecules to the left side of the reaction, we disrupt the equilibrium and drive the reaction to the right until a new equilibrium is established. Similarly, removing CO_2 molecules from the left side "pulls" the reaction to the left. In other words, adding or subtracting CO_2 molecules drives the reaction either toward the H^+ and HCO_3^- side or toward the CO_2 and H_2O side of the reaction.

CONCEPT QUESTION 9-1

What effect does removing CO_2 molecules through increased ventilation have on the H^+ concentration of the blood?

Relationship between Dissolved Carbon Dioxide and Carbonic Acid Concentrations

All gases dissolve in water to some extent, as discussed in previous chapters. According to Henry's law, the amount of CO_2 dissolving in plasma is proportional to the PCO_2 to which the plasma is exposed. In other words, CO_2 in the gaseous phase establishes equilibrium with CO_2 in the aqueous phase. In the lung, gaseous CO_2 in the alveoli establishes equilibrium with dissolved CO_2 in capillary blood plasma. The concentration of CO_2 in alveolar gas is expressed in terms of its partial pressure (mm Hg). The concentration of dissolved CO_2 in plasma is proportional to P_ACO_2 and is measured in millimoles per liter (mmol/L) rather than in milliliters per deciliter (mL/dL), as it is for oxygen content.

At 37° C, 0.03 mmol of CO_2 dissolves in 1 L of plasma for each mm Hg PCO_2; that is, mmol/L (CO_2) = 0.03 mmol/L/ mm Hg × PCO_2. (The derivation of the conversion factor [0.03] to change PCO_2 to millimoles per liter of dissolved CO_2 is shown in Box 9-1.) Thus, if plasma PCO_2 is 40 mm Hg, the concentration of dissolved CO_2 in plasma is as follows: 40 mm Hg × 0.03 mmol/L/mm Hg = 1.2 mmol/L, which is the normal amount of dissolved CO_2 in arterial blood. Figure 9-1 summarizes the relationship between gaseous CO_2, dissolved CO_2, and H_2CO_3. The slow uncatalyzed reaction between CO_2 and H_2O theoretically requires about 400 molecules of dissolved CO_2 to produce 1 molecule of H_2CO_3.[2] In other words, an extremely small amount of H_2CO_3 in plasma is in equilibrium with a relatively large pool of dissolved CO_2. The reaction in Figure 9-1 shows that an increased alveolar PCO_2 increases plasma PCO_2, which increases the dissolved CO_2 and H_2CO_3 concentration (**law of mass action**). Conversely, a decrease in

Conversion Factors for Dissolved Carbon Dioxide: Millimoles per Liter and Milliliters per Deciliter

1. 1 mole CO_2 = 22.3 L at STP; 1 mmol CO_2 = 22.3 mL at STP
2. CO_2 sol coeff = 0.592 mL CO_2/mL plasma/760 mm Hg PCO_2
3. mL CO_2 dissolving per mL plasma per mm Hg PCO_2 is as follows: 0.592/760 mm Hg = 0.00078 mL CO_2/mL plasma/mm Hg
4. mL CO_2 dissolving per 100 mL plasma (mL/dL) = 0.078 mL
5. mL CO_2 dissolving per L (1000 mL) plasma per mm Hg PCO_2 is as follows:
   0.00078× 1000 = 0.78 mL CO_2/L plasma/mm Hg
6. mmol CO_2 dissolving per L plasma per mm Hg PCO_2 is as follows: 0.78 mL CO_2/22.3 mL CO_2 per mmol = 0.03498 mmol CO_2/L/mm Hg
   $$PCO_2 \times 0.03 = mmol/L \text{ dissolved } CO_2$$
7. Factor to convert mmol/L to mL/dL (from steps 4 and 6) = 0.078/0.03498 = 2.23:
   $$mmol/L\ CO_2 \times 2.23 = mL/dL\ CO_2$$
   $$mL/dL\ CO_2/2.23 = mmol/L\ CO_2$$

STP, Standard temperature and pressure; *sol coeff*, soluble coefficient.

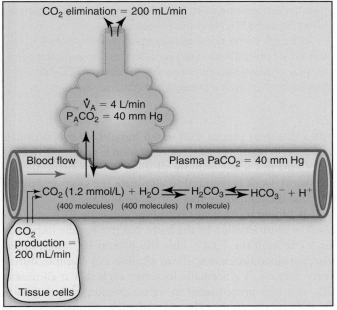

Figure 9-1 Equilibrium between gaseous CO_2, dissolved CO_2, and H_2CO_3. A trace amount of H_2CO_3 is in equilibrium with a relatively large amount of dissolved CO_2, which is in equilibrium with a plasma PCO_2 of 40 mm Hg. Normal resting conditions are shown.

alveolar PCO_2 forces the hydration reaction to the left, decreasing the plasma H_2CO_3 concentration. Because it is in equilibrium with CO_2 gas, H_2CO_3 is called a **volatile acid**. Plasma PCO_2 is an important marker of the blood's volatile acid content and the adequacy of alveolar ventilation.

What effect does inadequate $\dot{V}_A$ have on plasma PCO_2 and volatile acid content?

Although the concentration of dissolved CO_2 in plasma is not equal to the concentration of plasma H_2CO_3, its concentration is in direct proportion to the concentration of H_2CO_3; this makes it possible to treat CO_2 as if it were the acid instead of H_2CO_3. Because dissolved CO_2 and H_2CO_3 are indistinguishable from each other by chemical analysis,[4] dissolved CO_2, which can be easily measured, is commonly substituted for the concentration of H_2CO_3 in clinical acid-base equations (see Chapter 10).

Role of Ventilation in Regulating Arterial Carbon Dioxide Pressure and Volatile Acid

Changes in alveolar PCO_2 ultimately change the plasma H_2CO_3 concentration (see Figure 9-1). (Chapter 4 discusses the reciprocal relationship between $\dot{V}_A$ and $PaCO_2$.) Figure 9-2 shows the chemical events that occur during hypoventilation. In Figure 9-2, $\dot{V}_A$ is halved, causing P_ACO_2 to double. Subsequently, $PaCO_2$ and dissolved CO_2 double, pushing the hydration reaction to the right. The doubling of CO_2 molecules on the left side of the reaction drives the reaction to the right to a new equilibrium point (Le Chatelier's principle). Figure 9-2 shows that at equilibrium, the amount of H_2CO_3 molecules doubles, but the ratio of CO_2 to H_2CO_3 molecules stays the same.

At the outset of hypoventilation, the rate of CO_2 production momentarily exceeds the rate of alveolar CO_2 elimination, causing alveolar and blood CO_2 levels to increase. However, CO_2 levels cannot continually increase; instead, a new equilibrium point (i.e., a new steady state) is reached at which CO_2 production and elimination rates are again equal, but at higher P_ACO_2 and $PaCO_2$ levels. In Figure 9-1, a normal $\dot{V}_A$ of 4 L per minute maintains a P_ACO_2 of 40 mm Hg and eliminates 200 mL of CO_2 per minute (an amount equal to its production rate). If the $\dot{V}_A$ suddenly decreases to 2 L per minute with no change in CO_2 production (see Figure 9-2), the $PaCO_2$ and dissolved CO_2 in the blood increase temporarily until a new steady state is reached, at which time CO_2 production and elimination rates are again equal. However, for this steady state to occur at a $\dot{V}_A$ of 2 L per minute, P_ACO_2 and $PaCO_2$ must increase to 80 mm Hg, and dissolved plasma CO_2 must increase to 2.4 mmol/L (80 × 0.03) (see Figure 9-2). A proportionate increase in H_2CO_3 levels is produced, increasing the blood's acidity. This new steady state requires less ventilatory work to eliminate the same amount of CO_2; for this reason, people with limited ventilatory capacity adopt this ventilatory strategy, but the "tradeoff" is increased blood acid levels.

Hyperventilation also disrupts the chemical equilibrium of the hydration reaction (Figure 9-3). Hyperventilation pulls the reaction leftward to a new equilibrium point. At the new equilibrium, the ratio between dissolved CO_2 and H_2CO_3 is preserved, while plasma H_2CO_3 concentration is decreased. In Figure 9-3, $\dot{V}_A$ suddenly doubles from 4 L per minute to 8 L

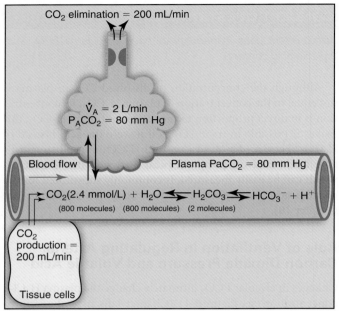

Figure 9-2 Hypoventilation. Alveolar and blood levels of CO_2 increase, creating more carbonic acid. A new equilibrium is established in which CO_2 elimination again equals CO_2 production but at higher alveolar and blood CO_2 levels.

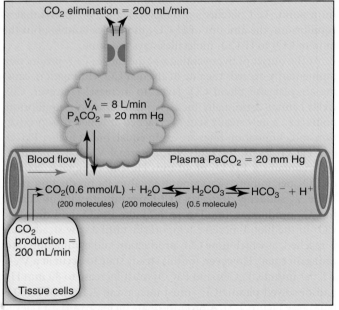

Figure 9-3 Hyperventilation. Alveolar and blood levels of CO_2 decrease, reducing carbonic acid concentration. A new equilibrium is established in which CO_2 elimination again equals CO_2 production but at lower alveolar and blood CO_2 levels.

per minute, whereas CO_2 production stays constant at 200 mL per minute. The CO_2 elimination rate temporarily exceeds the CO_2 production rate until a new equilibrium is established in which production and elimination rates are equal again. To eliminate only 200 mL of CO_2 per minute at a $\dot{V}_A$ of 8 L per minute, the P_ACO_2 must be at 20 mm Hg, which is associated

CLINICAL FOCUS 9-1

Hypercapnia as a Desirable Ventilatory Strategy in Severe Obstructive Airway Disease

Your patient with severe chronic obstructive pulmonary disease (COPD) is resting comfortably in bed. Arterial blood gas results show a $PaCO_2$ of 62 mm Hg. Why does this patient's body accept hypercapnia (high carbon dioxide levels) rather than increase pulmonary ventilation to restore a normal $PaCO_2$?

Discussion

Patients with severe COPD develop major ventilation-perfusion ($\dot{V}/\dot{Q}$) abnormalities over many years. A large amount of alveolar dead space develops, requiring the patient to increase minute ventilation to maintain a normal $PaCO_2$. Because of the deranged lung mechanics in COPD, the increased ventilatory work required to maintain a normal $PaCO_2$ becomes too great. To conserve energy, these patients are forced to reduce their ventilation, which reduces work of breathing and allows the P_ACO_2 to increase. Alveolar and blood PCO_2 values equilibrate, creating a new steady state in which the $PaCO_2$ is elevated (see Figure 9-2). Less ventilatory work is required to maintain this higher level of CO_2. Because CO_2 increases gradually, the body's kidneys have time to compensate by increasing plasma bicarbonate levels, keeping the pH in the normal range.

Although these patients may breathe with relative comfort at rest, they have limited ventilatory reserve capacity and may be unable to accommodate the increased CO_2 production associated with increased physical activity.

with a dissolved plasma CO_2 of 0.6 mmol/L. A proportionate reduction in plasma H_2CO_3 concentration is produced, making the plasma less acidic or more alkaline. In this situation, more ventilatory work is required to eliminate the same amount of CO_2 that is eliminated under normal conditions.

It is important that normal lungs eliminate CO_2 at a rate equal to its production by the body, but it is equally important for $\dot{V}_A$ to keep the P_ACO_2 near the 40-mm Hg range; otherwise, the blood becomes acidic or alkaline. For example, during heavy exercise, $\dot{V}_A$ normally increases such that it eliminates CO_2 at a rate proportional to its production; this maintains the P_ACO_2 near 40 mm Hg and maintains normal blood acid (H_2CO_3) levels. An elaborate neurochemical control system (see Chapter 11) is responsible for regulating $\dot{V}_A$ in this manner.

CONCEPT QUESTION 9-3

Explain how the increased CO_2 production of heavy exercise affects the blood's volatile acid level.

In some circumstances, the body does not maintain P_ACO_2 at 40 mm Hg, even when lung airways are normal. The lack of oxygen at high altitudes creates a chemical stimulus for ventilation, overriding the regulatory system that normally maintains a P_ACO_2 of 40 mm Hg. In such circumstances, the increased ventilation drives P_ACO_2 and $PaCO_2$ below 40 mm Hg, reducing the blood H_2CO_3 concentration; this creates a state of arterial alkalemia.

Ventilation also increases in response to abnormally high levels of nonvolatile (noncarbonic) acids in the blood (acidemia). Acids increase the blood's H^+ concentration, which chemically stimulates ventilation, eliminating more CO_2 and decreasing $PaCO_2$. These events pull the hydration reaction to the left, which decreases blood H_2CO_3 levels and offsets the blood's high levels of nonvolatile acids. These events constitute an important compensatory mechanism. The opposite compensatory response occurs for abnormally low blood levels of nonvolatile acids; the normal acidic stimulus to ventilation is reduced, decreasing the $\dot{V}_A$. These events drive the hydration reaction to the right, increasing blood H_2CO_3 concentration; this counteracts the effects of an abnormally low nonvolatile acid level. (These important compensatory ventilatory responses to nonrespiratory acid-base disturbances are discussed in detail in Chapter 10.)

HOW BLOOD CARRIES CARBON DIOXIDE

As with oxygen, CO_2 is transported in blood plasma and erythrocytes. However, CO_2 transport is more complex than oxygen transport. CO_2 is carried in the following three major forms in the plasma and erythrocyte: (1) dissolved CO_2 in the plasma, (2) plasma HCO_3^-, and (3) protein compounds (carbamino compounds). Figure 9-4 illustrates all modes of transport. CO_2 transport is intimately related to the blood's acid-base status because CO_2 reacts with water to form H_2CO_3.

Dissolved Carbon Dioxide

As illustrated in Figure 9-4, when CO_2 diffuses out of the tissues into the blood, a small portion physically dissolves in the plasma, but most diffuses into the erythrocyte. The small amount of dissolved CO_2 in the plasma is in equilibrium with the plasma PCO_2, which determines the direction and rate of CO_2 diffusion at both tissue and alveolar levels. CO_2 dissolves according to its solubility coefficient ($PCO_2 \times 0.03 = $ mmol/L dissolved CO_2). Thus, venous blood, with a PCO_2 of about 46 mm Hg, contains 1.38 mmol/L of dissolved CO_2 ($46 \times 0.03 = 1.38$). This converts to about 3 mL/dL of dissolved CO_2 in venous blood.

As the following equation shows, water hydrates a minuscule amount of plasma CO_2 to form H_2CO_3:

$$CO_2 + H_2O \rightarrow H_2CO_3$$

The rate of this reaction is quite slow in the plasma; no enzyme is present, as it is in the erythrocyte, to catalyze and speed up the reaction. The amount of CO_2 carried as H_2CO_3 in the plasma is infinitesimally small because at the pH of normal body fluids, H_2CO_3 instantly dissociates into HCO_3^- and H^+.[4] Because dissolved CO_2 reacts with H_2O to form H_2CO_3, dissolved CO_2 plays a key role in determining the blood pH (see Chapter 10).

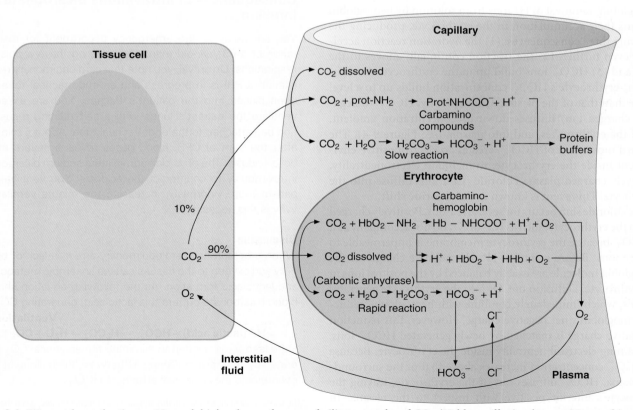

Figure 9-4 CO_2 uptake at the tissues. Hemoglobin's release of oxygen facilitates uptake of CO_2 (Haldane effect), whereas CO_2 combined with hemoglobin enhances release of oxygen (Bohr effect).

Bicarbonate

Most CO_2 diffusing into the blood from tissue cells enters the erythrocyte rather than remaining in the plasma. Several reactions occur in the erythrocyte, ultimately generating large amounts of HCO_3^-, which diffuse into the plasma (see Figure 9-4).

The reaction between CO_2 and H_2O occurs about 13,000 times faster in the erythrocyte than in the plasma because of the intracellular enzyme **carbonic anhydrase**.[4] When CO_2 enters the red blood cell, it is instantly converted into H_2CO_3 and its products, HCO_3^- and H^+. An extremely small amount of CO_2 remains dissolved in the erythrocyte fluid; this explains why most of the CO_2 molecules diffusing into the blood enter the erythrocyte rather than linger in the plasma. The rapid conversion of dissolved CO_2 to HCO_3^- and H^+ creates a concentration gradient that continually draws more plasma CO_2 into the erythrocyte.

CONCEPT QUESTION 9-4

Theoretically, what effect would a lack of carbonic anhydrase in the erythrocyte have on plasma PCO_2?

Chloride Shift

When the catalyzed hydration reaction forms H^+ and HCO_3^- ions in the erythrocyte, hemoglobin immediately buffers the H^+ ions, removing them from solution (see Figure 9-4). H^+ buffering occurs at the same time hemoglobin releases oxygen; deoxygenated hemoglobin is a more effective buffer than oxygenated hemoglobin. Removal of H^+ ions from solution by hemoglobin prevents their accumulation in the erythrocyte, producing the following three consequences: (1) the hydration reaction accelerates even further, (2) the reaction continually moves to the right, and (3) HCO_3^- ions build up in the erythrocyte. Eventually, the erythrocyte's HCO_3^- concentration builds up to a level higher than that of the plasma. Consequently, HCO_3^- (a negatively charged ion) diffuses down its concentration gradient, out of the erythrocytes, and into plasma (see Figure 9-4). The outward movement of HCO_3^- creates an electropositive environment inside the erythrocyte; to maintain electroneutrality, negatively charged plasma chloride (Cl^-) ions diffuse into the erythrocyte. This event is known as the **chloride shift**.

The chloride shift occurs for several reasons. Positively charged ions in the erythrocyte, such as Na^+ or K^+, do not accompany exit of HCO_3^- because the erythrocyte membrane is impermeable to positive ions. Before it buffers H^+, the negative charges of the hemoglobin molecule are exactly balanced by the positive ions in the erythrocyte. Diffusion of CO_2 into the erythrocyte generates H^+ ions, which immediately combine with hemoglobin, reducing hemoglobin's net negative charge. However, this reduction in negative charge is matched by newly generated HCO_3^- ions, maintaining electrical neutrality inside the erythrocyte. Because the HCO_3^- concentration increases above that of the surrounding plasma, HCO_3^- diffuses out of the erythrocyte, leaving the erythrocyte's interior positive with respect to the plasma. In response to this electrostatic gradient, the most abundant negatively charged ion in the plasma, Cl^-, moves into the erythrocyte

in exchange for HCO_3^- (see Figure 9-4). Hamburger, a Dutch physiologist, first described the chloride shift, which explains why it is also known as the Hamburger phenomenon.

Most CO_2 is transported from the tissues to the lungs in the form of plasma HCO_3^-, most of which is generated in the erythrocyte; this helps explain why the plasma HCO_3^- concentration is so much greater than the plasma H^+ concentration. The plasma HCO_3^- does not arise from the plasma hydration reaction, which creates equal amounts of H^+ and HCO_3^- ions; rather, it originates from the erythrocyte hydration reaction, where buffering of H^+ by hemoglobin allows HCO_3^- to accumulate and diffuse into the plasma.

All the reactions involving CO_2 are reversed in the lungs (Figure 9-5). CO_2 diffuses out of the blood into alveoli because of its partial pressure gradient. According to the law of mass action, as CO_2 leaves the blood, the hydration reaction in the erythrocyte shifts to the left. This shift causes HCO_3^- and H^+ to rapidly form CO_2 and H_2O, quickly depleting the erythrocyte HCO_3^- and H^+ concentrations. Consequently, plasma HCO_3^- diffuses into the cell and hemoglobin releases H^+. The CO_2 produced from these reactions diffuses into ventilated alveoli and is exhaled to the atmosphere.

CLINICAL FOCUS 9-2

Consequences of Intravenous Bicarbonate Ion Infusion

You are called to the emergency department for resuscitation of a 63-year-old man who does not have a pulse or respirations. On arrival, you note that cardiopulmonary resuscitation (CPR) is in progress and an endotracheal tube has been placed into the patient's trachea. You are asked to ventilate the patient's lungs with a self-inflating resuscitation bag attached to the endotracheal tube. About 5 minutes after the start of CPR, blood gases reveal a severe metabolic acidosis. The physician administers sodium bicarbonate intravenously to counteract the acidosis. You ventilate the patient more vigorously, increasing the minute ventilation. Why is this necessary?

Discussion

When a person has cardiopulmonary arrest, a lack of blood flow and oxygen to the tissues causes anaerobic metabolism and lactic acid formation. As the following equation shows, blood bicarbonate buffers this lactic acid, generating CO_2:

$$\text{Ventilation}$$
$$H^+ \text{(lactic acid)} + HCO_3^- \rightarrow H_2CO_3 \rightarrow H_2O + CO_2 \uparrow$$

Increased $\dot{V}_A$ is needed to eliminate the additional CO_2 generated by lactic acid buffering. Otherwise, the buildup of CO_2 counteracts the beneficial effects of HCO_3^-.*

*The use of sodium bicarbonate in this situation is not recommended, given the current understanding of emergency resuscitation. Nevertheless, this example is given here to illustrate the important concept that the buffering action of bicarbonate generates CO_2.

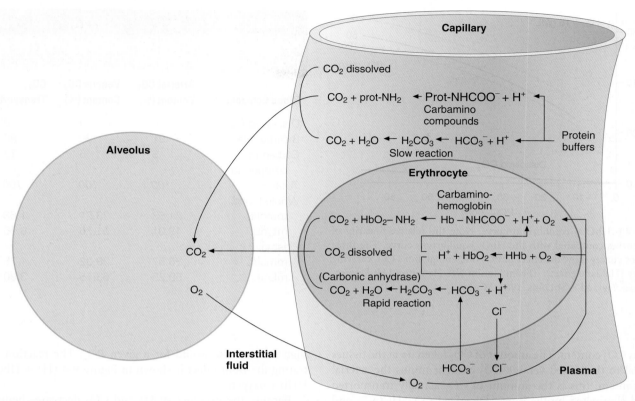

Figure 9-5 CO_2 release at the alveolus. Uptake of oxygen facilitates hemoglobin's release of CO_2 (Haldane effect), whereas release of CO_2 augments oxygen uptake (Bohr effect).

Carbamino Compounds

Plasma Carbamino Compounds

As illustrated in Figure 9-4, a small amount of CO_2 reacts with the free amino groups (NH_2) of plasma proteins to form carbamino compounds. This rapid reaction requires no catalyst ($CO_2 + $ prot-$NH_2 \rightarrow$ prot-$NHCOO^- + H^+$). Prot-NH_2 represents a protein molecule with a free amino group. When CO_2 combines with the amino group, it displaces a H^+ ion; a millimole of H^+ is released for each millimole of carbamino compound (prot-$NHCOO^-$) formed. These H^+ ions and the H^+ ions produced by the plasma hydration reaction are buffered by other plasma proteins (see Figure 9-4). (By convention, the carbamino compound amino group–CO_2 combination is written as $NHCOO^-$ rather than $NHCO_2^-$.)

Erythrocyte Carbamino Compounds: Carbaminohemoglobin

As with plasma proteins, CO_2 combines with the hemoglobin protein molecule at free amino sites. This reaction is rapid, requiring no catalyst ($CO_2 + HbO_2$-$NH_2 \rightarrow$ Hb-$NHCOO^- + H^+$). The resulting compound of hemoglobin and CO_2 is called carbaminohemoglobin (Hb-$NHCOO^-$). A millimole of H^+ is released for each millimole of Hb-$NHCOO^-$ formed. These H^+ ions are buffered by the hemoglobin molecule, along with H^+ ions formed by the rapid hydration reaction in the erythrocyte (see Figure 9-4). The hemoglobin molecule carries oxygen and CO_2 but not at the same binding site. Oxygen combines

with the heme groups (see Chapter 8), whereas CO_2 combines with the amino groups of α and β globin (protein) chains. However, the affinity of hemoglobin for CO_2 is greater when it is not combined with oxygen, a phenomenon known as the **Haldane effect**. The presence of oxygen on the heme portion hinders carbaminohemoglobin formation. Conversely, carbaminohemoglobin has a decreased affinity for oxygen (Bohr effect). Oxygenated blood carries less CO_2 for a given PCO_2 than deoxygenated blood. Figure 9-6 shows the CO_2 dissociation curve at different PO_2 values. For a given PCO_2, more CO_2 is carried at lower PO_2 values (lower saturations).

The CO_2 dissociation curve is essentially linear over the physiological range (see Figure 9-6), in contrast to the sigmoid-shaped oxygen-hemoglobin dissociation curve (see Chapter 8). Thus, a change in alveolar ventilation is much more effective in changing arterial CO_2 content than O_2 content; that is, a doubling of the alveolar ventilation in a healthy person cuts the CO_2 content in half but changes arterial O_2 content very little because the hemoglobin is already nearly 100% saturated with normal ventilation.

Relative Contribution of Carbon Dioxide Transport Mechanisms

In discussing how much each blood mechanism contributes to CO_2 transport, a distinction should be made between the amount of tissue CO_2 taken up by venous blood and the total

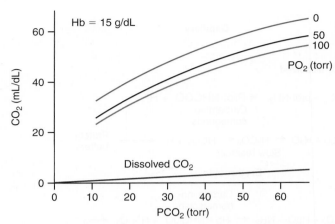

Figure 9-6 $HbCO_2$ equilibrium curve. Note the relative linearity of these curves compared with the HbO_2 equilibrium curve. The three different curves show the effect of PO_2 on hemoglobin's CO_2 carrying capacity (Haldane effect). (From Slonim NB, Hamilton LH: *Respiratory physiology*, ed 5, St Louis, 1987, Mosby.)

TABLE 9-1

Percentage Contribution of Blood Components to Carbon Dioxide Content and Transport

Blood Component	Arterial CO₂ Content (%)	Venous CO₂ Content (%)	CO₂ Transport (%)
Dissolved CO_2	4	5	8
Bicarbonate	91	90	80
Carbamino compounds	5	5	12
Total	*100*	*100*	*100*
Whole blood			
mmol/L	21.53	23.21	1.68
mL/dL	48.01	51.76	3.75
Plasma			
mmol/L	26.57	28.32	1.75
mL/dL	59.25	63.15	3.90

venous CO_2 content. The amount of CO_2 taken up at the tissues is equal to the mixed venous CO_2 content minus the arterial CO_2 content; this is the amount of CO_2 actually transported to and eliminated by the lungs. Dissolved CO_2, HCO_3^-, and carbamino compounds are responsible for 8%, 80%, and 12% of CO_2 transport.[4] Table 9-1 shows the percentage contribution of each major blood mechanism to CO_2 content and CO_2 transport.[4] (The percentage H_2CO_3 contributes is so small that it is not included in Table 9-1.) The milliliters per deciliter concentrations of CO_2 are calculated by multiplying millimoles per liter by the conversion factor, 2.23. The CO_2 concentration in plasma alone (see Table 9-1) is greater than that of whole blood (plasma plus erythrocytes) because the concentration of CO_2 in erythrocytes is considerably less than that in the plasma. The erythrocyte volume (about 40% of the whole blood volume) represents a dilute solution of CO_2, which when mixed with plasma, produces a lower CO_2 concentration in whole blood (millimoles per liter) than exists in plasma alone.

Complementary Interaction between Oxygen and Carbon Dioxide Transport: Bohr and Haldane Effects

Haldane and Bohr effects are mutually enhancing. While CO_2 is taken up at the tissues by various blood components, oxygen is diffusing down its partial pressure gradient from the blood plasma to the tissue cells (see Figure 9-4). Oxygen molecules dissociate from hemoglobin in response to decreasing plasma PO_2. The dissociation of oxygen from hemoglobin is augmented by the following two simultaneous processes: (1) CO_2 enters the erythrocyte and binds with the globin chains' amino acid groups, and (2) H^+ ions are formed by the rapid hydration of CO_2 (see Figure 9-4). Both processes shift the oxyhemoglobin equilibrium curve to the right, decreasing hemoglobin's affinity for oxygen (Bohr effect). Hemoglobin releases more oxygen

than it otherwise would for a given PO_2. The reaction illustrating the Bohr effect is shown in Figure 9-4 ($H^+ + HbO_2 \rightleftharpoons HHb + oxygen$).

Because the presence of H^+ and CO_2 decreases hemoglobin's affinity for oxygen, the presence of oxygen on the hemoglobin molecule must decrease hemoglobin's affinity for H^+ and CO_2. As it releases oxygen at the tissue level, hemoglobin more effectively takes up (buffers) the H^+ produced by the CO_2 hydration reaction. This buffering action promotes the production of HCO_3^-, increasing this mode of CO_2 transport. Because deoxygenated hemoglobin combines with CO_2 more readily than oxygenated hemoglobin, CO_2 transport by this mode (carbaminohemoglobin) is also enhanced. Thus, decreased oxygenation of the hemoglobin increases the blood's capacity for CO_2 at any given PCO_2 (Haldane effect). Haldane and Bohr effects enhance one another in a similar fashion in the lungs.

POINTS TO REMEMBER

- Aerobic metabolic activity of body tissues produces the blood CO_2.
- Alveolar ventilation normally eliminates CO_2 at the same rate that tissues produce it, maintaining a P_ACO_2 and $PaCO_2$ of about 40 mm Hg.
- CO_2 combines with water in the blood to form H_2CO_3, which subsequently dissociates into H^+ and HCO_3^- ions.
- The hydration reaction is reversible, allowing H_2CO_3 to be converted to its gaseous component, CO_2.
- Adding CO_2 molecules to the hydration reaction causes the reaction to move rightward (more H^+ and HCO_2^- production), and subtracting them causes the reaction to move leftward (less H^+ and HCO_2^- production).
- Because $\dot{V}_A$ controls blood CO_2 levels, it controls blood H_2CO_3 and hydrogen ion levels.

- The adequacy of alveolar ventilation is indicated by arterial PCO_2 levels.
- Hypoventilation and hyperventilation are associated with acidemia and alkalemia, respectively.
- Most CO_2 diffusing into the blood is converted to HCO_3^- ions in the erythrocyte.
- Blood carries CO_2 in three major forms—dissolved CO_2, HCO_3^-, and carbamino compounds—of these, HCO_3^- is the most predominant.
- Hemoglobin's affinity for CO_2 increases as oxygen dissociates from hemoglobin at the tissue level (Haldane effect).
- Alveolar ventilation changes arterial CO_2 content much more effectively than arterial O_2 content.

References

1. Boron WF: Acid-base physiology. In Boron WF, Boulpaep EL, editors: *Medical physiology*, ed 2, Philadelphia, 2009, Saunders.
2. Boron WF: The transport of oxygen and carbon dioxide in the blood. In Boron WF, Boulpaep EL, editors: *Medical physiology*, ed 2, Philadelphia, 2009, Saunders.
3. Bettelheim FA, Landesberg JM: The law of chemical equilibrium and Le Chatelier's Principle. In: *Laboratory experiments for introduction to general, organic and biochemistry*, ed 7, Florence, KY, 2009, Cengage Learning.
4. Klocke RA: Carbon dioxide transport. In Fishman AP, et al: *Handbook of physiology, section 3: the respiratory system, volume IV, gas exchange*, Bethesda, MD, 1987, American Physiological Society.

CHAPTER 10

Acid-Base Regulation

OBJECTIVES

After reading this chapter, you will be able to:

- Explain how hydrogen ion concentration [H^+] affects cellular enzyme activity
- Define acid and base according to the Brønsted-Lowry classification scheme
- Describe how the strength of an acid and its equilibrium or ionization constant are related
- Explain the relationship between the concept of pH and [H^+]
- Explain how isohydric buffering in the blood prevents large pH changes when carbon dioxide (CO_2) reacts with water to form carbonic acid
- Show why bicarbonate and nonbicarbonate buffer systems differ in their ability to buffer volatile and fixed acids
- Derive the Henderson-Hasselbalch (H-H) equation from the ionization constant for carbonic acid

- Explain why the body's open and closed buffer systems differ in their ability to buffer fixed and volatile acids
- Use the H-H equation to predict the change in ventilation required to produce a given arterial pH
- Use the H-H equation to calculate the pH, bicarbonate ion concentration ([HCO_3^-]), and carbon dioxide pressure (PCO_2)
- Use arterial blood gas values to distinguish between primary respiratory and primary metabolic acid-base disturbances
- Predict the body's compensatory responses to primary respiratory and metabolic acid-base disturbances
- Explain why acute changes in PCO_2 affect blood levels of HCO_3^-

KEY TERMS

anions
buffer base
buffers
cations
closed buffer systems
conjugate base
equilibrium constant
fixed acids
isohydric buffering

isohydric principle
metabolic acidosis
metabolic alkalosis
open buffer system
pH
pK
respiratory acidosis
respiratory alkalosis

BASIC CONCEPTS

Importance of Regulating Hydrogen Ions

Acid-base balance refers to physiological mechanisms that keep the hydrogen ion concentration ($[H^+]$) of blood and body fluids in a range compatible with life. The body's metabolic processes continually generate hydrogen ions; therefore, regulation is vital.

Hydrogen ions react with the negatively charged regions of protein molecules much more strongly than do other **cations** (positively charged ions). Protein molecules are large nondiffusible **anions** (negatively charged ions); they are too large to diffuse through cell membranes. Protein molecules are effective **buffers**; that is, they readily combine with hydrogen ions, removing them from solution. This process causes the protein molecule to change its physical shape. Proteins are the structural components of catalytic enzymes vital for normal cell function; a change in the shape of an enzyme molecule renders it inactive. In this way, even slight changes in $[H^+]$ can inactivate essential enzymes and cause normal metabolic processes to fail. The precise regulation of body fluid $[H^+]$ is extremely important.

Definition of Acid and Base

According to the widely accepted Brønsted-Lowry theory, an acid is any substance that donates a proton (H^+) to an aqueous solution; a base is any substance that accepts a proton, removing it from solution. By this definition, an H^+ donor is an acid and an H^+ acceptor is a base.

Body fluids are acidic if they have an abnormally high $[H^+]$. Increased $[H^+]$ in the blood is called acidemia. Acidosis refers to a general condition characterized by the accumulation of H^+ in body fluids.

The term alkali is synonymous with base. Originally, alkali referred to strong bases formed by metallic hydroxides, such as sodium hydroxide (NaOH) and potassium hydroxide (KOH). In medicine, the term alkali refers to any base (i.e., any H^+ acceptor). Body fluids are alkaline (or basic) if they contain abnormally high amounts of base or if they contain abnormally low amounts of H^+ compared with base. Therefore a body fluid can be alkaline even if the absolute concentration of base is normal. Increased base or reduced H^+ in the blood is called alkalemia; alkalosis refers to an alkaline condition of body fluids.

Acids and bases dissociate or ionize in solution to form their component ions:

$$\text{Acid: } HCl \leftrightarrows H^+ + Cl^-$$
$$\text{Base: } NaOH \leftrightarrows Na^+ + OH^-$$

The double arrows mean that this process is reversible; equilibrium is rapidly established between undissociated molecules and their dissociated ions.

Acids and bases react with one another in an aqueous solution to form a salt and water, neutralizing one another (i.e., the products are neither acidic nor basic), as the following reaction shows:

$$H^+Cl^- + Na^+OH^- \leftrightarrows Na^+Cl^- + H_2O$$

In this reaction, hydrogen chloride (HCl) (hydrochloric acid) donates H^+, which is accepted by the base component (OH^-) of NaOH. A neutral salt, sodium chloride (NaCl), and water (H_2O) are the results of this reaction.

Strong and Weak Acids and Bases: Equilibrium Constants

Strong acids and bases ionize almost completely in an aqueous solution; weak acids and bases ionize only to a slight extent. An example of a strong acid is HCl; nearly 100% of HCl molecules dissociate to form H^+ and Cl^-, as the following reaction shows:

1. $$HCl \rightarrow H^+ + Cl^-$$

At equilibrium, the concentration of HCl is extremely small compared with the concentration of H^+ and Cl^-. No arrow points to the left, emphasizing that HCl ionizes almost completely.

In contrast, a weak acid dissociates only partially as the following shows:

2. $$HA \leftrightarrows HA^+ + A^-$$

In this reaction, HA is a generic representation of an undissociated weak acid; H^+ and A^- represent the dissociated components of the weak acid. The short arrow pointing to the right indicates that at equilibrium the concentration of undissociated HA molecules is far greater than the concentrations of A^- or H^+.

The **equilibrium constant** of an acid is a measure of the extent to which the acid molecules dissociate (ionize). The law of mass action states that the velocity of a reaction is proportional to the product of the concentrations of the reactants. The following dissociation of the generic weak acid HA illustrates this concept:

3. $$[HA] \underset{v_1}{\overset{v_2}{\leftrightarrows}} [A^-] + [H^+]$$

Velocity 1 (V_1) is proportional to $[HA]$, and velocity 2 (V_2) is proportional to $[A^-]$ multiplied by $[H^+]$. At equilibrium, the number of HA molecules dissociating is equal to the number of A^- and H^+ associating (i.e., V_1 and V_2 are equal). In this state, no further net change occurs in $[HA]$, $[A^-]$, or $[H^+]$. The following equation represents conditions at equilibrium:

4. $$\frac{[A^-] \times [H^+]}{[HA]} = K_A \text{ (small)}$$

In equation 4, K_A represents the equilibrium constant for HA. (K_A is also known as the acid's ionization or dissociation constant.) In this example, the weak acid HA has an extremely small K_A because the denominator $[HA]$ is quite large with respect to the numerator ($[H^+]$ multiplied by $[A^-]$). At a given temperature, the value of K_A is always the same for this particular weak acid (HA) regardless of its initial concentration. Each acid has its own unique ionization constant.

A strong acid, such as HCl, has a large K_A because the denominator $[HCl]$ is extremely small compared with the numerator ($[H^+]$ multiplied by $[Cl^-]$). This is shown as follows:

5. $$\frac{[H^+] \times [Cl^-]}{[HCl]} = K_A \text{ (large)}$$

As shown by equations 4 and 5, K_A indicates an acid's strength; the greater the value of K_A, the stronger the acid—that is, the more completely it dissociates.

Carbonic acid (H_2CO_3)—the product of the reaction between CO_2 and H_2O—is often described as a weak acid, when in reality it is a moderately strong acid. In the pH environment of the blood, H_2CO_3 dissociates instantly and almost completely as soon as it is formed.[1] The idea that H_2CO_3 is a weak acid comes from the fact that the reaction between dissolved CO_2 and H_2O is quite slow in blood plasma, and from the fact that the sum of dissolved CO_2 and H_2CO_3 is commonly lumped together and treated as the undissociated acid. This practice is sensible because H_2CO_3 and dissolved CO_2 are indistinguishable from one other by chemical analysis (see Chapter 9). Even though H_2CO_3 is a relatively strong acid, (1) its treatment as being synonymous with dissolved CO_2 and (2) its slow formation make it appear to be a weak acid.[1]

Measuring Hydrogen Ion Concentration: The Concept of pH

$[H^+]$ in body fluids is extremely small (normally about 40×10^{-9} mol/L, or 40 billionths of 1 mole per liter [0.000000040 mol/L]). The prefix "nano" means billionths; therefore, $[H^+]$ of body fluids is about 40 nmol/L. In clinical medicine, acidity is generally expressed in terms of **pH** rather than nmol/L$[H^+]$.

The concept of pH was developed by Sørenson in 1909. The pH scale ranges from 0 to 14 pH units. The dissociation of pure water molecules (H_2O, or HOH) helps explain this concept:

6. $$HOH \underset{\rightarrow}{\leftarrow} H^+ + OH^-$$

The dissociation of H_2O is extremely slight. Therefore, water's K_A is exceedingly small, as the following shows:

7. $$\frac{[H^+] \times [OH^-]}{[HOH]} = K_A$$

Equation 7 can be rearranged to yield the following:

8. $$[H^+] \times [OH^-] = [HOH]K_A$$

In practical terms, [HOH] is constant because of its extremely slight dissociation. Therefore, the right side of equation 8 can be considered constant:

9. $$[HOH] K_A = K_W$$

In equation 9, K_w represents the dissociation constant of water. Equation 8 then becomes the following:

10. $$[H^+] \times [OH^-] = K_W$$

The numerical value of K_w is about 10^{-14}. At equilibrium, pure water contains 10^{-7} mol/L of H^+ and 10^{-7} mol/L of OH^-. If the value of $[H^+]$ is known, the value of $[OH^-]$ can be calculated because of the reciprocal relationship between $[H^+]$ and $[OH^-]$. For example, if $[H^+]$ equals 10^{-3} mol/L, $[OH^-]$ equals 10^{-11} mol/L.

pH is defined as the negative logarithm, or exponent (to the base 10), of $[H^+]$; this is shown as follows:

11. $$pH = -\log[H^+]$$

Water's pH ($[H^+] = 10^{-7}$ mol/L) is calculated as follows:

$$pH = -\log(10^{-7})$$

12. $$pH = -(-7)$$
$$pH = 7$$

A pH of 7 corresponds to $[H^+]$ of 100 nmol/L:

$$10^{-7} \text{mol/L} = 0.0000001 \text{ mol/L} = 0.000000100 \text{ mol/L}$$

Because pH is the negative logarithm of $[H^+]$, a decrease in pH indicates an increase in $[H^+]$ (Box 10-1).

A chemically neutral solution (neither acidic nor basic) has a pH of 7.0. To the chemist, a solution with a pH less than 7.0 is acidic, and a solution with a pH greater than 7.0 is alkaline (see Box 10-1). By this standard, body fluids are slightly alkaline, as the following shows:

Body fluid $[H^+] = 40 \times 10^{-9}$ mol/L
$$pH = -\log(40 \times 10^{-9})$$
$$pH = -\log 40 + (-\log 10^{-9})$$
$$pH = -1.6 + (-[-9])$$
$$pH = -1.6 + 9$$
$$pH = 7.40$$

Because pH is a logarithmic scale, a change of one pH unit corresponds to a 10-fold change in $[H^+]$ (Figure 10-1). $[H^+]$ at a pH of 7.0 (100 nmol/L) is 10 times the $[H^+]$ at a pH of 8.0 (10 nmol/L). Figure 10-1 shows that the relationship between pH and $[H^+]$ is linear in the normal physiological range of body fluids (pH = 7.35 to 7.45). Table 10-1 shows that in the physiological range, a 1-nmol/L change in $[H^+]$ produces a 0.01 change in pH. The pH-to-$[H^+]$ relationship maintains some degree of linearity between pH values of 7.20 and 7.55. However, below a pH of 7.20, linearity deteriorates rapidly (see Figure 10-1).

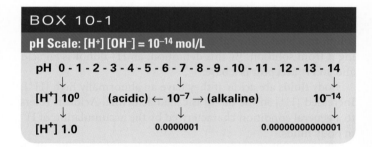

BOX 10-1

pH Scale: $[H^+] [OH^-] = 10^{-14}$ mol/L

pH 0 - 1 - 2 - 3 - 4 - 5 - 6 - 7 - 8 - 9 - 10 - 11 - 12 - 13 - 14

$[H^+]$ 10^0 (acidic) ← 10^{-7} → (alkaline) 10^{-14}

$[H^+]$ 1.0   0.0000001   0.00000000000001

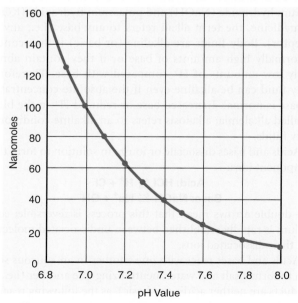

Figure 10-1 Relationship between pH and H^+ ion concentration (nmol/L). (From Wilkins RL, Stoller JK, Kacmarek RM: *Egan's fundamentals of respiratory care,* ed 9, St Louis, 2009, Mosby.)

CLINICAL FOCUS 10-1

Comparison of Blood [H⁺] Changes When pH Decreases 0.1 Unit: 7.4 to 7.3 and 7.1 to 7.0

A patient develops an acidosis in which the blood pH decreases from 7.40 to 7.30. Another patient, already acidotic, has a pH reduction from 7.10 to 7.00. Both patients experienced a decrease of 0.1 pH unit. Did both patients gain the same amount of [H⁺] in the blood? (*Hint*: See Table 10-1.)

Discussion

Table 10-1 shows that a decrease in pH from 7.40 to 7.30 is associated with [H⁺] gain measuring 10 nmol/L. The patient whose pH decreased from 7.10 to 7.00 gained more [H⁺] than the first patient because [H⁺] increased from 79 nmol/L to 100 nmol/L, a gain of 21 nmol/L. These findings show the nonlinear relationship between pH and [H⁺], which is most pronounced at the extremes of the physiological range (see Figure 10-1). In other words, pH is a logarithmic scale. Patients with a preexisting acidosis experience more serious consequences from a decrease in pH than patients who have the same pH reduction in the normal physiological range.

TABLE 10-1

Approximate Relationship between pH and [H⁺]

pH	[H⁺] nmol/L
6.80	158
6.90	126
7.00	100
7.10	79
7.15	71
7.20	63
7.25	56
7.30	50
7.35	**45**
7.40	**40**
7.45	**35**
7.50	32
7.55	28
7.60	25
7.70	20
7.80	16
8.00	10

Note: Bold values indicate normal range.

CONCEPT QUESTION 10-1

What is the pH of a solution if [H⁺] equals 10^{-6} mol/L? Does this solution contain more or fewer hydrogen ions per liter than a solution with a pH of 7.0?

Overview of Hydrogen Ion Regulation in Body Fluids

The body continually produces hydrogen ions, but the pH of body fluids varies minimally between 7.35 and 7.45 (45 to 35 nmol/L [H⁺]). As noted previously, this rigid control is necessary to sustain vital cellular enzyme activity. Hydrogen ions formed in the body arise from either volatile acids or nonvolatile acids, or **fixed acids**. Volatile acids in the blood arise from and are in equilibrium with a dissolved gas. The only volatile acid of physiological significance in the body is carbonic acid (H_2CO_3), which is in equilibrium with dissolved CO_2. Normal aerobic metabolism generates about 13,000 mM of CO_2 each day, producing an equal amount of H⁺:

$$CO_2 + H_2O \rightarrow H_2CO_3 \rightarrow HCO_3^- + H^+$$
$$\uparrow$$
Aerobic metabolism

In a process called **isohydric buffering**,[1] most of the hydrogen ions produced cause no pH change at the tissue level because newly forming deoxygenated hemoglobin immediately combines with the hydrogen ions (see Chapter 9). When blood reaches the lungs, hemoglobin releases these hydrogen ions, which combine with plasma bicarbonate ion (HCO_3^-) to form CO_2:

Ventilation
$$\uparrow$$
$$CO_2 + H_2O \leftarrow H_2CO_3 \leftarrow HCO_3^- + H^+$$
$$\uparrow$$
$$HHb \rightarrow H^+ + Hb^-$$

Ventilation eliminates carbonic acid (CO_2), keeping pace with its production. Isohydric buffering and ventilation are the two major mechanisms responsible for maintaining a stable pH in the face of massive CO_2 production.[2]

Catabolism of proteins continually produces fixed acids such as sulfuric and phosphoric acids. In addition, anaerobic metabolism produces lactic acid, another fixed acid. In contrast to carbonic acid, these fixed acids are nonvolatile and are not in equilibrium with a gaseous component. Therefore, the hydrogen ions of fixed acids must be buffered by bases in the body or eliminated in the urine by the kidneys. Compared with daily CO_2 production, fixed acid production is small, averaging only about 50 to 70 mEq per day.[3] Certain diseases, such as untreated diabetes, increase fixed acid production. The resulting hydrogen ions stimulate the respiratory centers in the brain, increasing ventilation and CO_2 elimination, pulling the CO_2 hydration reaction to the left:

Increased $\dot{V}_A$
$$\uparrow$$
$$CO_2 + H_2O \leftarrow H_2CO_3 \leftarrow HCO_3^- + H^+$$
$$\uparrow$$
Fixed acid H⁺

Thus, the respiratory system compensates for fixed acid accumulation, preventing a significant increase in [H⁺].

BODY BUFFER SYSTEMS

Function of a Buffer

A buffer solution resists changes in pH when an acid or a base is added to it. A buffer solution is a mixture of an acid and its corresponding base component. The acid component is the H^+ cation, formed when a weak acid dissociates in solution. The base component is the remaining anion portion of the acid molecule, known as the **conjugate base**. An example of one of the most important blood buffer systems is a solution of carbonic acid and its conjugate base, HCO_3^-:

$$H_2CO_3 \text{ (acid)} \leftrightharpoons HCO_3^- \text{ (conjugate base)} + H^+$$

In the blood, the bicarbonate ions combine with sodium ions (Na^+), forming sodium bicarbonate ($NaHCO_3$). If HCl (a strong acid) is added to the H_2CO_3/NaH_2CO_3 buffer solution, bicarbonate ions react with the added hydrogen ions to form more weak carbonic acid molecules and a neutral salt:

$$HCl + H_2CO_3 / Na^+ HCO_3^- \rightarrow H_2CO_3 + NaCl$$

The strong acidity of HCl is converted to the relatively weak acidity of H_2CO_3, preventing a large decrease in pH.

Similarly, if NaOH, a strong base, is added to this buffer solution, it reacts with the carbonic acid molecule to form the weak base, sodium bicarbonate, and water:

$$NaOH + H_2CO_3 / NaHCO_3 \rightarrow NaHCO_3 + H_2O$$

The strong alkalinity of NaOH is changed to the relatively weak alkalinity of $NaHCO_3$. The pH change is minimized.

CONCEPT QUESTION 10-2

Why is a solution of HCl and its conjugate base not an effective buffer system?

Bicarbonate and Nonbicarbonate Buffer Systems

Blood buffers are classified as either bicarbonate or nonbicarbonate buffer systems. The bicarbonate buffer system consists of carbonic acid (H_2CO_3) and its conjugate base, HCO_3^-. The nonbicarbonate buffer system consists mainly of phosphates and proteins, including hemoglobin. The blood **buffer base** is the sum of bicarbonate and nonbicarbonate bases, measured in millimoles per liter of blood.

The bicarbonate system is called an **open buffer system** because H_2CO_3 is in equilibrium with dissolved CO_2, which is readily removed by ventilation. That is, when HCO_3^- buffers H^+, the product, H_2CO_3, is broken down into CO_2 and H_2O; ventilation continually removes CO_2 from the reaction, preventing it from reaching equilibrium. As long as ventilation is adequate, buffering activity continues without being slowed or stopped:

$$HCO_3^- + H^+ \rightarrow H_2CO_3 \rightarrow H_2O + CO_2 \text{ (exhaled gas)}$$

Nonbicarbonate buffers are **closed buffer systems** because all components of acid-base reactions remain in the system. (In the following discussions, nonbicarbonate buffer systems are collectively represented as *HBuf/Buf⁻*, where HBuf is the weak acid, and Buf⁻ is the conjugate base.) When Buf⁻ buffers H^+, the

TABLE 10-2

Classification of Whole Blood Buffers

Open System	Closed System
Bicarbonate	**Nonbicarbonate**
Plasma	Hemoglobin
Erythrocyte	Organic phosphates
	Inorganic phosphates
	Plasma proteins

TABLE 10-3

Individual Buffer Contributions to Whole Blood Buffering

Buffer Type	Percent of Total Buffering
Bicarbonate	
Plasma bicarbonate	35
Erythrocyte bicarbonate	18
Total bicarbonate buffering	53
Nonbicarbonate	
Hemoglobin	35
Organic phosphates	3
Inorganic phosphates	2
Plasma proteins	7
Total nonbicarbonate buffering	47
Total	**100**

product, HBuf, builds up and eventually reaches equilibrium with the reactants, preventing further buffering activity:

$$Buf^- + H^+ \leftrightharpoons HBuf$$

Table 10-2 summarizes the characteristics and components of bicarbonate and nonbicarbonate buffer systems.

Open and closed buffer systems differ in their ability to buffer fixed and volatile acids. They also differ in their ability to function in wide-ranging pH environments. Both systems are physiologically important, each playing a unique and essential role in maintaining pH homeostasis. Table 10-3 summarizes the approximate contributions of various blood buffers to the total buffer base. The bicarbonate buffer system has the greatest buffering capacity because it is an open system.

Bicarbonate and nonbicarbonate buffer systems do not function in isolation from one another; they are intermingled in the same solution (whole blood) and are in equilibrium with the same [H^+] (Figure 10-2). As Figure 10-2 shows, increased ventilation increases the CO_2 removal rate, ultimately causing nonbicarbonate buffers (HBuf) to release H^+. Conversely, cessation of ventilation reverses the reaction; CO_2 builds up, more H^+ is generated, and, ultimately, more HBuf is formed.

pH of a Buffer System and Henderson-Hasselbalch Equation

Physiological buffer solutions consist mostly of undissociated acid molecules and only a small amount of H^+ and conjugate

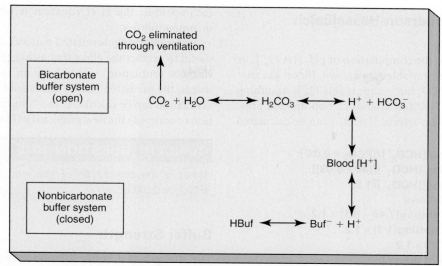

Figure 10-2 Bicarbonate and nonbicarbonate buffer systems. The two systems coexist in the blood and are in equilibrium with each other.

base anions. The $[H^+]$ of a buffer solution can be calculated if the concentrations of its components and the acid's equilibrium constant are known. Consider the bicarbonate buffer system:

$$H_2CO_3 \overset{\longrightarrow}{\leftharpoonup} H^+ + HCO_3^- \text{ (slight dissociation)}$$

The equilibrium constant (K_A) for H_2CO_3 is as follows:

$$K_A = \left[\frac{[H^+] \times [HCO_3^-]}{[H_2CO_3]} \right]$$

$[H^+]$ can be isolated through the following algebraic rearrangement of this equation:

$$[H^+] = K_A \times \left[\frac{[H_2CO_3]}{[HCO_3^-]} \right]$$

The $[H^+]$ is determined by the ratio between undissociated acid molecules $[H_2CO_3]$ and base anions $[HCO_3^-]$.

Henderson-Hasselbalch Equation

The foregoing concept is the basis for the Henderson-Hasselbalch (H-H) equation. The H-H equation is specific for calculating the pH of the blood's bicarbonate buffer system, which is the same as the pH of the plasma. That is, because all buffer systems in the blood are in equilibrium with the same pH, the pH of any one buffer system is equal to the pH of the entire plasma solution (the **isohydric principle**).[2]

The H-H equation is derived from the equilibrium constant for H_2CO_3:

$$\left[\frac{[H^+] \times [HCO_3^-]}{[H_2CO_3]} \right] = K_A$$

To express $[H^+]$ in terms of pH, the logarithm of both sides of the equation is determined:

$$\log \left[\frac{[H^+] \times [HCO_3^-]}{[H_2CO_3]} \right] = \log K_A$$

This equation is algebraically equivalent to the following:

$$\log[H^+] + \log \left[\frac{[HCO_3^-]}{[H_2CO_3]} \right] = \log K_A$$

Transposing:

$$\log[H^+] = \log K_A - \log \left[\frac{[HCO_3^-]}{[H_2CO_3]} \right]$$

Multiplying both sides of the equation by −1 produces the following:

$$-\log[H^+] = -\log K_A + \log \left[\frac{[HCO_3^-]}{[H_2CO_3]} \right]$$

The pH (i.e., $-\log [H^+]$) is now on the left side of the equation; the negative logarithm of K_A is the definition of **pK**, which is the pH of the buffer system when H_2CO_3 is exactly 50% dissociated. Substituting, the equation becomes the following:

$$pH = pK + \log \left[\frac{[HCO_3^-]}{[H_2CO_3]} \right]$$

The H-H equation substitutes dissolved CO_2 ($PCO_2 \times 0.03$ mmol/L/mm Hg) for $[H_2CO_3]$. This is legitimate because dissolved CO_2 is in equilibrium with and directly proportional to the blood's $[H_2CO_3]$, as explained in Chapter 9. In contrast to H_2CO_3, dissolved CO_2 is easily calculated from the blood's carbon dioxide pressure (PCO_2). For these reasons, dissolved CO_2 is treated as though it were the acid instead of H_2CO_3. The H-H equation is as follows:

$$pH = pK' + \log \left[\frac{[HCO_3^-]}{(PCO_2 \times 0.03)} \right]$$

The substitution of ($PCO_2 \times 0.03$) for $[H_2CO_3]$ produces a different pK—hence the term pK'. The pK' for the $(HCO_3^-)/(PCO_2 \times 0.03)$ system is 6.1, which is a different value than the pK of the HCO_3^-/H_2CO_3 system. (Using the pK' of 6.1 is incorrect if H_2CO_3 is used in the equation's denominator.) The clinical form of the H-H equation is as follows:

$$pH = 6.1 + \log \left[\frac{[HCO_3^-]}{(PCO_2 \times 0.03)} \right]$$

Clinical Use of Henderson-Hasselbalch Equation

The H-H equation allows the computation of pH, [HCO$_3^-$], or PCO$_2$ if two of these three variables are known. Blood gas analyzers measure pH and PCO$_2$ but compute [HCO$_3^-$]. Assuming a normal arterial pH of 7.40 and arterial carbon dioxide pressure (PaCO$_2$) of 40 mm Hg, arterial [HCO$_3^-$] can be calculated as follows:

$$pH = 6.1 + log[[HCO_3^-]/(PCO_2 \times 0.03)]$$
$$7.40 = 6.1 + log[[HCO_3^-]/[40 \times 0.03]]$$
$$7.40 = 6.1 + log[[HCO_3^-]/1.2]$$

[HCO$_3^-$] is solved as follows:

$$[HCO_3^-] = antilog(7.40 - 6.1) \times 1.2$$
$$= antilog(1.3) \times 1.2$$
$$= 20 \times 1.2$$
$$= 24\ mEq/L$$

The different forms of the H-H equation needed to calculate pH, PCO$_2$, and HCO$_3^-$ are shown in Box 10-2.

The H-H equation is useful for checking a clinical blood gas report to determine whether the pH, PCO$_2$, and [HCO$_3^-$] values are compatible with one another. In this way, transcription errors (which are common) can be detected. Experienced clinicians can often spot combinations of blood gas values that seem incompatible; the H-H equation is helpful in verifying such incompatibilities.

In mechanically ventilated patients, it also may be clinically useful to predict the effect that a change in tidal volume or rate (minute ventilation) would have on the arterial pH. In other words, the predicted PaCO$_2$ that would result from a change in ventilation can be calculated and "plugged in" to the H-H equation to compute the new projected pH (see Clinical Focus 10-2).

CONCEPT QUESTION 10-3

What is the blood's pH if the ratio between [HCO$_3^-$] and (PCO$_2$ × 0.03) is 25:1?

Buffer Strength

The strength of a buffer solution is determined by measuring the number of hydrogen ions that must be added to or taken away from the solution to change its pH by one unit. A buffer solution's strength varies, depending on its initial pH, before hydrogen ions are added or subtracted. A given buffer solution has its own unique pH range in which it most effectively resists pH changes. The titration curve for the bicarbonate buffer system, HCO$_3^-$/(PCO$_2$ × 0.03), illustrates this point (Figure 10-3).

This titration curve shows the degree to which pH changes when hydrogen ions are added to or subtracted from a bicarbonate buffer solution. The upper right side of the graph shows a hypothetical condition in which the solution's concentration of HCO$_3^-$ is 100% and that of dissolved CO$_2$ is 0% (i.e., no H$^+$ ions exist in this imaginary solution). As H$^+$ ions are added to the solution, the pH decreases rapidly at first. The amount of H$^+$ needed to change the buffer solution's pH one unit, from 7.9 to 6.9, is represented by the width of the orange-shaded band at the upper left corner of the graph. Progressively greater amounts of H$^+$ are required to reduce the pH by one unit as the buffer solution's pH decreases. As H$^+$ ions are added, the decrease in the buffer solution's pH follows the S-shaped titration curve (see Figure 10-3) from right to left. The curve is steepest when the buffer solution contains 50% dissolved CO$_2$ and 50% HCO$_3^-$, which corresponds to a solution pH of 6.1. At this point, the

---

BOX 10-2

Using the Henderson-Hasselbalch Equation

1. *Known:* PCO$_2$ and [HCO$_3^-$]; *calculate* pH as follows:

$$pH = 6.1 + log\left[\frac{[HCO_3^-]}{[PCO_2 \times 0.03]}\right]$$

2. *Known:* PCO$_2$ and pH; *calculate* [HCO$_3^-$] as follows:
$$[HCO_3^-] = antilog(pH - 6.1) \times (PCO_2 \times 0.03)$$

3. *Known:* pH and [HCO$_3^-$]; *calculate* PCO$_2$ as follows:

$$PCO_2 = \left[\frac{[HCO_3^-]}{(antilog[pH - 6.1]) \times 0.03}\right]$$

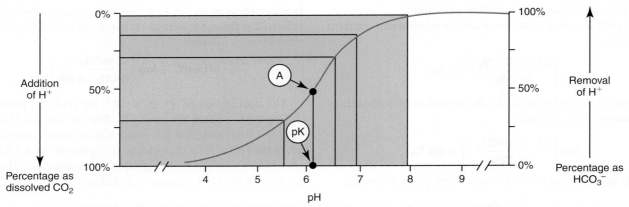

Figure 10-3 Titration curve for the HCO$_3^-$/dissolved CO$_2$ buffer system. Buffering is most effective when the solution contains 50% acid and 50% base, or when the solution's pH equals the buffer's pK. (Redrawn from Beachey WD: *Curr Rev Respir Ther* 8:92, 1986.)

solution's ability to resist a pH change is at its maximum. A relatively large amount of H^+ must be added to decrease the solution's pH by one unit, from 6.5 to 5.5; it takes a much smaller amount of H^+ to cause the pH to decrease from 7.9 to 6.9. (Compare the widths of the orange-shaded bands on the left side of the graph.) The buffer solution's pH at its maximal buffering power (point *A* on the steepest part of the titration curve) is known as the pK, which is 6.1 for the HCO_3^-/dissolved CO_2 system. A given buffer solution is most effective in resisting pH changes when it operates in a pH environment near its pK.

Physiological Importance of Bicarbonate Buffer System

The HCO_3^-/dissolved CO_2 system would appear to be an ineffective buffer in humans because the system's pK of 6.1 is well out of the physiological pH range for body fluids. Why then is the bicarbonate buffer system so effective in the blood? The answer is simply that HCO_3^-/dissolved CO_2 is an open buffer system; that is, one of its components, CO_2, is continually removed through ventilation:

$$HCO_3^- + H^+ \rightarrow H_2CO_3 \rightarrow H_2O + CO_2 \uparrow \text{ (exhaled gas)}$$

HCO_3^- is able to continue buffering H^+ as long as ventilation continues to remove CO_2 effectively; hypothetically, this buffering activity could continue until all body sources of HCO_3^- are used up in binding H^+ ions.

To understand the effectiveness of the open bicarbonate buffer system in the body, it is helpful to visualize what would happen if this system were closed, as illustrated in Figure 10-4. In this figure, containers *A* and *B* have a bicarbonate buffer dissolved in 1 L of solution. Initially, the buffer solution has HCO_3^- and dissolved CO_2 concentrations equal to the concentrations of normal blood plasma, and the pH is 7.40, according to the H-H equation (see Figure 10-4, *A*). When 12 mM of a strong acid (HCl) is added, 12 mM of HCO_3^- is converted to 12 mM of CO_2, which decreases the HCO_3^- concentration from 24 mM to 12 mM and increases the dissolved CO_2 from 1.2 mM to

13.2 mM (see Figure 10-4, *B*). Because the CO_2 produced by this reaction cannot escape from the system, the denominator of the H-H equation (dissolved CO_2) is increased, causing pH to decrease to 6.06 (see Figure 10-4, *B*).

Figure 10-5 illustrates why the open bicarbonate buffer system is more effective in resisting pH changes produced by the addition of 12 mM of HCl. To simulate normal ventilation, a gas with a PCO_2 of 40 mm Hg is continuously bubbled through the bicarbonate buffer solution in Figure 10-5. This keeps the PCO_2 of the solution at 40 mm Hg, and keeps the dissolved CO_2 concentration constant at 1.2 mM/L (40 mm Hg $\times$ 0.03 = 1.2 mM/L). Figure 10-5, *A*, represents normal plasma values for HCO_3^-, dissolved CO_2, and pH. As in the closed system (see Figure 10-4), adding 12 mM of HCl converts an equal amount of HCO_3^- to dissolved CO_2. HCO_3^- decreases from 24 mM to 12 mM, but the simultaneously generated 12 mM of CO_2 is bubbled out of the solution to the atmosphere (see Figure 10-5, *B*). This keeps the denominator of the H-H equation (dissolved CO_2) constant at 1.2 mM/L. As shown in Figure 10-5, *B*, the pH decreased to only 7.07 because CO_2 cannot build up in the solution, as it did in the closed system. Thus, the bicarbonate buffer system is effective in buffering fixed acid even though it operates in a pH environment of 7.40 rather than its pK of 6.1. However, the effectiveness of the bicarbonate buffering system depends on the ability of the lungs to produce adequate ventilation.

CONCEPT QUESTION 10-4

Why is the patient's ability to increase ventilation critical to the effectiveness of the bicarbonate buffer system?

Physiological Roles of Bicarbonate and Nonbicarbonate Buffer Systems

The functions of bicarbonate and nonbicarbonate buffer systems are summarized in Table 10-4.

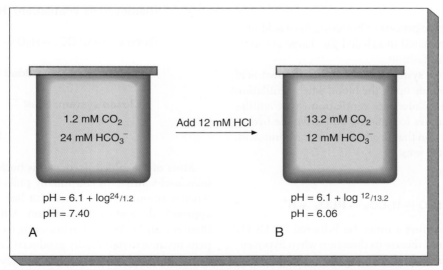

A

$$pH = 6.1 + \log{^{24}/1.2}$$
$$pH = 7.40$$

B

$$pH = 6.1 + \log{^{12}/13.2}$$
$$pH = 6.06$$

1.2 mM CO_2
24 mM HCO_3^-

Add 12 mM HCl

13.2 mM CO_2
12 mM HCO_3^-

Figure 10-4 Bicarbonate buffering of fixed acid in a closed system. (Redrawn from Beachey WD: *Curr Rev Respir Ther* 8:93, 1986.)

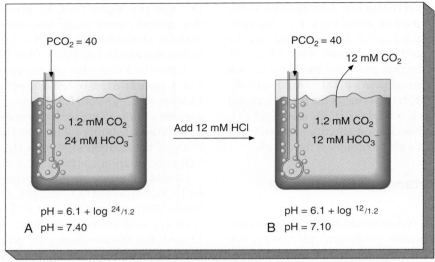

Figure 10-5 Bicarbonate buffering of fixed acid in an open system. (Redrawn from Beachey WD: *Curr Rev Respir Ther* 8:94, 1986.)

TABLE 10-4

Buffering Functions

Buffer	Type of System	Acids Buffered
Bicarbonate	Open	Fixed (nonvolatile)
Nonbicarbonate	Closed	Volatile (carbonic) Fixed

Bicarbonate Buffer System

The bicarbonate buffer system can buffer only fixed acids. An increased fixed acid load in the body reacts with HCO_3^- of the bicarbonate buffer system in the following way:

$$\underset{\underset{\textbf{Fixed acid}}{\uparrow}}{H^+} + HCO_3^- \rightarrow H_2CO_3 \rightarrow H_2O + \underset{\underset{\textbf{Ventilation}}{\uparrow}}{CO_2}$$

This reaction shows that the process of buffering fixed acid produces CO_2, which is eliminated in exhaled gas. Large amounts of acid are buffered in this fashion.

The bicarbonate buffer system cannot buffer its own acid (carbonic acid), which builds up in the blood when ventilation is inadequate. As long as inadequate ventilation (hypoventilation) persists, CO_2 continues to build up and drive the hydration reaction in the direction that produces more carbonic acid, hydrogen, and bicarbonate ions:

$$\underset{\downarrow}{\textbf{Hypoventilation}}$$
$$CO_2 + H_2O \rightarrow H_2CO_3 \rightarrow HCO_3^- + H^+$$

H^+ created in this manner cannot be buffered by HCO_3^- because the reaction cannot reverse its direction when hypoventilation is present. H^+ arising from increased blood levels of CO_2 must be buffered by the nonbicarbonate (closed) buffer system.

Nonbicarbonate Buffer System

Table 10-3 lists the nonbicarbonate buffers in the blood. Of these, hemoglobin is the most important because it is the most abundant. These buffers are the only ones available to buffer carbonic acid. However, they can buffer H^+ produced by any acid, fixed or volatile. Because nonbicarbonate buffers (HBuf/Buf$^-$) function in closed systems, the products of their buffering activity build up, slowing or stopping further buffering activity:

$$H^+ + Buf^- \leftrightarrows HBuf$$

This means not all of the Buf$^-$ is available for buffering activity. At equilibrium (denoted by the double arrow), Buf$^-$ still exists in the solution but cannot combine further with H^+. In contrast, virtually all of the HCO_3^- in the bicarbonate buffer system is available for buffering activity because it functions in an open system where equilibrium between reactants and products never occurs. Both open and closed systems function in a common fluid compartment (blood plasma) as the following reactions illustrate:

$$\textbf{(Removed by ventilation)} \quad \textbf{(HCO}_3^-\textbf{ stores)}$$
$$\uparrow \qquad\qquad\qquad \downarrow$$
$$\textbf{Open system: } CO_2 + H_2O \leftarrow H^+ + HCO_3^-$$
$$\uparrow$$
$$\textbf{Added fixed acid}$$
$$\downarrow$$
$$\textbf{Closed system: } HBuf \leftrightarrows H^+ + Buf^-$$
$$\uparrow$$
$$\textbf{(Buf}^-\textbf{ stores)}$$

Most of the added fixed acid is buffered by HCO_3^- because increased ventilation continually pulls the reaction to the left. Smaller amounts of H^+ react with Buf$^-$ because equilibrium is approached, slowing this reaction. Although all HCO_3^- could theoretically be depleted in buffering fixed acids, this never happens because metabolically produced CO_2 provides a continual source of HCO_3^-; that is, at the tissue level, CO_2 diffuses into the erythrocyte where it reacts with H_2O to form H^+ and HCO_3^-;

hemoglobin's subsequent buffering of H^+ causes HCO_3^- to be continuously generated, as described in Chapter 9.

CONCEPT QUESTION 10-5

Normal arterial [HCO_3^-] is about 24 mEq/L, and normal $PaCO_2$ is about 40 mm Hg. How much does [HCO_3^-] need to increase above normal to maintain a pH of 7.40 if $PaCO_2$ increases to 60 mm Hg?

ACID EXCRETION

Bicarbonate and nonbicarbonate buffer systems are the mechanisms whereby the body immediately neutralizes accumulated acids. However, if the body had no mechanism for ridding itself of acids, these buffers would soon be exhausted, and the pH of body fluids would quickly decrease to life-threatening levels. The lungs and kidneys are the primary acid-excreting organs. The lungs excrete only volatile acid (i.e., the CO_2 arising from dissociated H_2CO_3), whereas the kidneys excrete primarily fixed acids. The lungs can excrete large quantities of CO_2 in minutes, whereas the kidneys remove fixed acids at a much slower pace (hours to days). These two organs complement one another in their acid-excreting function; the failure of one organ can usually be offset by a compensatory response in the other.

Lungs

Normal oxidative (aerobic) metabolism produces CO_2, forming more than 10,000 mEq of H_2CO_3 per day.[4] Because H_2CO_3

CLINICAL FOCUS 10-2

Using the Henderson-Hasselbalch Equation to Predict Arterial pH for a Given Change in Arterial Carbon Dioxide Pressure

A patient with acute respiratory distress syndrome whose lungs are mechanically ventilated is in the intensive care unit. Current arterial blood gas values are as follows:

pH = 7.34
$PaCO_2$ = 50 mm Hg
HCO_3^- = 26 mEq/L

The patient's lungs have such low compliance that dangerously high pressures are required to maintain normal tidal volumes and alveolar ventilation ($\dot{V}_A$). The respiratory therapist and attending physician decide to decrease the tidal volume delivered by the ventilator to prevent structural damage to lung tissue. In this way, alveolar pressures and the risk of alveolar rupture can be decreased. However, the decrease in tidal volume will cause the $PaCO_2$, which is already above normal, to increase further, decreasing the arterial pH even more. Nevertheless, some degree of hypercapnia and acidemia is acceptable if the detrimental effect of pressure-induced alveolar trauma (barotrauma) is avoidable. The respiratory therapist and physician decide they will not allow the pH to decrease below 7.25.

The patient's lungs are being ventilated with a tidal volume of 700 mL at a frequency of 10 breaths per minute for a $\dot{V}_E$ of 7 L per minute. How high can the $PaCO_2$ be allowed to increase without decreasing the arterial pH below 7.25, and how much should the tidal volume be decreased to accomplish this?

Discussion

First, the $PaCO_2$ that will produce a pH of 7.25 needs to be calculated as follows, using known values:

$$PaCO_2 = \frac{26 \text{ mEq/L}}{0.03 \times \text{antilog}(7.25 - 6.1)}$$

$$PaCO_2 = \frac{26}{0.03 \times 14.13} = \frac{26}{0.42}$$

$$PaCO_2 = 61.9 \text{ or } 62 \text{ mm Hg}$$

A $PaCO_2$ of 62 mm Hg will produce a pH of about 7.25.*

Next, $\dot{V}_E$ required to produce a $PaCO_2$ of 62 mm Hg must be calculated. Chapter 9 indicated that $\dot{V}_E$ is inversely proportional to $PaCO_2$, as the following equation shows:

$$(\dot{V}_E)_1 \times (PaCO_2)_1 = (\dot{V}_E)_2 \times (PaCO_2)_2$$

In this equation, subscripts 1 and 2 represent current and future values. The solution for $(\dot{V}_E)_2$ is as follows:

$$7 \text{ L/min} \times 50 \text{ mm Hg} = (\dot{V}_E)_2 \times 62 \text{ mm Hg}$$

$$(7 \times 50)/62 = (\dot{V}_E)_2$$

$$5.65 \text{ L/min} = (\dot{V}_E)_2$$

Decreasing $\dot{V}_E$ from the current value of 7 L per minute to 5.65 L per minute produces a $PaCO_2$ of approximately 62 mm Hg and a pH of 7.25. The newly calculated $\dot{V}_E$ of 5.65 L per minute is divided by the respiratory frequency (10 breaths per minute) to calculate the new tidal volume (V_T = 5.65 L/min ÷ 10 = 0.565 L or 565 mL). A tidal volume of 565 mL at a respiratory rate of 10 breaths per minute should produce a pH of about 7.25 in the patient. This example is more theoretical than it is practical; in the clinical setting, the patient's minute ventilation would be gradually reduced over time to allow the kidneys to compensate (retain HCO_3^- ions) and keep the pH closer to the normal range.

---

*This calculation is an oversimplification because of the CO_2 hydration effect: An increased $PaCO_2$ causes a small increase in [HCO_3^-]. A decrease in V_T without changing the respiratory rate would directly decrease alveolar ventilation without affecting anatomical dead space ventilation; this would increase the V_D/V_T ratio, resulting in a higher $PaCO_2$ than predicted by this calculation.

is in equilibrium with dissolved CO_2, the lungs can lower blood H_2CO_3 concentration by eliminating CO_2 in exhaled gas. Neurochemical mechanisms control ventilation in such a way that CO_2 elimination matches CO_2 production while keeping $PaCO_2$ and pH near 40 mm Hg and 7.40.

In addition to production of H_2CO_3 via aerobic metabolism, H_2CO_3 and ultimately CO_2 are generated by the reaction between fixed acids and HCO_3^- buffers. The lung eliminates CO_2 from both sources. In this way, the lung can eliminate large amounts of volatile acid (H_2CO_3) in seconds, producing rapid pH changes. CO_2 elimination by the lungs does not physically remove H^+ from the body, but its removal causes the hydration reaction to proceed in the direction that converts H^+ ions to harmless H_2O molecules, as follows:

$$H^+ + HCO_3^- \rightarrow H_2CO_3 \rightarrow H_2O + CO_2$$

Kidneys (Renal System)

The kidneys physically remove hydrogen ions from the body; the amount eliminated depends on the blood level of hydrogen ions—the higher the blood levels, the more hydrogen ions excreted. Blood hydrogen ions may originate from H_2CO_3 (when $PaCO_2$ is high) or from a buildup of fixed acids. The kidneys excrete less than 100 mEq of fixed acid per day, a relatively small amount compared with the lung's excretion of volatile H_2CO_3. Besides excreting H^+, the kidneys also influence blood pH by reabsorbing HCO_3^- from the filtrate into the blood or by eliminating HCO_3^- in the urine. If $PaCO_2$ is high (creating high levels of H_2CO_3), the kidneys not only excrete greater amounts of H^+, but they also return all of the kidney filtrate's HCO_3^- to the blood. The opposite happens when $PaCO_2$ is low—the kidneys excrete less H^+ but more HCO_3^-. In this way, the kidneys work to maintain a normal blood pH when the lungs fail to maintain normal CO_2 levels. Compared with the lung's ability to change the $PaCO_2$ in seconds, the renal process is slow, requiring hours to days. Renal regulation of acid-base and electrolyte balance is discussed in detail in Chapter 22.

ACID-BASE DISTURBANCES

In healthy individuals, the buffer systems of the lungs, kidneys, and body work together to maintain acid-base homeostasis under various conditions.

Normal Acid-Base Balance

Normally, alveolar ventilation maintains a $PaCO_2$ of about 40 mm Hg, whereas the kidneys maintain a plasma HCO_3^- concentration of about 24 mEq/L. These normal values produce an arterial pH of 7.40, as the H-H equation shows:

$$pH = 6.1 + \log\left[\frac{[HCO_3^-]}{(PCO_2 \times 0.03)}\right]$$
$$pH = 6.1 + \log\left[\frac{24}{(40 \times 0.03)}\right]$$
$$pH = 6.1 + \log(20)$$
$$pH = 6.1 + 1.3 = 7.40$$

The pH is determined by the ratio of $[HCO_3^-]$ to dissolved CO_2, not by the absolute concentrations of these substances. As long as the ratio of $[HCO_3^-]$ to dissolved CO_2 is 20:1, the pH is normal at 7.40. Because the kidneys control the plasma $[HCO_3^-]$ and the lungs control blood CO_2 levels, the H-H equation can be conceptually rewritten as follows:

$$pH = \left[\frac{\textbf{Kidney control of } [HCO_3^-]}{\textbf{Lung control of PCO}_2}\right]$$

From this relationship, it is apparent that an increase in $[HCO_3^-]$ or a decrease in PCO_2 (hyperventilation) increases the pH, leading to alkalemia. Both situations produce an $[HCO_3^-]$-to-$(PCO_2 \times 0.03)$ ratio greater than 20:1 (e.g., 25:1). Similarly, a decreased $[HCO_3^-]$ or an increased PCO_2 (hypoventilation) decreases the pH, leading to acidemia; this produces an $[HCO_3^-]$-to-$(PCO_2 \times 0.03)$ ratio less than 20:1 (e.g., 15:1). The normal ranges for arterial pH, PCO_2, and $[HCO_3^-]$ are as follows:

$$pH = 7.35 \text{ to } 7.45$$
$$PaCO_2 = 35 \text{ to } 45 \text{ mm Hg}$$
$$[HCO_3^-] = 22 \text{ to } 26 \text{ mEq/L}$$

Alkalemia is defined as a blood pH greater than 7.45; acidemia is defined as a blood pH less than 7.35. Hyperventilation is defined as a $PaCO_2$ less than 35 mm Hg; hypoventilation is defined as a $PaCO_2$ greater than 45 mm Hg.

Primary Respiratory Disturbances

$PaCO_2$ abnormalities that cause abnormal arterial pH values are called primary respiratory disturbances because alveolar ventilation controls the PCO_2 of arterial blood. Respiratory disturbances affect the denominator of the H-H equation. An elevated $PaCO_2$ increases dissolved CO_2, decreasing the pH:

$$\downarrow pH \propto \left[\frac{\rightarrow HCO_3^-}{\uparrow PaCO_2}\right]$$

In this equation, $\downarrow$ represents a decrease, $\rightarrow$ represents no change, and $\uparrow$ represents an increase. Respiratory disturbances causing acidemia produce **respiratory acidosis**. A low $PaCO_2$ decreases dissolved CO_2, increasing the pH. This is called **respiratory alkalosis**:

$$\uparrow pH \propto \left[\frac{\rightarrow HCO_3^-}{\downarrow PaCO_2}\right]$$

Hypoventilation leads to respiratory acidosis, whereas hyperventilation leads to respiratory alkalosis.

Primary Metabolic (Nonrespiratory) Disturbances

Nonrespiratory processes change the arterial pH by changing $[HCO_3^-]$; these processes are called primary metabolic disturbances. The term metabolic in this context is arbitrary, but by convention it refers to all nonrespiratory acid-base disturbances. These disturbances involve a gain or loss of either fixed acids or HCO_3^-. Such processes affect the numerator of the H-H equation. For example, an accumulation of fixed acid in the body is buffered by bicarbonate, lowering the plasma $[HCO_3^-]$ and decreasing the pH:

$$\downarrow pH \propto \left[\frac{\downarrow HCO_3^-}{\rightarrow PaCO_2} \right]$$

Exactly the same effect is created by a loss of HCO_3^-. Nonrespiratory processes causing acidemia produce metabolic acidosis.

In contrast, the ingestion of too much alkali (e.g., $NaHCO_3$ or other antacids) raises $[HCO_3^-]$, increasing pH:

$$\uparrow pH \propto \left[\frac{\uparrow HCO_3^-}{\rightarrow PaCO_2} \right]$$

Plasma $[HCO_3^-]$ can be increased either by its addition (as in the previous example) or by its generation (as occurs when fixed acid is lost from the body). For example, HCl is lost after a person vomits large amounts of gastric secretions. Nasogastric suction catheters, often placed in critically ill patients, also deplete gastric HCl. A loss of HCl generates HCO_3^-, as the following reaction shows:

Body CO_2 stores $\rightarrow CO_2 + H_2O \rightarrow H^+ + HCO_3^-$

Vomiting $\leftarrow$ HCl $\leftarrow H^+ + Cl^- \leftarrow$ body Cl^- stores

Processes that increase the arterial pH by losing fixed acid or gaining HCO_3^- produce a condition called **metabolic alkalosis**. Because HCO_3^- can be added or lost through mechanisms not related to metabolism (alkali ingestion or vomiting), the term metabolic acidosis is misleading. Similarly, acid not produced by metabolism (e.g., salicylic acid [aspirin]) can be ingested, producing so-called **metabolic acidosis**. The term metabolic has been entrenched by tradition and continues to be used. Table 10-5 shows the four primary acid-base disturbances causing alkalemia and acidemia.

CONCEPT QUESTION 10-6

In metabolic (nonrespiratory) acidosis, what must the lungs do to bring the pH back to normal?

Compensation: Restoring pH to Normal

When any primary acid-base defect occurs, the organ system not responsible immediately initiates a compensatory process, counteracting the primary defect. For example, if reduced ventilation is the primary defect (respiratory acidosis), the kidneys work to restore the pH to normal by returning HCO_3^- to the blood. In contrast, the compensatory renal response to hyperventilation (respiratory alkalosis) is the urinary elimination of HCO_3^- (bicarbonate diuresis).

Similarly, if a nonrespiratory process increases or decreases $[HCO_3^-]$, the lungs compensate for this defect by eliminating CO_2 (hyperventilating) or retaining CO_2 (hypoventilating), restoring the pH to the normal range. Consider the example of pure (uncompensated) respiratory acidosis in which $PaCO_2$ increases to 60 mm Hg, creating an $[HCO_3^-]$-to-dissolved CO_2 ratio of about 13:1, as shown:

$$pH = 6.1 + log \left[\frac{24 \text{ mEq/L}}{60 \text{ mm Hg} \times 0.03} \right]$$
$$pH = 6.1 + log(13.3)$$
$$pH = 7.22$$

The kidneys compensate, restoring the $[HCO_3^-]$-to-dissolved CO_2 ratio by actively reabsorbing HCO_3^- into the blood:

$$pH = 6.1 + log \left[\frac{34 \text{ mEq/L}}{60 \text{ mm Hg} \times 0.03} \right]$$
$$pH = 6.1 + log(18.9)$$
$$pH = 7.38$$

By increasing the plasma $[HCO_3^-]$ level to 34 mEq/L in this example, the kidneys brought the $[HCO_3^-]$-to-dissolved CO_2 ratio back to about 19:1, restoring the pH to the normal range (7.35 to 7.45); the PCO_2 remains abnormally elevated. The elevated plasma $[HCO_3^-]$ brought about by the kidneys' compensatory response should not be misconstrued as metabolic alkalosis. Compensatory HCO_3^- retention is a normal secondary response to the primary event of respiratory acidosis.

The lungs normally compensate quickly for metabolic acid-base defects because ventilation can change $PaCO_2$ in seconds. The kidneys require more time to retain or excrete significant amounts of HCO_3^-, and they compensate for respiratory defects at a much slower pace. Table 10-6 summarizes the four primary

---

TABLE 10-5

Primary Acid-Base Disturbances

pH Change	Main Abnormality	Designation
Alkalemia (pH >7.45)	Decreased PCO_2	Respiratory alkalosis
	Increased HCO_3^-	Metabolic (nonrespiratory alkalosis)
Acidemia (pH <7.35)	Increased PCO_2	Respiratory acidosis
	Decreased HCO_3^-	Metabolic (nonrespiratory acidosis)

TABLE 10-6

Primary Acid-Base Disorders and Compensatory Responses

Acid-Base Disorder	Primary Defect	Compensatory Response
Respiratory acidosis	$\left[\frac{\rightarrow HCO_3^-}{\uparrow PaCO_2} \right] = \downarrow pH$	$\left[\frac{\uparrow HCO_3^-}{\uparrow PaCO_2} \right] = \rightarrow pH$
Respiratory alkalosis	$\left[\frac{\rightarrow HCO_3^-}{\downarrow PaCO_2} \right] = \uparrow pH$	$\left[\frac{\downarrow HCO_3^-}{\downarrow PaCO_2} \right] = \rightarrow pH$
Metabolic acidosis	$\left[\frac{\downarrow HCO_3^-}{\rightarrow PaCO_2} \right] = \downarrow pH$	$\left[\frac{\downarrow HCO_3^-}{\downarrow PaCO_2} \right] = \rightarrow pH$
Metabolic alkalosis	$\left[\frac{\uparrow HCO_3^-}{\rightarrow PaCO_2} \right] = \uparrow pH$	$\left[\frac{\uparrow HCO_3^-}{\uparrow PaCO_2} \right] = \rightarrow pH$

$\rightarrow$, No change, or normal; $\downarrow$, decrease; $\uparrow$, increase.

acid-base disturbances and the body's compensatory responses. (Primary and compensatory responses appear in bold font.)

Effect of Carbon Dioxide Hydration Reaction on Bicarbonate Ion Concentration

In the foregoing examples of pure (uncompensated) respiratory acidosis and alkalosis, it was assumed that $[HCO_3^-]$ did not change when $PaCO_2$ increased or decreased. This simplification was made to emphasize that $PaCO_2$, not HCO_3^-, is the primary abnormality in respiratory acidosis or alkalosis. However, arterial $[HCO_3^-]$ does slightly increase as $PaCO_2$ increases secondary to HCO_3^- generation in the erythrocyte through the hydration reaction. As explained in Chapter 9, the hydration reaction occurs primarily in the red blood cell because the catalytic enzyme carbonic anhydrase is present. This is shown as follows:

$$CO_2 + H_2O \text{ (carbonic anhydrase)} \rightarrow H_2CO_3 \rightarrow H^+ + HCO_3^-$$

As H^+ and HCO_3^- are rapidly produced, hemoglobin immediately buffers H^+, generating HCO_3^- in the process:

$$CO_2 + H_2O \rightarrow H_2CO_3 \rightarrow H^+ + HCO_3^- \text{ (HCO}_3^- \text{ generation)}$$
$$\downarrow$$
$$Hb^- + H^+ \rightarrow HHb \text{ (Hb buffering of H}^+\text{)}$$

The extent to which $[HCO_3^-]$ increases for a given increase in $PaCO_2$ depends on how much nonbicarbonate buffer (mainly hemoglobin) is present to accept the hydrogen ions produced by the hydration reaction. In other words, the increase in the number of plasma bicarbonate ions is exactly equal to the number of hydrogen ions buffered by the nonbicarbonate buffers. Generally, when the nonbicarbonate buffer concentration is normal, an acute $PaCO_2$ increase of 10 mm Hg causes $[HCO_3^-]$ to increase by about 1 mEq/L; this is a clinically useful rule of thumb. A slight increase in $[HCO_3^-]$ is a natural consequence of an acute increase in $PaCO_2$. This small increase in $[HCO_3^-]$

should not be confused with compensatory renal HCO_3^- retention.

Figure 10-6 illustrates what would happen if the blood contained no nonbicarbonate buffers. In Figure 10-6, *A*, the solution's PCO_2 is 40 mm Hg, the $[HCO_3^-]$ is 24 mEq/L, and the pH is 7.40. If the PCO_2 of gas bubbling through the solution suddenly increases to 80 mm Hg (see Figure 10-6, *B*), dissolved CO_2 ($PCO_2 \times 0.03$) increases to 2.4 mM/L, and the pH decreases to 7.10. These events are recorded on the pH-$[HCO_3^-]$ diagram in Figure 10-7. The conditions shown in Figure 10-6, *A*, are represented by point *A* on the pH-$[HCO_3^-]$ diagram. (The curved lines are PCO_2 isobars, constructed by maintaining the PCO_2 of the gas bubbling through the solution constant while adding or subtracting a strong acid.) $[HCO_3^-]$ did not change when the PCO_2 increased to 80 mm Hg (from point *A* to point *B* in Figure 10-7). The lack of a perceptible change might seem odd because an increase in PCO_2 from 40 mm Hg to 80 mm Hg would double the H_2CO_3 concentration, which means that $[HCO_3^-]$ would increase to some extent when H_2CO_3 dissociates into bicarbonate and hydrogen ions. Any such increase in bicarbonate ions would have to be equal to the increase in hydrogen ions because each molecule of H_2CO_3 produces one H^+ and one HCO_3^-. As estimated from the decrease in pH from 7.40 to 7.10, the increase in $[H^+]$ is about 40 nmol/L (see Table 10-1), which means that the $[HCO_3^-]$ would also increase by about 40 nmol/L. This minuscule increase in $[HCO_3^-]$ cannot be accurately measured or plotted on the pH-$[HCO_3^-]$ diagram in Figure 10-7 and can be ignored.

The reason $[HCO_3^-]$ did not increase perceptibly in the example just described is that nonbicarbonate buffers were not present to accept the H^+ produced by the hydration reaction. In whole blood, nonbicarbonate buffers are plentiful. As described earlier, when they buffer H^+, HCO_3^- is generated. Figure 10-8 is a pH-$[HCO_3^-]$ diagram for whole blood. A normal status is represented by point *A* (PCO_2 of 40 mm Hg, pH of 7.40, and plasma $[HCO_3^-]$ of 24 mEq/L). An acute

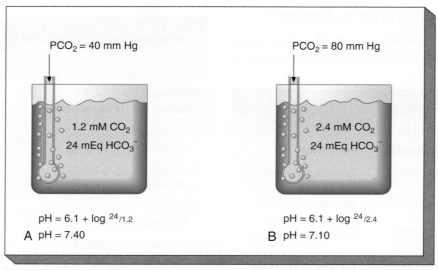

Figure 10-6 Bicarbonate buffering activity for an abrupt increase in PCO_2 from 40 mm Hg to 80 mm Hg in a hypothetical solution lacking nonbicarbonate buffers. (Redrawn from Beachey WD: *Curr Rev Respir Ther* 8:94, 1986.)

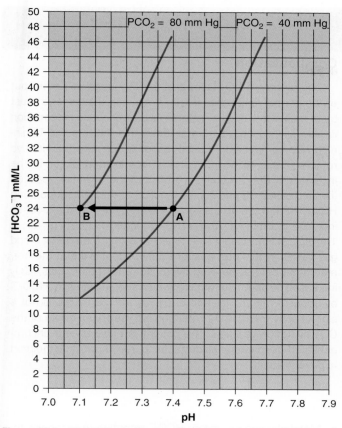

Figure 10-7 pH-[HCO_3^-] diagram illustrating the events shown in Figure 10-6 when PCO_2 abruptly increases from 40 mm Hg to 80 mm Hg. Points *A* and *B* correspond with diagrams *A* and *B* in Figure 10-6. Nonbicarbonate buffers are not present to accept H^+ generated by the increase in PCO_2; the [HCO_3^-] increase is undetectable, and pH decreases to 7.10.

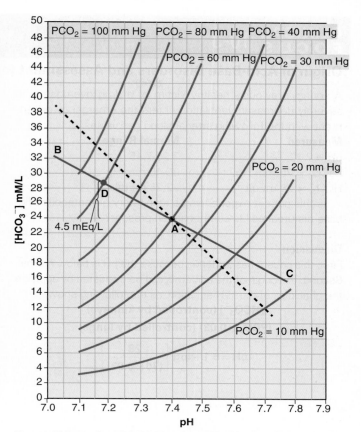

Figure 10-8 pH-[HCO_3^-] diagram illustrating events occurring in whole blood when PCO_2 abruptly increases from 40 to 80 mm Hg. Nonbicarbonate buffers (mostly hemoglobin) accept the H^+ produced by the CO_2 hydration reaction, generating about 4.5 mEq/L of HCO_3^- in the process (points *A* to *D*); this moderates the decrease in pH compared with Figure 10-7 where nonbicarbonate buffers were absent (pH decreases to 7.18 instead of 7.10). Line *BDAC* is the nonbicarbonate blood buffer line. The same 40-mm Hg increase in PCO_2 would generate a greater amount of HCO_3^- if the blood concentration of nonbicarbonate buffers were higher, producing a steeper buffer line (*dashed line*). (Data from Masoro EJ, Siegel PD: *Acid-base regulation: its physiology and pathophysiology*, Philadelphia, 1971, Saunders.)

increase in PCO_2 to 80 mm Hg proceeds along the nonbicarbonate blood buffer line (*BAC*) to point *D*, where the buffer line intersects the 80-mm Hg PCO_2 isobar. Point *D* indicates an increase in [HCO_3^-] of about 4.5 mEq/L, which is exactly the same as the amount of H^+ buffered by nonbicarbonate buffers. This corresponds to a pH of 7.18 compared with the pH of 7.10 in Figure 10-7, in which nonbicarbonate buffers are absent. The slope of *BAC* is a measure of the amount of nonbicarbonate buffer present; the slope is steeper if greater amounts of nonbicarbonate buffer are present. For example, if hemoglobin concentration increases, an acute increase in PCO_2 from point *A* (see Figure 10-8) to 80 mm Hg proceeds along a steeper line (*dashed line*); at the 80-mm Hg PCO_2 isobar, [HCO_3^-] and pH are higher because hemoglobin buffered greater amounts of H^+.

As a general rule, the hydration reaction, in the presence of normal nonbicarbonate buffer concentration, increases the plasma [HCO_3^-] about 1 mEq/L for every 10-mm Hg increase in PCO_2 greater than 40 mm Hg. However, this relationship is not linear; [HCO_3^-] is reduced about 1 mEq/L for every 5-mm Hg PCO_2 decrease less than 40 mm Hg.

POINTS TO REMEMBER

- Normal aerobic metabolism continually produces hydrogen ions, making their regulation necessary.
- The three major mechanisms that maintain [H^+] in a range compatible with life are (1) blood buffers, (2) alveolar ventilation, and (3) renal excretion of H^+ or retention of HCO_3^-.
- Blood buffers consist of bicarbonate (open) or nonbicarbonate (closed) systems; open system buffering reactions never proceed to equilibrium as they do in closed systems.
- Nonbicarbonate buffers are the only available system for buffering H^+ arising from hypoventilation.
- Bicarbonate buffers can buffer only fixed acids and then only if ventilation is not impaired.
- The bicarbonate buffer system has a much greater fixed acid buffering capacity than the nonbicarbonate system because the bicarbonate system is an open system.

CLINICAL FOCUS 10-3

Origin of Acid-Base Disorders and Assessment for Compensation

A young, previously healthy victim of a drug overdose with severely depressed ventilation enters the emergency department with the following arterial blood gas values:

Measured	Normal Range
pH = 7.22	7.35-7.45
$PaCO_2$ = 70 mm Hg	35-45 mm Hg
HCO_3^- = 28 mEq/L	22-26 mEq/L

Is this patient experiencing a respiratory or metabolic acid-base disturbance? Is compensation present?

Discussion

First, this patient has acidemia because the pH is below normal. Second, the origin of the acidemia can be evaluated by applying the principles of the H-H equation, as the following shows:

$$\frac{[HCO_3^-] \text{ (controlled by kidneys)}}{(PCO_2 \times 0.03) \text{ (controlled by lungs)}}$$

$$pH = 6.1 + \log\left[\frac{28}{(70 \times 0.03)}\right]$$

The dissolved CO_2 (controlled by the lungs) is further out of the normal range than $[HCO_3^-]$ meaning the acidosis must be of respiratory origin. The plasma bicarbonate concentration is also slightly above normal; does this indicate the beginning of a compensatory renal response (i.e., are the kidneys retaining base to counteract the increased acid), or is the increased $[HCO_3^-]$ merely an artifact of the hydration reaction (i.e., increased CO_2 drives the reaction to the right, generating HCO_3^-)? From the discussion in the text, we would expect an increase in PCO_2 of 10 mm Hg to increase HCO_3^- by about 1 mEq/L. It is probably safe to assume that the arterial blood gas values in this previously healthy patient were in the normal range before the drug overdose. This means that PCO_2 increased by about 30 mm Hg, which should increase $[HCO_3^-]$ by about 3 mEq/L. Therefore, $[HCO_3^-]$ of 28 mEq/L is not a sign of early renal HCO_3^- retention but merely an effect of the CO_2 hydration reaction. The patient is experiencing uncompensated respiratory acidosis as a result of drug-induced hypoventilation.

- Because $\dot{V}_A$ controls blood levels of CO_2, ventilation is intimately involved in acid-base regulation.
- The kidneys affect [H+] by excreting it or by conserving or eliminating HCO_3^-.
- The H-H equation can be used clinically to calculate pH, PCO_2, or HCO_3^- and to predict changes in one variable when the other two are changed.
- Processes that produce an abnormal arterial blood pH by changing the $PaCO_2$ are called respiratory acid-base disturbances.
- Processes that produce an abnormal arterial blood pH by changing the $[HCO_3^-]$ are called metabolic or nonrespiratory acid-base disturbances.
- A respiratory (PCO_2) acid-base imbalance usually elicits a compensatory renal response that changes $[HCO_3^-]$, restoring the pH to the normal range.
- A metabolic (HCO_3^-) acid-base imbalance usually elicits a compensatory respiratory response that changes the $PaCO_2$, restoring the pH to the normal range.

- Metabolic compensatory HCO_3^- retention in response to a primary respiratory acidosis should not be confused with a metabolic alkalosis.
- Blood buffering of H+ generated by the CO_2 hydration reaction causes $[HCO_3^-]$ to increase slightly when PCO_2 increases; this should not be confused with compensatory renal retention of HCO_3^-.

References

1. Klocke RA: Carbon dioxide transport. In Fishman AP, et al: *Handbook of physiology, section 3: the respiratory system, volume IV, gas exchange*, Bethesda, MD, 1987, American Physiological Society.
2. Masoro EJ, Siegel PD: *Acid-base regulation: its physiology and pathophysiology*, Philadelphia, 1971, Saunders.
3. Comroe JH: *Physiology of respiration*, ed 2, Chicago, 1974, Year Book Medical Publishers.
4. West JB: *Respiratory physiology: the essentials*, ed 8, Baltimore, 2008, Lippincott Williams & Wilkins.

Control of Ventilation

OBJECTIVES

After reading this chapter, you will be able to:

- Explain how the medullary respiratory center generates the basic breathing pattern
- Describe how the medullary respiratory neurons and pontine centers interact
- Explain how various reflexes and receptors affect ventilation, including the Hering-Breuer inflation reflex, J-receptors, proprioceptors, and muscle spindles
- Show how carbon dioxide (CO_2) indirectly stimulates the medullary chemoreceptors
- Explain why high arterial carbon dioxide pressure ($PaCO_2$) more readily stimulates the central chemoreceptors than high arterial levels of metabolically produced fixed acid

- Explain why $PaCO_2$ is a more appropriate controller of ventilation than arterial oxygen pressure (PaO_2)
- Explain why hypoxemia plays a more important role in regulating ventilation in patients with chronically high $PaCO_2$ than patients with normal $PaCO_2$
- Differentiate between the immediate and chronic effects of high altitude on ventilation and explain why they occur
- Describe two mechanisms whereby oxygen administration might induce hypercapnia in patients who have severe chronic obstructive pulmonary disease
- Explain how $PaCO_2$ affects the cerebral circulation and intracranial pressure

KEY TERMS

apneustic breathing
apneustic center
Biot's breathing
blood-brain barrier
central reflex hyperpnea
central reflex hypopnea
chemoreceptors

Cheyne-Stokes breathing
dorsal respiratory groups
Head's reflex
Hering-Breuer reflex
J-receptors
pneumotaxic center
ventral respiratory groups

Similar to the heartbeat, breathing is an automatic activity requiring no conscious awareness. Different from the heartbeat, breathing patterns can be consciously changed, although voluntary control is limited. Powerful neural control mechanisms overwhelm conscious control soon after one willfully stops breathing. The normal unconscious cycle of breathing is regulated by complex mechanisms that continue to elude complete understanding. The rhythmic cycle of breathing originates in the brainstem, mainly from neurons located in the medulla. Higher brain centers and many systemic receptors and reflexes modify the medulla's output. These different structures function in an integrated manner, precisely controlling ventilatory rate and depth to accommodate the body's gas exchange needs, whether at rest, during exercise, or in disease.

MEDULLARY RESPIRATORY CENTER

Rhythmic neural impulses responsible for ventilation originate in the medulla oblongata of the brainstem (Figure 11-1). Animal experiments show that transection of the brainstem just below the medulla (see level IV, Figure 11-1) stops all ventilatory activity. However, rhythmic breathing continues after the brainstem is transected just above the pons (see level I, Figure 11-1).

Physiologists previously thought that separate inspiratory and expiratory neuron "centers" in the medulla were responsible for the cyclical pattern of breathing. It was believed that inspiratory and expiratory neurons fired by self-excitation and that they mutually inhibited one another. It is now known that inspiratory and expiratory neurons are anatomically intermingled and do not necessarily inhibit one another.[1] These neurons are widely dispersed in the medulla; the **dorsal respiratory groups** (DRG) contain mainly inspiratory neurons, whereas the **ventral respiratory groups** (VRG) contain intermingled inspiratory and expiratory neurons.

Dorsal Respiratory Groups

As shown in Figure 11-1, the DRG consist of mainly inspiratory neurons located bilaterally in an area called the nucleus of the tractus solitarius. These neurons send impulses to the phrenic and external intercostal motor nerves in the spinal cord, providing the main stimulus for inspiration.[1] Many DRG nerves extend into the VRG, but few VRG fibers extend into the DRG. Thus, reciprocal inhibition is an unlikely explanation for rhythmic, spontaneous breathing.[1] The DRG consists of two neuron populations, one of which is inhibited by deep lung inflation (causing cessation of inspiratory effort), whereas the other is excited by lung inflation (causing continued inspiratory effort).[1] These neurons are involved in the Hering-Breuer and Head's reflexes described later in this chapter.

The vagus and glossopharyngeal nerves transmit many sensory impulses to the DRG from the lungs, airways, peripheral chemoreceptors, and joint proprioceptors. These impulses modify the basic breathing pattern generated in the medulla.

Ventral Respiratory Groups

VRG neurons are located bilaterally in the medulla in two separate nuclei that contain both inspiratory and expiratory neurons (see Figure 11-1). Some inspiratory VRG neurons send motor impulses through the vagus nerve to the laryngeal and pharyngeal muscles, abducting the vocal cords and increasing the diameter of the glottis. Other VRG inspiratory neurons transmit impulses to the diaphragm and external intercostal muscles. Still other VRG neurons have mostly expiratory discharge patterns and send impulses to the internal intercostal and abdominal expiratory muscles. The most rostral (toward the head) part of the VRG, Bötzinger's complex (see Figure 11-1), contains the only expiratory neurons known to inhibit the inspiratory VRG and DRG impulses.[2]

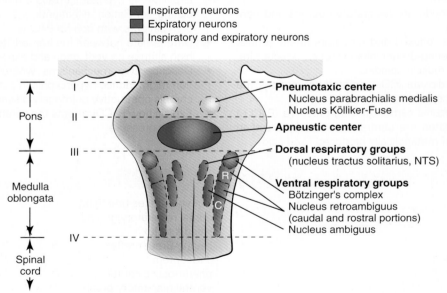

■ Inspiratory neurons
■ Expiratory neurons
□ Inspiratory and expiratory neurons

- **Pneumotaxic center**
  Nucleus parabrachialis medialis
  Nucleus Kölliker-Fuse
- **Apneustic center**
- **Dorsal respiratory groups**
  (nucleus tractus solitarius, NTS)
- **Ventral respiratory groups**
  Bötzinger's complex
  Nucleus retroambiguus
  (caudal and rostral portions)
  Nucleus ambiguus

Pons

Medulla oblongata

Spinal cord

I
II
III
IV

Figure 11-1 Dorsal view of the brainstem. Phases I to IV refer to transections at different levels.

CLINICAL FOCUS 11-1

Use of Dorsal Respiratory Group Neural Impulses to Trigger Mechanical Ventilation: Neurally Adjusted Ventilatory Assist

Critically ill patients in hospital intensive care units often cannot breathe adequately on their own and require mechanical ventilation. The electrical impulses of the DRG neurons can be used to adjust the mechanical ventilator's inspiratory gas flow to meet the patient's inspiratory demands precisely. One challenge of mechanical ventilation is to ensure that the patient and the ventilator are in synchrony, such that the ventilator senses the patient's slightest inspiratory effort and immediately provides gas flow to the patient in an amount proportional to the inspiratory effort.

Neurally adjusted ventilatory assist (NAVA) is a mode that accomplishes this task by measuring the diaphragm's electrical activity in response to phrenic nerve impulses; this kind of measurement is called electromyography (EMG). A specially designed thin tube (nasogastric tube) with a series of EMG electrodes at one end is inserted into the patient's esophagus by way of the nasal cavity and advanced until the electrodes are adjacent to the diaphragm. When the patient wants to take a breath, electrical impulses from the medulla's DRG neurons travel down the phrenic nerves to the diaphragm causing it to contract, which produces an electrical current proportional to the level of muscle activity. The nasogastric tube's EMG electrodes sense the electrical current and transmit this information to the ventilator's microprocessor, which instructs the ventilator to generate an inspiratory gas flow rate that is proportional to the signal strength. Through the ventilator's control panel, the clinician can set how much pressure the ventilator applies to the patient's airway for each millivolt of EMG activity. The ventilator assists the patient's inspiratory efforts in a way that is precisely matched to the EMG signal strength—that is, proportional to the patient's inspiratory effort. The greater the inspiratory effort, the more pressure the ventilator applies; with less effort, the less pressure is applied. In theory, NAVA should provide the patient with a more natural and comfortable mode of mechanical ventilation because it recognizes the inspiratory signal high up in the neural pathway that controls breathing.[14]

Respiratory Rhythm Generation

The exact origin of the basic rhythmic pattern of breathing is unknown; no single group of pacemaker cells have been identified. The Bötzinger complex and a structure located between it and the VRG, the pre-Bötzinger complex, are thought to be responsible for rhythmic breathing.[2] Two predominant theories of rhythm generation are the pacemaker hypothesis and the network hypothesis. The pacemaker hypothesis holds that certain medullary cells have intrinsic pacemaker properties—that is, rhythmic self-exciting characteristics—and that these cells drive other medullary neurons. The network hypothesis suggests that rhythmic breathing is the result of a particular pattern of interconnections between neurons dispersed throughout the rostral VRG, the pre-Bötzinger complex, and the Bötzinger complex. This hypothesis assumes that certain populations of inspiratory and expiratory neurons inhibit one another and that one of the neuron types fires in a self-limiting way, such that it becomes less responsive the longer it fires. There is no definitive proof of either hypothesis; the precise origin of respiratory rhythm generation remains elusive.

Inspiratory Ramp Signal

The dorsal and ventral inspiratory neurons do not send an abrupt burst of impulses to the inspiratory muscles; instead, their firing rate increases gradually after expiration ceases, creating a smoothly increasing ramp signal (Figure 11-2). This ramp signal leads to a progressively stronger contraction of inspiratory muscles, smoothly and gradually inflating the lungs instead of filling them in an abrupt inspiratory gasp. During

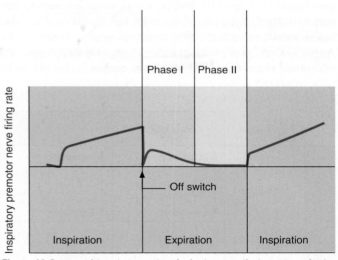

Figure 11-2 Neural inspiratory signals during ventilation. Note the inspiratory ramp signal (*left*) and braking action of inspiratory signals early in phase I of expiration. (Redrawn from Leff AR, Schumacker PT: *Respiratory physiology: basics and applications,* Philadelphia, 1993, Saunders.)

exercise, various peripheral reflexes and receptors influence the medullary neurons, steepening the inspiratory ramp signal and filling the lungs more rapidly.

As the inspiratory ramp signal strengthens, inhibitory neurons begin to fire with increasing frequency.[2] After approximately 2 seconds, these restraining impulses become strong enough to switch off the inspiratory signal abruptly. Expiration proceeds for about 3 seconds.[3] As expiration begins, inspiratory neurons fire briefly, "braking" the early phase of expiration by maintaining some inspiratory muscle tone (see Figure 11-2). Inspiratory neuronal activity completely stops in the last phase of expiration. The inhibitory neurons that switch off the inspiratory ramp arise from the pneumotaxic center and pulmonary stretch receptors, which are discussed in the next section.

CONCEPT QUESTION 11-1

What effect does the lack of pneumotaxic and stretch receptor neurons have on ventilation?

PONTINE CENTERS

If the brainstem is transected above the medulla (see Figure 11-1, level III), spontaneous respiration continues, although in a more irregular pattern; thus, the pons promotes rhythmic breathing by modifying the output of the medullary centers. Figure 11-1 shows two groups of neurons in the pons: (1) the apneustic center and (2) the pneumotaxic center.

Apneustic and Pneumotaxic Centers

The two respiratory centers in the pons (apneustic and pneumotaxic) have been identified through animal brain transection experiments. If the brainstem is severed at the midpons level (see Figure 11-1, level II), and the vagus nerves connecting this area with the lower parts of the brain and spinal cord are also cut, a breathing pattern called apneusis results (Figure 11-3). Apneusis consists of prolonged inspiratory gasps interrupted by occasional expirations. The **apneustic center** is thought to be in a region in the lower pons, but it has never been anatomically identified with certainty.[2] Its existence and function can be demonstrated only if its connections to the higher **pneumotaxic center** are severed and the vagus nerves are cut. Under these circumstances, the area in the lower pons (i.e., the apneustic center) sends signals to the DRG neurons, preventing the inspiratory ramp signal from being switched off.[3] Apparently, vagal and pneumotaxic center impulses hold the apneustic center's stimulatory effect on DRG neurons in check because apneusis does not occur if the vagus is left intact (see Figure 11-3).

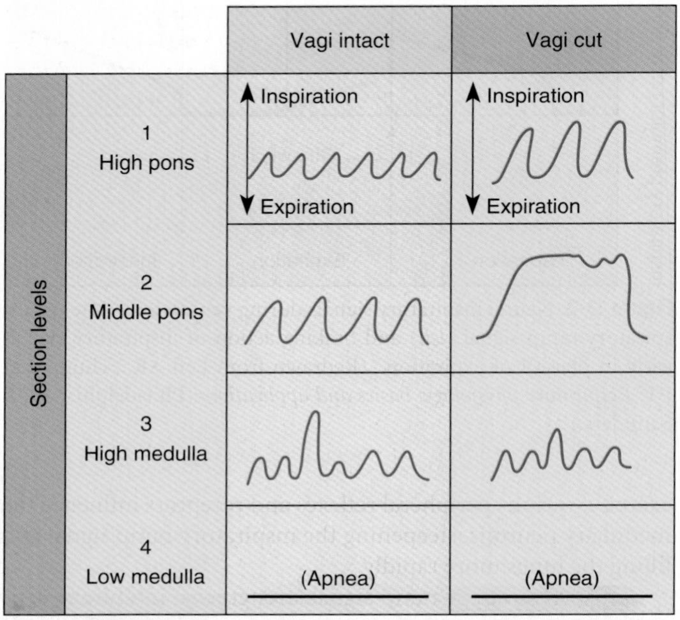

The pneumotaxic centers are bilateral groups of neurons in the upper pons (see Figure 11-1). These centers control the off-switch point of the DRG's inspiratory ramp signal, sending inhibitory impulses to medullary inspiratory neurons; thus, pneumotaxic signals control the length of inspiration. Strong pneumotaxic signals shorten the inspiratory time and increase the respiratory rate. Weak signals produce prolonged inspiration and large tidal volumes. The primary function of the pneumotaxic center is to limit inspiration and hold apneustic center impulses in check. The exact nature of the interaction between the apneustic and pneumotaxic centers remains poorly understood; they apparently work together to control the depth of inspiration.[3] The effect of the pontine centers on the lower medullary centers seems to be fine-tuning the respiratory pattern because the transection of the brainstem between the pons and medulla (see Figures 11-1, level III, and 11-3) results in an irregular breathing pattern.[1]

REFLEX CONTROL OF BREATHING

The central ventilatory drive arising from the medulla is modified by various inputs from peripheral sensors. These sensors are located in the lungs, muscles, and joints.

Hering-Breuer Inflation Reflex

The Hering-Breuer inflation reflex, described by Hering and Breuer in 1868, is generated by stretch receptors located in smooth muscle of large and small airways. These receptors are called slowly adapting receptors because their activity continues as long as the stimulus persists (see Chapter 2). When stretched, these receptors send inhibitory impulses through the vagus nerve to the DRG neurons, stopping further inspiration. Thus, the **Hering-Breuer reflex** has an effect similar to that of the pneumotaxic center.[3] The Hering-Breuer reflex in adults is activated only at large tidal volumes ($\geq$800 to 1000 mL) and is apparently not an important control mechanism in quiet breathing. However, this reflex is important in regulating the respiratory rate and depth during moderate to strenuous exercise.[2]

Diseases associated with low lung compliance (i.e., strong elastic retractive forces) may stimulate the inflation stretch receptors by increasing the mechanical stress acting on the airways during inspiratory efforts.[2] This stimulation tends to increase the respiratory rate because it sends an early inhibitory signal, shortening the inspiratory phase.

Various combinations of respiratory rate and tidal volume can produce the level of ventilation needed to meet metabolic

	Vagi intact	Vagi cut
1 High pons	↑ Inspiration ↓ Expiration	↑ Inspiration ↓ Expiration
2 Middle pons		
3 High medulla		
4 Low medulla	(Apnea)	(Apnea)

Section levels

Figure 11-3 Breathing patterns produced by transections of the brainstem at different levels. These levels correspond with phases I to IV shown in Figure 11-1. (From Berne RM, Levy MN: *Principles of physiology*, ed 2, St Louis, 1996, Mosby.)

gas exchange demands, but there is always a specific combination that results in the least work. The information stretch receptors send to the medullary centers, which can be consciously sensed, probably helps to establish this optimal combination. The sensation of dyspnea is thought to be produced when the medullary centers demand a level of ventilation greater than the actual ventilation achieved.[2]

Hering-Breuer Deflation Reflex

Hering and Breuer also observed that sudden collapse of the lung stimulates strong inspiratory efforts and increases the respiratory rate. This deflation reflex may be the result of decreased stretch receptor activity, or it may be caused by the stimulation of other receptors, such as the irritant receptors and J-receptors (discussed later). Although it is unclear which receptors are involved, it is clear that the vagus nerve is the pathway (as it is for the Hering-Breuer reflex) and that the effect is hyperpnea.[1] The deflation reflex is probably responsible for the hyperpnea observed with pneumothorax.

Head's Paradoxical Reflex

In 1889, Head observed that if the Hering-Breuer reflex is partially blocked by cooling the vagus nerve, lung hyperinflation causes a further increase in inspiratory effort, opposite of the Hering-Breuer reflex. The receptors for this paradoxical reflex are called rapidly adapting receptors because they stop firing promptly after a volume change occurs. **Head's reflex** may help maintain large tidal volumes during exercise and may be involved in periodic deep sighs during quiet breathing. Periodic sighs help prevent alveolar collapse or atelectasis. This reflex also may be involved in stimulating the first breaths of a newborn infant.[1]

Irritant Receptors

Rapidly adapting irritant receptors in the epithelium of the larger conducting airways have vagal sensory nerve fibers. When stimulated by inhaled irritants or by mechanical factors, they cause reflex bronchoconstriction, coughing, sneezing, tachypnea, and narrowing of the glottis. Some of these reflexes, called vagovagal reflexes, have both sensory and motor vagal components; sensory nerve stimulation results in motor reflexes that cause laryngospasm, bronchospasm, coughing, and slowing of the heartbeat. Endotracheal intubation, airway suctioning, and bronchoscopy readily elicit vagovagal reflexes. Physical stimulation of the conducting airways, as with suctioning or bronchoscopy, may cause a severe case of bronchospasm, coughing, and laryngospasm.

J-Receptors

C-fibers in the lung parenchyma near pulmonary capillaries are called juxtacapillary receptors, or **J-receptors** (see Chapter 1). They are stimulated by alveolar inflammatory processes (pneumonia), pulmonary vascular congestion (congestive heart failure), and edema. J-receptor stimulation causes rapid, shallow breathing; a sensation of dyspnea; and expiratory narrowing of the glottis. Expiratory narrowing of the glottis causes grunting on expiration, especially in infants.

Peripheral Proprioceptors

Proprioceptors (positional sensors) in muscles, tendons, and joints, and pain receptors in muscles and skin send stimulatory impulses to the medullary centers, increasing inspiratory activity and hyperpnea.[2] For this reason, moving the limbs, slapping the skin, and other painful stimuli stimulate ventilation in patients who have respiratory depression. Splashing cold water on the skin has a similar effect.

Proprioceptors in joints and tendons may be important in initiating and maintaining increased ventilation at the beginning of exercise. Passive limb movement around a joint increases the breathing rate in anesthetized animals and unanesthetized humans.[3]

Muscle Spindles

Muscle spindles in the diaphragm and intercostal muscles are part of a reflex arc that helps the muscles adjust to an increased load. Muscle spindles are stretch-sensing elements located on intrafusal muscle fibers, which are arranged in parallel with the main extrafusal muscle fibers (Figure 11-4). The extrafusal skeletal muscle fibers that elevate the ribs (see Figure 11-4) are innervated by different motor fibers (alpha motor fibers) than the intrafusal spindle fibers (gamma motor fibers). As the main extrafusal muscle fiber and the intrafusal fibers contract together in parallel, the spindle-sensing element stretches and sends impulses over spindle afferent nerves directly to the spinal cord (see Figure 11-4). The number of impulses sent is proportional to the spindle's stretch. The spindle's afferent (sensory) nerve synapses directly with the same alpha motor neuron in the spinal cord that sends motor impulses back to the main extrafusal muscle fiber; this creates a single synapse reflex arc. When stimulated by the spindle's afferent nerve signal, the alpha motor neuron sends signals to only the main extrafusal muscle fibers, causing them to contract with greater force, which unloads and shortens the adjacent intrafusal muscle fibers. As a result, the stretch-sensitive spindle is unloaded, and its impulses cease. In this way, inspiratory muscle force automatically adjusts to the load imposed by decreased lung compliance or increased airway resistance.

CHEMICAL CONTROL OF VENTILATION

The body maintains the proper amounts of oxygen, carbon dioxide, and hydrogen ions in the blood, mainly by regulating ventilation. Physiological mechanisms that monitor these substances in the blood allow ventilation to respond appropriately to maintain homeostasis. An increase in blood H^+ concentration stimulates specialized nerve structures called **chemoreceptors**. Consequently, the chemoreceptors transmit impulses to the medulla, increasing ventilation. Centrally located chemoreceptors in

CLINICAL FOCUS 11-2

Vagovagal Reflex Stimulation during Endotracheal Suctioning

Patients who have endotracheal tubes in place have impaired cough effectiveness because they cannot close the glottis to generate the necessary high intrapulmonary pressure. A suction catheter is frequently inserted into the endotracheal tube and trachea to remove excess secretions. The tip of the catheter often enters the mainstem bronchi during suctioning.

Consider a situation in which you are suctioning the airway of a patient whose lungs are being mechanically ventilated; the cardiac monitoring screen at the patient's bedside shows a sudden decrease in heart rate and blood pressure. On withdrawing the catheter and manually ventilating the patient's lungs with 100% oxygen, you note that the heart rate and blood pressure return to their previous levels. What is the explanation for your patient's response?

Discussion

The suction catheter mechanically stimulated tracheal and bronchial irritant receptors, eliciting a vagovagal reflex. The heart responds to vagal (parasympathetic) stimulation by slowing its rate (bradycardia). Severe bradycardia decreases the cardiac output. Consequently, blood pressure decreases.

Irritation from the suction catheter also stimulates cough receptors in the trachea and carina, eliciting vigorous cough efforts. Such coughing may increase intrathoracic pressure enough to reduce momentarily the venous blood return to the heart, reducing the blood pressure momentarily. These complications of endotracheal suctioning are best avoided by using the following technique:

1. Use a manual resuscitator with 100% oxygen to preoxygenate and reoxygenate intermittently between suctioning attempts.
2. When the suction catheter meets resistance on insertion, do not force the catheter down farther; instead, withdraw it slightly before applying suction.
3. As you withdraw the catheter, applying suction, never jab the catheter in an up-and-down motion; instead, rotate the catheter by twirling it between your thumb and forefinger.
4. Limit each pass of the suction catheter to 10 seconds or less.

The vagovagal reflex is also often elicited during endotracheal intubation. A local anesthetic sprayed into the pharynx and applied to the endotracheal tube helps blunt this reflex.

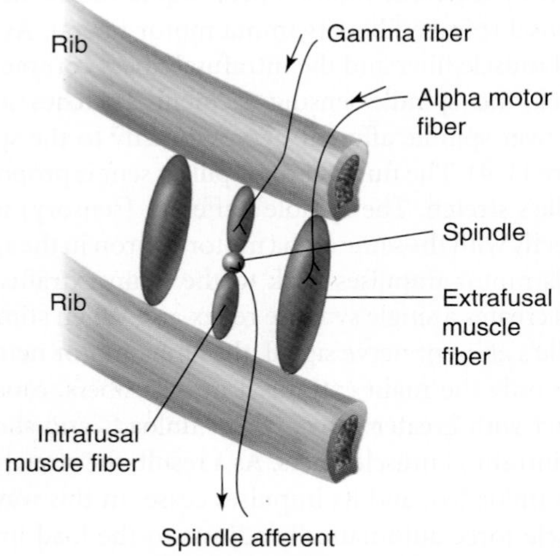

Figure 11-4 Stretch-sensitive muscle spindle of intercostal muscle fibers. Spindle afferent fibers synapse with alpha motor fibers in the spinal cord, creating a single synapse reflex arc. (From Berne RM, Levy MN: *Physiology*, ed 3, St Louis, 1993, Mosby.)

the medulla respond to H^+, which normally arises from the reaction between dissolved CO_2 and H_2O in the cerebrospinal fluid (CSF). Peripherally located chemoreceptors in the fork of the common carotid arteries and the aortic arch are also sensitive to H^+ and thus are indirectly sensitive to CO_2. In addition, peripheral chemoreceptors are indirectly sensitive to hypoxemia because hypoxemia increases their sensitivity to hydrogen ions.[2]

Central (Medullary) Chemoreceptors

Hydrogen ions, not CO_2 molecules, stimulate highly responsive chemosensitive nerve cells, located bilaterally in the medulla. Nevertheless, these central chemoreceptors are extremely responsive to CO_2 because the $[H^+]$ surrounding them is dependent on the reaction between CO_2 and H_2O in their local environment. The chemoreceptors are not in direct contact with arterial blood. Instead, they are bathed in the cerebral spinal fluid, separated from the blood by a semipermeable membrane called the **blood-brain barrier**. This membrane is almost impermeable to H^+ and HCO_3^-, but it is freely permeable to CO_2. When the $PaCO_2$ rises, CO_2 diffuses rapidly through the blood-brain barrier into the CSF. In the CSF, CO_2 reacts with H_2O to form hydrogen ions (Figure 11-5); this stimulates the central chemoreceptors, which in turn stimulate the medullary inspiratory neurons. Because CSF contains no protein buffers, CO_2 diffusion from the blood into the CSF increases $[H^+]$ almost instantly, exciting the central chemoreceptors within seconds. Through this mechanism, alveolar ventilation increases by approximately 2 to 3 L/min for each millimeter of mercury increase in $PaCO_2$.[4] In this indirect fashion, $PaCO_2$ is the principal minute-to-minute stimulus for ventilation mediated through the central chemoreceptors.

CONCEPT QUESTION 11-2

Which of the following stimulates the central chemoreceptors more quickly and elicits the most rapid increase in ventilation: elevated blood PCO_2 or elevated blood $[H^+]$? Explain.

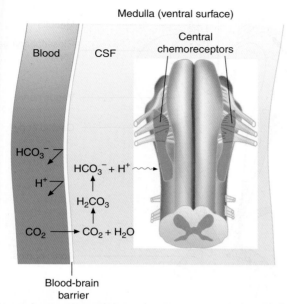

Figure 11-5 CO_2 stimulation of medullary central chemoreceptors via formation of hydrogen ions. The blood-brain barrier is fairly impermeable to H^+ and HCO_3^- but freely permeable to CO_2. *CSF,* Cerebrospinal fluid.

Figure 11-6 compares the ventilatory response to increased $PaCO_2$ with the ventilatory response to increased arterial $[H^+]$ arising from fixed acid accumulation (i.e., acidemia from a non-respiratory cause). A great change in ventilation occurs between $PaCO_2$ values of 40 mm Hg and 80 mm Hg compared with a relatively small change in ventilation caused by a fixed acid–induced fall in arterial pH from 7.40 to 7.00 (see Figure 11-6).

Hydrogen ions in the arterial blood do not readily diffuse across the blood-brain barrier and thus cannot stimulate the medullary chemoreceptors to any great extent; the effect of hydrogen ions is mediated mainly through the less responsive peripheral chemoreceptors, which are discussed in the next section.

The stimulatory effect of CO_2 on the central chemoreceptors gradually declines over 1 to 2 days because of renal compensatory responses. The kidneys increase blood bicarbonate ion $[HCO_3^-]$ concentration in response to respiratory acidosis (see Chapter 10), which returns blood pH to the normal range. The increased number of bicarbonate ions in the blood eventually diffuses across the blood-brain barrier into the CSF where they buffer H^+ and bring the CSF pH back to normal; this removes the stimulus to the chemoreceptors, and ventilation decreases. Although an increase in $PaCO_2$ has an extremely powerful effect on ventilation, its effect is greatly weakened after 1 or 2 days of adaptation.

CONCEPT QUESTION 11-3

The chronically high $PaCO_2$ in patients with advanced chronic obstructive pulmonary disease (COPD) who have compensated respiratory acidosis does not stimulate the central chemoreceptors. Why is this?

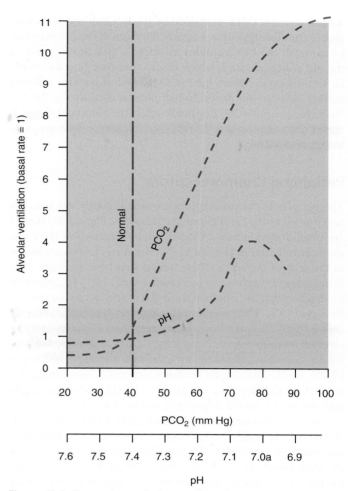

Figure 11-6 Comparison of the ventilatory response to increased $PaCO_2$ and decreased arterial pH. (Redrawn from Guyton AC: *Textbook of medical physiology,* ed 8, Philadelphia, 1991, Saunders.)

Unimportance of Oxygen as a Primary Controller of Ventilation

Although it would seem that oxygen should play an important role in controlling ventilation, oxygen molecules have no effect on the medullary chemoreceptors. Ventilation does not control arterial PO_2 or hemoglobin oxygen saturation with any degree of precision. If an individual's normal resting ventilation is cut in half, PaO_2 decreases from 100 mm Hg to about 60 mm Hg, which still produces an oxygen hemoglobin saturation of about 90% (see Chapter 8). If ventilation then increases, and a normal PaO_2 of 100 mm Hg is restored, oxyhemoglobin saturation increases to about 98%; in other words, an increase in ventilation that raises the PaO_2 from 60 mm Hg to 100 mm Hg adds only marginally more oxygen to the blood. Even maximal hyperventilation cannot raise the PaO_2 higher than 125 to 130 mm Hg (refer to the alveolar air equation in Chapter 7). This degree of hyperventilation (which increases the PaO_2 from 100 mm Hg to 130 mm Hg) increases the hemoglobin saturation by only 1.5%. Thus, in healthy individuals under normal conditions, ventilation ranging from about half normal to many times normal produces very little change in arterial oxygen content; this is explained by the fact that the oxyhemoglobin equilibrium curve is nearly flat from 60 to 125 mm Hg. In contrast, the CO_2 equilibrium curve is practically linear in the physiological range, which means that doubling the alveolar ventilation decreases the $PaCO_2$ to half of normal, whereas cutting alveolar ventilation to half normal doubles the $PaCO_2$. Such changes in $PaCO_2$ drastically affect the blood pH. Thus, it makes sense that carbon dioxide (not oxygen) is the main controller of ventilation.

Peripheral Chemoreceptors

The peripheral chemoreceptors are small, highly vascular tissues known as the carotid and aortic bodies. The carotid bodies are small organs located bilaterally in bifurcations of the common carotid arteries (Figure 11-7). The aortic bodies are found in the arch of the aorta. These neural structures increase their firing rates in response to increased arterial [H$^+$] regardless of its origin—that is, whether from fixed acid accumulation or increased CO_2. The carotid bodies contain far more chemoreceptors than the aortic bodies; they send their impulses over the glossopharyngeal nerve to medullary DRG and VRG, whereas the aortic bodies send their impulses over the vagus nerve (see Figure 11-7). The carotid bodies exert much more influence over the respiratory centers than do the aortic bodies, especially with respect to arterial hypoxemia and acidemia.[1]

The carotid bodies receive an extremely high blood flow, about 20 times their weight each minute.[3] This extremely high flow rate means the carotid bodies have little time to remove oxygen from the blood, so the venous blood leaving the carotid bodies has almost the same oxygen content as the arterial blood entering them. The carotid bodies are exposed at all times to arterial (not venous) blood, and they sense arterial (not venous) [H$^+$].

Response to Decreased Arterial Oxygen
Traditionally, it was believed that the carotid bodies directly sensed decreased PaO_2 levels, implying that arterial hypoxemia represents an independent drive to breathe—the so-called hypoxic drive. Although peripheral chemoreceptors fire more frequently in the presence of arterial hypoxemia, they do so only because hypoxemia makes them more sensitive to hydrogen ions.[2] That is, in the presence of hypoxemia, carotid body sensitivity to a given [H$^+$] increases; in this way, hypoxia increases ventilation for any given pH. Conversely, a very high PO_2 (hyperoxia) decreases carotid body sensitivity to [H$^+$]. Thus, the carotid bodies respond to arterial hypoxemia but only because hypoxia makes them more sensitive to [H$^+$]; this implies that if the arterial [H$^+$] is extremely low, as in severe alkalemia, hypoxemia has little effect on the carotid bodies.[2] Simply stated, the ultimate effect of hypoxemia is to increase the neural firing rate of the peripheral chemoreceptors, which increases minute ventilation.

Because carotid body tissues have extremely high blood flow rates, they respond to decreased PaO_2 (in the indirect way just described) rather than to an actual decrease in arterial oxygen content. That is, the carotid bodies' extraction of oxygen from each unit of rapidly flowing blood is so small that their oxygen needs are met entirely by dissolved oxygen in the plasma. This is

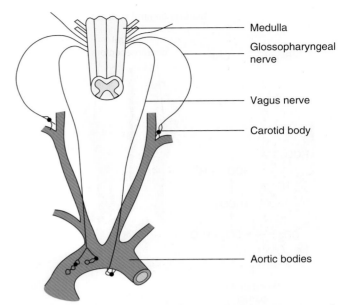

Figure 11-7 Control of respiration by peripheral chemoreceptors: the carotid and aortic bodies. (Redrawn from Guyton AC: *Textbook of medical physiology,* ed 8, Philadelphia, 1991, Saunders.)

why conditions associated with low arterial oxygen content but normal PaO_2 (e.g., anemia and carbon monoxide poisoning) do not stimulate ventilation.[4]

When pH and $PaCO_2$ are normal (i.e., pH = 7.40 and $PaCO_2$ = 40 mm Hg), the carotid bodies' rate of nerve impulse transmission does not increase significantly until PaO_2 decreases to about 60 mm Hg.[4] As PaO_2 decreases from 60 mm Hg to 30 mm Hg, the rate of impulse transmission increases sharply and linearly because hypoxemia makes the carotid bodies much more sensitive to a pH of 7.40 (Figure 11-8). A decrease in PaO_2 from 60 mm Hg to 30 mm Hg corresponds to the sharpest decrease in oxygen content on the oxygen-hemoglobin equilibrium curve—that is, the steepest part of the curve. Arterial hypoxemia does not stimulate ventilation greatly until the PaO_2 decreases to values less than 60 mm Hg; this is why ventilation increases as one ascends to high altitudes. Decreased barometric pressure at high altitudes decreases inspired and arterial PO_2 values, which increases the sensitivity of peripheral chemoreceptors to hydrogen ions. However, the resulting increase in ventilation is less than expected because hyperventilation increases arterial pH by decreasing $PaCO_2$ and subsequently, blood [H$^+$]. The increase in arterial pH depresses the medullary respiratory center, counteracting the excitatory effect of decreased PaO_2 on peripheral chemoreceptors. However, lung mechanics in certain conditions, such as advanced chronic obstructive pulmonary disease, are so deranged that the stimulatory effect of hypoxemia on ventilation fails to decrease $PaCO_2$ regardless of the patient's effort. In such instances, there is no alkalosis to counteract stimulatory effects of hypoxemia on ventilation.

Response to Increased Arterial Carbon Dioxide Pressure and Hydrogen Ions
Similar to the central chemoreceptors, the peripheral chemoreceptors are directly sensitive to hydrogen ions and indirectly

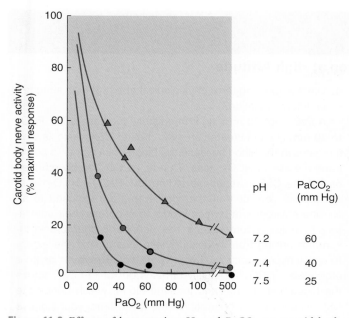

Figure 11-8 Effects of hypoxemia, pH, and $PaCO_2$ on carotid body nerve activity. A decrease in PaO_2 less than 60 mm Hg elicits significantly more nerve activity for a given pH or $PaCO_2$ value. (Redrawn from Taylor AE, et al: *Clinical respiratory physiology*, Philadelphia, 1989, Saunders; modified from Hornbein TF: The relation between stimulus to chemoreceptors and their response. In Torrance RW, editor: *The proceedings of the Wates Foundation Symposium on Arterial Chemoreceptors*, Oxford, 1968, Blackwell Science.)

sensitive to PCO_2. That is, ventilation controls arterial $[H^+]$ by controlling $PaCO_2$ (which generates H^+ through the hydration reaction), and in this way, the peripheral chemoreceptors are sensitive to $PaCO_2$. Increased $PaCO_2$ increases blood $[H^+]$, directly exciting the carotid bodies and stimulating ventilation. However, this increase in ventilation is far less than the increase produced by the central chemoreceptors when they are stimulated by CO_2-generated H^+. The peripheral chemoreceptors account for only 20% to 30% of the ventilatory response to hypercapnia.[4] However, the peripheral chemoreceptors respond to a fixed acid-induced rise in arterial $[H^+]$ about five times more quickly than the central chemoreceptors.[3] In contrast to the central chemoreceptors, the carotid bodies are directly exposed to arterial blood. Thus, the initial ventilatory response to fixed acid accumulation is quick, offsetting the fact that hydrogen ions cross the blood-brain barrier with great difficulty.

As stated earlier, hypoxemia increases the sensitivity of the peripheral chemoreceptors to hydrogen ions and thus indirectly to $PaCO_2$. Conversely, an excessively high PaO_2 (hyperoxia) decreases the peripheral chemoreceptors' $PaCO_2$ sensitivity to almost zero.[2] Thus, when PaO_2 is increased, the ventilatory response to $PaCO_2$ is mainly mediated by the central chemoreceptors, which are unaffected by hypoxemia.

The fact that the only effect of hypoxia on the peripheral chemoreceptors is to increase their sensitivity to arterial $[H^+]$ and subsequently to $PaCO_2$ means that (1) high PO_2 renders the peripheral chemoreceptors almost unresponsive to PCO_2, and (2) decreased $PaCO_2$ (low arterial $[H^+]$) renders the peripheral chemoreceptors almost unresponsive to hypoxemia.[2] Coexisting arterial hypoxemia, acidemia, and high $PaCO_2$ (i.e., asphyxia) maximally stimulate the peripheral chemoreceptors (see Figure 11-8).

Control of Breathing during Chronic Hypercapnia

A sudden increase in $PaCO_2$ causes an immediate increase in ventilation because CO_2 rapidly diffuses from the blood into the CSF, increasing $[H^+]$ surrounding the central chemoreceptors. On the other hand, if $PaCO_2$ increases gradually over many years, as might occur in the development of severe COPD and steadily worsening lung mechanics, the kidneys compensate by increasing the plasma bicarbonate concentration, keeping the arterial pH within normal limits (see Chapter 10). As plasma bicarbonate levels increase, these ions slowly diffuse across the blood-brain barrier, keeping CSF pH in its normal range. Because the central chemoreceptors respond to $[H^+]$, not the CO_2 molecule, they sense a normal pH environment, even though the $PaCO_2$ is abnormally high.

This adaptation explains why chronically elevated $PaCO_2$ in patients with severe COPD does not overly stimulate ventilation. Instead, the hypoxemia that accompanies chronic hypercapnia becomes the minute-to-minute breathing stimulus in the roundabout way discussed previously: Hypoxemia increases the peripheral chemoreceptors' sensitivity to $[H^+]$, increasing the nerve impulses they transmit to the medulla, stimulating ventilation. Patients with severe COPD are invariably hypoxemic when breathing room air because their lungs have severe mismatches in ventilation and blood flow. It stands to reason that breathing supplemental oxygen would increase the PaO_2 and make the carotid bodies less sensitive to $[H^+]$, which would decrease ventilation further and thus increase $PaCO_2$.

Oxygen-Associated Hypercapnia

An acute increase in $PaCO_2$ sometimes occurs after oxygen is given to patients with severe COPD who are chronically hypoxemic and hypercapnic; the reason for this phenomenon continues to be a subject of much debate and misunderstanding. The traditional explanation has been that oxygen breathing removes hypoxemia's stimulatory effect on the peripheral chemoreceptors. As explained in the previous section, the ventilatory stimulus of the peripheral chemoreceptors increases significantly when the PaO_2 decreases to less than 60 mm Hg; this is true in hypoxemic patients with or without a history of chronic hypercapnia. If breathing supplemental oxygen increases the PaO_2 to levels greater than 60 mm Hg, it stands to reason that the stimulatory effect of the peripheral chemoreceptors on ventilation would diminish, which would decrease ventilation and increase $PaCO_2$. This explanation for the increase in $PaCO_2$ after oxygen administration is widely accepted in reference to hypoxemic patients without COPD—for example, a patient with pneumonia whose hypoxemia is corrected by O_2 administration; it seems to be challenged only in reference to patients with COPD who are chronically hypercapnic. The major reason

CLINICAL FOCUS 11-3

Chronic Physiological Effect of Low Inspired Oxygen at High Altitude

You and some friends decide to vacation in the mountains of Colorado and climb a 14,000-foot peak (barometric pressure = 460 mm Hg). You are currently at sea level. You drive to your destination in 1 day, and the next morning you hike to the peak of the 14,000-foot mountain and set up camp for the night.

Questions and Discussion

1. At the top of the mountain, what is the inspired PO_2 (P_IO_2) in your trachea?

$$P_IO_2 = 0.21(460 - 47) = 87 \text{ mm Hg}$$

2. What is your alveolar PO_2 (P_AO_2) if your ventilation does not change and P_ACO_2 remains at 40 mm Hg?

$$P_AO_2 = 0.21(460 - 47) - (40 \times 1.2) = 39 \text{ mm Hg}$$

PaO_2 would be a few millimeters of mercury lower than this because of a normal $P(A\text{-}a)O_2$ difference (secondary to normal anatomical shunting). Actually, your ventilation does not remain the same; hypoxia makes your peripheral chemoreceptors more sensitive, which stimulates ventilation quite strongly at this PaO_2.

3. If your ventilation increases enough to reduce your $PaCO_2$ to 20 mm Hg, what is your P_AO_2?

$$P_AO_2 = 0.21(460 - 47) - (20 \times 1.2) = 63 \text{ mm Hg}$$

(Because of the normal $P(A\text{-}a)O_2$, PaO_2 would be in the upper 50s.)

4. What is the long-term physiological effect of high altitude on your ventilation?

A $PaCO_2$ of 20 mm Hg immediately decreases CSF PCO_2 to 20 mm Hg and creates an even greater CSF alkalosis than it creates in the blood because the blood-brain barrier is nearly impermeable to HCO_3^- ions. That is, as CO_2 rapidly diffuses out of the CSF in response to the low $PaCO_2$, HCO_3^- cannot follow. Your central chemoreceptors are exposed to an alkaline environment, which works to suppress their ventilatory stimulus, counteracting the peripheral chemoreceptor stimulus arising from hypoxia. These events limit the extent to which hypoxia increases your ventilation. However, as time progresses, HCO_3^- gradually diffuses out of the CSF across the blood-brain barrier and into the blood, which brings the CSF pH back toward normal. At the same time, your kidneys compensate for the hyperventilation-induced alkalemia by excreting HCO_3^- ions; over the next 24 hours, this brings your blood pH back toward normal—even though the $PaCO_2$ is still low. With the inhibiting effects of an alkalotic CSF removed, the hypoxic stimulus gradually increases ventilation again. On arriving at the mountaintop, about 24 hours pass before your minute ventilation increases to its maximum level. This considerable increase in ventilation greatly improves your ability to tolerate the low P_IO_2.

---

why alternative explanations have been sought is that the reduction in minute ventilation after oxygen breathing in patients with advanced COPD is not always severe enough to account for the increased $PaCO_2$.[5,6]

The question is not whether hypoxemia heightens peripheral chemoreceptor sensitivity to $[H^+]$ in hypercapnic patients with COPD (it does) but whether oxygen administration decreases this sensitivity sufficiently to account for the observed increase in $PaCO_2$. An additional pertinent question is whether an acute increase in $PaCO_2$ on top of already elevated $PaCO_2$ stimulates the medullary chemoreceptors in these patients as it does in healthy patients.

Several investigators have suggested that oxygen breathing worsens the lungs' ventilation-perfusion ($\dot{V}/\dot{Q}$) relationships, creating more dead space.[5,6] Other investigators suggested that oxygen-induced hypercapnia is caused by the combined effects of hypoxic stimulus removal and redistribution of $\dot{V}/\dot{Q}$ relationships in the lungs.[7-9]

$\dot{V}/\dot{Q}$ relationships may worsen in the lungs after oxygen administration because improved oxygenation abolishes hypoxic pulmonary vasoconstriction in poorly ventilated lung regions. The resulting reduction in vascular resistance shifts more blood flow to these underventilated areas, drawing blood flow away from well-ventilated regions (Figure 11-9). As poorly ventilated regions receive more blood flow, they become even less ventilated as oxygen-rich inspired gas

washes out resident nitrogen gas, making alveoli more subject to absorption atelectasis; that is, oxygen may be absorbed by the pulmonary circulation more rapidly than the slowed ventilation can replenish it (notice the further decreased $\dot{V}$ in Figure 11-9, *B*). As a result, inspired gas flows preferentially to the already well-ventilated alveoli (see Figure 11-9, *B*), increasing their $\dot{V}/\dot{Q}$ ratios. The increased $\dot{V}/\dot{Q}$ in these alveoli is further exaggerated because they lose some blood flow to the poorly ventilated regions, which now have lower vascular resistance owing to oxygen breathing. In the end, more blood flow is directed to poorly ventilated alveoli, which takes blood flow away from well-ventilated alveoli. The key point is that when already underventilated alveoli receive additional blood flow, arterial blood PCO_2 increases further. These events occur without a decline in overall minute ventilation.

Although some investigators believe the mechanisms just described explain why oxygen administration induces hypercapnia in patients with COPD, other studies support an equally important role for oxygen suppression of the hypoxic ventilatory stimulus.[7-9] These studies demonstrated that in exacerbated, chronically hypercapnic patients with COPD, oxygen administration significantly reduced their ventilation[8,9] and elevated the $PaCO_2$ level required to stimulate ventilation via the medullary chemoreceptors.[7]

The diagnosis of COPD on a patient's medical record does not automatically mean the patient has a chronically increased

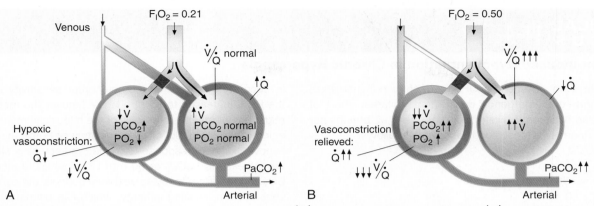

Figure 11-9 Oxygen-induced hypercapnia in severe COPD through the $\dot{V}/\dot{Q}$ mismatch mechanism. **A,** The low $\dot{V}/\dot{Q}$ unit (*left*) is hypoxic and hypercapnic, inducing pulmonary vasoconstriction. **B,** Oxygen breathing further decreases the $\dot{V}/\dot{Q}$ of the poorly ventilated unit, while increasing the $\dot{V}/\dot{Q}$ of the normal unit (*right*). Oxygen breathing (1) predisposes the poorly ventilated unit to absorption atelectasis and (2) improves blood flow to the poorly ventilated unit. Both of these factors further decrease the $\dot{V}/\dot{Q}$ of the poorly ventilated unit and increase the alveolar PCO_2 (**B,** *left*).

PaCO₂ or that hypercapnia will follow oxygen administration. These characteristics are present only in patients with severe end-stage disease, which includes only a small percentage of patients with the diagnosis of COPD; therefore, concern about oxygen-induced hypercapnia and acidemia is not warranted in most patients with a diagnosis of COPD. In any event, the fear of inducing hypoventilation and hypercapnia is never a justifiable rationale for withholding oxygen from acutely hypoxemic patients with COPD. Tissue oxygenation is an overriding priority; oxygen must never be withheld for any reason from hypoxemic COPD patients experiencing exacerbations of their disease. The clinician must be prepared to mechanically support the patient's ventilation if severe hypoventilation occurs.

Medullary Response to Acute Carbon Dioxide Increase in Chronic Hypercapnia

As discussed earlier, the kidneys compensate for the acidic effects of chronic hypercapnia by raising the plasma bicarbonate level, keeping the medullary chemoreceptor pH environment in the normal range. However, the medullary chemoreceptors can still respond to further acute increases in $PaCO_2$. A sudden rise in $PaCO_2$ means more CO_2 molecules immediately cross the blood-brain barrier into the CSF generating hydrogen ions that stimulate the medullary chemoreceptors.

The resulting ventilatory response is depressed for both chemical and mechanical reasons: (1) the blood's increased buffering capacity (high HCO_3^- level) in chronic hypercapnia prevents arterial pH from decreasing as sharply as it would in normal conditions, and (2) abnormal breathing mechanics impair the lungs' ability to increase ventilation appropriately. To illustrate the blood's changed buffering capacity, compare a healthy person (pH = 7.40; $PaCO_2$ = 40 mm Hg; HCO_3^- = 24 mEq/L) with a chronically hypercapnic patient (pH = 7.38; $PaCO_2$ = 60 mm Hg; HCO_3^- = 34 mEq/L). If $PaCO_2$ suddenly increases by 30 mm Hg in both individuals, the healthy person's arterial pH decreases to 7.21, and the hypercapnic patient's pH decreases to only 7.24. (These values are calculated using the Henderson-Hasselbalch equation, assuming a 1-mEq/L increase in plasma HCO_3^- concentration for each

acute 10-mm Hg increase in $PaCO_2$.) Thus, the chronically hypercapnic patient's central chemoreceptors experience less stimulation than the central chemoreceptors of the healthy person for the same increase in $PaCO_2$. Several investigators have confirmed the reduced ventilatory response to CO_2 in patients with chronic hypercapnia.[10,11]

VENTILATORY RESPONSE TO EXERCISE

During strenuous exercise, CO_2 production and oxygen consumption may increase 20-fold.[3] These increases are extremely well matched by ventilation and cardiac output. Ventilation keeps pace with CO_2 production, keeping $PaCO_2$, PaO_2, and arterial pH remarkably constant. What drives the greatly increased ventilation that accompanies exercise if arterial blood gases do not change?

The exact mechanisms responsible for increased ventilation during exercise are not well understood. Figure 11-10 illustrates the three stages of exercise: I, onset; II, period of adjustment; III, steady state. Especially mysterious is the abrupt increase in ventilation at the onset of exercise (stage I), long before any chemical or humoral changes can occur in the body. The two predominating theories are as follows: (1) when the cerebral motor cortex sends impulses to exercising muscles, it apparently sends collateral excitatory impulses to the medullary respiratory centers, and (2) exercising limbs moving around their joints stimulate proprioceptors, which transmit excitatory impulses to the medullary centers.[3] Evidence also suggests that the sudden increase in ventilation at the onset of exercise is a learned response.[3] In other words, with repeated experience, the brain learns to anticipate the proper amount of ventilation required to maintain normal blood gases during exercise.

ABNORMAL BREATHING PATTERNS

Common abnormal breathing patterns include (1) Cheyne-Stokes breathing, (2) Biot's breathing, (3) apneustic breathing, and (4) central reflex hypopnea and hyperpnea. In

CLINICAL FOCUS 11-4

Oxygen-Induced Hypoventilation in Chronic Hypercapnia

A patient with advanced COPD and chronic hypercapnia comes into the emergency department agitated, short of breath, and hypoxemic. His respiratory rate is 32 breaths per minute. Room air arterial blood gases are as follows:

pH = 7.34
PCO_2 = 65 mm Hg
HCO_3^- = 34 mEq/L
PaO_2 = 50 mm Hg

Emergency department personnel immediately administer oxygen by using an air-entrainment mask set to deliver 40% oxygen. Within 30 minutes, the patient is much less agitated, and the respiratory rate is 10 breaths per minute and shallow. The patient seems sleepy and does not respond in an alert manner to verbal questions. Arterial blood gases are drawn with the following results:

pH = 7.26
PCO_2 = 80 mm Hg
HCO_3^- = 35 mEq/L
PaO_2 = 95 mm Hg

What is the explanation for these blood gas results?

Discussion

Given this patient's history, chronic hypoxemia probably increases peripheral chemoreceptor sensitivity enough (via mechanisms explained in this chapter) to have an effect on his normal ventilation. His initial PaO_2 of 50 mm Hg is low enough to increase significantly peripheral chemoreceptor sensitivity to H^+. It stands to reason that the relatively high fractional concentration of oxygen in inspired gas (F_IO_2) of 0.40 played a role

in decreasing peripheral chemoreceptor sensitivity because the PaO_2 increased to 95 mm Hg. Whatever the mechanism might be (whether it is removal of the hypoxic stimulus, worsening of the $\dot{V}/\dot{Q}$ ratio, or a combination of both), this patient hypoventilated in response to oxygen therapy as is shown by the increase in $PaCO_2$ to 80 mm Hg. This acute increase in CO_2 and the accompanying acidemia depress the central nervous system, causing lethargy, which can ultimately lead to a coma. Aside from the causative mechanism, the clinically important fact is that uncontrolled oxygen therapy can lead to hypoventilation and acute acidemia in patients who are chronically hypercapnic. For this reason, spontaneously breathing, hypoxemic, chronically hypercapnic patients with COPD who are experiencing exacerbations are generally given low concentrations of oxygen (24% to 28%). Devices that produce a fixed F_IO_2 regardless of the patient's ventilatory pattern should be used. Initial oxygen therapy is monitored closely through arterial blood gases to detect acute CO_2 retention and acidemia. Low levels of inspired oxygen often increase the arterial oxygen content quite effectively in these patients because their blood PO_2 is on the steep part of the oxygen-hemoglobin equilibrium curve (see Chapter 8). In other words, small increases in PaO_2 produce relatively large increases in oxygen content. However, concern about inducing hypoventilation, hypercapnia, and acidemia is never a justifiable reason for withholding oxygen from a patient with tissue hypoxia; tissue hypoxia has a far greater potential to be life threatening than hypercapnia and acidemia. The clinician must be prepared to mechanically ventilate these patients as necessary.

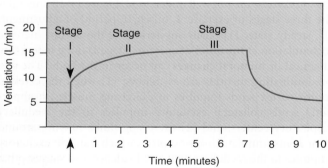

Figure 11-10 Three stages of ventilatory response to exercise. (From Berne RM, Levy MN: *Physiology*, ed 3, St Louis, 1993, Mosby.)

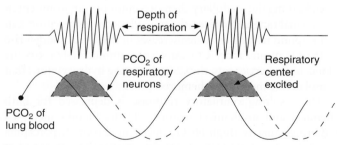

Figure 11-11 Cheyne-Stokes breathing pattern. (From Guyton AC: *Textbook of medical physiology*, ed 8, Philadelphia, 1991, Saunders.)

Cheyne-Stokes breathing, the respiratory rate and tidal volume gradually increase and then gradually decrease to complete apnea (absence of ventilation), which may last several seconds. The tidal volume and breathing frequency gradually increase again, repeating the cycle (Figure 11-11). This pattern occurs when cardiac output is low, as in congestive heart failure, which

delays the blood transit time between the lungs and the brain.[3] As shown in Figure 11-11, changes in respiratory center PCO_2 lag behind changes in $PaCO_2$. When increasing $PaCO_2$ reaches the medullary neurons, ventilation is stimulated, decreasing the arterial blood PCO_2. When this blood, now low in $PaCO_2$, eventually reaches the medulla, it inhibits ventilation, but it is so slow to reach the medullary neurons that hyperventilation persists for an inappropriately long time. When the blood from the lung

CLINICAL FOCUS 11-5

Mechanical Hyperventilation of a Patient with Head Trauma

An automobile accident victim, previously healthy, sustained a closed head injury with accompanying high ICP. Mechanical ventilation in the intensive care unit is required. In ventilating this patient's lungs, you can control the $PaCO_2$. What is your goal in establishing an appropriate $PaCO_2$?

Discussion

Clinical investigators showed more than 40 years ago that the volume of the swollen brain could be reduced by decreasing $PaCO_2$. Since then, mechanical hyperventilation has been a cornerstone in managing elevated ICP associated with TBI.[12] Hyperventilation decreases ICP by causing cerebral vasoconstriction, ultimately reducing cerebral blood volume. This subject is not without controversy; hyperventilation-induced cerebral vasoconstriction has the potential to reduce CBF to levels that cause cerebral hypoxia (ischemia). Over the last decade, this concern has dampened enthusiasm for hyperventilation in cases of TBI. Both the proponents and the opponents of hyperventilation recognize that TBI poses an ischemic threat to the brain; proponents believe that the reduction of CBF ultimately improves cerebral oxygenation by reducing the ICP, which helps sustain the cerebral perfusion pressure. Opponents point out that no other hypoxic organ in the body is treated by reducing its blood flow and oxygen supply. (Hyperventilation in this context is generally defined as a $PaCO_2$ <35 mm Hg.[12])

The debate centers around the question of whether a hyperventilation-induced decrease in CBF creates an additional hypoxic insult to the already ischemic brain and whether patients managed in this way have better clinical outcomes than patients in whom hyperventilation is not instituted. A comprehensive review of this subject published in 2005 concluded that no advantage in long-term clinical outcome could be shown in TBI, whether or not hyperventilation was used.[12] The authors concluded that in TBI, hyperventilation therapy should be considered only for patients with high ICPs; no benefit can be expected if ICP is normal. They further concluded that hyperventilation is most appropriate the second or third day after injury because CBF is lowest in the first 24 hours after injury, and the risk of inducing ischemia through hyperventilation is greatest in this time frame. The authors advised against hyperventilating TBI patients to a $PaCO_2$ less than 30 mm Hg because this increases the danger of cerebral ischemia. Finally, it is important to remember that hyperventilation is effective for only about 24 to 48 hours because compensatory renal elimination of bicarbonate restores the acid-base balance, negating the vasoconstrictive effect of hypocapnia.[12] What is not controversial is that hypoventilation in patients with head trauma and increased ICPs is especially dangerous because hypercapnia dilates cerebral vessels and increases ICP further. Even opponents of hyperventilation generally maintain $PaCO_2$ of patients with TBI in the low-normal range around 35 mm Hg.

finally reaches the medullary centers, its decreased $PaCO_2$ greatly depresses ventilation to the point of apnea. $PaCO_2$ then increases, but an increase in medullary center PCO_2 is delayed because of the low blood flow rate. The brain eventually receives the high $PaCO_2$ signal, and the cycle is repeated. Cheyne-Stokes breathing also may be caused by brain injuries in which the respiratory centers overrespond to changes in PCO_2. In this situation, slight increases in PCO_2 cause exaggerated increases in ventilation, and low PCO_2 may completely turn off the medullary centers.[3]

Biot's breathing is similar to Cheyne-Stokes breathing except tidal volumes have essentially the same depth. The mechanism for this pattern is unclear; it occurs in patients with lesions of the pons.[13]

Apneustic breathing (discussed previously) also indicates damage to the pons.[13] **Central reflex hyperpnea** (formerly known as central neurogenic hyperventilation) is continuous deep breathing driven by abnormal neural stimuli. It is related to midbrain and upper pons damage that may occur with head trauma, severe brain hypoxia, or lack of blood flow to the brain.[13] Conversely, in **central reflex hypopnea** (formerly known as central neurogenic hypoventilation), the respiratory centers do not respond appropriately to ventilatory stimuli such as CO_2. Central reflex hypopnea is associated with head

trauma, brain hypoxia, and narcotic suppression of the respiratory center.[2]

Carbon Dioxide and Cerebral Blood Flow

CO_2 plays an important role in regulating cerebral blood flow (CBF). Its effect is mediated through the formation of hydrogen ions by CO_2.[12] Increased PCO_2 dilates cerebral vessels, increasing CBF, whereas decreased PCO_2 constricts cerebral vessels and reduces CBF. In patients with traumatic brain injury (TBI), the brain swells acutely; this increases the intracranial pressure (ICP) in the rigid skull to such high levels that blood supply to the brain might be cut off, causing cerebral hypoxia (ischemia)—increased ICP may exceed cerebral arterial pressure and stop blood flow. Normal ICP is less than 10 mm Hg; a pressure of 20 mm Hg places the brain at risk for ischemia and requires active treatment to reduce the ICP.[12] The brain has a high oxygen requirement; it accounts for about 20% of the entire body's resting oxygen consumption. To meet this oxygen demand, the body maintains a constant CBF of about 50 to 60 mL per 100 g of brain tissue per minute; CBF less than 18 mL/100 g/min is the threshold for cerebral ischemia.[18] To sustain the CBF, cerebral perfusion pressure (CPP) of about

60 mm Hg must be maintained. CPP is the difference between mean arterial pressure and ICP; cerebral ischemia is likely to occur if CPP decreases to less than 55 mm Hg.[12]

Mechanical hyperventilation has been used for many years in TBI to reduce $PaCO_2$ and reduce CBF and ICP. In patients with TBI, a cerebral blood volume reduction of only 0.5 to 0.7 mL decreases ICP by 1 mm Hg; on the other hand, for every 1-mm Hg acute reduction in $PaCO_2$ (between 20 mm Hg and 60 mm Hg), there is a 3% reduction in CBF.[12] Thus, although an acute reduction in $PaCO_2$ reduces ICP, it also reduces CBF and potentially causes cerebral ischemia. In any event, hypoventilation in a patient with head trauma and a preexisting elevated ICP is especially dangerous because the resulting hypercapnia dilates cerebral vessels and elevates ICP even more.

POINTS TO REMEMBER

- The respiratory center responsible for the basic spontaneous breathing pattern consists of inspiratory and expiratory neurons located in the medulla of the brainstem.
- Impulses from higher pontine centers and medullary chemoreceptors alter the basic breathing pattern, producing a smooth, cyclical ventilatory rhythm.
- The respiratory center receives many neural inputs from peripherally located chemoreceptors, stretch receptors, irritant pain receptors, and the cerebral cortex.
- Arterial blood CO_2 is the primary stimulus driving ventilation minute to minute; its effect on medullary chemoreceptors is mediated through the formation of hydrogen ions in the CSF.
- If a state of high arterial and CSF PCO_2 persists, renal compensatory mechanisms conserve bicarbonate ions, returning the pH to which the central chemoreceptors are exposed into the acidic end of the normal range.
- Hypoxemia makes the peripheral chemoreceptors located in the carotid bodies become more sensitive to hydrogen ions, indirectly driving ventilation.
- The effect of hypoxemia on ventilation is not significant until PaO_2 decreases to less than 60 mm Hg.
- Oxygen administration in patients with chronic hypercapnia might cause hypoventilation, further elevation of $PaCO_2$, and acidemia, which means the clinician must be prepared to mechanically assist ventilation in such circumstances.

- Increased $PaCO_2$ dilates cerebral vessels, increasing blood flow and ICP; acutely decreasing $PaCO_2$ has the opposite effect.
- Mechanical hyperventilation to decrease ICP in patients with TBI has unproven long-term beneficial effects.

References

1. Levitzky MG: *Pulmonary physiology*, ed 7, New York, 2007, McGraw-Hill Medical.
2. Philipson EA, Duffin J: Hypoventilation and hyperventilation syndromes. In Mason RJ, et al, editors: *Murray and Nadel's textbook of respiratory medicine*, ed 5, Philadelphia, 2010, Saunders.
3. Hall JE: *Guyton and Hall textbook of medical physiology*, ed 12, Philadelphia, 2010, Saunders.
4. West JB: *Respiratory physiology: the essentials*, ed 8, Philadelphia, 2008, Lippincott Williams & Wilkins.
5. Crossley DJ, et al: Influence of inspired oxygen concentration on deadspace, respiratory drive, and $PaCO_2$ in intubated patients with chronic obstructive pulmonary disease, *Crit Care Med* 25(9):1522, 1997.
6. Gomersall CD, et al: Oxygen therapy for hypercapnic patients with chronic obstructive pulmonary disease and acute respiratory failure: a randomized, controlled pilot study, *Crit Care Med* 30(1):113, 2002.
7. Dunn WF, Nelson SB, Hubmayr RD: Oxygen-induced hypercapnia in obstructive pulmonary disease, *Am Rev Respir Dis* 144(3 Pt 1):526, 1991.
8. Robinson TD, et al: The role of hypoventilation and ventilation-perfusion redistribution in oxygen-induced hypercapnia during acute exacerbations of chronic obstructive pulmonary disease, *Am J Respir Crit Care Med* 161(5):1524, 2000.
9. Calverley PM: Oxygen-induced hypercapnia revisited (editorial), *Lancet* 356(9241):1538, 2000.
10. Heyer L, et al: Carbon dioxide respiratory response during positive inspiratory pressure in COPD patients, *Respir Physiol* 109(1):29, 1997.
11. Scano G, et al: Carbon dioxide responsiveness in COPD patients with and without chronic hypercapnia, *Eur Respir J* 8(1):78, 1995.
12. Stocchetti N, et al: Hyperventilation in head injury: a review, *Chest* 127(5):2005, 1812.
13. Bleck TP: Levels of consciousness and attention. In Goetz CG, editor: *Textbook of clinical neurology*, ed 2, Philadelphia, 2003, Saunders.
14. Kacmarek RM: Proportional assist ventilation and neurally adjusted ventilatory assist, *Respir Care* 56(2):140, 2011.

Ventilation-Perfusion Relationships

OBJECTIVES

After reading this chapter, you will be able to:

- Explain why alveolar ventilation ($\dot{V}_A$) and pulmonary capillary blood flow ($\dot{Q}_C$) determine alveolar oxygen pressure (P_AO_2)
- Use the oxygen–carbon dioxide diagram to characterize absolute shunt and absolute dead space
- Explain why there is an alveolar-to-arterial oxygen pressure difference ($P(A-a)O_2$) in the normal lung
- Show why $P(A-a)O_2$ increases as fractional concentration of inspired oxygen (F_IO_2) increases
- Explain why high $\dot{V}_A/\dot{Q}_C$ lung regions can compensate for the hypercapnia but not the hypoxemia of low $\dot{V}_A/\dot{Q}_C$ regions
- Differentiate between general hypoventilation, shunt, and $\dot{V}_A/\dot{Q}_C$ mismatch as causes of hypoxemia

- Explain why absolute shunt is not responsive to oxygen therapy
- Describe the major pathological defects involved in shunt-producing and dead space–producing diseases
- Differentiate between the effects absolute shunt and absolute dead space have on arterial blood gases
- Identify which of the following shunt indicators is the most clinically accurate and reliable: $P(A-a)O_2$, PaO_2/F_IO_2 ratio, or PaO_2/P_AO_2 ratio
- Use the classic physiological shunt equation to calculate the fraction of shunted cardiac output
- Explain why changes in cardiac output affect PaO_2 in a patient with abnormally high intrapulmonary shunt

KEY TERMS

A-a gradient
a-A ratio
absolute dead space
absolute shunt
continuous positive airway pressure (CPAP)

refractory hypoxemia
relative dead space
relative shunt
venous admixture

OVERALL $\dot{V}_A/\dot{Q}_C$ RATIO

Normal gas exchange between air and blood can occur only if pulmonary blood flow perfuses ventilated alveoli. Thus the $\dot{V}_A/\dot{Q}_C$ ratio is critical in maintaining normal gas exchange. The $\dot{V}_A/\dot{Q}_C$ ratio may refer to ventilation and blood flow in a single alveolus, all alveoli in a single lobe, or all 300 million plus alveoli in the lung. The average resting $\dot{V}_A$ (alveolar ventilation) for the lung is about 4 L per minute, and the resting $\dot{Q}_C$ (pulmonary capillary blood flow) is about 5 L per minute. The overall average $\dot{V}_A/\dot{Q}_C$ is about 0.8 for the lung as a whole.[1] However, the overall $\dot{V}_A/\dot{Q}_C$ ratio reveals little about the lung's ability to function as a gas-exchange organ. For example, consider the hypothetical extreme situation in which

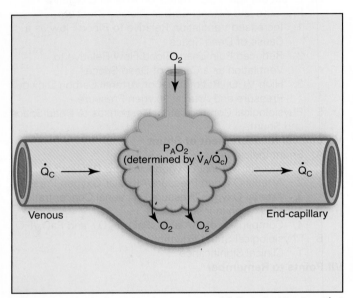

Figure 12-1 The balance between oxygen added to the alveolus ($\dot{V}_A$) and oxygen removed from it ($\dot{Q}_C$), or the $\dot{V}_A/\dot{Q}_C$ ratio, determines P_AO_2.

5 L per minute of pulmonary blood perfuses a nonventilated left lung and 4 L per minute of gas ventilates a nonperfused right lung. The overall average $\dot{V}_A/\dot{Q}_C$ would be normal (4 L/min ÷ 5 L/min = 0.8), but gas exchange would be impossible.

CONCEPT QUESTION 12-1

What effect does a decrease in $\dot{V}_A$ with respect to $\dot{Q}_C$ (low $\dot{V}_A/\dot{Q}_C$ ratio) have on P_ACO_2?

$\dot{V}_A/\dot{Q}_C$ RATIO AS A DETERMINANT OF ALVEOLAR PO_2

The model of the lung and its pulmonary blood flow in Figure 12-1 shows that ventilation continually adds atmospheric oxygen to the alveoli, whereas pulmonary blood flow continually removes oxygen from the alveoli. If blood flow ceases and ventilation continues, oxygen builds up in the alveoli until alveolar PO_2 equals the inspired PO_2. If ventilation ceases and blood flow continues, P_AO_2 decreases until it is equal to the PO_2 of venous blood. Thus, the balance between the addition of oxygen ($\dot{V}_A$) and its removal ($\dot{Q}_C$) determines P_AO_2. Decreased $\dot{V}_A$ relative to $\dot{Q}_C$ decreases the $\dot{V}_A/\dot{Q}_C$ ratio and reduces P_AO_2 (blood removes oxygen more rapidly than it is replenished). Decreased $\dot{Q}_C$ relative to $\dot{V}_A$ increases the $\dot{V}_A/\dot{Q}_C$ ratio and increases P_AO_2 (ventilation adds oxygen more rapidly than it is removed). In the same way, the $\dot{V}_A/\dot{Q}_C$ ratio also determines P_ACO_2. In this instance, blood flow adds carbon dioxide to alveoli, whereas ventilation removes it.

ALVEOLAR OXYGEN–CARBON DIOXIDE DIAGRAM

Figure 12-2 is a theoretical model of three alveoli with three different $\dot{V}_A/\dot{Q}_C$ relationships. The inspired PO_2 and PCO_2 for all alveoli are 150 mm Hg and 0 mm Hg (breathing room air

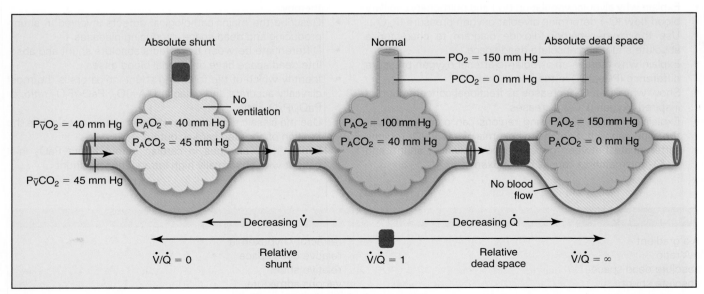

Figure 12-2 Shunt–dead space continuum.

at sea level). The middle alveolus has a normal $\dot{V}_A/\dot{Q}_C$ ratio, maintaining a P_AO_2 equal to 100 mm Hg and a P_ACO_2 equal to 40 mm Hg. Incoming mixed venous blood with a PO_2 of 40 mm Hg and a PCO_2 of 45 mm Hg takes on alveolar PO_2 and PCO_2 values as diffusion and equilibrium occur between the blood and alveolar gas pressures.

If ventilation gradually decreases with no change in blood flow, the $\dot{V}_A/\dot{Q}_C$ ratio decreases until it eventually equals 0 when ventilation ceases (left alveolus, Figure 12-2). This condition is called **absolute shunt**. Because no ventilation exists, P_AO_2 and P_ACO_2 levels eventually equalize with the levels of mixed venous blood (i.e., P_AO_2 becomes 40 mm Hg, and P_ACO_2 becomes 45 mm Hg). This condition is called shunt because blood leaving unventilated alveoli is identical in composition to the mixed venous blood entering the alveoli, as though blood flow took a detour around the lung, bypassing it altogether. (In reality, a completely blocked alveolus would collapse because blood flow would continually absorb oxygen and shrink the alveolus until it collapsed.)

The alveolus on the right (see Figure 12-2) shows the other extreme. Blood flow is completely blocked, but ventilation persists unchanged. Because no carbon dioxide can enter the alveolus and no oxygen can be taken up by the blood, P_ACO_2 and P_AO_2 take on values identical to room air. This alveolus has exactly the same PO_2 and PCO_2 as the conducting airways (i.e., the anatomical dead space). This alveolus represents **absolute dead space**; the $\dot{V}_A/\dot{Q}_C$ equals ∞ (infinity) because blood flow is zero. The horizontal double arrow below the three alveolar units represents a $\dot{V}_A/\dot{Q}_C$ continuum of all possibilities ranging from absolute shunt to absolute dead space (from $\dot{V}_A/\dot{Q}_C = 0$ to $\dot{V}_A/\dot{Q}_C = 8$).

CONCEPT QUESTION 12-2

Referring to Figure 12-2, on which side of the $\dot{V}/\dot{Q}$ continuum is hyperventilation located?

These three hypothetical alveolar units do not represent the only possibilities. Alveolar $\dot{V}_A/\dot{Q}_C$ ratios may be located anywhere on the continuum, representing $\dot{V}_A/\dot{Q}_C$ relationships that are lower than normal or higher than normal. Alveoli with abnormally high $\dot{V}/\dot{Q}$ ratios, but still less than infinity, produce **relative dead space**; blood flow is present but is abnormally low with respect to ventilation. Alveoli with abnormally low $\dot{V}/\dot{Q}$ ratios, but still greater than zero, produce **relative shunt**; ventilation is present but is abnormally low with respect to blood flow. A high $\dot{V}/\dot{Q}$ ratio generally implies a blood flow deficiency, whereas a low $\dot{V}/\dot{Q}$ ratio generally implies a ventilatory deficiency. The terms relative dead space and relative shunt are equivalent to the terms dead space effect and shunt effect, or simply high $\dot{V}/\dot{Q}$ and low $\dot{V}/\dot{Q}$. Either way, these terms refer to conditions in which blood flow or ventilation is low but not completely absent.

Figure 12-3 illustrates the positions of the three hypothetical alveoli in Figure 12-2 on the oxygen–carbon dioxide diagram.[1] P_ACO_2 is plotted on the vertical (y) axis, and P_AO_2 is plotted on the horizontal (x) axis. Gas pressures in the normal alveolus ($\dot{V}/\dot{Q} = 1$) are represented by a point on the oxygen–carbon dioxide diagram where P_AO_2 and P_ACO_2 are 100 mm Hg and 40 mm Hg. This point also indicates PO_2 and PCO_2 values for end-capillary blood leaving the normal alveolus because capillary blood equilibrated with alveolar gas. The absolute shunt alveolus ($\dot{V}/\dot{Q} = 0$) takes on P_AO_2 values identical to values of

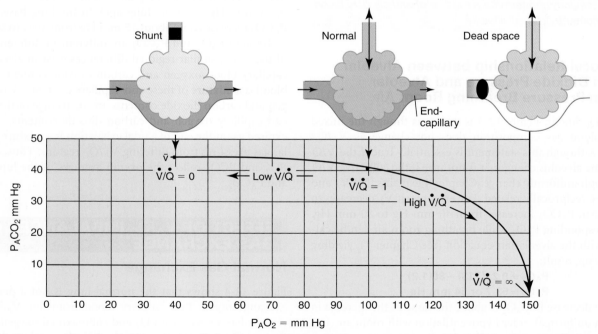

Figure 12-3 Oxygen–carbon dioxide diagram. The $\dot{V}/\dot{Q}$ line represents all possible P_AO_2-P_ACO_2 combinations from absolute shunt to absolute dead space in a single alveolus. The $\dot{V}/\dot{Q}$ line also represents end-capillary PO_2 and PCO_2 values. $\bar{v}$, Mixed venous blood composition; *I,* inspired tracheal gas composition.

mixed venous blood (note the mixed venous symbol, $\bar{v}$). Gas pressures in this alveolus are plotted on the oxygen–carbon dioxide diagram showing that PO_2 equals 40 mm Hg and PCO_2 equals 45 mm Hg. The absolute dead space alveolus ($\dot{V}/\dot{Q} = \infty$) takes on a P_AO_2 equal to 150 mm Hg and a P_ACO_2 equal to 0 mm Hg, values identical to inspired atmospheric gas (note the inspired symbol, I, on the x axis). The curved line passing through these three points is the $\dot{V}_A/\dot{Q}_C$ line. It represents all possible gas compositions in a single alveolus (breathing room air) supplied by mixed venous blood with a PO_2 equal to 40 mm Hg and a PCO_2 equal to 45 mm Hg. Because end-capillary blood leaving the alveoli equilibrated with alveolar gas, the $\dot{V}_A/\dot{Q}_C$ line also represents all possible PO_2 and PCO_2 combinations of end-capillary blood from a single alveolus.

Figure 12-3 shows that a P_AO_2 of 50 mm Hg and P_ACO_2 of 80 mm Hg cannot coexist in a single alveolus while the patient is breathing room air because this point does not lie on the $\dot{V}_A/\dot{Q}_C$ line. However, this alveolar gas composition can exist if the mixed venous blood composition changes greatly, creating a new $\dot{V}_A/\dot{Q}_C$ line passing through different points. For example, a greatly increased metabolic rate would produce more carbon dioxide, increasing $P\bar{v}CO_2$ and decreasing $P\bar{v}O_2$, especially if cardiac output cannot increase appropriately. A new $\dot{V}_A/\dot{Q}_C$ line would be created, beginning at much higher carbon dioxide and lower oxygen values on the left end (see Figure 12-3) but curving down to the same inspired point ($PCO_2 = 0$ mm Hg and $PO_2 = 150$ mm Hg) on the right end. The gas composition of any single alveolus and thus of its end-capillary blood depends on the PO_2 and PCO_2 of its mixed venous blood and its $\dot{V}/\dot{Q}$ ratio.

CONCEPT QUESTION 12-3

What is the common term for a mixture of end-capillary blood oxygen contents from all alveoli?

Reciprocal Relationship between Alveolar Carbon Dioxide Pressure and Alveolar Oxygen Pressure Breathing Room Air

The $\dot{V}_A/\dot{Q}_C$ line in Figure 12-3 is drawn as though the mixed venous blood gas composition does not change as $\dot{V}_A/\dot{Q}_C$ changes. Although this statement is essentially true if the $\dot{V}/\dot{Q}$ of only one alveolus changes, it is not true if the collective $\dot{V}/\dot{Q}$ of all alveoli uniformly change. Chapter 4 explains that $\dot{V}_A$ and P_ACO_2 are reciprocally related. For example, if $\dot{V}_A$ decreases to half normal, P_ACO_2 increases from 40 mm Hg to 80 mm Hg. The corresponding P_AO_2 while breathing room air can be calculated with the alveolar air equation (see Chapter 7), yielding the following result:

$$P_AO_2 = 0.21(713) - 80(1.2)$$
$$P_AO_2 = 53.7 \text{ or } 54 \text{ mm Hg}$$

Thus, the decrease in P_AO_2 is about the same as the increase in P_ACO_2 in uniform alveolar hypoventilation with room air (i.e., P_ACO_2 and P_AO_2 are reciprocally related).

This reciprocal relationship is not shown on the oxygen–carbon dioxide diagram in Figure 12-3 because this diagram

represents a hypothetical change in the $\dot{V}/\dot{Q}$ of one alveolus out of millions of alveoli; a $\dot{V}/\dot{Q}$ change in one alveolus would not affect mixed venous blood composition. (The P_AO_2 of 54 mm Hg and P_ACO_2 of 80 mm Hg in the example do not define a point on the $\dot{V}/\dot{Q}$ curve.) In reality, mixed venous blood gases do change when the entire lung hypoventilates. For example, if all 300 million alveoli uniformly hypoventilate, the average P_ACO_2 increases, producing an equal increase in the average end-capillary PCO_2. As a result, arterial PCO_2 increases. When this arterial blood with an increased PCO_2 passes through tissue capillaries, tissue PCO_2 builds up until a diffusion gradient from tissues to blood is created; this increases mixed venous PCO_2. By increasing P_ACO_2, overall hypoventilation ultimately also increases the mixed venous PCO_2. The end result is a new P_ACO_2-P_AO_2 combination, identifying a point on a new $\dot{V}_A/\dot{Q}_C$ line in the oxygen–carbon dioxide diagram. The important point illustrated by Figure 12-3 is that the gas composition of any alveolus is determined by its incoming venous gas composition and $\dot{V}/\dot{Q}$ ratio.

$\dot{V}_A/\dot{Q}_C$ RATIO DISTRIBUTION IN NORMAL LUNG

Chapter 6 describes why the $\dot{V}_A/\dot{Q}_C$ ratio increases from the lung base to the lung apex (see Figure 6-11). Similar to blood flow, ventilation is greatest in the lung base and least in the apex. However, from the base to apex, blood flow decreases at a more rapid rate than ventilation, which means that apical regions are relatively overventilated with respect to blood flow (high $\dot{V}_A/\dot{Q}_C$), whereas basal regions are relatively underventilated with respect to blood flow (low $\dot{V}_A/\dot{Q}_C$). Figure 12-4 illustrates these regional differences in $\dot{V}_A/\dot{Q}_C$ with respect to the oxygen–carbon dioxide diagram. (In this figure, P_AO_2 decreases by 40 mm Hg from the lung apex to the lung base, whereas P_ACO_2 increases only about 15 mm Hg from apex to base.[2])

Because P_AO_2 and P_ACO_2 are different in different regions of the lungs, similar regional differences exist in alveolar end-capillary blood oxygen and carbon dioxide contents. Arterial blood is a mixture of these end-capillary contents. Arterial oxygen and carbon dioxide contents are an average of the alveolar end-capillary oxygen and carbon dioxide contents. Similarly, expired gas at the end of a tidal exhalation is a mixture of alveolar gas pressures from differing $\dot{V}_A/\dot{Q}_C$ regions. Thus, end-tidal PO_2 and PCO_2 reflect the overall averages of the lungs' P_AO_2 and P_ACO_2.

EFFECT OF $\dot{V}_A/\dot{Q}_C$ IMBALANCES ON GAS EXCHANGE

Normal Gas Exchange

Figure 12-4 shows that the normal lung is not a perfect gas-exchange organ. End-capillary blood from *low* $\dot{V}_A/\dot{Q}_C$ basal regions has a decreased PO_2 and submaximal oxygen content. End-capillary blood from *normal* $\dot{V}_A/\dot{Q}_C$ regions has near-maximal oxygen content ($PO_2 = 100$ mm Hg; hemoglobin saturation = 98.5%). Blood from *high* $\dot{V}_A/\dot{Q}_C$ apical regions carries

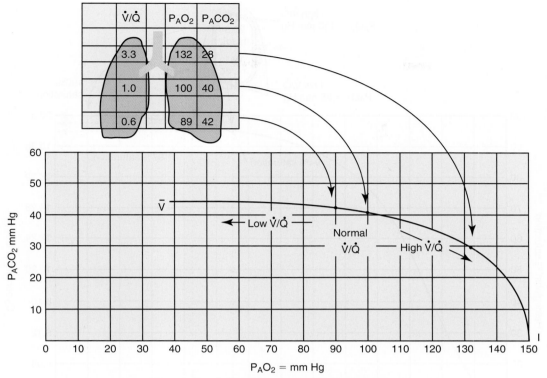

Figure 12-4 $\dot{V}/\dot{Q}$ distribution in the normal lung.

only slightly more oxygen per 100 mL than blood from normal units because blood from normal $\dot{V}_A/\dot{Q}_C$ regions already has near-maximal oxygen content.

Because end-capillary blood from low $\dot{V}_A/\dot{Q}_C$ regions is not maximally saturated with oxygen while room air is breathed, arterial blood is also never maximally saturated. This is true because arterial blood is a mixture of end-capillary blood from all $\dot{V}_A/\dot{Q}_C$ regions. As long as any low $\dot{V}_A/\dot{Q}_C$ regions exist, low end-capillary oxygen contents mix with and dilute maximally saturated end-capillary blood, causing submaximal arterial oxygen content.

CONCEPT QUESTION 12-4

Assuming no absolute shunting exists, does breathing 100% oxygen maximally saturate the hemoglobin of arterial blood?

Normal Alveolar-Arterial Oxygen Pressure Difference

To understand how the lung's normal $\dot{V}_A/\dot{Q}_C$ imbalances contribute to the normal $P(A-a)O_2$, one must understand what determines alveolar and arterial oxygen compositions. (Recall from Chapter 1 that another source of the normal $P(A-a)O_2$ is anatomical shunting, in which bronchial venous blood mixes with freshly oxygenated pulmonary venous blood.) Arterial blood is a mixture of the end-capillary blood from all $\dot{V}_A/\dot{Q}_C$ regions in the lungs. Alveolar gas, collected at the end of a tidal exhalation, is a mixture of alveolar gases from these same differing $\dot{V}_A/\dot{Q}_C$ regions. Although alveolar gas is in equilibrium with end-capillary blood, the average P_AO_2 is not the same as the average end-capillary blood PO_2. The oxygen-hemoglobin

equilibrium curve illustrates this point (Figure 12-5). For the sake of simplicity, this illustration assumes that equal volumes of end-capillary blood from apical and basal lung regions mix to form arterial blood. (This is not actually true because the lung's bases receive more blood flow than the apices.) PaO_2 is not determined by an average of the mixed end-capillary PO_2 values; instead, PaO_2 is determined by an average of the mixed end-capillary oxygen contents.

For example, let us assume in Figure 12-5 that 100 mL of end-capillary blood from the lung apex is mixed with 100 mL of end-capillary blood from the lung base. Blood from the apex has a PO_2 equal to 130 mm Hg and an oxygen saturation (SaO_2) of 100%. Blood from the base has a PO_2 of 85 mm Hg and an SaO_2 of about 94%. With a hemoglobin concentration of 15 g/dL, the oxygen content in 100 mL of apical blood is as follows:

$$(15 \times 1.34 \times 1.0) + (130 \times 0.003) = 20.5 \text{ mL}$$

The oxygen content in 100 mL of basal blood is as follows:

$$(15 \times 1.34 \times 0.94) + (85 \times 0.003) = 19.1 \text{ mL}$$

Mixing these two samples produces 200 mL of blood containing 39.6 mL of oxygen, or 19.8 mL of oxygen per 100 mL of blood (19.8 mL/dL), corresponding to about 97% saturation on the oxyhemoglobin equilibrium curve (see Figure 12-5). This mixture produces a PaO_2 of about 96 to 97 mm Hg, which is obviously not the average of apical and basal PO_2 values. High $\dot{V}_A/\dot{Q}_C$ apical units cannot negate the desaturating effect that low $\dot{V}_A/\dot{Q}_C$ basal units have on mixed end-capillary blood. The desaturating effects of basal alveolar units are even more pronounced than illustrated in this example because basal regions actually receive more blood flow and contribute proportionally more to the arterial blood.

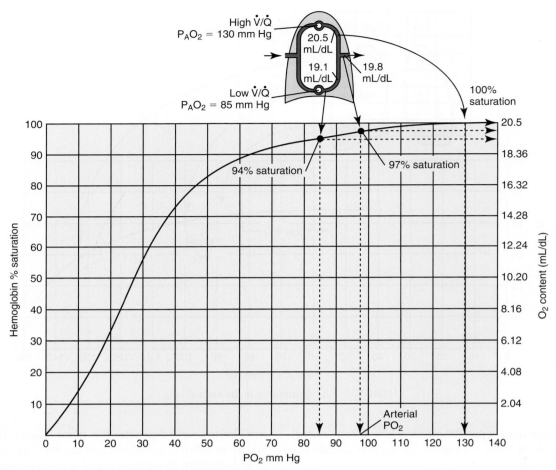

Figure 12-5 Determinants of mixed end-capillary oxygen content and PaO$_2$.

In contrast, mixed expired alveolar gas PO$_2$ is simply the average of the PO$_2$ values from all of the differing $\dot{V}_A/\dot{Q}_C$ regions in the lungs because no hemoglobin is involved. In the example just discussed, the average P$_A$O$_2$ is (130 + 85)/2 = 108 mm Hg, producing a P(A-a)O$_2$ of 12 mm Hg (P$_A$O$_2$ of 108 mm Hg − PaO$_2$ of 96 mm Hg). The differing $\dot{V}_A/\dot{Q}_C$ ratios in the lung create a normal P(A-a)O$_2$ of approximately 7 to 14 mm Hg, if room air is breathed (F$_I$O$_2$ = 0.21).[3] Severely diseased lungs have many abnormally low $\dot{V}_A/\dot{Q}_C$ regions; in such instances, the P(A-a)O$_2$ is even higher.

CONCEPT QUESTION 12-5

Why does absolute shunting affect P(A-a)O$_2$?

Why Alveolar-Arterial Oxygen Pressure Difference Increases When Fractional Concentration of Oxygen in Inspired Gas Increases

P(A-a)O$_2$ increases from about 10 mm Hg when room air is breathed to greater than 50 mm Hg when 100% oxygen is breathed. The shape of the oxygen-hemoglobin equilibrium curve helps explain this phenomenon. Figure 12-6 shows the oxygen-hemoglobin curve extended to a PO$_2$ of 663 mm Hg, which compresses the sigmoid shape of the curve into the

extreme left side of the diagram. At PO$_2$ values between 100 mm Hg and 663 mm Hg, the curve is practically flat because the hemoglobin is essentially saturated to capacity between these two points; the small increase in oxygen content is due to increased dissolved oxygen. The diagram of the lung indicates a small, normal amount of shunt—about 2% to 5% of the cardiac output does not perfuse ventilated alveoli. This shunted blood is venous in composition (PO$_2$ = 40 mm Hg; saturation = 75%; oxygen content = 15 mL/dL). Figure 12-6 shows the effects of adding this small, fixed amount of desaturated venous blood to arterial blood when 100% oxygen is breathed (P$_A$O$_2$ = 663 mm Hg, lower right of the graph) and while room air is breathed (P$_A$O$_2$ = 100 mm Hg, lower left of the graph). Because the amount of shunted blood is fixed, the same decrease in arterial oxygen content occurs whether room air or 100% oxygen is breathed. For the sake of illustration, let us assume this reduction in arterial oxygen content is 0.5 mL/dL in both instances (see Figure 12-6). As shown, this 0.5-mL/dL decrease produces a much greater decrease in PaO$_2$ when 100% oxygen compared to 21% oxygen is breathed because of the flatness of the curve at high PO$_2$ values. The breathing of 100% oxygen increases the P(A-a)O$_2$, not because it somehow impairs gas transfer from the alveolus to the blood, but simply because of the unique way hemoglobin binds to O$_2$ molecules.

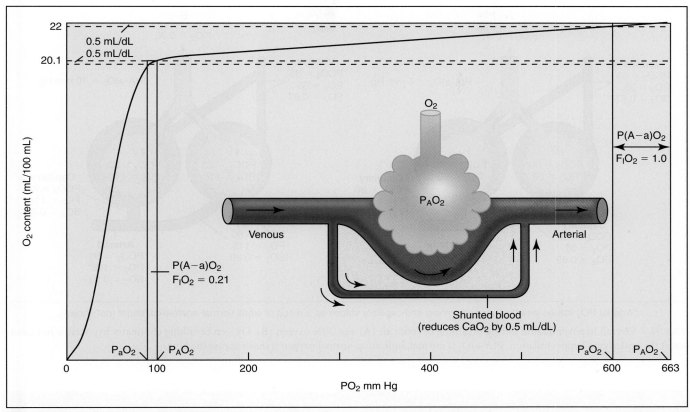

Figure 12-6 The reason $P(A\text{-}a)O_2$ increases when F_IO_2 increases. A fixed amount of shunt, resulting in a 0.5-mL/dL decrease in CaO_2, reduces the PaO_2 much more when F_IO_2 equals 1.0 (flat part of the curve) than when F_IO_2 equals 0.21 (steeper part of the curve).

Abnormal Gas Exchange

The small imbalance normally present between ventilation and perfusion is greatly exaggerated in various diseases affecting the lung. Low $\dot{V}_A/\dot{Q}_C$ ratios produce hypoxemia. Carbon dioxide elimination may also be hindered, but the effect on oxygenation is usually much greater, as discussed later. The major $\dot{V}_A/\dot{Q}_C$ imbalance mechanisms causing hypoxemia are (1) overall hypoventilation, (2) absolute shunt, and (3) $\dot{V}_A/\dot{Q}_C$ mismatch. By convention, the term $\dot{V}_A/\dot{Q}_C$ mismatch generally refers to a low $\dot{V}_A/\dot{Q}_C$ ratio (<0.8). From this point on in this chapter, $\dot{V}_A/\dot{Q}_C$ mismatch means a low $\dot{V}_A/\dot{Q}_C$ ratio.

Hypoventilation

Overall hypoventilation increases P_ACO_2; P_AO_2 consequently decreases in a reciprocal fashion (Figure 12-7, *A*). This kind of hypoxemia points to a ventilation problem, not an oxygen transfer problem; in other words, if ventilation is restored to normal, hypoxemia resolves. Figure 12-7 shows that the $P(A\text{-}a)O_2$ is within normal limits when either room air or 30% oxygen is breathed, indicating normal oxygen transfer across the lung. (PaO_2 is less than PO_2 of the blood in either capillary in Figure 12-7 because a normal shunt of 2% to 5% [not illustrated] decreases arterial oxygen content and PO_2.) Causes of general hypoventilation include muscle paralysis or weakness and drug-induced respiratory center depression (Table 12-1).

The logical corrective treatment for patients experiencing general hypoventilation and hypoxemia involves therapy that increases ventilation. At the extreme, intubation and mechanical ventilation may be needed. Hypoventilation-induced hypoxemia can be corrected with oxygen therapy (see Figure 12-7, *B*), but oxygen therapy does not correct the underlying cause of hypoxemia.

CONCEPT QUESTION 12-6

Why is $P(A\text{-}a)O_2$ essentially normal in overall hypoventilation?

Absolute Shunt

Absolute shunt occurs when deoxygenated mixed venous blood bypasses ventilated alveoli and mixes directly with oxygenated, ventilated arterial blood. For this reason, shunting is often called **venous admixture**. In absolute shunt, blood moves from the right, or venous, side of the circulation to the left, or arterial, side of the circulation without contacting alveolar gas; thus, shunts that produce arterial hypoxemia are called right-to-left shunts.

Right-to-left shunting occurs in three different conditions, two of which are anatomical shunts. Anatomical shunting occurs when mixed venous blood flows through a normal or abnormal anatomical channel, physically bypassing the alveoli and mixing with arterial blood. An example of a normal anatomical shunt is the bronchial systemic veins (carrying deoxygenated blood)

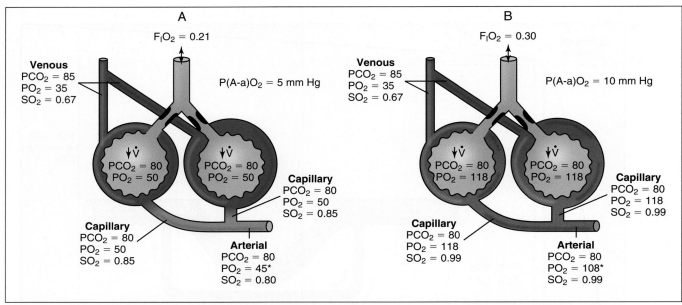

*Arterial PO₂ values less than average mixed end-capillary values as a result of small normal anatomical shunt (not shown).

Figure 12-7 Overall hypoventilation during breathing of room air (**A**) and 30% oxygen (**B**). Oxygen breathing eliminates hypoxemia but cannot correct the underlying hypoventilation. $P(A-a)O_2$ is normal, indicating normal oxygen transfer across the lung.

TABLE 12-1

Respiratory Causes of a Low Arterial PO₂

Cause	Mechanism	P(A-a)O₂	PaO₂ Response to Oxygen	Examples
Hypoventilation	Decreased $\dot{V}_A$; increased P_ACO_2	Normal	Good response	Drug overdose Muscle paralysis
Shunt (intrapulmonary)	Venous blood mixing with arterial blood (venous admixture)	Increased	Extremely poor response	Atelectasis Pneumonia
Ventilation-perfusion mismatch	Underoxygenated blood mixing with arterial blood (venous admixture)	Increased	Good response	Partial airway obstruction: asthma, obstructive lung diseases Nonuniform distribution of compliance

emptying directly into the pulmonary veins (carrying freshly oxygenated blood). An abnormal anatomical shunt occurs in the heart if the septum separating the right and left ventricles has a large hole (ventricular septal defect), allowing deoxygenated right ventricular blood to mix with oxygenated left ventricular blood.

Physiological, or intrapulmonary, shunting occurs when mixed venous blood flows through the pulmonary capillaries of airless, unventilated alveoli (Figure 12-8, *A*). Venous blood does not physically bypass the lung, but the effect is the same; shunted blood can neither take up oxygen nor release carbon dioxide (i.e., the blood remains venous in composition). Any abnormal process that prevents alveolar ventilation produces physiological shunt (see Table 12-1). Examples include alveolar filling

processes, such as pneumonia or pulmonary edema, and processes causing alveolar collapse, such as pulmonary surfactant abnormalities, pneumothorax, and major bronchial occlusion.

An increase in the percentage of oxygen (the gas) breathed by patients with shunting disease does little to improve arterial oxygenation because shunted venous blood cannot contact inspired gas (see Figure 12-8, *B*). Thus, the hallmark of intrapulmonary shunting is hypoxemia that responds poorly to oxygen therapy (**refractory hypoxemia**). An increase in F_IO_2 can increase the PO_2 of only ventilated alveoli, but this adds little oxygen to the already saturated blood of these alveolar capillaries. (Compare capillary blood saturations in Figure 12-8, *A* and *B*.) Even increasing the F_IO_2 to 1.0 does not improve PaO₂ significantly because arterial oxygen content (CaO_2) or saturation

CLINICAL FOCUS 12-1

Hypoventilation as a Cause of Hypoxemia

A 61-year-old man with known myasthenia gravis (a disorder that causes muscular weakness and may reduce ventilatory capacity) was brought to the emergency department. The patient stated that he has become progressively weaker and short of breath. You obtain arterial blood gases and measure the vital capacity and maximum inspiratory force.

Arterial blood gas values (on room air; barometric pressure = 760 mm Hg) are as follows:

PaO_2 = 59 mm Hg
$PaCO_2$ = 63 mm Hg
pH = 7.22
HCO_3^- = 25 mEq/L

Vital capacity and maximum inspiratory force are below normal. From a previous hospitalization that year, you know his normal room air arterial blood gas values are as follows:

PaO_2 = 80 mm Hg
$PaCO_2$ = 40 mm Hg
pH = 7.39
HCO_3^- = 24 mEq/L

What is the reason for this patient's hypoxemia? Is he having greater oxygen-transfer (lung to blood) problems compared with earlier normal blood gas values?

Discussion

This man is experiencing an acute respiratory acidosis (i.e., he is hypoventilating). $PaCO_2$ has increased about 23 mm Hg above his normal, stable value, and PaO_2 has decreased by about 21 mm Hg. This reciprocal relationship between $PaCO_2$ and PaO_2 indicates that the observed hypoxemia is a consequence of hypoventilation. If ventilation were restored to normal, the hypoxemia would be resolved. Is there a worsening oxygen-transfer problem? $P(A-a)O_2$ is a good indicator of oxygen-transfer efficiency. Using the alveolar air equation, calculate the $P(A-a)O_2$ for the stable, normal arterial blood gas values:

$$P_AO_2 = F_IO_2(P_B - 47) - PaCO_2 \times 1.2$$
$$P_AO_2 = 0.21(713) - 40 \times 1.2$$
$$P_AO_2 = 102 \text{ mm Hg}$$
$$P(A-a)O_2 = 102 - 80 = 22 \text{ mm Hg}$$

Calculate the $P(A-a)O_2$ for the current arterial blood gas values:

$$P_AO_2 = 0.21(713) - 63 \times 1.2$$
$$P_AO_2 = 74 \text{ mm Hg}$$
$$P(A-a)O_2 = 74 - 59 = 15 \text{ mm Hg}$$

Oxygen-transfer efficiency did not worsen. The origin of hypoxemia is hypoventilation. This is primarily a ventilation problem, not an oxygenation problem.

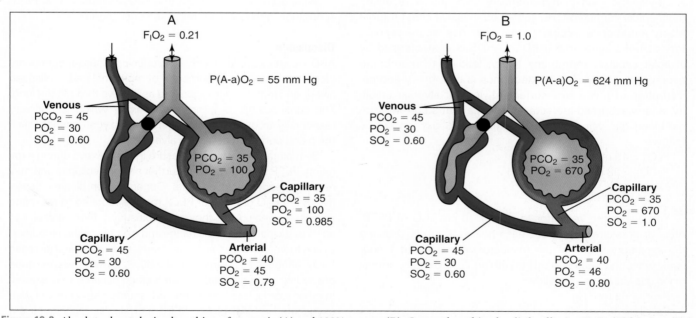

Figure 12-8 Absolute shunt during breathing of room air (**A**) and 100% oxygen (**B**). Oxygen breathing has little effect on PaO_2 (**B**) because (1) it cannot reach blood in collapsed alveoli, and (2) blood from ventilated units is already near maximum saturation. The increased $P(A-a)O_2$ indicates impaired oxygen transfer across the lung.

is determined by the mixed oxygen saturations of end-capillary blood. The resulting arterial oxygen saturation determines PaO_2 (see earlier discussion regarding Figure 12-5). The difference between P_AO_2 and PaO_2 values is increased in absolute shunt when either room air or 100% oxygen is breathed (see Figure 12-8). This alveolar-arterial difference indicates impaired oxygen transfer across the lung. The magnitude of $P(A-a)O_2$ is an indicator of the severity of shunt.

CONCEPT QUESTION 12-7

What is the basic defect of a disease that causes intrapulmonary shunting?

In Figure 12-8, $PaCO_2$ remains normal, around 40 mm Hg because arterial hypoxemia sensitizes the peripheral chemoreceptors, increasing the ventilation of normal alveoli such that the PCO_2 of their capillary blood is decreased to 35 mm Hg; this balances the PCO_2 of 45 mm Hg in the blood coming from the shunt unit, producing a final normal $PaCO_2$ of 40 mm Hg. Such an increase in ventilation of the normal alveoli cannot similarly create a normal PaO_2.[1] This phenomenon is explained later in this chapter.

The corrective treatment for intrapulmonary shunting is to restore ventilation to the airless alveoli. This procedure may involve special mechanical ventilatory support techniques that prevent alveolar pressure from decreasing to atmospheric pressure, even during expiration. These techniques include positive end expiratory pressure (PEEP) **and continuous positive airway pressure (CPAP).** If alveolar collapse is caused by pneumothorax, treatment may involve inserting a chest tube into the intrapleural space to evacuate pleural air and reexpand the lung.

Ventilation-Perfusion Mismatch

$\dot{V}_A/\dot{Q}_C$ mismatch ($\dot{V}_A/\dot{Q}_C$ <1 but >0) is the most common cause of hypoxemia.[2] Low $\dot{V}_A/\dot{Q}_C$ ratios are sometimes called relative shunt because they produce a shuntlike effect. In other words, they produce hypoxemia and increase the $P(A-a)O_2$. As discussed previously, normal lungs have a small degree of $\dot{V}_A/\dot{Q}_C$ mismatch, producing a normal $P(A-a)O_2$ gradient. However, this mismatch involves such a small number of alveoli that normal PaO_2 and $PaCO_2$ can easily be maintained.

Unlike intrapulmonary shunt, blood perfusing low $\dot{V}_A/\dot{Q}_C$ alveoli is exposed to some ventilation. However, this blood receives inadequate ventilation, producing an increased end-capillary PCO_2 and decreased PO_2 (Figure 12-9, *A*). In contrast to overall hypoventilation, $\dot{V}_A/\dot{Q}_C$ mismatch is a localized regional hypoventilation and does not usually produce an increased $PaCO_2$ (see Figure 12-9, *A*). $\dot{V}_A/\dot{Q}_C$ mismatch must be quite extensive throughout the lungs before hypercapnia occurs (e.g., severe chronic obstructive pulmonary disease [COPD]). In most conditions involving $\dot{V}_A/\dot{Q}_C$ mismatch, normally

---

CLINICAL FOCUS 12-2

Treating Hypoxemia Caused by Intrapulmonary Shunt

A 28-year-old man in the intensive care unit is receiving mechanical ventilation. He sustained massive chest trauma in an automobile accident and now has acute respiratory distress syndrome (ARDS). ARDS is characterized by alveolar capillary membrane injury, leading to membrane hyperpermeability. The consequence is pulmonary edema, disruption of pulmonary surfactant, loss of alveolar stability, and widespread atelectasis. This patient's current arterial blood gas values while breathing 50% oxygen are as follows:

 PaO_2 = 45 mm Hg
 $PaCO_2$ = 38 mm Hg
 pH = 7.41
 SaO_2 = 0.79

You adjust the ventilator to deliver 10 cm H_2O of PEEP. Alveolar pressure cannot decrease below 10 cm H_2O during the expiratory phase of the respiratory cycle. About 1 hour later, while the patient is still breathing 50% oxygen, arterial blood gas values are as follows:

 PaO_2 = 65 mm Hg
 $PaCO_2$ = 36 mm Hg
 pH = 7.42
 SaO_2 = 0.92

What accounts for the fact that PaO_2 increased after PEEP application, although F_IO_2 remained unchanged?

Discussion

ARDS is an example of a shunt-producing disease; pulmonary blood perfuses large numbers of nonventilated, collapsed alveoli and remains unoxygenated as it flows through the lung. The consequence is arterial hypoxemia, which is not very responsive to oxygen therapy; inspired oxygen cannot reach the blood perfusing collapsed alveoli.

By maintaining positive pressure in the airways during expiration, PEEP tends to prevent further alveolar collapse and may reopen already collapsed units. Depending on disease severity, 15 cm H_2O or more of PEEP may be required to reexpand collapsed alveoli. After they are reexpanded, these alveoli can again participate in gas exchange and oxygenate the blood perfusing them. PEEP can prevent or reduce shunting and increase PaO_2. Although F_IO_2 remained at 0.50, PaO_2 improved because previously unoxygenated, shunted blood became oxygenated. In other words, less unoxygenated, shunted blood mixed with oxygenated arterial blood. PEEP and similar techniques are the cornerstone of therapy in diseases characterized by widespread alveolar instability and atelectasis.

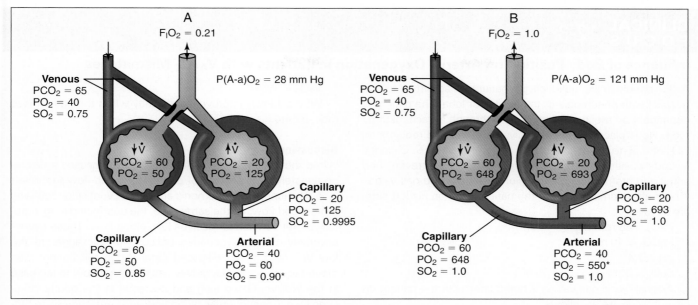

A
$F_IO_2 = 0.21$

Venous
$PCO_2 = 65$
$PO_2 = 40$
$SO_2 = 0.75$

$P(A-a)O_2 = 28$ mm Hg

$\downarrow \dot{V}$
$PCO_2 = 60$
$PO_2 = 50$

$\uparrow \dot{V}$
$PCO_2 = 20$
$PO_2 = 125$

Capillary
$PCO_2 = 20$
$PO_2 = 125$
$SO_2 = 0.9995$

Capillary
$PCO_2 = 60$
$PO_2 = 50$
$SO_2 = 0.85$

Arterial
$PCO_2 = 40$
$PO_2 = 60$
$SO_2 = 0.90*$

B
$F_IO_2 = 1.0$

Venous
$PCO_2 = 65$
$PO_2 = 40$
$SO_2 = 0.75$

$P(A-a)O_2 = 121$ mm Hg

$\downarrow \dot{V}$
$PCO_2 = 60$
$PO_2 = 648$

$\uparrow \dot{V}$
$PCO_2 = 20$
$PO_2 = 693$

Capillary
$PCO_2 = 20$
$PO_2 = 693$
$SO_2 = 1.0$

Capillary
$PCO_2 = 60$
$PO_2 = 648$
$SO_2 = 1.0$

Arterial
$PCO_2 = 40$
$PO_2 = 550*$
$SO_2 = 1.0$

*Arterial PO_2 values less than average mixed end-capillary values as a result of small normal anatomical shunt (not shown).

Figure 12-9 $\dot{V}/\dot{Q}$ mismatch during breathing of room air (**A**) and 100% oxygen (**B**). Oxygen can enter the poorly ventilated unit and completely eliminate hypoxemia. The increased $P(A-a)O_2$ indicates impaired oxygen transfer across the lung.

ventilated alveoli can easily compensate for the increased PCO_2 of underventilated alveoli and maintain a normal or even low $PaCO_2$. (Note the increased ventilation of normal units in Figure 12-9; PCO_2 is decreased enough to balance the increased PCO_2 of underventilated units.) The reason increased ventilation cannot do the same for oxygen is explained in detail in the next section.

As with shunting, $\dot{V}_A/\dot{Q}_C$ mismatch increases the $P(A-a)O_2$, indicating impaired oxygen transfer across the lung (see Figure 12-9). In contrast to shunting, $\dot{V}_A/\dot{Q}_C$ mismatch responds well to oxygen therapy because oxygen can enter underventilated units and increase the PO_2 values to near-maximum (see Figure 12-9, *B*). Blood perfusing these underventilated units is maximally oxygenated, and the effect of venous admixture disappears. As in overall hypoventilation, PaO_2 values in Figure 12-9 are lower than the values derived from averaging the saturations of end-capillary blood. The normal 2% to 5% shunt (which is not illustrated) accounts for this disparity.

Table 12-1 summarizes the mechanisms and effects of overall hypoventilation, absolute shunt, and $\dot{V}_A/\dot{Q}_C$ mismatch on arterial blood. $\dot{V}_A/\dot{Q}_C$ mismatch is the most common mechanism causing hypoxemia and is seen in all lung diseases characterized by low $\dot{V}/\dot{Q}$ ratios. These diseases include not only diseases involving partial airway obstruction but also those involving regional variations in lung compliance. For example, in emphysema and fibrotic lung diseases, compliance of all alveoli is not uniformly abnormal, and ventilation is not uniformly distributed.

Variable Effect of $\dot{Q}_C$ Imbalance on Carbon Dioxide and Oxygen Exchange

Theoretically, low $\dot{V}_A/\dot{Q}_C$ ratios (<1 and >0) should cause hypoxemia and hypercapnia. Consider a situation in which carbon dioxide production and oxygen consumption remain constant while overall $\dot{V}_A/\dot{Q}_C$ decreases; if all other factors remain constant, this causes $PaCO_2$ to increase and PaO_2 to decrease. However, in the clinical setting, patients who are hypoxic because of $\dot{V}_A/\dot{Q}_C$ mismatches or shunt often have a normal or low $PaCO_2$.[1] The reason is not, as some individuals erroneously suppose, that carbon dioxide is more diffusible than oxygen. Rather, when the medullary chemoreceptors sense even a slight increase in $PaCO_2$, they increase the ventilatory drive[1]; this increases the ventilation of normal $\dot{V}_A/\dot{Q}_C$ units enough to offset the effects of low $\dot{V}_A/\dot{Q}_C$ units, keeping $PaCO_2$ in the normal range. A normal $PaCO_2$ can be maintained in this situation only by increasing total minute ventilation ($\dot{V}_E$) above that which would normally be required. If a low $\dot{V}_A/\dot{Q}_C$ ratio causes significant hypoxemia, $PaCO_2$ may actually be lower than normal. That is, hypoxemia sufficient to activate the peripheral chemoreceptors may increase the ventilation of normal $\dot{V}_A/\dot{Q}_C$ units enough to produce overall hyperventilation and respiratory alkalosis.

How can an increased $\dot{V}_E$ effectively decrease $PaCO_2$ without significantly increasing PaO_2? The differences in the shapes of the carbon dioxide and oxygen equilibrium curves answer this question. Figure 12-10 shows that the carbon dioxide equilibrium curve is almost a straight diagonal line in the physiological range, whereas the oxygen equilibrium curve is almost horizontal. Oxygen or carbon dioxide content is plotted on the vertical axis, and the partial pressure of either gas in arterial blood is plotted on the horizontal axis. The lung model to the right

CLINICAL FOCUS 12-3

Influence of Body Position on Arterial Oxygenation in Patients with $\dot{V}_A/\dot{Q}_C$ Mismatches

A 35-year-old male quadriplegic patient is admitted to the hospital with pneumonia of the left lower lobe. The patient is dependent on mechanical ventilation through a tracheostomy tube. He is placed in the intensive care unit and requires an F_IO_2 of 0.55 to maintain the SaO_2 greater than 90%. Changes in body position are ordered every 2 hours to prevent bed sores and promote lung expansion. Arterial blood gas values 1 hour after admission, with the patient lying on his left side, are as follows:

PaO_2 = 68 mm Hg
$PaCO_2$ = 40 mm Hg
pH = 7.43
SaO_2 = 92%

Arterial blood gas values 2 hours later with the patient on his right side are as follows:

PaO_2 = 110 mm Hg
$PaCO_2$ = 40 mm Hg
pH = 7.42

SaO_2 = 99%

Why did PaO_2 improve significantly when the patient was moved onto his right side?

Discussion

When the patient is on his left side, gravity causes a disproportionately large amount of pulmonary blood flow to the left lung. The lung with pneumonia and poorer ventilation receives more blood flow. At the same time, the unaffected lung, naturally better ventilated, receives less blood flow. These events adversely affect oxygenation because they exaggerate the low $\dot{V}/\dot{Q}$ ratio in the diseased lung. When the patient was moved to his right side, gravity caused blood flow to increase in the well-ventilated lung and decrease in the poorly ventilated lung. Consequently, blood flow and ventilation were better matched, and oxygenation improved. For this reason, the general rule is to place a patient with unilateral lung disease in a "good lung down" position.

CLINICAL FOCUS 12-4

Differentiating among Hypoventilation, Shunt, and $\dot{V}_A/\dot{Q}_C$ Mismatch as the Cause of Hypoxemia

A 22-year-old patient with asthma is admitted to the hospital with the following room air arterial blood gas values:

PO_2 = 60 mm Hg
PCO_2 = 35 mm Hg
pH = 7.46
SaO_2 = 90%

Bronchodilator treatments are started, and oxygen is administered via a nasal cannula at 2 L per minute. Arterial blood gas values 1 hour later are as follows:

PO_2 = 90 mm Hg
PCO_2 = 38 mm Hg
pH = 7.42
SaO_2 = 96%

Was this patient's hypoxemia caused by hypoventilation, shunt, or $\dot{V}_A/\dot{Q}_C$ mismatch?

Discussion

Table 12-1 is helpful in analyzing the cause of this patient's hypoxemia. Hypoventilation can be dismissed immediately on the basis of the low-normal $PaCO_2$. Apparently, hypoxemia is stimulating the peripheral chemoreceptors, increasing this patient's ventilation and decreasing $PaCO_2$. Shunt is not the cause because PaO_2 increased significantly when oxygen was administered. (Increasing PO_2 in nonventilated alveoli is impossible.) The cause of this patient's hypoxemia must be a ventilation-perfusion mismatch. Airway narrowing associated with asthma results in underventilation of some lung units, whereas ventilation to other lung units remains normal (see Figure 12-9). Breathing supplemental oxygen increases PO_2 in normal and underventilated alveoli, increasing PaO_2.

illustrates low and high $\dot{V}_A/\dot{Q}_C$ ratios. These $\dot{V}_A/\dot{Q}_C$ ratios are plotted on both equilibrium curves, showing their respective contents and partial pressures. Point *a* on each curve represents normal arterial contents and partial pressures. (Low $\dot{V}_A/\dot{Q}_C$ ratios produce high carbon dioxide contents and PCO_2 values but low oxygen contents and PO_2 values.)

The mixing of equal blood volumes from high and low $\dot{V}_A/\dot{Q}_C$ units produces a final carbon dioxide content determined by averaging high and low $\dot{V}_A/\dot{Q}_C$ points, represented by point *a* on the carbon dioxide curve. (Point *a* denotes a PCO_2

of about 35 mm Hg.) Using the same method, the averaging of high and low $\dot{V}_A/\dot{Q}_C$ points on the much flatter oxygen curve (half the vertical distance between these two points) produces a final oxygen content, denoted by point *X*. The corresponding PO_2 is slightly less than 60 mm Hg, well below the normal arterial point designated by *a* on the oxygen curve.

The shapes of the oxygen and carbon dioxide equilibrium curves dictate that high $\dot{V}_A/\dot{Q}_C$ units can effectively decrease the end-capillary carbon dioxide contents and PCO_2 values but cannot significantly increase the end-capillary oxygen contents

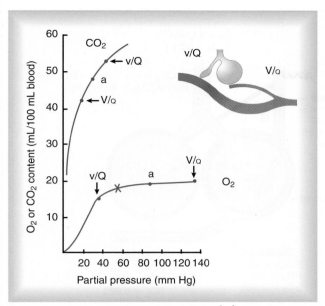

Figure 12-10 Increased ventilation of normal $\dot{V}/\dot{Q}$ units compensates for increased PCO_2 of low $\dot{V}/\dot{Q}$ units but cannot do so for decreased PO_2 of low $\dot{V}/\dot{Q}$ units. (From Martin L: *Pulmonary physiology in clinical practice,* St Louis, 1987, Mosby.)

(i.e., end-capillary oxygen contents are already maximal). Overventilated alveoli can compensate for the increased PCO_2 values produced by underventilated areas, but overventilated alveoli cannot compensate for the decreased PO_2 values of underventilated regions.

If ventilation-perfusion mismatch involves a large number of the lung's alveoli, as it does in advanced COPD, patients may be unable to increase their overall alveolar ventilation enough to sustain a normal $PaCO_2$. These patients cannot ventilate their small amount of normal lung tissues enough to compensate for the high PCO_2 values in their diseased lung tissue. Consequently, these patients must adapt to less ventilation and allow $PaCO_2$ values to increase. Thus, $\dot{V}_A/\dot{Q}_C$ imbalance is not only the most common cause of hypoxemia but also the most common cause of chronic hypercapnia.

Effect of High $\dot{V}_A/\dot{Q}_C$ Ratios on Arterial PO_2 and Arterial PCO_2

Increased Ventilation Relative to Blood Flow as a Cause of Dead Space

The discussion so far has focused mainly on the effect of low $\dot{V}_A/\dot{Q}_C$ ratios on gas exchange. It was briefly mentioned that high $\dot{V}_A/\dot{Q}_C$ ratios are produced in the normal alveoli of lungs with shunt and $\dot{V}_A/\dot{Q}_C$ mismatch (see Figures 12-8 and 12-9). However, these units do not produce hypoxemia or hypercapnia in the end-capillary blood; instead, they increase P_AO_2 and decrease P_ACO_2 because their ventilation is high with respect to their blood flow. These units constitute relative dead space, or a dead space effect. Overall ventilation must increase in the lung to maintain a normal $PaCO_2$, which is a hallmark of dead space. In this situation, increased dead space ventilation occurs because ventilation is increased out of proportion to blood flow.

Generally, however, dead space–producing diseases are diseases in which reduced blood flow is the primary defect.

Reduced Pulmonary Blood Flow Relative to Ventilation as a Cause of Dead Space

Pulmonary blood flow may be reduced or stopped by vessel obstruction (pulmonary emboli), low blood pressure and flow (shock), or alveolar overdistention as might occur in mechanical ventilation with high alveolar inflation pressures or as a result of auto-PEEP (air trapping resulting from inadequate exhalation time). Shock may be caused by blood loss, cardiac pump failure, or inappropriate massive vasodilation.

Whatever its cause, alveolar dead space is produced when blood flow is diminished or absent in ventilated alveoli. Ventilation of a nonperfused alveolus is useless, or wasted, because alveolar gas cannot contact blood. Ventilation of normally perfused alveoli must increase to maintain adequate gas exchange, which means the ventilation of nonperfused, dead space alveoli must also increase. This type of ventilation is inefficient because overall $\dot{V}_E$ must increase greatly to sustain a normal-range $PaCO_2$. Increased work of breathing and $\dot{V}_E$ out of proportion with $PaCO_2$ are the major characteristics of increased alveolar dead space.

CONCEPT QUESTION 12-9

What effect does increased alveolar dead space have on mixed expired gas PCO_2?

Effect of High $\dot{V}_A/\dot{Q}_C$ on Arterial PCO_2 and Arterial PO_2

Figure 12-11, *A*, illustrates the effect of cutting off blood flow to one lung while the lung continues to ventilate. Assuming both lungs had originally received equal blood flows, blood is redirected to the normal lung, doubling its flow. If ventilation of the normal lung remains constant, a low $\dot{V}_A/\dot{Q}_C$ ratio is created (i.e., perfusion increases while ventilation stays the same). Such conditions would produce increased $PaCO_2$ and decreased PaO_2 (see Figure 12-11, *A*).

However, ventilation normally does not remain constant when dead space develops. At the same instant $PaCO_2$ increases, medullary chemoreceptors stimulate an increase in $\dot{V}_E$ (see Figure 12-11, *B*). Ventilation increases as much as necessary to maintain normal $PaCO_2$. Figure 12-11, *B*, represents the usual response to alveolar dead space; ventilation of the perfused lung increases to match its increased blood flow, preserving normal blood gases at the expense of greatly increased $\dot{V}_E$ and work of breathing.

Arterial hypoxemia is not an inherent feature of dead space disease unless the ability to increase overall ventilation is impaired, as might be the case in patients with severe obstructive lung disease. Also, P_ACO_2 of mixed alveolar gases is decreased because the nonperfused lung has a P_ACO_2 of 0 mm Hg. This situation creates an alveolar-to-arterial carbon dioxide pressure difference ($P[a-A]CO_2$) which is a diagnostic indicator of increased dead space. Alveolar dead space also creates an increased difference between $PaCO_2$ and mixed expired PCO_2 ($P_{\bar{E}}CO_2$). This difference is the basis for the Bohr dead space

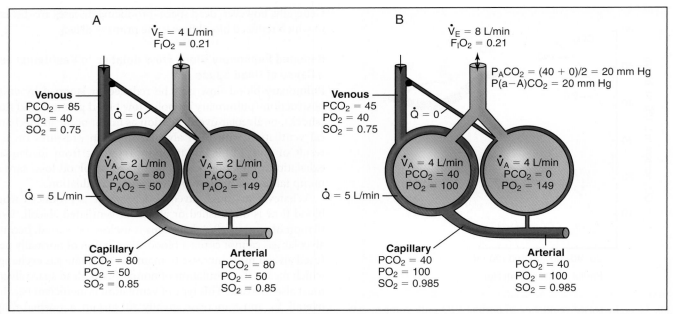

Figure 12-11 Dead space disease without compensatory increased $\dot{V}_E$ (**A**) and with increased $\dot{V}_E$ (**B**). Alveolar dead space leads to a disproportionately increased $\dot{V}_E$ with respect to $PaCO_2$ (**B**) and increases $P(a-A)CO_2$.

equation explained in Chapter 4. The Bohr equation is used to calculate the dead space-to-tidal volume ratio (V_D/V_T). If V_D/V_T is known and $\dot{V}_E$ is measured, $\dot{V}_A$ can be calculated.

Physiological Compensatory Responses to Dead Space and Shunt

The lung has two compensatory responses that help restore abnormal $\dot{V}_A/\dot{Q}_C$ ratios toward normal. Figures 12-8, 12-9, and 12-11 are oversimplified because they do not take these responses into account. In shunt, the decreased PO_2 of blood passing through unventilated alveoli causes localized hypoxic pulmonary vasoconstriction (see Chapter 6). This vasoconstriction redistributes blood flow to well-ventilated alveoli. Poorly ventilated units receive less blood flow, which improves their $\dot{V}_A/\dot{Q}_C$ ratios and reduces their effect on arterial blood. With regard to alveolar dead space, the low PCO_2 values of alveoli with little or no blood flow cause local alveolar duct constriction, increasing airways resistance and decreasing ventilation in these regions; this helps create a better match between ventilation and blood flow, reducing the adverse blood gas effects of the $\dot{V}_A/\dot{Q}_C$ imbalance.

CLINICAL MEASUREMENT OF SHUNT

Shunt Indicators

Indicators of shunt are clinically valuable because they provide a tool to evaluate the oxygen-transfer efficiency of the lung. This evaluation helps differentiate among various causes of hypoxemia. For example, overall hypoventilation causes hypoxemia, but the alveoli can still efficiently transfer their reduced amount of oxygen into the blood. Shunt indicators allow one to identify

processes that decrease ventilation of perfused alveoli. Shunt measurements help clinicians make informed decisions about therapy options and provide a way to monitor the effectiveness of therapy.

Alveolar-Arterial Oxygen Pressure Difference

$P(A-a)O_2$ has been discussed extensively in earlier sections. $P(A-a)O_2$, often called the **A-a gradient**, is probably the best-known index of oxygen-transfer efficiency. In the complete absence of shunt, no difference would exist between P_AO_2 and PaO_2 values (see Figure 12-6); arterial blood would be identical to end-capillary blood of the ventilated alveolus. Thus, an increased $P(A-a)O_2$ indicates increased physiological shunting. The normal $P(A-a)O_2$ is about 7 to 14 mm Hg during breathing of room air and 50 to 60 mm Hg when breathing 100% oxygen.[3] These normal values increase with age as the lung becomes more inefficient. The variability of $P(A-a)O_2$ with F_IO_2 limits its usefulness as a shunt indicator when F_IO_2 is changed.

Calculation of $P(A-a)O_2$ is straightforward. The ideal alveolar gas equation is used to compute P_AO_2, and arterial blood gas analysis provides PaO_2. At F_IO_2 values ≤0.60, P_AO_2 is calculated as follows (see Chapter 7):

$$P_AO_2 = F_IO_2(P_B - 47) - PaCO_2 \times 1.2$$

At F_IO_2 values > 0.60, the factor 1.2 is eliminated, as the following equation shows:

$$P_AO_2 = F_IO_2(P_B - 47) - PaCO_2$$

Arterial PO₂/Alveolar PO₂

The PaO_2/P_AO_2 index (**a-A ratio**) represents the percentage of the alveolar PO_2 that is transferred to the arterial blood. In theory, the percentage of P_AO_2 transferred across the lung stays constant as long as lung function (whether normal or abnormal)

CLINICAL FOCUS 12-5

Using the Bohr Dead Space Equation to Determine Dead Space and Alveolar Ventilation

You are conducting tests to determine whether your patient receiving mechanical ventilation is ready to be removed from the ventilator and breathe spontaneously. In addition to performing various other tests, you wish to evaluate the efficiency of your patient's ventilation. To do this, you need to know the amount of your patient's total ventilation that does not participate in gas exchange. You can then calculate the degree to which ventilation participates in gas exchange. You have the following information:

$\dot{V}_E$ = 10 L/min
pH = 7.39
$PaCO_2$ = 43 mm Hg
HCO_3^- = 25 mEq/L
$P_{\bar{E}}CO_2$ = 17 mm Hg
PaO_2 = 70 mm Hg
F_IO_2 = 0.35

Discussion

The Bohr dead space equation calculates V_D/V_T, which is the fraction of the tidal volume used to ventilate nonperfused airspace, as the following shows:

$$V_D/V_T = PaCO_2 - \frac{P_{\bar{E}}CO_2}{PaCO_2}$$

$\dot{V}_D / \dot{V}_E$ can be substituted for V_D/V_T to calculate the fraction of total $\dot{V}_E$ that is devoted to dead space ventilation. Using the appropriate data as provided, you can determine the following:

$$\dot{V}_D/\dot{V}_E = \frac{43 - 17}{43}$$
$$\dot{V}_D/\dot{V}_E = \frac{26}{43}$$
$$\dot{V}_D/\dot{V}_E = 0.6$$

This means 0.6, or 60%, of the $\dot{V}_E$ is dead space ventilation, leaving 40% for $\dot{V}_A$. Specifically, the following equation is true:

$$\dot{V}_D = 0.6(10 \text{ L/min}) = 6 \text{ L/min}$$
$$\dot{V}_A = 0.4(10 \text{ L/min}) = 4 \text{ L/min}$$

A normal V_D/V_T or $\dot{V}_D / \dot{V}_E$ is about 0.25 to 0.40. An abnormally high amount of this patient's $\dot{V}_E$ is used to ventilate nonperfused dead space. Ventilation is relatively inefficient; a high $\dot{V}_E$ is required to maintain a normal $PaCO_2$ of 43 mm Hg (see previous patient data). The patient may have difficulty breathing spontaneously because the work of breathing required to sustain a normal $PaCO_2$ is abnormally high.

---

stays constant. Thus, PaO_2/P_AO_2 is more stable than $P(A-a)O_2$ when F_IO_2 changes.[3] The lower normal limit for PaO_2/P_AO_2 is about 0.75. That is, at least 75% of P_AO_2 is normally transferred to the arterial blood. Because there is always some degree of $P(A-a)O_2$ present, PaO_2/P_AO_2 can never be 1.0.

Because of its stability, PaO_2/P_AO_2 is useful in following a patient's lung function as F_IO_2 is changed. Its stability also means PaO_2/P_AO_2 can be used to predict the F_IO_2 required to achieve a desired PaO_2.

Arterial PO₂/Fractional Concentration of Inspired Oxygen

The PaO_2/F_IO_2 ratio is another measure of oxygenation efficiency. A normal range is about 380 to 475 (i.e., when PaO_2 is 80 to 100 mm Hg on F_IO_2 of 0.21). PaO_2/F_IO_2 is easy to calculate because it does not require calculation of P_AO_2. However, its usefulness as a shunt indicator is limited. A major problem with PaO_2/F_IO_2 is that changes in $PaCO_2$ affect it. For example, if $PaCO_2$ increases from 40 mm Hg to 80 mm Hg during general hypoventilation, PaO_2 decreases by about the same amount (i.e., from 90 mm Hg to 50 mm Hg). If the patient is breathing room air, PaO_2/F_IO_2 is 50/0.21 = 238. This low value implies that oxygen-transfer efficiency is impaired when it is not; $P(A-a)O_2$ does not change in this situation. For this reason, PaO_2/F_IO_2 is the least accurate indicator of shunt, especially at low F_IO_2 values when the effect of $PaCO_2$ is greatest.

Comparison of P(A-a)O₂, PaO₂/P_AO₂, and PaO₂/F_IO₂

None of the indicators discussed previously consider the fact that in abnormally high shunt conditions mixed venous oxygen content ($C\bar{v}O_2$) affects CaO_2 and PaO_2. This is true because shunted blood is composed of mixed venous blood, which eventually becomes part of the arterial blood. As was explained in Chapter 8, a decrease in cardiac output can decrease $C\bar{v}O_2$. Thus, a nonpulmonary factor (cardiac output) can decrease PaO_2. In this respect, shunt indicators sensitive to only pulmonary factors are inaccurate in reflecting the efficiency of the lung's oxygen-transfer ability.

Consider a patient in whom 20% of the cardiac output (venous blood) is shunted through capillaries of nonventilated alveoli; this produces abnormal $P(A-a)O_2$, PaO_2/P_AO_2, and PaO_2/F_IO_2 values because the shunted venous blood reduces the PaO_2. Now assume that the cardiac output decreases to half normal, decreasing $C\bar{v}O_2$ significantly. The same 20% shunted blood is now more profoundly deoxygenated, and further decreases CaO_2 and PaO_2. In this situation, each shunt indicator would show a greater degree of abnormality, although the percentage of shunted cardiac output and oxygen-transfer efficiency did not change. Therefore, these shunt indicators must be cautiously interpreted in patients with cardiovascular instability.

Assuming that cardiovascular function is constant, PaO_2/P_AO_2 is the most reliable shunt indicator.[3] It varies least with

CLINICAL FOCUS 12-6

Calculation of Fractional Concentration of Inspired Oxygen Required to Achieve Acceptable Arterial PO₂

A 29-year-old woman has been admitted to the hospital. She complains of severe shortness of breath. Her room air arterial blood gas values are as follows:

$PaO_2 = 65$ mm Hg
$PaCO_2 = 30$ mm Hg
pH = 7.45
$HCO_3^- = 20$ mEq/L
$F_IO_2 = 0.21$
$P_B = 760$ mm Hg

How much oxygen is needed to achieve a PaO_2 of 90 mm Hg? What F_IO_2 should be used?

Discussion

The equation used to calculate a F_IO_2 required for a desired PaO_2 is as follows:

$$F_IO_2 \text{ required} = \frac{[\text{Desired } PaO_2/([PaO_2/P_AO_2])] + PaCO_2 \times 1.2}{(P_B - 47)}$$

This equation is a rearrangement of the alveolar air equation. The following shows the alveolar air equation solved for F_IO_2:

1    $P_AO_2 = F_IO_2(P_B - 47) - PaCO_2 \times 1.2$
2    $F_IO_2(P_B - 47) = P_AO_2 + PaCO_2 \times 1.2$
3    $F_IO_2 = P_AO_2 + PaCO_2 \times 1.2/P_B - 47$

Equation 3 is similar to the "F_IO_2 required" equation. In fact, equation 3 can be used to calculate the F_IO_2 required. The P_AO_2 in the numerator of equation 3 is the P_AO_2 needed to produce the desired PaO_2. This needed P_AO_2 can be calculated as follows if the original PaO_2/P_AO_2 ratio is known:

Needed P_AO_2 = Desired PaO_2 / (PaO_2 / P_AO_2)

The term "desired $PaO_2/(PaO_2/P_AO_2)$" in the numerator of the "F_IO_2 required" equation is merely a way to calculate the P_AO_2 needed to achieve the PaO_2 desired. The PaO_2/P_AO_2 ratio can be calculated from the current measured PaO_2, and the P_AO_2 can be calculated from the current F_IO_2.

First, the patient's PaO_2/P_AO_2 ratio is calculated from current data. This ratio indicates the fraction of the P_AO_2 that entered the arterial blood. Dividing the desired PaO_2 by this fraction provides the P_AO_2 that must exist in the alveoli to produce the desired PaO_2 in the arterial blood. Using the patient's current data, you can determine the following:

Current $P_AO_2 = 0.21(760 - 47) - (30 \times 1.2) = 113.73$ mm Hg
Current $PaO_2 = 65$ mm Hg
$PaO_2/P_AO_2 = 65/113.73 = 0.57$

This means 0.57, or 57%, of the P_AO_2 enters the blood. Therefore, the desired PaO_2 of 90 mm Hg must be 0.57 of the needed P_AO_2, as the following shows:

90 mm Hg = 0.57 × needed P_AO_2
90 mm Hg/0.57 = 157.9 mm Hg =
needed P_AO_2 to achieve PaO_2 of 90 mm Hg

Referring to the "F_IO_2 required" equation at the beginning, the appropriate numbers are inserted to arrive at the following solution:

$$F_IO_2 \text{ required} = \frac{\text{Desired } PaO_2/(PaO_2/P_AO_2) + PaCO_2 \times 1.2}{P_B - 47}$$
$$F_IO_2 = \frac{157.8 + (30 \times 1.2)}{(760 - 47)}$$
$$F_IO_2 = \frac{193.8}{713}$$
$$F_IO_2 = 0.27$$

An F_IO_2 of 0.27 should produce a PaO_2 of about 90 mm Hg.

---

changes in F_IO_2, is not affected by $PaCO_2$, and can be used to compute the F_IO_2 necessary to achieve a desired PaO_2.

Physiological Shunt Equation

The physiological shunt equation takes into account the effects of both pulmonary and nonpulmonary factors (e.g., cardiac output) that influence arterial oxygenation. With this equation, the true fraction of cardiac output that is shunted through non-ventilated airspace can be calculated. The shunt equation takes both anatomical and intrapulmonary shunting into account (i.e., physiological shunt [$\dot{Q}_s$]). Shunt calculated by this method is the only accurate way to measure physiological shunting when cardiac output is unstable and is the most reliable method to assess oxygen-transfer efficiency. $\dot{Q}_s$ is calculated as a fraction of the total cardiac output ($\dot{Q}_T$), or the shunt fraction, as the following shows:

$$\frac{\dot{Q}_s}{\dot{Q}_T} = \frac{C\acute{c}O_2 - CaO_2}{C\acute{c}O_2 - C\bar{v}O_2}$$

In this equation, $\dot{Q}_s/\dot{Q}_T$ represents the physiological shunt fraction, $Cc'O_2$ represents the end-capillary oxygen content from ideal alveoli, CaO_2 represents the arterial oxygen content, and $C\bar{v}O_2$ represents the mixed venous oxygen content.

Figure 12-12 helps illustrate the rationale for the shunt equation. The ($Cc'O_2 - C\bar{v}O_2$) is equal to the total oxygen uptake by the capillary blood. The ($Cc'O_2 - CaO_2$) is the amount of oxygen lost from the $Cc'O_2$ as a result of mixing with poorly oxygenated $\dot{Q}_s$. In other words, the greater the amount of shunted blood ($\dot{Q}_s$), the greater the amount of oxygen lost from the $Cc'O_2$ when it mixes with $\dot{Q}_s$. The shunt equation expresses this oxygen loss as a fraction of the total oxygen uptake:

$\dfrac{(C\acute{c}O_2 - CaO_2)}{(C\acute{c}O_2 - C\bar{v}O_2)}$ = Oxygen lost from mixing with Q_s
= Total amount of oxygen uptake

It should be apparent that this fraction is equal to the shunt fraction ($\dot{Q}_s/\dot{Q}_T$).

A mixed venous blood sample must be available to use the shunt equation in the clinical setting. Mixed venous blood is

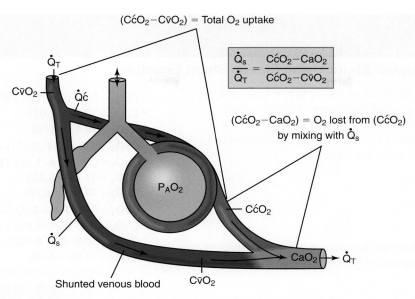

Figure 12-12 Schematic concept of classic shunt equation.

available only when a pulmonary artery catheter is in place (see Chapter 6). In addition, because end-capillary blood cannot be directly sampled, the $Cc'O_2$ is calculated as follows:

$$C\acute{c}O_2 = (Hb \times 1.34 \text{ g / dL} \times S\acute{c}O_2) + (P_AO_2 \times 0.003 \text{ mL/dL})$$

In reference to Figure 12-12, the $Pc'O_2$ is of necessity equal to P_AO_2 because alveolar gas and end-capillary blood are in equilibrium. $Pc'O_2$ is calculated from the alveolar air equation.

Virtually all patients requiring shunt measurements breathe supplementary oxygen. Because even low concentrations of inspired oxygen result in P_AO_2 values greater than 150 mm Hg, the assumption is that capillary blood oxygen saturation is 1.0 when the patient breathes any amount of supplementary oxygen. The $Sc'O_2$ term of the shunt equation is generally ignored in calculating $Cc'O_2$.

CONCEPT QUESTION 12-10

Which part of the classic shunt equation—the numerator or denominator—is most affected by atelectasis? Which is affected most by decreased cardiac output?

Clinical Significance

The periodic assessment of $\dot{Q}_s$ in patients with oxygenation difficulties is clinically important. Increased shunting indicates an increase in nonventilated alveoli.

The effect of increased shunt on CaO_2 is magnified by a low cardiac output. As discussed previously, low cardiac output decreases $C\bar{v}O_2$, exaggerating the desaturating effect of shunted venous blood on CaO_2. A low cardiac output and decreased

TABLE 12-2

Clinical Significance of Shunt

Shunt Fraction Percentage	Clinical Significance
<10%	Clinically compatible with normal lungs
10-19%	Intrapulmonary abnormality; seldom requires significant ventilatory support
20-29%	Significant abnormality; requires ventilatory assistance with PEEP or CPAP
≥30%	Severe disease; life threatening; requires aggressive mechanical support with PEEP

CPAP, Continuous positive airway pressure; *PEEP,* positive end expiratory pressure.

$C\bar{v}O_2$ do not affect arterial oxygenation in people with normal shunt because shunt units contribute very little desaturated blood to the arterial stream.

Calculated shunt fractions of 10% or less have no significant clinical effect. Table 12-2 summarizes the clinical significance of shunting.[4]

Because shunting involves loss of airspace in the lung (i.e., alveolar collapse or fluid-filled alveoli), it is associated with decreased lung compliance, which increases the work of breathing. The severe hypoxemia of shunting combined with associated low lung compliance may place such high work demands on the respiratory system that mechanical ventilation is required.

CLINICAL FOCUS 12-7

Calculating Physiological Shunt Using Classic Shunt Equation

A 36-year-old woman is admitted to the intensive care unit with diffuse bilateral pneumonia. Because of severe hypoxia (PaO_2 = 40 mm Hg), the patient is intubated and placed on a mechanical ventilator with an F_IO_2 of 1.0. Arterial blood gases are drawn 1 hour later and show the following:

PaO_2 = 145 mm Hg

$PaCO_2$ = 42 mm Hg

pH = 7.39

SaO_2 = 1.0

Hb = 13 g/dL

A catheter is placed into the patient's pulmonary artery, and the following blood gas values are obtained:

$P\overline{v}O_2$ = 34 mm Hg

$S\overline{v}O_2$ = 0.63

Using the classic shunt equation, calculate this patient's $\dot{Q}_s$ fraction.

Discussion

$$\frac{\dot{Q}_s}{\dot{Q}_T} = \frac{C\acute{c}O_2 - CaO_2}{C\acute{c}O_2 - C\overline{v}O_2}$$

To calculate shunt, first calculate $Cc'O_2$, CaO_2, and $C\overline{v}O_2$:

$$C\acute{c}O_2 = (Hb \times 1.34 \times S\acute{c}O_2) + (P_AO_2 \times 0.003)$$
$$C\acute{c}O_2 = (13 \times 1.34 \times 1.0) + (P_AO_2 - 0.003)$$

$$P_AO_2 = P_IO_2 - PaCO_2$$
$$P_AO_2 = F_IO_2(760 - 47) - PaCO_2$$
$$P_AO_2 = 1.0(713) - 42$$
$$P_AO_2 = 671 \text{ mm Hg (this } PO_2 \text{ yields } ScO_2 = 1.0)$$

$$C\acute{c}O_2 = (13 \times 1.34 \times 1.0) + (671 \times 0.003)$$
$$C\acute{c}O_2 = 17.42 + 2.013$$
$$C\acute{c}O_2 = 19.43 \text{ mL/dL}$$
$$CaO_2 = (Hb \times 1.34 \times SaO_2) + (PaO_2 \times 0.003)$$
$$CaO_2 = (13 \times 1.34 \times 1.0) + (145 \times 0.003)$$
$$CaO_2 = 17.42 + 0.435$$
$$CaO_2 = 17.855 \text{ mL/dL}$$
$$C\overline{v}O_2 = (Hb \times 1.34 \times S\overline{v}O_2) + (P\overline{v}O_2 \times 0.003)$$
$$C\overline{v}O_2 = (13 \times 1.34 \times 0.63) + (34 \times 0.003)$$
$$C\overline{v}O_2 = 10.9746 + 0.102$$
$$C\overline{v}O_2 = 11.08 \text{ mL/dL}$$

The following calculations are made:

$$\frac{\dot{Q}_s}{\dot{Q}_T} = \frac{19.43 - 17.855}{19.43 - 11.08}$$
$$\frac{\dot{Q}_s}{\dot{Q}_T} = \frac{1.575}{8.35}$$
$$\frac{\dot{Q}_s}{\dot{Q}_T} = 0.19 \text{ or } 19\% \text{ shunt}$$

This means 19% of the cardiac output flows through non-ventilated alveoli and receives no oxygen from the lungs. Normal $\dot{Q}_s$ is less than 5%. This patient's severe pneumonia fills many alveoli with inflammatory debris, rendering them airless. Venous blood perfusing these alveoli cannot take up oxygen and ultimately mixes with arterial blood. To correct the resulting arterial hypoxemia, you must find ways to re-aerate the diseased alveoli; possible measures include secretion mobilization and removal techniques or PEEP with mechanical ventilation.

CLINICAL FOCUS 12-8

Effect of Low Cardiac Output on Arterial Oxygenation When Shunt Is High

Consider again the case presented in Clinical Focus 12-7. The patient is a 36-year-old woman with severe bilateral pneumonia, which fills many alveoli with fluid, creating a $\dot{Q}_s$ of 21%. Her cardiac output decreases from 6.0 L per minute to 3.0 L per minute. Arterial blood gases are drawn and reveal the following:

	Cardiac Output 6.0 L/min	Cardiac Output 3.0 L/min
F_IO_2 =	1.0	1.0
PaO_2 =	145 mm Hg	82 mm Hg
$PaCO_2$ =	42 mm Hg	45 mm Hg
pH =	7.39	7.34

Examine the effect that decreased cardiac output had on this patient's arterial oxygenation.

Discussion

Arterial oxygenation worsened with a decrease in cardiac output because low cardiac output results in low $C\overline{v}O_2$.

Blood that moves more slowly spends more time giving up oxygen to the tissues, decreasing $C\overline{v}O_2$. Blood perfusing nonventilated alveoli is now even more hypoxic than before, and when mixed with arterialized blood, it decreases the PaO_2 and arterial oxygen content even more. If you estimated this patient's shunt by examining the $P(A-a)O_2$, PaO_2/P_AO_2 ratio, or PaO_2/F_IO_2 ratio, you would incorrectly assume that PaO_2 is decreased because of increased shunting. In other words, these estimators do not consider the effect of $C\overline{v}O_2$ on PaO_2. The classic shunt equation reflects the effect of pulmonary and cardiac factors on PaO_2 and is the most accurate way to estimate $\dot{Q}_s$ in patients with unstable cardiac output. This case illustrates that cardiac output changes can affect PaO_2, although F_IO_2 remains unchanged.

- Gas exchange between air and blood can occur only if pulmonary blood flow perfuses ventilated alveoli.
- The overall lung $\dot{V}_A/\dot{Q}_C$ ratio reveals little about gas-exchange efficiency; the distribution of individual alveolar $\dot{V}_A/\dot{Q}_C$ ratios determines the match between air and blood flow.
- The range of $\dot{V}_A/\dot{Q}_C$ abnormalities extends from absolute shunt (ratio = zero) to absolute dead space (ratio = infinity).
- Low $\dot{V}_A/\dot{Q}_C$ ratios (<1) always cause hypoxemia but not always hypercapnia.
- Shunting disease is frequently associated with low $PaCO_2$ because shunt-produced hypoxemia sensitizes the peripheral chemoreceptors, inducing hyperventilation.
- High $\dot{V}_A/\dot{Q}_C$ ratios produce relative or absolute dead space and abnormally high ventilation to maintain normal $PaCO_2$.
- Hypoxemia associated with low $\dot{V}_A/\dot{Q}_C$ ratios is separated into three categories: (1) hypoventilation, (2) $\dot{V}_A/\dot{Q}_C$ mismatch, and (3) shunt.
- $\dot{V}_A/\dot{Q}_C$ mismatch responds well to oxygen therapy, whereas shunt produces hypoxemia refractory to oxygen therapy.
- The hallmark of shunt is refractory hypoxemia and reduced lung compliance, and the hallmark of dead space is high $\dot{V}_E$ out of proportion with $PaCO_2$.

- $\dot{V}_A/\dot{Q}_C$ abnormalities are much more likely to create hypoxemia than hypercapnia.
- High $\dot{V}_A/\dot{Q}_C$ regions can compensate for the hypercapnic effects of low $\dot{V}_A/\dot{Q}_C$ units but cannot do the same for the hypoxemic effects of low $\dot{V}_A/\dot{Q}_C$ units.
- Of the various shunt indicators, PaO_2/P_AO_2 is the most stable and clinically useful, although $P(A-a)O_2$ is probably the most popular and familiar.
- The actual measurement of shunt, determined by use of the classic shunt equation, is the only accurate shunt indicator when cardiac output is unstable.

References

1. Wagner PD, Powell FL, West JB: Ventilation, blood flow, and gas exchange. In Mason RJ, et al, editors: *Murray and Nadel's textbook of respiratory medicine*, ed 5, Philadelphia, 2010, Saunders.
2. West JB: *Respiratory physiology: the essentials*, ed 8, Philadelphia, 2008, Lippincott Williams & Wilkins.
3. Hess D, Maxwell C: Which is the best index of oxygenation—$P(A-a)O_2$, PaO_2/P_AO_2, or PaO_2/F_IO_2, *Respir Care* 30(4):961, 1985. (editorial).
4. Wandrup JH: Quantifying pulmonary oxygen transfer deficits in critically ill patients, *Acta Anaesthesiol Scand Suppl* s107(9):34, 1995.

CHAPTER 13

Clinical Assessment of Acid-Base and Oxygenation Status

OBJECTIVES

After reading this chapter, you will be able to:
- Differentiate between arterial blood gas classification and interpretation
- Apply a systematic arterial blood gas classification method
- Differentiate between oxygenation and ventilation defects
- Describe the basis for compensatory activity in all acid-base disturbances
- Explain how the anion gap computation can help the clinician differentiate the causes of metabolic acidosis
- Explain why acute changes in $PaCO_2$ affect plasma $[HCO_3^-]$
- Explain how acid-base disturbances affect plasma $[K^+]$ and $[Cl^-]$
- Explain why the standard bicarbonate and base excess measurements more accurately reflect purely metabolic acid-base disturbances than plasma $[HCO_3^-]$

OBJECTIVES—cont'd

- Differentiate between the traditional Henderson-Hassel-balch approach and Stewart's strong ion approach to acid-base physiology
- Distinguish between pulmonary and cardiovascular factors that affect tissue oxygenation

- Classify the causes and severity of oxygenation defects
- Interpret various pulmonary and cardiovascular tissue oxygenation indicators

KEY TERMS

acute acidemia
acute alkalemia
anion gap
base excess (BE)
chronic acidemia
chronic alkalemia
hypercapnia

hypocapnia
Kussmaul's respiration
standard bicarbonate (SB)
strong ion
strong ion difference
tetany

CLASSIFICATION VERSUS INTERPRETATION

Chapter 10 discusses the concept of respiratory and metabolic acid-base disturbances and the compensatory responses they elicit. This chapter introduces a systematic method for the classification, or categorization, of arterial blood gases in terms of acid-base balance and oxygenation status. Classification is the first essential step in the development of a rational therapeutic basis for correcting acid-base and oxygenation problems. The classification process focuses attention on the general problem areas and provides a starting point for interpretation, or the in-depth exploration and comprehension of the underlying disorder.

Arterial blood gas interpretation entails the evaluation of blood gases in the context of the patient's total clinical picture. The patient's medical history, physical examination findings, current therapy, and other clinical diagnostic information must be integrated with blood gas results to arrive at a sound interpretation. Respiratory therapists not only must comprehend the processes that led to the current blood gases but also must anticipate future blood gas changes. Only then can an informed, definitive arterial blood gas interpretation be made; only then can the respiratory therapist arrive at a rational basis for therapeutic intervention.

CLASSIFICATION OF ACID-BASE DISTURBANCES

Acid-base disturbances and oxygenation problems should be evaluated separately as two distinct entities. Although these two problems are sometimes interrelated, evaluating them separately helps identify these relationships.

The relevant arterial blood gas components in evaluating acid-base status are pH, PCO_2, and $[HCO_3^-]$. Arterial pH reflects hydrogen ion activity of extracellular fluid (plasma), which generally correlates with intracellular fluid pH. Chapter 10 emphasizes the importance of regulating the pH from

a cellular enzyme standpoint. Abnormal pH values also affect the central nervous system, causing the clinical manifestations shown in Figure 13-1. Generally, a low arterial pH (acidemia) depresses neuronal excitability, whereas a high pH (alkalemia) has the opposite effect (greatly increased excitability).[1] An extremely low pH (pH <7.00) causes a coma, whereas an extremely high pH (pH >7.80) causes convulsions and **tetany** (a state of sustained muscle spasm). Low arterial pH values (pH <7.10) also predispose patients to ventricular arrhythmias and reduce heart muscle contractility.[2]

Systematic Classification

The most consistent, reliable results are achieved when an orderly, systematic, unvarying approach is used to analyze acid-base problems. If exactly the same step-by-step approach is used for each problem, confusion and premature conclusions can be

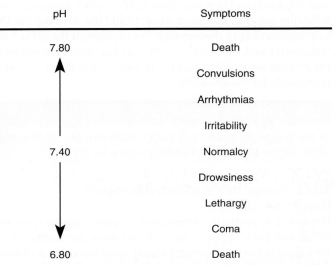

pH	Symptoms
7.80	Death
	Convulsions
	Arrhythmias
	Irritability
7.40	Normalcy
	Drowsiness
	Lethargy
	Coma
6.80	Death

Figure 13-1 Symptoms associated with pH abnormalities. (Modified from Malley WJ: *Clinical blood gases: assessment and intervention,* St Louis, 2005, Saunders.)

avoided. A systematic approach also helps identify inconsistencies and errors in blood gas data. Box 13-1 outlines four steps in acid-base classification. The order of steps 1 through 3 is not as important as following the same sequence for each situation.

Step 1: Classify pH

The normal limits for arterial pH in humans are 7.35 to 7.45. This range is not affected by age or gender. An arterial pH greater than 7.45 is called alkalemia, and a pH less than 7.35 is called acidemia. If the pH is classified as abnormal, one determines whether the abnormality is of respiratory or nonrespiratory (metabolic) origin.

Step 2: Analyze Respiratory Involvement ($PaCO_2$)

The $PaCO_2$ is controlled by alveolar ventilation and is thus the indicator of respiratory involvement. The normal range for $PaCO_2$ in humans is 35 to 45 mm Hg and is not affected by age or gender; high and low $PaCO_2$ values are called **hypercapnia** and **hypocapnia**. The $PaCO_2$ is analyzed, keeping the pH (step 1) in mind. A $PaCO_2$ greater than 45 mm Hg means blood H^+ levels (from dissociated carbonic acid) are abnormally high; this is compatible with acidemia and hypoventilation. A $PaCO_2$ less than 35 mm Hg has the opposite meaning; it is compatible with alkalemia and hyperventilation. If the pH is abnormal, the following question should be asked: Could the observed $PaCO_2$ help explain the pH abnormality? For example, if the pH is 7.50 (alkalemia) and the $PaCO_2$ is 30 mm Hg (hyperventilation), the respiratory system must be at least partly, if not entirely, responsible for the alkalemia.

Step 3: Analyze Nonrespiratory (Metabolic) Involvement ($[HCO_3^-]$)

Because it is primarily determined by nonrespiratory, or so-called metabolic factors, plasma bicarbonate concentration is the logical indicator of nonrespiratory involvement in acid-base disturbances. The normal range for arterial plasma $[HCO_3^-]$ in humans is 22 to 26 mEq/L and is unaffected by age or gender. Bicarbonate is a chemical base; high plasma bicarbonate

(>26 mEq/L) is compatible with alkalemia, and low plasma bicarbonate (<22 mEq/L) is compatible with acidemia.

Plasma $[HCO_3^-]$ is not as specific and accurate in indicating metabolic acid-base disturbances as $PaCO_2$ is in indicating respiratory disturbances. The reason is that plasma bicarbonate responds slightly to pure respiratory (i.e., PCO_2) changes. The carbon dioxide hydration reaction explains this phenomenon. As explained in Chapter 10, an acute increase in $PaCO_2$ of 10 mm Hg increases $[HCO_3^-]$ by about 1 mEq/L. Thus, the plasma $[HCO_3^-]$ must be evaluated with caution; if it falls outside of the normal range but the abnormality can be explained by the effect of the carbon dioxide hydration reaction, the $[HCO_3^-]$ level is not responsible for any existing acid-base disorder.

Keeping the foregoing limitation in mind, the $[HCO_3^-]$ is inspected and compared with the pH. If the pH is abnormal, one must ask: Can the observed $[HCO_3^-]$ explain the pH abnormality? For example, if the arterial pH is 7.25 (acidemia) and $[HCO_3^-]$ is low (18 mEq/L), this is compatible with acidemia. Therefore, metabolic (nonrespiratory) factors are at least partly, if not entirely, responsible for the acidosis.

Step 4: Assess for Compensation

When the acid-base abnormality has been identified as either respiratory or metabolic, the degree of compensation present, if any, must be determined. In other words, if a respiratory acidosis exists (increased $PaCO_2$), have the kidneys compensated by elevating the plasma $[HCO_3^-]$? Conversely, if a metabolic acidosis exists (decreased HCO_3^-), have the lungs compensated by hyperventilating and lowering the $PaCO_2$?

If the pH has been restored to the normal range (7.35 to 7.45), full compensation has occurred even though pH remains on the acid or alkaline side of the range. Compensation is partial if the pH is still outside of the normal range but the noncausative component (either $PaCO_2$ or HCO_3^-) is also abnormal in a way that brings the pH back toward the normal range. A compensated acid-base disturbance is sometimes referred to as a **chronic acidemia** or **chronic alkalemia** because a certain amount of time is required to bring about compensation. Partial compensation means compensatory activity has begun but has not had enough time to restore the pH to normal. The term uncompensated means the acid-base disturbance is of such recent origin that compensatory activity has not yet started. Therefore, an uncompensated condition is sometimes called an **acute acidemia** or **acute alkalemia**.

It is assumed that compensation for a primary acid-base disorder is never truly complete in the sense of restoring arterial pH all the way to 7.40.[3] In a compensated disorder, the pH is on the acid or alkaline side of the normal range, depending on whether the primary causative disorder created an acidosis or an alkalosis. That is, if the pH is on the acid side of normal (<7.40 but at least ≥7.35), the main cause of the original acid-base imbalance is the component ($PaCO_2$ or HCO_3^-) that, by itself, would cause

TABLE 13-1

Acid-Base and Ventilatory Classification

Component	Classification	Ranges
pH (arterial)	Normal status	7.35-7.45
	Acidemia	<7.35
	Alkalemia	>7.45
PaCO₂ (mm Hg)	Normal ventilatory status	35-45
	Respiratory acidosis (hypoventilation)	>45
	Respiratory alkalosis (hyperventilation)	<35
[HCO₃⁻] (mEq/L)	Normal metabolic status	22-26
	Metabolic acidosis	<22
	Metabolic alkalosis	>26

TABLE 13-2

Degrees of Acid-Base Compensation

Compensating (Noncausative) Component	pH	Classification
Within normal range	Abnormal	Noncompensated (acute)
Out of normal range in the expected direction	Abnormal	Partially compensated
Out of normal range in the expected direction	Normal	Compensated (chronic)

an acidosis. For example, if the pH is 7.36, PaCO₂ is 80 mm Hg, and HCO₃⁻ is 44 mEq/L, compensation is present because the pH is in the normal range, although it is on the acid side of normal. The primary cause of the original acid-base disturbance (before compensatory activity started) must be the factor that would produce acidemia (i.e., the increased PaCO₂ of 80 mm Hg). Thus, this set of blood gases would be classified as compensated (chronic) respiratory acidosis. The primary disturbance is of respiratory origin, and the increased [HCO₃⁻] is a secondary metabolic compensatory response. The reason the pH is on the acid side of the normal range is that the body generally does not overcompensate; it does not increase the [HCO₃⁻] so much that it converts the previously acidotic environment to one with a pH on the alkaline side of normal. Conversely, if the pH is 7.15, PaCO₂ is 80 mm Hg, and HCO₃⁻ is 26 mEq/L, no compensation has occurred; that is, HCO₃⁻ is still normal, not elevated as would be expected if compensatory action were underway.

Compensatory activity does not *correct* the primary acid-base disturbance; the primary defect is still present. Compensatory activity merely works to restore the pH to the normal range. Table 13-1 summarizes acid-base and ventilatory classification. Table 13-2 classifies the degree of compensation for acid-base disturbances.

Respiratory Acidosis (Inadequate Ventilation)

Any physiological process causing an increased PaCO₂ (>45 mm Hg) produces respiratory acidosis. The increased PaCO₂ (hypercapnia) decreases the arterial pH because dissolved carbon dioxide produces carbonic acid and hydrogen ions, as the following reaction shows:

$$CO_2 + H_2O \rightarrow H_2CO_3 \rightarrow HCO_3^- + H^+$$

Therefore, hypercapnia is synonymous with respiratory acidosis.

Causes

Hypoventilation causes hypercapnia, which implies inadequate ventilation. Any process that hinders alveolar ventilation can

CLINICAL FOCUS 13-1

Acute (Uncompensated) Respiratory Acidosis

A 21-year-old previously healthy man is brought to the emergency department. He was unconscious when found by his girlfriend and had apparently taken an overdose of prescription narcotic medication. He is breathing shallowly and slowly. You obtain the following arterial blood gas results:

pH = 7.27
PaCO₂ = 58 mm Hg
[HCO₃⁻] = 26 mEq/L

Step 1: Categorize the pH
The pH is below normal, indicating acidemia.

Step 2: Determine Respiratory Involvement
PaCO₂ is above normal, consistent with the low pH. Hypoventilation is the cause of this patient's hypercapnia and is partly, if not totally, responsible for the acidemia.

Step 3: Determine Metabolic Involvement
[HCO₃⁻] is normal and not contributing to the acidemia.

Step 4: Assess for Compensation
In compensating for this acidemia, the expectation is that [HCO₃⁻] will increase above the normal range. [HCO₃⁻] is in the normal range; no compensation is present.

Conclusion
Acute (uncompensated) respiratory acidosis secondary to narcotic-induced hypoventilation: Therapy involves mechanically assisted ventilation and drugs to reverse the effects of the narcotic.

cause respiratory acidosis. Chronic obstructive pulmonary disease (COPD) is the most frequent cause of respiratory acidosis, mostly because the airways resistance of a patient with severe COPD is so high that the patient cannot sustain the ventilatory work required to maintain a normal $PaCO_2$.[3] Central nervous system depression (drug-induced), extreme obesity (impaired diaphragmatic movement), and neuromuscular disorders (spinal cord lesions, paralytic neuromuscular diseases) are other causes of hypoventilation and respiratory acidosis. Hypercapnia may occur in different ways. A person may have an absolute decrease in ventilation because of drug-induced central nervous system depression, or a patient with COPD and a limited ventilatory reserve may sustain a normal $PaCO_2$ at rest but may not accommodate the increased carbon dioxide production associated with increased physical activity.

Uncompensated hypercapnia implies the presence of acute ventilatory failure; the resulting respiratory acidosis is manifested by a low arterial pH, increased $PaCO_2$, and normal or slightly high $[HCO_3^-]$. In this situation, a slightly increased $[HCO_3^-]$ is not a sign that the kidneys have started compensatory activity; it merely reflects the effect of the carbon dioxide hydration reaction on $[HCO_3^-]$ (see Chapter 10).

Compensation

Renal (kidney) compensation for respiratory acidosis begins as soon as $PaCO_2$ increases. The kidney reclaims HCO_3^- from the renal tubular filtrate, returning it to the blood. The arterial pH is brought into the normal range because the $[HCO_3^-]$-dissolved carbon dioxide ratio is restored near its normal 20:1 range (see Chapter 10). However, this process cannot keep pace with an acutely increasing $PaCO_2$. Full compensation may take several days.

Over the course of developing COPD, a person's $PaCO_2$ increases gradually, allowing the compensatory process enough time to keep pace with the rising $PaCO_2$. The arterial pH is thus maintained in the normal range. Partly compensated respiratory acidosis is characterized by increased $PaCO_2$, increased $[HCO_3^-]$, and an acid pH still not quite in the normal range. A compensated respiratory acidosis is characterized by a pH on the acid side of the normal range (<7.40 but at least ≥7.35), increased $PaCO_2$, and increased $[HCO_3^-]$. The high $[HCO_3^-]$ in the presence of a high $PaCO_2$ is a sign that the $PaCO_2$ has been elevated for a considerable time (i.e., the kidneys have had sufficient time to compensate). Thus, compensated respiratory acidosis is synonymous with chronic ventilatory inadequacy. Although the pH is in the normal range, the underlying pathological process that produces hypercapnia is still present; the kidneys simply mask the problem by maintaining a normal pH range. Because hypercapnia persists, the term acidosis is retained in classifying this condition (compensated respiratory acidosis). This term emphasizes that lung function is still abnormal and has the potential to produce an acidosis.

Clinical Manifestations

Patients with neuromuscular weakness or mechanical breathing difficulties usually breathe shallowly and rapidly and are short of breath; they are often anxious and in obvious distress. Drug-induced central nervous system depression produces slow, shallow breathing and possibly apnea. Acute respiratory acidosis produces

more serious physiological consequences than chronic respiratory acidosis. Rapidly increasing $PaCO_2$ causes cerebral vasodilation and increased intracranial pressure (ICP), possibly leading to retinal venous distention and retinal hemorrhages; in addition, the patient may develop myoclonus (spasmodic muscle jerks), asterixis (a hand-flapping tremor in which the patient cannot keep the wrists flexed with the arms extended), and mental confusion.[3] An abrupt onset of hypercapnia in which $PaCO_2$ rises beyond 70 mm Hg can lead to coma, although patients with chronic hypercapnia can tolerate much higher $PaCO_2$ values.[3] Hypercapnia increases the cardiac output and dilates peripheral vessels, often resulting in a bounding pulse and warm, flushed skin.

Correction

The corrective action in acute respiratory acidosis is to restore alveolar ventilation. Various respiratory therapy modalities ranging from secretion mobilization and bronchodilator drugs to endotracheal intubation and mechanical ventilation may be

---

CLINICAL FOCUS 13-2

Partially Compensated Respiratory Acidosis

A 58-year-old woman is admitted to the hospital with muscle weakness and increasing respiratory distress. Tests confirm a diagnosis of amyotrophic lateral sclerosis, a progressive neuromuscular disease. An arterial blood gas analysis reveals the following:

pH = 7.33
$PaCO_2$ = 59 mm Hg
$[HCO_3^-]$ = 30 mEq/L

Step 1: Categorize the pH
The pH is below the normal range, indicating acidemia.

Step 2: Determine Respiratory Involvement
$PaCO_2$ is above normal, consistent with the low pH. Hypoventilation must be a contributing factor to the acidemia.

Step 3: Determine Metabolic Involvement
$[HCO_3^-]$ is above normal; by itself, this would cause alkalemia. The low pH must be of respiratory origin alone. The slightly elevated $[HCO_3^-]$ cannot be explained by the hydration reaction and is probably a compensatory response by the kidneys.

Step 4: Assess for Compensation
The increased $[HCO_3^-]$ is consistent with the expected compensatory response by the kidneys but has not yet increased the pH to the normal range.

Conclusion
Partially compensated respiratory acidosis: This represents persistent hypoventilation secondary to muscular weaknesses with early renal compensatory activity. One must be prepared to mechanically assist ventilation if necessary.

needed to restore ventilation. However, if hypoventilation is chronic and compensation has restored arterial pH to the normal range, corrective action aimed at reducing the $PaCO_2$ is inappropriate and possibly harmful. In this situation, a rapidly decreasing $PaCO_2$ induces a sudden alkalosis because of renal compensation and elevated blood HCO_3^- levels.

CLINICAL FOCUS 13-3

Fully Compensated Respiratory Acidosis

You are asked to assess a stable 60-year-old man with a long-standing history of cigarette smoking; he was diagnosed with severe COPD. Arterial blood gas values are as follows:

pH = 7.37
$PaCO_2$ = 59 mm Hg
$[HCO_3^-]$ = 33 mEq/L

Step 1: Categorize the pH
The pH is normal, but it is on the acid side of the normal range (<7.40).

Step 2: Determine Respiratory Involvement
$PaCO_2$ is increased, indicating hypoventilation is present.

Step 3: Determine Metabolic Involvement
$[HCO_3^-]$ is elevated; this would increase the pH and is the expected compensatory response of the kidneys to increased $PaCO_2$.

Step 4: Assess for Compensation
The increased $[HCO_3^-]$ is the kidneys' appropriate compensatory response to chronic respiratory acidosis (increased $PaCO_2$). Over the years, the kidneys have reclaimed HCO_3^- from the tubular filtrate and returned it to the blood; this process has kept pace with the increasing $PaCO_2$ and has kept the pH in the normal range. Because the pH is on the acid side of the normal range, the component that would produce acidosis (i.e., $PaCO_2$ of 59 mm Hg) is the cause of the original acid-base imbalance.

Conclusion
Completely compensated (chronic) respiratory acidosis: This represents chronic hypoventilation secondary to poor ventilatory mechanics of COPD; full renal compensation has occurred. Therapy generally includes inhaled medication to dilate the airways and reduce airway inflammation. The patient must be educated about the nature of his disease, signs of respiratory infection, and worsening respiratory status; he also must be instructed on the proper technique for self-administering inhaled medications. Home oxygen therapy might be indicated. The emphasis of therapy is on education about self-care and self-monitoring to prevent acute exacerbations and visits to the hospital emergency department.

CONCEPT QUESTION 13-4

What is the difference between compensation and correction in the context of acid-base disturbances?

Respiratory Alkalosis (Alveolar Hyperventilation)

Any physiological process causing a decreased $PaCO_2$ (<35 mm Hg) produces respiratory alkalosis. The decreased $PaCO_2$ (hypocapnia) forces the hydration reaction to the left, decreasing H^+ concentration and increasing the pH, as the following reaction shows:

$$CO_2 + H_2O \leftarrow H_2CO_3 \leftarrow HCO_3 + H^+$$

Therefore, hypocapnia is synonymous with respiratory alkalosis.

Causes

Hyperventilation causes hypocapnia. Any process in which ventilatory elimination of carbon dioxide exceeds its production causes respiratory alkalosis. Causes can be divided into three categories: (1) hypoxia, (2) pulmonary diseases, and (3) central nervous system diseases. Probably the most common cause of hyperventilation in patients with pulmonary disease is arterial hypoxemia, mediated through the peripheral chemoreceptors.[3] Hypoxia-induced respiratory alkalosis can be caused by high altitude or pulmonary diseases characterized by intrapulmonary shunting (e.g., pneumonia, pulmonary edema). Other pulmonary diseases associated with hyperventilation and respiratory alkalosis include interstitial fibrosis, pulmonary embolism, and acute asthma. J-receptor stimulation in the lung parenchyma may be involved in interstitial diseases, pneumonia, and pulmonary edema. The feeling of dyspnea from high airways resistance and resulting anxiety is a probable mechanism for respiratory alkalosis in acute asthma. General anxiety, fever, stimulating drugs, pain, and injuries of the central nervous system are other possible causes of hyperventilation.

Hyperventilation and respiratory alkalosis also may be iatrogenically induced (i.e., induced by health care personnel). Iatrogenic hyperventilation is most commonly associated with overly aggressive mechanical ventilation; it may also be associated with aggressive deep breathing and lung-expanding respiratory therapy procedures. Acute respiratory alkalosis is characterized by decreased $PaCO_2$, a high pH, and normal-range $[HCO_3^-]$. An extremely slight decrease in $[HCO_3^-]$ is expected to be present as a result of the hydration reaction's effect.

CONCEPT QUESTION 13-5

Explain why arterial hypoxemia might lead to respiratory alkalosis.

Clinical Manifestations

An early sign of acute respiratory alkalosis (hypocapnia) is paresthesia, a numb or tingling sensation in the extremities; light-headedness may also occur. Severe hyperventilation and alkalosis is associated with hyperactive reflexes, muscle

CLINICAL FOCUS 13-4

Acute (Uncompensated) Respiratory Alkalosis

A 45-year-old woman enters the emergency department, complaining of severe back pain occurring after a fall from a ladder. The patient appears to be anxious; is taking rapid, deep breaths; and tells you she feels numbness and tingling in her hands and feet. An arterial blood gas analysis reveals the following:

pH = 7.57
$PaCO_2$ = 25 mm Hg
$[HCO_3^-]$ = 22 mEq/L

Step 1: Categorize the pH
The pH is above the normal range, indicating alkalemia.

Step 2: Determine Respiratory Involvement
$PaCO_2$ is quite low, consistent with the high pH. Hyperventilation is partly, if not completely, responsible for the alkalemia.

Step 3: Determine Metabolic Involvement
$[HCO_3^-]$ is in the normal range and is not contributing to the alkalemia.

Step 4: Assess for Compensation
The expectation is that the kidneys will eliminate HCO_3^- to compensate for this alkalemia. The $[HCO_3^-]$ is normal, so renal compensation is not present.

Conclusion
Acute (uncompensated) respiratory alkalosis: This represents acute alveolar hyperventilation secondary to pain and anxiety. Therapy includes pain-relieving drugs.

cramping of the hands or feet (carpopedal spasm), and possibly tetanic convulsions (a fusion of many muscle spasms producing a sustained contraction without relaxation). The low $PaCO_2$ level may constrict cerebral vessels enough to impair cerebral circulation, causing light-headedness, dizziness, and syncope (fainting). If respiratory alkalosis is anxiety-induced, the patient may show signs of panic and express feelings of impending doom. Vision may become impaired (tunnel vision), and speaking may become difficult.[3]

Compensation
The kidneys compensate for respiratory alkalosis by excreting HCO_3^- in the urine (bicarbonate diuresis). This activity brings the arterial pH down toward the normal range because the $[HCO_3^-]$-dissolved carbon dioxide ratio is restored near its normal 20:1 range. However, renal compensation rarely causes $[HCO_3^-]$ to fall below 18 mEq/L.[3] Renal compensation is a relatively slow process; it may take days until the compensation process is finally completed.

Partially compensated respiratory alkalosis is characterized by decreased $PaCO_2$, decreased $[HCO_3^-]$, and an alkaline pH that is still not quite down in the normal range. Compensated respiratory alkalosis is characterized by decreased $PaCO_2$, decreased $[HCO_3^-]$, and pH on the alkaline side of normal (pH >7.40 but ≤7.45). Compensated respiratory alkalosis is sometimes called chronic respiratory alkalosis or chronic alveolar hyperventilation. The underlying hyperventilation and hypocapnia are still present. Thus, the term alkalosis is used in classifying this condition, although the pH is in the normal range.

Correction
Respiratory alkalosis is corrected by removing the stimulus causing the hyperventilation. If hypoxemia is the stimulus, oxygen therapy is administered. If the cause is iatrogenic, the therapy causing the hyperventilation is reduced or eliminated. In patients with severe anxiety, reassurance and rebreathing exhaled air (breathing into a paper bag) to increase $PaCO_2$ may be effective.

Alveolar Hyperventilation Superimposed on Compensated Respiratory Acidosis
A patient with advanced but stable COPD and compensated respiratory acidosis may exhibit the following arterial blood gas values:

pH = 7.38
$PaCO_2$ = 58 mm Hg
HCO_3^- = 33 mEq/L

The HCO_3^- level is high because of renal compensatory activity. If the person now experiences an acute exacerbation of disease and becomes severely hypoxic, this may stimulate the peripheral chemoreceptors enough to increase alveolar ventilation and acutely decrease $PaCO_2$ despite the patient's deranged lung mechanics.

In this case, let us assume that the patient was incapable of hyperventilating enough to decrease $PaCO_2$ all the way down into the normal range. Although $PaCO_2$ is still above normal, the acute lowering of the $PaCO_2$ coupled with the preexisting high compensatory level of HCO_3^- causes the pH to swing from the acidic to the alkalotic side of normal, as the following values illustrate:

pH = 7.44
$PaCO_2$ = 50 mm Hg
HCO_3^- = 33 mEq/L

If one pays attention to only the blood gas data and applies the strict criteria for interpretation as outlined earlier in this chapter, one would arrive at the completely incorrect interpretation of compensated metabolic alkalosis. This interpretation would lead the novice to conclude that the patient is hypoventilating to compensate for a preexisting primary metabolic alkalosis; in light of this patient's medical history, this would be an absurd conclusion. This example illustrates the fact that blood gas data alone are an insufficient basis for rational acid-base assessment. The patient's medical history, the physical examination, and the nature of the current problem are vital in accurately evaluating blood gas abnormalities. The above-listed blood gases are correctly described as acute

CLINICAL FOCUS 13-5

Partially Compensated Respiratory Alkalosis Progressing to Completely Compensated (Chronic) Alkalosis

Initial Evaluation

A 38-year-old athlete is admitted to the hospital with a diagnosis of asthma. The patient complains of shortness of breath and a tight feeling in his chest and appears near panic. Breathing is labored, and the respiratory rate is high. An arterial blood gas analysis reveals the following:

pH = 7.48
$PaCO_2$ = 25 mm Hg
$[HCO_3^-]$ = 18 mEq/L

Step 1: Categorize the pH

The pH is high, indicating alkalemia.

Step 2: Determine Respiratory Involvement

The $PaCO_2$ is significantly below normal, consistent with a high pH. Hyperventilation must be a contributing factor to the high pH.

Step 3: Determine Metabolic Involvement

$[HCO_3^-]$ is substantially below normal, which by itself would decrease the pH. The high pH must be of respiratory origin alone. The low $[HCO_3^-]$ is consistent with a compensatory response by the kidneys.

Step 4: Assess for Compensation

$[HCO_3^-]$ is significantly decreased, which is the expected compensatory response by the kidneys. Because the pH is still above the normal range, not enough time has elapsed for complete compensation to occur.

Conclusion

Partially compensated respiratory alkalosis: This represents persistent alveolar hyperventilation secondary to feelings of panic and shortness of breath and possibly hypoxemia (enhanced peripheral chemoreceptor sensitivity). Therapy consists of bronchodilators, antiinflammatory drugs, and oxygen.

Reevaluation

This patient is treated with bronchodilators, inhaled steroids, and oxygen therapy. His condition slowly improves over the next 3 days, although he is still quite short of breath. Arterial blood gases, drawn on day 3 of hospitalization, reveal the following:

pH = 7.44
$PaCO_2$ = 26 mm Hg
$[HCO_3^-]$ = 17 mEq/L

Step 1: Categorize pH

The pH is in the normal range, although it is on the high (alkaline) side (>7.40).

Step 2: Determine Respiratory Involvement

$PaCO_2$ remains low, indicating hyperventilation is still present. The decreased $PaCO_2$ tends to increase the pH and helps explain the reason the pH is in the high-normal range.

Step 3: Determine Metabolic Involvement

$[HCO_3^-]$ is now even lower than before. The decreased $[HCO_3^-]$ would decrease the pH and is consistent with a compensatory response of the kidneys to the chronically low $PaCO_2$.

Step 4: Assess for Compensation

The low $[HCO_3^-]$ is the kidney's expected compensatory response to respiratory alkalosis (low $PaCO_2$). Enough time has passed for the kidneys to decrease the $[HCO_3^-]$ sufficiently to bring the pH down into the normal range. Because the pH is on the alkaline side of the normal range, the component that would produce alkalosis (i.e., $PaCO_2$ of 26 mm Hg) is the cause of the original acid-base imbalance.

Conclusion

Completely compensated (chronic) respiratory alkalosis: This represents chronic alveolar hyperventilation secondary to feelings of shortness of breath.

---

hyperventilation superimposed on compensated respiratory acidosis.

CONCEPT QUESTION 13-6

What are the clinical treatment consequences of misinterpreting acute hyperventilation superimposed on compensated respiratory acidosis as a metabolic alkalosis?

Metabolic (Nonrespiratory) Acidosis

Any process that lowers plasma $[HCO_3^-]$ is called metabolic acidosis. A reduction in the $[HCO_3^-]$ decreases the blood pH

because the amount of base relative to the amount of acid (dissolved CO_2) in the blood is reduced. The $[HCO_3^-]$-dissolved carbon dioxide ratio becomes less than 20:1 (e.g., 15:1 or 10:1). According to the Henderson-Hasselbalch equation, this produces an acid pH.

Causes

Metabolic acidosis can occur in two general ways: (1) the accumulation of fixed (nonvolatile) acid in the blood or (2) an excessive loss of HCO_3^- from the body. For example, a lack of blood flow leads to tissue hypoxia, anaerobic metabolism, and production of lactic acid (a fixed acid). The resulting accumulation of hydrogen ions reacts with bicarbonate ions, lowering the blood $[HCO_3^-]$, producing nonrespiratory or metabolic acidosis. Another example is severe diarrhea, in which large stores of HCO_3^- are lost from the bowel, again producing nonrespiratory acidosis.

Because of their different causative mechanisms, these two types of metabolic acidosis are treated differently; the identification of the underlying mechanism is necessary to treat metabolic acidosis effectively. The analysis of plasma electrolytes—specifically, the so-called **anion gap**—is helpful in determining whether metabolic acidosis was caused by a gain of fixed acids or by a loss of base.

Anion Gap

The law of electroneutrality states that the total number of positive charges in the body fluids must equal the total number of negative charges. Plasma cations (positively charged ions) are exactly balanced by anions (negatively charged ions); that is, the plasma has no net electrical charge. The routinely measured plasma electrolytes (cations and anions) in clinical medicine include only Na^+, K^+, Cl^-, and HCO_3^-, although body fluids contain many other cations and anions. The normal plasma concentrations of these routinely measured electrolytes are such that the cations (Na^+ and K^+) outnumber the anions (Cl^- and HCO_3^-), causing what seems to be an anion gap. Generally, K^+ is ignored in calculating the anion gap because of its very low concentration:

Anion gap (mEq/L) = $[Na^+]-([Cl^-] + [HCO_3^-])$

The "anion gap" can be thought of as a measure of the concentrations of other anions in the plasma besides Cl^- and HCO_3^-. Figure 13-2, *A*, shows that normal concentrations of the routinely measured electrolytes in the plasma are about 140 mEq/L for Na^+, 105 mEq/L for Cl^-, and 24 mEq/L for HCO_3^-, producing an apparent anion gap of 11 mEq/L ($140 - [105 + 24] = 11$). The normal range for the anion gap is 8 to 16 mEq/L.[3] Because $[Na^+]$ exceeds ($[Cl^-] + [HCO_3^-]$), the unmeasured anions must outnumber the unmeasured cations (see Figure 13-2, *A*). Therefore, the anion gap also can be thought of as the difference between the unmeasured anions and unmeasured cations:

Anion gap = unmeasured anions − unmeasured cations

If total anion and cation concentrations each equal 154 mEq/L (see Figure 13-2, *A*), there are normally 14 mEq/L of unmeasured cations and 25 mEq/L of unmeasured anions. Figure 13-2, *A*, shows that the anion gap is 11 mEq/L:

Anion gap = 25 (unmeasured anions) −
14 (unmeasured cations) = 11 mEq/L

Metabolic acidosis caused by an accumulation of fixed acids in the body increases the anion gap (>16 mEq/L). The hydrogen ions of these fixed acids react with HCO_3^-, lowering its concentration in the plasma. This leads to an increased number of unmeasured anions; that is, when HCO_3^- buffers the fixed acid's H^+, the anion portion of the fixed acid remains in the plasma, increasing the unmeasured anion concentration (see Figure 13-2, *B*). Therefore, a high anion gap indicates the fixed acid concentration has increased in the body. The patient's clinical history and current status help clarify which type of acid this may be. For example, in severe shock, tissue hypoxia may generate lactic acid. A history of diabetes is consistent with ketoacid formation. A history of kidney failure is consistent with uremic acidosis.

CONCEPT QUESTION 13-7

Why does the accumulation of fixed acids in the body create a high anion gap?

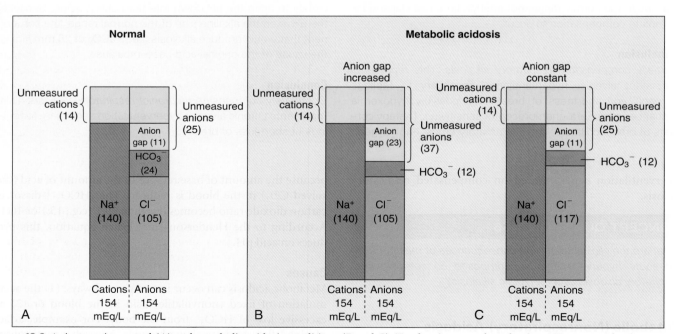

Figure 13-2 Anion gap in normal (**A**) and metabolic acidosis conditions (**B** and **C**). Total cations equal total anions. Unmeasured anions exceed unmeasured cations in all conditions. **A**, Normal anion gap. **B**, Increased anion gap in metabolic acidosis, reflecting an accumulation of fixed acid. **C**, Normal anion gap in metabolic acidosis, reflecting a loss of HCO_3^- from the body.

Metabolic acidosis caused by HCO_3^- loss from the body does not produce an increased anion gap because HCO_3^- loss is accompanied by Cl^- gain, keeping the anion gap within normal limits (see Figure 13-2, *C*). The law of electroneutrality helps explain the reciprocal nature of $[HCO_3^-]$ and $[Cl^-]$ in this situation. With a constant cation concentration, the loss of HCO_3^- means another anion must be gained to maintain electroneutrality. In this situation, the kidney increases its reabsorption of the most abundant anion in the tubular filtrate, Cl^-. (This disturbance in electroneutrality does not occur when fixed acids accumulate and are buffered by HCO_3^- because no anions are actually lost from the body in that situation.) The type of metabolic acidosis in which HCO_3^- is lost from the body is sometimes called hyperchloremic acidosis because of the characteristic increase in plasma $[Cl^-]$ that occurs. Examples of conditions in which HCO_3^- is lost or Cl^- is gained include severe diarrhea and pancreatic fistulas. A fistula is an abnormal tubelike channel connecting one body cavity to another (in this situation, abnormally connecting the pancreas to the intestinal tract). Pancreatic juice is fairly alkaline, as are all intestinal fluids below the stomach.[2] Thus much bicarbonate can be lost during prolonged diarrhea. Box 13-2 summarizes causes of anion gap and non–anion gap metabolic acidosis.

Compensation

Hyperventilation is the essential compensatory mechanism for metabolic acidosis. Plasma HCO_3^- buffers the increased plasma $[H^+]$ of metabolic acidosis, depleting the plasma $[HCO_3^-]$. In response, HCO_3^- diffuses out of the cerebrospinal fluid (CSF) into the blood, lowering the CSF pH, which stimulates the central chemoreceptors. Peripheral chemoreceptors are also directly stimulated by increased plasma $[H^+]$. The end result is increased ventilation and lowered volatile acid (H_2CO_3) and dissolved carbon dioxide levels in the blood. The $[HCO_3^-]$-dissolved carbon dioxide ratio is thus restored toward a normal 20:1 ratio, normalizing the pH. The peripheral chemoreceptor response to metabolic acidosis is rapid. Uncompensated metabolic acidosis is therefore rare, and its presence implies a ventilatory defect; that is, metabolic acidosis accompanied by a normal $PaCO_2$ means the lungs are unable to respond appropriately to chemoreceptor stimulation. The defect may lie in nerve impulse transmission, the respiratory muscles, or the lungs.

Clinical Manifestations

Metabolic acidosis generally causes a great increase in minute ventilation. Patients may complain of dyspnea and, in extreme acidosis, may descend into a stupor and coma.[3] Hyperpnea (increased tidal volume depth) is a common finding on physical examination. In severe metabolic acidosis (e.g., diabetic ketoacidosis), an extremely deep, gasping type of breathing develops, called **Kussmaul's respiration**.

Arterial pH values less than 7.00 to 7.10 predispose the heart to potentially fatal ventricular arrhythmias and can reduce not only heart muscle contractility but also the heart's ability to increase its contractile force in response to the body's secretion of catecholamines, such as epinephrine.[3] Neurological symptoms range from lethargy to coma in severe metabolic acidosis (see Figure 13-1).

Correction

The initial goal in treating severe acidemia is to raise the arterial pH above 7.2, a level at which serious cardiac arrhythmias are less likely, contractility is restored, and responsiveness to catecholamines improves.[2] If increased ventilation maintains the pH at or above this level, immediate corrective action is usually not indicated. Treatment should be focused on correction of the underlying metabolic disorder. For example, in diabetic acidosis, insulin is given; in shock-induced lactic acidosis, measures are taken to improve blood pressure and cardiac output.

Historically, sodium bicarbonate ($NaHCO_3$) was routinely infused during cardiac arrest to combat the lactic acidosis of tissue hypoxia; this practice has generally been discontinued. The 2010 American Heart Association (AHA) Guidelines for Cardiopulmonary Resuscitation and Emergency Cardiovascular Care recommend against the routine use of $NaHCO_3$ in cardiac arrest because of the lack of evidence showing improved survival, and because of the negative side effects of $NaHCO_3$, which include intracellular acidosis, cardiac arrhythmias, and inhibited hemoglobin release of oxygen.[4] The AHA maintains that rapid return of spontaneous circulation (ROSC) through effective cardiopulmonary resuscitation is the mainstay of restoring acid-base balance during cardiac arrest. Rapid correction of arterial pH to values greater than 7.20 by $NaHCO_3$ infusion can be harmful for the following reasons: when HCO_3^- buffers H^+, the hydration reaction moves to the left, rapidly producing carbon dioxide, which quickly diffuses across the blood-brain barrier into the CSF. Because blood HCO_3^- cannot follow carbon dioxide across the blood-brain barrier, the CSF rapidly becomes more acidic, possibly aggravating the neurological

---

BOX 13-2

Causes of Anion Gap and Non–Anion Gap Metabolic Acidosis

High Anion Gap
Metabolically produced gain of acid
    Lactic acidosis
    Ketoacidosis
    Renal failure (e.g., retained sulfuric acid)
Ingestion of acids
    Salicylate intoxication (aspirin)
    Methanol (formic acid)
    Ethylene glycol (oxalic acid)

Normal Anion Gap (Hyperchloremic Acidosis)
Gastrointestinal loss of HCO_3^-
    Diarrhea
    Pancreatic fistula
Renal tubular loss: failure to reabsorb HCO_3^-
    Renal tubular acidosis
Ingestion
    Ammonium chloride
    Hyperalimentation intravenous nutrition

symptoms (coma) of metabolic acidosis.[2] The decreased CSF pH increases central chemoreceptor stimulation, causing the successfully resuscitated patient to hyperventilate, which coupled with the prior $NaHCO_3$ infusion may rapidly swing the previously acidotic arterial pH into an alkalotic range. In the same way, carbon dioxide produced by the buffering action of $NaHCO_3$ diffuses rapidly across all cell membranes, including the cell membranes of the heart; this may precipitate cardiac arrhythmias.[3] Intracellular pH generally tends to decrease with the rapid infusion of $NaHCO_3$ because carbon dioxide diffuses across cell membranes into the cell much more rapidly than bicarbonate ions.[3] The 2010 AHA Guidelines list special circumstances in which $NaHCO_3$ infusion may be beneficial during cardiac arrest such as in patients with preexisting metabolic acidosis, and in patients with severe hyperkalemia (high plasma potassium concentration).

CONCEPT QUESTION 13-8

Why would intravenous administration of $NaHCO_3$ to a patient with severe metabolic acidosis during cardiopulmonary resuscitation require the rescuer to increase the minute ventilation?

Metabolic (Nonrespiratory) Alkalosis

Metabolic alkalosis is associated with increased plasma $[HCO_3^-]$ or the loss of H^+ ions. However, elevated $[HCO_3^-]$ is not diagnostic of a primary metabolic alkalosis because it may represent renal compensation for respiratory acidosis. An increased $[HCO_3^-]$ relative to the dissolved plasma carbon dioxide raises the blood pH because it increases the $[HCO_3^-]$-dissolved carbon dioxide ratio.

Causes

Metabolic alkalosis can occur in two general ways: (1) loss of fixed acids or (2) gain of blood buffer base. Both processes produce an increased plasma $[HCO_3^-]$. It is easy to understand why plasma $[HCO_3^-]$ increases if it is ingested or administered

intravenously. It is not as apparent why $[HCO_3^-]$ increases when fixed acids are lost from the body. For an explanation of this phenomenon, consider a situation in which vomiting or nasogastric suction removes gastric hydrochloric acid (HCl) from the body (Figure 13-3). In response to HCl loss, H^+ diffuses out of the gastric cell, accompanied by Cl^- from the blood. The loss of H^+ forces the carbon dioxide hydration reaction in the gastric cell to the right, which generates HCO_3^-; the HCO_3^- ion diffuses into the blood in exchange for Cl^-. Thus, the plasma gains a bicarbonate ion for each chloride ion (or hydrogen ion) lost (see Figure 13-3).[5]

Box 13-3 summarizes the causes of metabolic alkalosis. Increased HCO_3^- ingestion rarely causes metabolic alkalosis because the normal kidney can rapidly excrete large amounts of HCO_3^- in the urine.[2] Metabolic alkalosis is most often caused by the loss of gastric acid through protracted vomiting or continuous nasogastric suctioning.[3] It is also caused by hypochloremia (low plasma $[Cl^-]$) and hypokalemia (low plasma $[K^+]$). Metabolic alkalosis is quite common in acutely ill patients and probably the most complicated acid-base imbalance to treat because it involves fluid and electrolyte imbalances. Many causes of metabolic alkalosis are iatrogenic, resulting from the use of diuretics, low-salt diets, and nasogastric drainage.

The mechanisms by which volume depletion, hypokalemia, and hypochloremia produce alkalosis are discussed in Chapter 22. Briefly, the kidney's strong stimulus to reabsorb Na^+ from the renal tubule filtrate is predominant over its need to maintain chloride, potassium, or acid-base balance. A low plasma $[Cl^-]$ (hypochloremia) produces a low tubular filtrate Cl^- concentration; this presents a special problem because chloride ions must accompany sodium ions when they are reabsorbed from the tubular filtrate. If chloride ions are scarce (as may be induced by diuretic therapy, low-salt diets, or gastric HCl loss), the kidney reabsorbs Na^+ by secreting abnormally large amounts of H^+ and K^+ into the filtrate. In other words, these ions are secreted in exchange for Na^+ to maintain electroneutrality of the filtrate. This process leads to alkalosis (H^+ loss) and hypokalemia

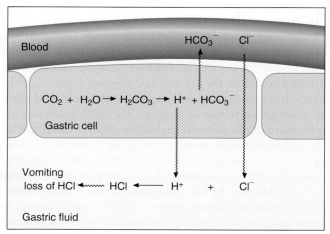

Figure 13-3 Generation of plasma HCO_3^- by gastric H^+ loss. For each H^+ lost, one HCO_3^- is generated, increasing plasma HCO_3^- and causing metabolic alkalosis.

BOX 13-3

Causes of Metabolic Alkalosis (Increased Plasma $[HCO_3^-]$)

Loss of Hydrogen Ions
Gastrointestinal loss
  Vomiting
  Nasogastric drainage
Renal loss
  Diuretics (loss of chloride, potassium, fluid volume)
  Hypochloremia (increased H^+ secretion and HCO_3^- reabsorption)
  Hypokalemia (increased H^+ secretion and HCO_3^- reabsorption)
  Hypovolemia (increased H^+ secretion)

Retention of Bicarbonate Ions
$NaHCO_3$ infusion or ingestion

CLINICAL FOCUS 13-6

Partially Compensated Metabolic Acidosis

A 17-year-old girl enters the emergency department. She is conscious and breathing rapidly and deeply. She has a history of diabetes. Arterial blood gas values are as follows:

pH = 7.10
$PaCO_2$ = 20 mm Hg
$[HCO_3^-]$ = 6 mEq/L
$[Cl^-]$ = 105 mEq/L
$[Na^+]$ = 145 mEq/L

Step 1: Categorize the pH
The pH is well below the normal range, indicating severe acidemia.

Step 2: Determine Respiratory Involvement
The $PaCO_2$ is far below normal. A $PaCO_2$ at this level indicates severe hyperventilation. The decreased $PaCO_2$ by itself would cause alkalemia. Considering the severe acidemia, the decreased $PaCO_2$ is probably a compensatory response to a primary metabolic acidosis, although it is not low enough to raise the pH to the normal range.

Step 3: Determine Metabolic Involvement
$[HCO_3^-]$ is severely reduced, consistent with the low pH. The low $[HCO_3^-]$ must be responsible for the low pH in this patient; acidosis must be of metabolic origin.

Step 4: Assess for Compensation
The decreased $PaCO_2$ represents severe hyperventilation, an expected compensatory response to the severe metabolic acidosis. However, compensation is incomplete, as evidenced by the low pH.

Conclusion
*Partially compensated metabolic acidosis**: The $PaCO_2$ of 20 mm Hg represents extreme alveolar hyperventilation in an attempt to compensate for severe diabetes-induced metabolic acidosis. Corrective therapy includes infusion of insulin. The apparent anion gap is greatly increased: 145 − (105 + 6) = 34 mEq/L. This increased anion gap is consistent with the gain of abnormal ketoacids seen in untreated diabetes; that is, plasma $[HCO_3^-]$ decreases in the process of buffering these acids.

*One could argue that the severe acidemia (pH of 7.10) represents uncompensated metabolic acidosis; however, if the $PaCO_2$ were normal, the pH would be even lower.

CLINICAL FOCUS 13-7

Compensated Metabolic Acidosis

A 15-year-old girl has had diarrhea for a week. She told her mother that she has been taking laxatives in an attempt to lose weight. Arterial blood gas values are as follows:

pH = 7.36
$PaCO_2$ = 22 mm Hg
$[HCO_3^-]$ = 12 mEq/L

Step 1: Categorize the pH
The pH is in the normal range, although it is on the acid side.

Step 2: Determine Respiratory Involvement
The $PaCO_2$ is below normal. A decreased $PaCO_2$ indicates hyperventilation, which by itself can cause alkalemia. However, alkalemia is not present. The decreased $PaCO_2$ is consistent with a compensatory response to low $[HCO_3^-]$.

Step 3: Determine Metabolic Involvement
$[HCO_3^-]$ is below normal, which by itself would cause a low pH. Considering the coexisting low $PaCO_2$ and the pH on the acid side, the low $[HCO_3^-]$ must be the primary cause of the acid-base disturbance.

Step 4: Assess for Compensation
The decreased $PaCO_2$ (hyperventilation) is the expected compensatory response to metabolic acidosis (decreased $[HCO_3^-]$). Hyperventilation is sufficient to bring the pH up to the normal range. Because the pH is on the acid side of the normal range, the component that would produce an acidosis (i.e., $[HCO_3^-]$ of 12 mEq/L) is the cause of the original acid-base imbalance.

Conclusion
Completely compensated metabolic acidosis: This represents chronic hyperventilation to compensate for metabolic acidosis secondary to severe diarrhea and loss of HCO_3^-.

occurs because alkalemia eventually leads to CSF alkalosis, decreasing the stimulation of central chemoreceptors. During hypoventilation, the increase in $PaCO_2$ increases the plasma carbonic acid concentration, offsetting the metabolically generated alkalosis. On average, the $PaCO_2$ increases about 0.7 mm Hg for every 1-mEq/L increase in plasma $[HCO_3^-]$.[6]

Traditionally, the belief was that the hypoxemia induced by hypoventilation limited respiratory compensation for metabolic alkalosis. In other words, as P_ACO_2 increases during hypoventilation, P_AO_2 decreases, leading to hypoxemia, which would stimulate peripheral chemoreceptors and counteract compensatory hypoventilation. However, more recent evidence contradicts this theory; alkalosis blunts the sensitivity of the carotid bodies to hypoxemia (see Chapter 11). Alkalemic patients with

(K^+ loss). Volume depletion (hypovolemia) induced by diuretics exaggerates alkalosis and hypokalemia because hypovolemia profoundly increases the kidney's Na^+ reabsorption stimulus.

Compensation
The expected respiratory response to metabolic alkalosis is hypoventilation and carbon dioxide retention. This response

PaO_2 values less than 50 mm Hg may hypoventilate to $PaCO_2$ values much greater than 60 mm Hg.[6]

Underlying pulmonary disease may also limit compensatory hypoventilation in metabolic alkalosis. Pulmonary edema, fibrosis, vascular congestion, and inflammatory processes such as pneumonia stimulate intrapulmonary irritant receptors in airway walls and J-receptors in the alveolar interstitium. Such stimulation causes tachypnea and hyperventilation, which may limit compensatory hypoventilation and carbon dioxide retention.[2,6] Other factors that tend to limit compensatory hypoventilation for metabolic alkalosis include anxiety, pain, infection, and fever.

Symptoms

Symptoms directly related to metabolic alkalemia are most likely related to causative factors (e.g., volume depletion [weakness and dizziness on standing] and hypokalemia [muscle weakness and high urine output]). As with respiratory alkalosis, patients may exhibit hyperactive reflexes, muscle cramping, and possibly tetanic convulsions.[3] Similar to acidosis, severe alkalosis may also induce cardiac arrhythmias. Alkalosis, whether of respiratory or metabolic origin, promotes the movement of K^+ into the cells, creating a hypokalemia that also can contribute to cardiac arrhythmias.

Correction

Corrective action is aimed at the underlying causes of metabolic alkalosis (e.g., restoring normal fluid volume, potassium, and chloride levels). After these fluids and electrolytes are restored to normal levels, the kidney can reabsorb Na^+ normally (i.e., Cl^- can be reabsorbed with Na^+). The kidney does not need to reabsorb HCO_3^- with Na^+ as it did when Cl^- was scarce; this allows excess HCO_3^- to be excreted in the urine. Restoring plasma K^+ levels causes K^+ to diffuse into the red blood cells in exchange for H^+, which moves out of the cell into the plasma. This reciprocal shift of K^+ and H^+ helps bring the plasma pH back toward normal.[2]

In extremely severe metabolic alkalosis (pH >7.55), acidifying agents such as dilute HCl or ammonium chloride may be infused intravenously.[3] (The liver metabolizes NH_4Cl, producing HCl.)

CLINICAL FOCUS 13-8

Uncompensated Metabolic Alkalosis

A 68-year-old man is admitted to the hospital for treatment of dehydration. The man's son states that his father has been vomiting for 36 hours and is unable to keep clear liquids down. An arterial blood gas analysis reveals the following:

pH = 7.57
$PaCO_2$ = 45 mm Hg
$[HCO_3^-]$ = 40 mEq/L

Step 1: Categorize the pH
The pH is high, indicating the presence of an alkalemia.

Step 2: Determine Respiratory Involvement
$PaCO_2$ is in the normal range. It cannot be contributing to the high pH.

Step 3: Determine Metabolic Involvement
$[HCO_3^-]$ is elevated, consistent with a high pH. The increased $[HCO_3^-]$ must be responsible for the high pH because $PaCO_2$ is in the normal range.

Step 4: Assess for Compensation
The lungs would be expected to hypoventilate (increase $PaCO_2$) to compensate for the metabolic alkalosis. However, $PaCO_2$ is still in the normal range.

Conclusion
Uncompensated metabolic alkalosis, secondary to dehydration and loss of H^+ from prolonged vomiting.

CLINICAL FOCUS 13-9

Compensated Metabolic Alkalosis

A 57-year-old woman in the intensive care unit has a nasogastric tube placed through her nose and into her stomach. This tube is attached to a suction device that empties her gastric contents. Her arterial blood gases reveal the following:

pH = 7.44
$PaCO_2$ = 49 mm Hg
$[HCO_3^-]$ = 32 mEq/L

Step 1: Categorize pH
The pH is in the normal range, although on the alkalotic side.

Step 2: Determine the Respiratory Involvement
The $PaCO_2$ is above normal, which by itself would cause acidemia. Because acidemia is not present, the elevated $PaCO_2$ is consistent with a compensatory response to the increased $[HCO_3^-]$.

Step 3: Determine Metabolic Involvement
$[HCO_3^-]$ is elevated, which by itself would cause alkalemia. Considering the coexisting high $PaCO_2$ and the pH on the alkaline side of the normal range, the factor that would cause alkalemia (increased $[HCO_3^-]$) must be the primary acid-base disturbance.

Step 4: Assess for Compensation
Hypoventilation (increased $PaCO_2$) is the expected compensatory response to metabolic alkalosis. In this case, hypoventilation was sufficient to bring pH down into the normal range. The pH is on the alkaline side of the normal range. The component that would cause alkalosis ($[HCO_3^-]$ of 32 mEq/L) was the cause of the original acid-base imbalance.

Conclusion
Completely compensated metabolic alkalosis: The original alkalosis was caused by loss of gastric HCl owing to continuous nasogastric suction.

Metabolic Acid-Base Disturbance Indicators

As discussed previously, plasma [HCO_3^-] is the indicator for metabolic acid-base disturbances. However, [HCO_3^-] has its shortcomings in this regard because it is affected to some extent by respiratory changes (i.e., changes in $PaCO_2$). (The effect of the carbon dioxide hydration reaction on plasma [HCO_3^-] was discussed earlier.) Thus, [HCO_3^-] is not a pure index of metabolic acid-base disturbances.

Standard Bicarbonate

The **standard bicarbonate (SB)** laboratory procedure was developed to eliminate the respiratory component's ($PaCO_2$) effect on [HCO_3^-]. SB is defined as the plasma [HCO_3^-] measured at 37° C after a laboratory blood sample has been exposed to and equilibrated with a gas having a PCO_2 of 40 mm Hg; this eliminates the effect of an abnormal $PaCO_2$ on [HCO_3^-]. If an abnormal [HCO_3^-] (<22 mEq/L or >26 mEq/L) persists in the presence of a PCO_2 of 40 mm Hg, a metabolic acid-base disturbance is theoretically present.

SB has shortcomings as a purely metabolic index. The laboratory (in vitro) process of bringing the blood sample's PCO_2 to 40 mm Hg creates an artificial condition not present in the patient's body (in vivo conditions). For example, if a patient has an increased $PaCO_2$, this would increase plasma [HCO_3^-] slightly as a result of the hydration reaction. This increased plasma [HCO_3^-] would establish equilibrium with the fluid outside of the blood capillaries (extravascular fluid). The fluid outside of the capillaries would develop an equally increased [HCO_3^-]. If the patient increased the alveolar ventilation, bringing the $PaCO_2$ back down to 40 mm Hg, the hydration reaction would reverse directions, and the plasma [HCO_3^-] would decrease slightly. Consequently, the extravascular HCO_3^- would diffuse back into the capillary until equilibrium is reestablished between intravascular and extravascular [HCO_3^-]. These exchanges between intravascular and extravascular fluid cannot take place in laboratory conditions. When PCO_2 of a laboratory blood sample is artificially lowered to 40 mm Hg, plasma [HCO_3^-] decreases, as it would in the body, but extravascular HCO_3^- is not present and cannot diffuse into the plasma as it does in the body; this in vivo–in vitro discrepancy is a limitation of the SB measurement.

CONCEPT QUESTION 13-9

Is the SB measurement (in vitro) falsely low or falsely high compared with the true [HCO_3^-] in the body (in vivo)?

Base Excess

Similar to the SB measurement, the **base excess (BE)** is also obtained by exposing a blood sample in the laboratory to a gas with a constant PCO_2 of 40 mm Hg at 37° C. When the blood sample PCO_2 is brought to 40 mm Hg, the sample pH changes. In the next step of the procedure, the blood gas machine calculates the milliequivalents of acid or base needed to bring the blood sample pH to 7.40, holding the pH constant at 40 mm Hg.

The first step (bringing the blood sample PCO_2 to 40 mm Hg) theoretically eliminates any respiratory contribution to the acid-base imbalance, whereas the second step quantifies the amount of base that must be removed or added to the blood to bring its pH to 7.40. If the pH of the original blood sample rose above 7.40 (became alkalotic) after the sample PCO_2 was brought to 40 mm Hg, a nonrespiratory (metabolic) process must be responsible for the alkalosis. The milliequivalents of strong acid required to bring the blood pH to 7.40 is exactly equal to the milliequivalents of excess base the original blood sample contained. This calculated BE is reported in milliequivalents per liter (mEq/L). If the blood sample pH fell after it was exposed to a PCO_2 of 40 mm Hg, the blood gas machine computes the quantity of strong base needed to bring the blood pH up to 7.40, which would be exactly equal to the amount of base the original blood sample lacked (base deficit).

By convention, BE is reported as either a positive or a negative number; a positive BE indicates an alkalosis of metabolic origin, and a negative BE indicates an acidosis of metabolic origin. Normal BE is ±2 mEq/L. The BE determination has the same limitations as the SB; in vitro conditions differ from in vivo conditions, and the same discrepancy occurs.

The use of BE to determine whether acid-base disturbances are metabolic in origin can be easily misinterpreted. For example, in a patient with compensated respiratory acidosis, the arterial blood has a high $PaCO_2$, which is compensated by a high [HCO_3^-] that keeps arterial pH in the normal range. In determining the BE, high $PaCO_2$ of this patient's blood sample is abruptly reduced to 40 mm Hg in the laboratory, which produces an alkalotic pH because the blood [HCO_3^-] is still high; large amounts of acid must be titrated to bring the blood sample pH to 7.40. This process may lead some clinicians to believe that too much base is present in the blood, which might be incorrectly interpreted as a primary metabolic alkalosis that requires treatment. The high BE in this case would simply be a reflection of secondary renal compensation, not a primary metabolic alkalosis.

Expected pH Relationships

Table 13-3 illustrates acute $PaCO_2$ and pH relationships. If $PaCO_2$ changes suddenly as a result of an acute ventilatory change, the subsequent change in pH must be caused by the change in $PaCO_2$ (i.e., a respiratory change). The expected pH for a given acute change in $PaCO_2$ can be precisely predicted

TABLE 13-3
Acute Arterial Carbon Dioxide Pressure–pH Relationship

PaCO₂ Change	pH Change
Decrease	Increase
1 mm Hg	0.01
10 mm Hg	0.10
Increase	Decrease
1 mm Hg	0.006
10 mm Hg	0.06

using the Henderson-Hasselbalch equation. Table 13-3 illustrates this relationship. If PCO_2 acutely increases by 20 mm Hg, the pH should decrease by (20 × 0.006), or 0.12 units, producing an expected pH of 7.28 (i.e., [7.40 − 0.12] = 7.28). This calculated expected pH differs from the actual measured blood pH only if a metabolic acid-base disturbance is present. For example, if the actual measured pH is more acidic than the calculated expected pH, nonrespiratory metabolic factors are causing the acidosis. Likewise, if the actual measured pH is more alkalotic than the expected pH, the alkalosis must be of metabolic origin. The following pH formulas can be derived from Table 13-3 and used to determine whether a measured abnormal pH is strictly due to the abnormal PCO_2 or whether the abnormal pH is partly due to nonrespiratory (metabolic) factors:

- If measured $PaCO_2$ is less than 40 mm Hg, the following is true:

  Expected pH = 7.40 + (40 mm Hg − measured $PaCO_2$) 0.01

- If measured $PaCO_2$ is greater than 40 mm Hg, the following is true:

  Expected pH = 7.40 − (measured $PaCO_2$ − 40 mm Hg) 0.006

If expected and measured pH values are identical, the metabolic status must be normal. If the two pH values are not equal, metabolic factors must be involved in the acid-base imbalance. A normal metabolic status is present if the measured and calculated pH values are within ±0.03 units of each other.

Combined Acid-Base Disturbances

A combined acid-base disturbance is one in which respiratory and metabolic factors join to promote the same type of acid-base disturbance. Consider the following blood gas results:

pH = 7.10
$PaCO_2$ = 50 mm Hg
HCO_3^- = 15 mEq/L

The acidotic pH is caused by both respiratory ($PaCO_2$) and metabolic (HCO_3^-) factors. Two primary disturbances coexist in this example. In combined acid-base disturbances the concept of compensation does not apply. These blood gases may occur in a cardiopulmonary arrest. Lack of ventilation leads to respiratory acidosis, and lack of blood flow leads to tissue hypoxia and lactic acidosis.

Stewart's Strong Ion Approach to Acid-Base Balance

In the early 1980s, Stewart, a mathematician and biophysicist, introduced the **strong ion** approach to the study of acid-base physiology. Stewart's physicochemical perspective is controversial because it refutes the time-honored Henderson-Hasselbalch approach. Although the Henderson-Hasselbalch approach to acid-base analysis is appropriate from a practical clinical standpoint, a basic overview of the strong ion approach is presented here to acquaint the reader with the concepts involved.

In the strong ion approach, substances that affect acid-base balance in body fluids are classified into three groups, based on their degree of dissociation in aqueous solution: strong ions, weak ions, and nonelectrolytes. Strong ions (e.g., Na^+ and Cl^-) are always fully dissociated, existing only as ions in aqueous solutions. (The term "strong" means strongly dissociated.) In other words, the number of strong ions in body fluids can never be changed by conversion back to the parent compound (e.g., NaCl or KCl), as occurs with weak ions. Weak ions are produced from compounds that only partially (weakly) dissociate in solution, including volatile CO_2-related carbonic acid ions (HCO_3^- and H^+) and nonvolatile acid ions such as phosphates and proteins.[8] Weak acids dissociate until they reach equilibrium with their component ions, each in accordance with its unique equilibrium constant (see Chapter 10). The nonvolatile weak acids include proteins (chiefly albumin) and inorganic phosphates. Nonelectrolytes are substances that never dissociate in solution but contribute to the solution's osmotic pressure; thus they affect the movement of ions and water across biological membranes that separate body fluids.

Independent Variables That Affect [H^+]: [SID], [A_{TOT}], and [CO_2]

Stewart distinguished between independent and dependent variables involved in [H^+] regulation. He showed through a series of complex equations that the [H^+] of a solution is a dependent variable determined solely by three independent variables:[9] (1) **strong ion difference** [SID]; (2) total concentration of nonvolatile weak acids [A_{TOT}]; and (3) dissolved [CO_2], which is a function of PCO_2. The [SID] is the summative difference between the concentrations of all strong cations (positively charged ions) and all strong anions (negatively charged ions) in body fluids; for clinical purposes, [SID] = ([Na^+] + [K^+] + [Ca^{++}] + [Mg^{++}]) − ([Cl^-] + [unidentified strong anions]).[8,9] Normal body fluids contain more strong cations than strong anions[8]; the [SID] thus represents a net positive charge that must be balanced by weak anions in solution, as explained in the following paragraphs. The kidneys are responsible for maintaining a normal [SID] of about 40 to 42 mEq/L, primarily by excreting or reabsorbing Na^+, K^+, and Cl^- ions.

Stewart's theory of acid-base assessment rests on three basic assumptions about physiological solutions:[3] (1) All solutions must obey the powerful principle of electrical neutrality; that is, the sum of all strong and weak cations must equal the sum of all strong and weak anions. (2) All weak nonvolatile acids in body fluids attain equilibrium with their dissociated ions according to their equilibrium constants (law of mass action). (3) The total amount of a substance in solution must remain constant unless it is added, removed, generated, or destroyed (conservation of mass).

The principle of electrical neutrality demands that the normal [SID] of body fluids, which represents a net positive charge, must be equal to the net negative charge of all weak anions in solution, that is, anions contributed by volatile and nonvolatile weak acids.[8] This principle means that normally the [SID] is equal to [HCO_3^-] + [A^-], or, stated differently, the [SID] is equal to the sum of the bicarbonate [HCO_3^-] and nonbicarbonate [A^-] buffers, or the total buffer base (see Chapter 10). The number of weak anions supplied by volatile acid (i.e., HCO_3^- originating from H_2CO_3) is determined by the independent variable, PCO_2, which is controlled by ventilation. The number of weak anions supplied by all nonvolatile weak acids is determined by the dissociation constant (temperature dependent) of the independent variable $[A_{TOT}]$. The total amount of nonvolatile weak acid present ($[A_{TOT}]$) at any given time is constant, such that $[A_{TOT}] = [H^+] + [A^-]$, where the universal symbols H^+ and A^- represent dissociated weak acid molecules. All weak acids in the plasma can be treated as a single acid because they are in equilibrium with the same solution; the dissociation of this combined weak acid group is represented by $HA \leftrightharpoons H^+ + A^-$, which has an *apparent* dissociation constant that determines the number of weak anions contributed by $[A_{TOT}]$ in balancing the positive [SID].

At any given time, $PaCO_2$ is determined by ventilation, and the dissociation of $[A_{TOT}]$ is determined by its apparent dissociation constant. With these two independent variables predetermined, a change in the [SID] generates powerful electrochemical forces that cause H_2O molecules to dissociate or reassociate in a way that maintains electrical neutrality. In this way, changes in the [SID] affect the solution's $[H^+]$; a decrease in the [SID] (a decrease in net positive charges) increases H_2O dissociation, liberating more H^+ to maintain electrical neutrality, whereas an increase in the [SID] (an increase in net positive charges) has the opposite effect.[8] (This is consistent with a decrease or increase in total buffer base.)

Determinants of Metabolic Acid-Base Balance: [SID] and [A$_{TOT}$]

In Stewart's system, metabolic (nonrespiratory) acid-base disturbances can be caused only by changes in [SID] and nonvolatile weak acid concentration $[A_{TOT}]$, not by changes in $[HCO_3^-]$. Stewart asserts that $[HCO_3^-]$ and $[H^+]$ are dependent variables, that is, dependent on the [SID], $[A_{TOT}]$, and PCO_2. In this scheme, the kidneys manipulate the [SID] to change the plasma $[H^+]$ by excreting or reabsorbing Na^+, K^+, and Cl^-. The kidneys place priority on keeping $[Na^+]$ constant to maintain intravascular volume. $[K^+]$, $[Ca^{++}]$, and $[Mg^{++}]$ do not vary enough to affect the [SID] significantly; the kidneys change the [SID] primarily by excreting or reabsorbing Cl^- ions.[8] With a constant $[Na^+]$, an increase in plasma $[Cl^-]$ reduces the [SID], causing hyperchloremic acidosis, whereas a decrease in plasma $[Cl^-]$ causes hypochloremic alkalosis; these changes cause equal magnitude losses and gains in $[HCO_3^-]$. Thus, in responding to metabolic acid-base disturbances, the kidney does not manipulate the HCO_3^- ion; instead it regulates the [SID], primarily by controlling $[Cl^-]$.

This perspective is a departure from the Henderson-Hasselbalch concept of acid-base balance in which $[HCO_3^-]$ is treated as though it varies independently of dissolved $[CO_2]$, independently influencing pH or $[H^+]$. However, in reality, $[HCO_3^-]$ and $[CO_2]$ cannot vary independently of each other as the CO_2 hydration reaction clearly shows; instead, both $[HCO_3^-]$ and $[H^+]$ depend on $[CO_2]$:[9]

$$CO_2 + H_2O \leftrightharpoons H_2CO_3 \leftrightharpoons HCO_3^- + H^+$$

Changes in $[HCO_3^-]$ cannot cause changes in $[H^+]$; changes in $[HCO_3^-]$ and $[H^+]$ are merely correlated with each other. Therefore, it would seem that $[HCO_3^-]$ cannot be a valid indicator of metabolic acid-base disturbances.

Clinical Practicality of Strong Ion Approach

The complex nature of the equations involved in Stewart's strong ion approach make this method clinically unwieldy; knowledge of protein and phosphate concentrations is required for accurate acid-base assessment. PCO_2 and pH can be easily and directly measured in the clinical setting, and $[HCO_3^-]$ can be calculated with sufficient precision using the Henderson-Hasselbalch equation; there is no need to calculate $[HCO_3^-]$ and pH from the concentrations of electrolytes and weak acids, which are often unknown.[3] Although the strong ion approach is a more conceptually correct approach, it is not sufficiently superior to the Henderson-Hasselbalch approach in the clinical context to merit its universal adoption. It is reasonable and clinically appropriate to explain metabolic acid-base physiology in terms of $[H^+]$ and $[HCO_3^-]$ from the Henderson-Hasselbalch perspective.[3,8,10] Hence, the traditional approach is retained in this book.

ASSESSMENT AND TREATMENT OF HYPOXIA

When room air is breathed, a low PaO_2 can coexist with a normal or low $PaCO_2$; that is, poor oxygenation can coexist with ventilation that adequately eliminates CO_2. However, hypoventilation cannot coexist with normal oxygenation while breathing room air because hypoventilation always leads to an increased P_ACO_2, which mandates a reciprocal decrease in P_AO_2. For this reason, oxygenation should be evaluated separately from ventilation; adequate ventilation does not imply adequate oxygenation.

Tissue oxygenation cannot be adequately evaluated by examining only the PaO_2 and SaO_2 (see Chapter 8). The focus in evaluating oxygenation must always be on oxygen delivery to the tissues. This process involves the breathing of an adequate concentration of oxygen (F_IO_2), the efficient transfer of oxygen from the alveolus to arterial blood (P_AO_2-PaO_2 relationship), the maintenance of an adequate blood oxygen-carrying capacity (hemoglobin concentration), and adequate oxygen transport to all body tissues (blood flow or cardiac output). The clinician must consider all of these factors to assess oxygenation status adequately.

Classifying Tissue Hypoxia

Traditionally, the causes of tissue hypoxia have been classified arbitrarily into four categories: *h*ypoxic hypoxia, *a*nemic hypoxia, *s*tagnant (hypoperfusion) hypoxia, and *h*istotoxic hypoxia; the acronym *HASH* helps one recall these categories. Table 13-4 summarizes the characteristics of these four different types of hypoxia. One can make appropriate, effective treatment decisions only if one understands the root causes of hypoxia.

Hypoxic Hypoxia (Decreased P$_A$O$_2$)

Hypoxic hypoxia refers to mechanisms that decrease the alveolar PO_2 (see Table 13-4). These mechanisms (hypoventilation, shunt, $\dot{V}/\dot{Q}$ mismatch, and high-altitude breathing) were

TABLE 13-4
Classification of Hypoxia

Category	Mean P_AO_2	PaO_2	CaO_2	$C\bar{v}O_2$	Oxygen Delivery	Helped by Higher F_IO_2?
Hypoxic hypoxia						
Hypoventilation	Low	Low	Low	Low	Low	Yes
High altitude	Low	Low	Low	Low	Low	Yes
Absolute shunt	Low	Low	Low	Low	Low	Limited*
$\dot{V}/\dot{Q}$ mismatch	Low	Low	Low	Low	Low	Yes
Anemic hypoxia						
Low hemoglobin	Normal	Normal	Low	Low	Low	No*
Carbon monoxide poisoning	Normal	Normal	Low	Low	Low	Yes
Stagnant (hypoperfusion)						
Shock (heart failure)	Normal	Normal	Normal	Low	Low	No*
Histotoxic hypoxia						
Cyanide poisoning	Normal	Normal	Normal	High	Normal	No
Diffusion defect	Normal	Low	Low	Low	Low	Yes

*Although its effectiveness is limited, oxygen therapy is generally administered in these clinical conditions. The small gains in CaO_2 may be critical in severely hypoxic patients, especially patients with myocardial hypoxia and cardiac arrest.

discussed in detail in Chapter 12. In shunt, the PO_2 of collapsed or otherwise airless alveoli is effectively 0 mm Hg, reducing the overall average P_AO_2. Likewise, in $\dot{V}/\dot{Q}$ mismatch, P_AO_2 of underventilated lung regions is low, reducing the mean P_AO_2. Alveolar hypoxia produces low PaO_2 values, leading to low arterial oxygen content and reduced oxygen delivery to the tissues. As discussed in Chapter 12, the effectiveness of oxygen therapy is limited in shunt because the added oxygen cannot reach collapsed alveoli. Treatment in this situation must be aimed at reopening and ventilating collapsed alveoli.

Anemic Hypoxia (Decreased Hemoglobin Concentration)
Anemia refers to low amounts of functional hemoglobin in the blood; this can be caused by the loss of hemoglobin (hemorrhage), decreased red blood cell production, abnormal hemoglobin production, or inability of the hemoglobin molecule to bind chemically with oxygen. All forms of anemia reduce the blood's oxygen-carrying capacity and reduce oxygen delivery to the tissues. Carbon monoxide poisoning produces a functional anemia by aggressively binding with the hemoglobin molecule, rendering it unable to bind oxygen.

Carbon monoxide poisoning occurs in the setting of smoke inhalation from house fires, automobile exhaust, or poorly ventilated charcoal fires or gas furnaces. Oxygen therapy cannot add much oxygen to the blood because the available functional hemoglobin is already almost 100% saturated with room air breathing. Nevertheless, oxygen breathing hastens the displacement of carbon monoxide from the hemoglobin molecule, and the administration of 100% inspired oxygen is extremely important in treating carbon monoxide poisoning. The ideal treatment of this condition involves hyperbaric oxygen therapy, in which the individual's body is placed in an oxygen-enriched environment pressurized above atmospheric pressure (i.e., a hyperbaric oxygen chamber). In this way, PaO_2 and the amount of oxygen dissolved in the plasma can be raised far above values achievable while breathing 100% oxygen at atmospheric pressure; this significantly increases the total amount of oxygen the blood can carry. In addition, the extremely high plasma oxygen pressure facilitates the release of carbon monoxide by the hemoglobin molecule, shortening the half-life of carbon monoxide. Severe anemia caused by blood loss or decreased red blood cell production may be treated by blood transfusion (see Chapter 8).

Stagnant Hypoxia (Decreased Blood Flow)
Low blood flow and blood pressure—that is, low oxygen-delivery rate—are general features of shock. Low blood flow may be caused by cardiac (pump) failure or by low blood volume (hypovolemia) caused by hemorrhage or severe dehydration. In such instances, lung function and arterial oxygen content may be completely normal, but reduced blood flow greatly decreases oxygen transport to the tissues. Oxygen therapy is of little benefit because arterial oxygen content is almost at its maximal level while the patient is breathing room air; that is, the only possible increase in blood oxygen content is the small additional amount that dissolves in the plasma. However, in patients with coronary artery disease and myocardial tissue hypoxia (ischemia), this small increase in dissolved oxygen may be critical in preventing myocardial tissue death (infarction); thus, oxygen therapy is always given to patients in cardiogenic shock. An extreme example of stagnant hypoxia is cardiac arrest. In cardiac arrest, even a small increase in arterial oxygen content is vitally important. Thus, 100% oxygen is routinely given during cardiopulmonary resuscitation. The focus in treating shock-induced tissue hypoxia is generally the restoration of adequate blood flow.

Histotoxic Hypoxia (Blocked Oxidative Metabolism)

Histotoxic hypoxia refers to poisoning of the cellular oxygen use mechanisms. Cyanide poisoning is the typical example of histotoxic hypoxia. Cyanide combines with and inactivates cellular enzymes necessary for oxidative metabolism. Cyanide poisoning often occurs with carbon monoxide poisoning in the setting of smoke inhalation from house fires.[11] High blood lactic acid levels with high mixed venous oxygen content are evidence that cellular oxygen consumption has been blocked and should raise the suspicion of cyanide poisoning. Treatment includes administration of 100% oxygen and inhaled amyl nitrite and intravenous sodium nitrite, which convert hemoglobin to methemoglobin; methemoglobin is an effective scavenger of free cyanide molecules.[11]

CONCEPT QUESTION 13-10

Explain why histotoxic hypoxia (e.g., cyanide poisoning) affects the $C\bar{v}O_2$ and $C(a\text{-}\bar{v})O_2$.

Diffusion Defects

Conditions that increase the diffusion pathway distance across the alveolar capillary membrane include pulmonary edema and processes leading to interstitial alveolar fibrosis. Normally, capillary blood and alveolar gas PO_2 values equilibrate in the first one third of the time required to travel through the alveolar capillary. Thickened membranes require longer equilibrium times, and during exercise, equilibrium may not occur, leading to arterial hypoxemia (see Chapter 7). The contribution of diffusion defects to arterial hypoxemia when the patient is at rest is uncertain; the major mechanism is probably uneven ventilation-perfusion relationships caused by regional differences in lung compliance secondary to nonuniform distribution of lung disease.[7] For this reason, some physiologists classify diffusion defects in the hypoxic hypoxia category. Increased F_IO_2 is helpful in treating diffusion defects because the increased diffusion gradient greatly enhances oxygen transfer across the alveolar capillary membrane into the blood.

Physiological Effects of Hypoxia

The tissue cells respond to the lack of oxygen by converting to anaerobic metabolism. A by-product of anaerobic metabolism is lactic acid. Lactic acid accumulation lowers the blood pH, creating a metabolic acidosis. The coexistence of metabolic acidosis and poor oxygen delivery to the tissues (i.e., low cardiac output, low arterial oxygen content) strongly suggests hypoxia-induced lactic acidosis. Blood lactate concentration may therefore be an indicator of tissue hypoxia.

The body's compensatory response to hypoxemia is increased cardiac output, improved tissue perfusion (as a result of capillary recruitment), and increased red blood cell production.[1] Increased cardiac output and perfusion are immediate responses, whereas increased red blood cell production is a response to chronic hypoxia. Increased cardiac output increases oxygen delivery to the tissues. Even if the blood is

BOX 13-4

Clinical Signs and Symptoms of Acute Hypoxemia

- Tachycardia
- Increased minute ventilation
- Restlessness and irritability
- Mild hypertension
- Peripheral vasoconstriction
- Muscular incoordination
- Confusion
- Cyanosis
- Bradycardia and arrhythmias
- Hypotension
- Loss of consciousness

hypoxemic, circulating it more rapidly supplies the tissues with greater amounts of oxygen per minute.

Clinical Signs and Symptoms

If hemoglobin concentration and cardiac output are normal, PaO_2 must acutely decrease to less than 50 to 60 mm Hg before clinical manifestations appear.[7] At this PaO_2, most people experience mild nausea, light-headedness, and dizziness. These symptoms do not necessarily occur in slowly progressing, chronic hypoxemia of equal severity. In chronic hypoxemia, the body compensates by producing more erythrocytes, increasing the CaO_2.

In acute hypoxemia in the range of 50 to 60 mm Hg, peripheral chemoreceptor stimulation increases minute ventilation, although dyspnea is generally not perceived. PaO_2 values from 35 to 50 mm Hg cause mental confusion; PaO_2 less than 35 mm Hg causes decreased renal blood flow and cardiac conduction disturbances. This level of hypoxemia causes maximal minute ventilation and severe lethargy. Loss of consciousness and respiratory center depression occur at PaO_2 values less than 25 mm Hg.[12] In the presence of anemia or cardiac insufficiency, these manifestations become apparent at higher PaO_2 values. Box 13-4 summarizes clinical signs and symptoms of acute hypoxemia from mild to severe conditions. Tissues with high oxygen consumption requirements, such as brain, heart, and kidney cells, are the most susceptible to hypoxia. A total lack of oxygen causes irreversible brain cell injury or death in minutes.

Normal and Abnormal Oxygenation Values

Normal PaO₂ Values

PaO_2 is the only blood gas value that normally changes with age. A general clinical rule for estimating a person's normal PaO_2 is as follows: A 10-year-old child has a normal PaO_2 of about 100 mm Hg at sea level. Normal PaO_2 decreases about 5 mm Hg for every 10 years of age up to 90 years. Using this criterion, a normal PaO_2 for a 30-year-old adult (breathing room air at sea level) is about 90 mm Hg and for an 80-year-old adult is about 65 mm Hg.

A more precise formula for calculating normal PaO_2 considers age and position (supine or standing). This formula is as follows:

$$\text{Supine: Normal } PaO_2 = 109 - (0.43 \times age) \pm 8 \text{ mm Hg}$$
$$\text{Standing: Normal } PaO_2 = 104 - (0.27 \times age) \pm 12 \text{ mm Hg}$$

A widely accepted normal range for PaO_2 in people 60 years old or younger (breathing room air at sea level) is 80 to 100 mm Hg.

Normal PaO₂ at High Altitude

Altitude also affects normal, expected PaO_2. High altitude decreases barometric pressure and therefore it decreases inspired PO_2. Up to an altitude of 10,000 feet above sea level, barometric pressure decreases about 24 mm Hg per 1000 feet of elevation.[1] For example, in Denver, Colorado, where the elevation is 5280 feet, barometric pressure is about 633 mm Hg. At 10,000 feet elevation, barometric pressure is only 523 mm Hg.

The general formula for changing observed sea-level PaO_2 values to PaO_2 values at a different barometric pressure is as follows:

$$\text{Expected } PO_2 \text{ at high altitude} = (\text{high altitude}$$
$$\text{barometric pressure} / 760 \text{ mm Hg}) \times \text{sea} - \text{level } PO_2$$

According to this calculation, if normal sea-level PaO_2 is 95 mm Hg, normal PaO_2 in Denver is about 79 mm Hg; at 10,000 feet elevation, normal PaO_2 is only 65 mm Hg.

Severity of Arterial Hypoxemia

Table 13-5 arbitrarily classifies the severity of arterial hypoxemia. Traditionally, only PaO_2 is classified in evaluating oxygenation. (Corresponding SaO_2 values are included in Table 13-5.) Both CaO_2 and cardiac output (i.e. oxygen delivery) are essential in evaluating oxygenation. (These factors are discussed later in this chapter.) Table 13-5 assumes a normal cardiac output and blood hemoglobin content.

Mild hypoxemia is generally well tolerated and not associated with tissue hypoxia; hemoglobin saturation is 90% or greater. Moderate hypoxemia requires an increased cardiac output to maintain adequate oxygen delivery to the tissues. A failing or compromised heart may be unable to meet this challenge, leading to tissue hypoxia. Even a normal heart and an increased cardiac output would probably not sustain adequate oxygen delivery to the tissues in severe hypoxemia (PaO_2 values <40 mm Hg). Hypoxemia in this range invariably leads to tissue hypoxia and lactic acidosis. Severe hypoxemia requires immediate therapy because at this level

of PaO_2, heart and brain cells may be permanently injured within minutes.

Evaluating Pulmonary Oxygenation Defects

F₁O₂-PaO₂ Relationship

Knowledge of PaO_2 without knowledge of F_IO_2 is diagnostically worthless. A PaO_2 of 100 mm Hg with adequate hemoglobin concentration and cardiac output implies adequate tissue oxygenation, but if F_IO_2 is 1.0, a severe pulmonary oxygenation defect (i.e., severe intrapulmonary shunting) is clearly present.

CONCEPT QUESTION 13-11

Explain why a normal PaO_2 of 100 mm Hg could still be associated with a severe tissue oxygenation defect.

At sea level, a 100% oxygen gas sample has a PaO_2 of 760 mm Hg. Thus, 1% oxygen represents a PO_2 of 7.6 mm Hg, and 10% oxygen represents a PO_2 of 76 mm Hg. An increase in F_IO_2 by 0.10 increases inspired PO_2 by 76 mm Hg; in the normal lung, after humidification and dilution with carbon dioxide, the same F_IO_2 increase raises P_AO_2 by about 60 mm Hg. Considering the normal $P(A-a)O_2$ (alveolar-to-arterial oxygen pressure difference) of about 10 mm Hg, PaO_2 increases by about 50 mm Hg in response to the 10% inspired oxygen increase. As a general rule, PaO_2 should increase by at least 50 mm Hg for every 10%

CLINICAL FOCUS 13-10

Normal PaO₂ for Denver Residents

In a Denver hospital, a 25-year-old patient with asthma has arterial blood gases drawn and analyzed in the pulmonary function laboratory. With the patient breathing room air, the PaO_2 is 75 mm Hg. Does this represent normal oxygenation?

Discussion

At sea level, P_AO_2 is about 100 mm Hg while a person breathes room air, as the following equation shows:*

$$P_AO_2 = 0.21 (760 - 47) - PaCO_2 \times 1.2 = 100 \text{ mm Hg}$$

At Denver's elevation, barometric pressure is about 633 mm Hg. Room air P_AO_2 is (633/760), or 0.83 of sea level P_AO_2, as the following shows:

$$\text{Denver } P_AO_2 = (633 / 760) \times 100 \text{ mm Hg}$$
$$= 0.83 \times 100 \text{ mm Hg}$$
$$\text{Denver } P_AO_2 = 83 \text{ mm Hg}$$

PaO_2 is always about 5 to 10 mm Hg less than P_AO_2 when breathing room air because of normal anatomical shunting. Assuming $P(A-a)O_2$ of 5 mm Hg, normal room air PaO_2 should be as follows: (83 − 5 mm Hg) = 78 mm Hg. A room air PaO_2 of 75 mm Hg for a patient with asthma is normal and does not represent an oxygenation problem. The healthiest person in Denver would have a similar PaO_2.

TABLE 13-5

Classifying Severity of Hypoxemia*

Classification	PaO₂ (mm Hg)	SaO₂ (%)
Normal	80-100	>95
Mild hypoxemia	60-79	90-94
Moderate hypoxemia	40-59	75-89
Severe	<40	<75

*Sea level, room air, <60 years of age.

*$PaCO_2$ is assumed to be normal at 40 mm Hg.

increase in inspired oxygen concentration. Beginning with a normal sea-level, room air PaO_2 of about 100 mm Hg, F_IO_2 of 0.30 should produce a minimum PaO_2 value of 150 mm Hg, F_IO_2 of 0.40 should produce a PaO_2 of at least 200 mm Hg, and F_IO_2 of 1.0 should produce a PaO_2 of at least 500 mm Hg. If a patient breathing oxygen has a PaO_2 less than the value predicted by these calculations, the patient will be hypoxemic while breathing room air.

Indicators of Oxygen Transfer Efficiency

$P(A-a)O_2$, PaO_2/P_AO_2, and PaO_2/F_IO_2 are indicators of the lung's efficiency in transferring oxygen from alveolar gas to capillary blood. The advantages and disadvantages of these indicators are reviewed in Chapter 12. All of these indicators are sensitive to the degree of intrapulmonary shunt present, although PaO_2/P_AO_2 is the most stable and reliable in this regard. Calculating the intrapulmonary shunt fraction using the classic shunt equation is the most accurate way to quantify the degree of shunt present (see Chapter 12).

The greater the shunt, the less effective oxygen therapy will be. Shunting leads to refractory hypoxemia, which means therapy must be focused on reopening and oxygenating airless alveoli.

Through observation of the PaO_2 response to increased F_IO_2, shunt can be differentiated from $\dot{V}_A/\dot{Q}_C$ mismatch as the major cause of hypoxemia (see Chapter 12). If PaO_2 is low but oxygenation efficiency indicators and shunt fraction are normal, overall hypoventilation may be the cause of hypoxemia; this would be confirmed by an increased $PaCO_2$, reciprocally related to PaO_2.

Evaluating Oxygenation Defects of Cardiovascular Origin

Oxygen Delivery to the Tissues

Arterial blood gases alone reveal nothing about the cardiovascular component of oxygenation. CaO_2 and cardiac output must be evaluated to estimate the most critical aspect of oxygenation status: oxygen delivery (O_2DEL) to the tissues. Oxygen transport, or O_2DEL, is equal to cardiac output ($\dot{Q}_T$) multiplied by CaO_2 (see Chapter 8), as the following equation shows:

$$O_2DEL = \dot{Q}_T \times (CaO_2 \times 10)$$

A normal cardiac output of 5 L per minute and a normal CaO_2 of 20 mL/dL produces a normal O_2DEL rate of 1000 mL per minute, as the following shows:

$$O_2DEL = 5 \text{ L/min} \times (200 \text{ mL oxygen/L})$$
$$O_2DEL = 1000 \text{ mL/min}$$

Resting oxygen consumption is about 250 mL per minute. The tissues normally use about one fourth of the oxygen delivered to them (i.e., oxygen-extraction ratio is about 0.25) (see Chapter 8).

Critically ill patients consume much greater quantities of oxygen per minute than healthy people. The body's major means of increasing oxygen delivery to the tissues is to increase the cardiac output by increasing the heart rate. Adequate cardiac reserves are critical for adequate tissue oxygenation, especially if pulmonary oxygenation defects decrease the CaO_2.

If cardiac output decreases to abnormally low levels, blood circulates more slowly through tissue capillary beds. However, tissue cells continue to extract oxygen from the blood at the same rate, regardless of blood flow. Slower circulation means blood has longer contact time with oxygen-consuming tissue cells. Therefore, more oxygen diffuses out of each milliliter of blood into the tissues. When blood leaves the tissue capillary beds and enters the venous system, its oxygen content is lower than normal (i.e., $C\bar{v}O_2$ is less than normal) (see Chapter 8). A low cardiac output increases $C(a-\bar{v})O_2$ (arterial venous oxygen-content difference).

The Fick cardiac output equation (see Chapter 8) illustrates the relationships among tissue oxygen consumption ($\dot{V}O_2$), $C(a-\bar{v})O_2$, and $\dot{Q}_T$. This is shown as follows:

$$\dot{Q}_T = \dot{V}O_2/[C(a-\bar{v})O_2 \times 10]$$

This equation shows that a reduction in $C\bar{v}O_2$ implies a decreased cardiac output.

Effect of Cardiac Output on PaO_2

Changes in cardiac output do not significantly affect PaO_2 or CaO_2 of individuals with a normal intrapulmonary shunt fraction (3% to 5%). However, as mentioned in Chapter 12, a decrease in cardiac output can significantly lower CaO_2 and PaO_2 in persons with increased shunt fractions because it lowers $C\bar{v}O_2$ and $P\bar{v}O_2$. Likewise, an increase in cardiac output can mask the hypoxemic effects of shunt by increasing $C\bar{v}O_2$ and $P\bar{v}O_2$.

The foregoing becomes clear when one considers the fact that arterial blood is a mixture of blood draining both normally oxygenated alveoli and airless alveoli (shunt units) (Figure 13-4, A and B). Shunted blood is actually unoxygenated venous blood. This blood mixes directly with the oxygenated blood that leaves ventilated alveoli. Low cardiac output reduces the mixed venous oxygen content and lowers the oxygen content of the shunted blood (see Figure 13-4, B). In this way, a reduced cardiac output decreases CaO_2 and PaO_2 as the more profoundly hypoxemic shunted blood mixes with arterial blood.

However, the normal response to increased shunting is an increase, not a decrease, in cardiac output. This increase in cardiac output increases $C\bar{v}O_2$, preventing a more severe decrease in CaO_2 than would occur if cardiac output remains normal. A sudden decrease in PaO_2 with a stable pulmonary oxygenation status (e.g., shunt fraction remains constant) suggests a reduction in cardiac output.

CONCEPT QUESTION 13-12

Why does an increase in cardiac output increase $C\bar{v}O_2$, with all other factors remaining constant?

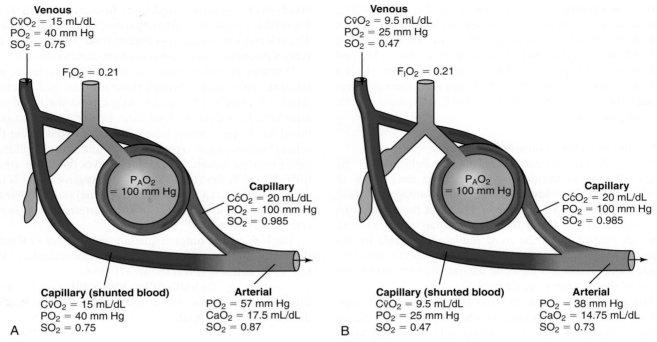

Figure 13-4 Effect of cardiac output on PaO_2 and CaO_2 in severe shunting. **A**, $P\bar{v}O_2$ and $C\bar{v}O_2$ are normal, implying appropriate cardiac output. **B**, Low cardiac output decreases $P\bar{v}O_2$ and $C\bar{v}O_2$, further reducing CaO_2.

CLINICAL FOCUS 13-11

Differentiating Pulmonary and Cardiovascular Oxygenation Defects

You are caring for two patients in the intensive care unit. Patient A is recovering from an emergency appendectomy and has a history of chronic bronchitis. Patient B has been admitted for management of an acute myocardial infarction (heart attack).

Patient A Data (Room Air)

PaO_2 = 50 mm Hg
$PaCO_2$ = 30 mm Hg
pH = 7.47
$[HCO_3^-]$ = 21 mEq/L
SaO_2 = 83%
Hb = 15 g/dL
CaO_2 = 16.8 mL oxygen/dL
$P(A-a)O_2$ = 63.7
CO = 4.8 L/min
$S\bar{v}O_2$ = 70%
$P\bar{v}O_2$ = 38 mm Hg
$C\bar{v}O_2$ = 14.2 mL oxygen/dL

Patient B Data (Room Air)

PaO_2 = 98 mm Hg
$PaCO_2$ = 40 mm Hg
pH = 7.38
$[HCO_3^-]$ = 23 mEq/L
SaO_2 = 99%

Hb = 15 g/dL
CaO_2 = 20.2 mL oxygen/dL
$P(A-a)O_2$ = 3.7
CO = 3.1 L/min
$S\bar{v}O_2$ = 55%
$P\bar{v}O_2$ = 29 mm Hg
$C\bar{v}O_2$ = 11.1 mL oxygen/dL

Discussion

At first glance, one notices that patient B has a higher PaO_2 and CaO_2 than patient A, breathing the same F_IO_2. Both patients have the same hemoglobin concentration. Pulmonary oxygenation defects are characterized by large $P(A-a)O_2$ differences, indicating impaired oxygen transfer from the lungs to the blood. Patient A has impaired oxygen transfer, whereas patient B's oxygen transfer is normal. (Patient A's hypoxemia is probably stimulating ventilation, creating a decreased $PaCO_2$ and respiratory alkalosis.) If the data are not examined further, the conclusion may be drawn (incorrectly) that patient B is better oxygenated than patient A.

The Fick equation is helpful in examining the amount of oxygen delivered to the tissues each minute by patient A and patient B:

Patient A:

$$O_2DEL = (16.8 \text{ mL oxygen/dL} \times 10) \times 4.8 \text{ L/min}$$
$$O_2DEL = 806 \text{ mL oxygen/min}$$

CLINICAL FOCUS 13-11

Differentiating Pulmonary and Cardiovascular Oxygenation Defects—cont'd

Patient B:

$$O_2DEL = (20.1 \text{ mL oxygen/dL} \times 10) \times 3.1 \text{ L/min}$$

$$O_2DEL = 623 \text{ mL/min}$$

Despite clearly superior PaO_2 and CaO_2, patient B delivers less oxygen to the tissues each minute than patient A. The key difference is the cardiac output. Although patient B does not have an oxygen-transfer problem in the lung, he has an oxygen-delivery problem. The low $P\overline{v}O_2$ of 29 mm Hg

and high arterial venous oxygen content difference of 9 mL oxygen/dL are signs of low cardiac output. In patient B, blood spends more time in tissue capillary beds and gives up more oxygen than in patient A. The important clinical point is that oxygenation involves pulmonary and cardiovascular systems; the contribution of each must be critically evaluated to assess overall oxygenation.

POINTS TO REMEMBER

- Classification of arterial blood gases is the first essential step in the interpretation and clinical treatment of acid-base and oxygenation problems.
- Arterial blood gases should be evaluated systematically in two distinctly separate steps: acid-base disturbances and oxygenation disturbances.
- With room air breathing, hypoxemia can coexist with normal ventilation, but hypoventilation cannot coexist with normal oxygenation.
- $PaCO_2$ is a reliable, accurate index of ventilatory status.
- $[HCO_3^-]$ is affected by ventilatory ($PaCO_2$) changes and is therefore not a pure indicator of metabolic acid-base disturbances.
- Respiratory acidosis and alkalosis refer to alveolar hypoventilation and hyperventilation, respectively.
- In compensated respiratory acidosis, plasma $[HCO_3^-]$ is elevated to compensate for increased $PaCO_2$ and does not mean metabolic alkalosis is present.
- The anion gap is used to determine the origin of metabolic acidosis.
- In metabolic acidosis, an increased anion gap means the body has gained nonvolatile acids, whereas a normal anion gap means the body has lost base.
- Metabolic alkalosis can occur in two ways: (1) loss of fixed acids or (2) gain of blood buffer base.
- In Stewart's strong ion theory, changes in $[H^+]$ can be caused only by changes in dissolved $[CO_2]$, the difference between strong cations and anions, and the total weak acid concentration; changes in $[HCO_3^-]$ cannot cause changes in $[H^+]$.
- Assessment of oxygenation involves evaluating pulmonary and cardiovascular factors: lung oxygen transfer efficiency ($P(A-a)O_2$, PaO_2/P_AO_2, and $\dot{Q}_S/\dot{Q}_T$) and oxygen delivery to the tissues (cardiac output, CaO_2, O_2DEL, and $C\overline{v}O_2$).

- Age and altitude affect the normal PaO_2 and must be considered in assessing oxygenation.
- A reduced cardiac output in the presence of abnormal intrapulmonary shunt causes arterial hypoxemia by reducing the oxygen saturation of mixed venous (shunted) blood.

References

1. Hall JE: *Guyton and Hall textbook of medical physiology*, ed 12, Philadelphia, 2011, Saunders.
2. Rose BD, Post TW: *Clinical physiology of acid-base and electrolyte disorders*, ed 5, New York, 2000, McGraw-Hill.
3. Effros RM, Swenson ER: Acid-base balance. In Mason RJ, et al, editors: *Murray and Nadel's textbook of respiratory medicine*, ed 5, Philadelphia, 2010, Saunders.
4. American Heart Association: Part 8: Adult advanced cardiovascular life support: 2010 American Heart Association Guidelines for Cardiopulmonary Resuscitation and Emergency Cardiovascular Care, *Circulation* 122(suppl 3):S729, 2010.
5. Filley GF: *Acid-base and blood gas regulation*, Philadelphia, 1971, Lea & Febiger.
6. Javaheri S, Kazemi H: Metabolic alkalosis and hypoventilation in humans, *Am Rev Respir Dis* 136(4):1011, 1987.
7. West JB: *Respiratory physiology: the essentials*, ed 8, Baltimore, 2008, Lippincott Williams & Wilkins.
8. Kellum JA: Determinants of blood pH in health and disease, *Crit Care* 4(1):6, 2000.
9. Morfei J: Stewart's strong ion difference approach to acid-base analysis, *Respir Care* 44(1):45, 1999.
10. Swenson ER: The strong ion difference approach: can a strong case be made for its use in acid-base analysis? *Respir Care* 44(1):26, 1999.
11. Mokhlesi B, et al: Adult toxicology in critical care: part II: specific poisonings, *Chest* 123(3):897, 2003.
12. Marini JJ, Wheeler AP: *Critical care medicine: the essentials*, Baltimore, 1989, Williams & Wilkins.

CHAPTER 14

Physiological Basis for Oxygenation and Lung Protection Strategies

OBJECTIVES

After reading this chapter, you will be able to:

- Explain why monitoring arterial carbon dioxide pressure ($PaCO_2$) is an important consideration when monitoring oxygen therapy in patients with chronic obstructive pulmonary disease (COPD) who are chronically hypercapnic
- Explain why a change in body position might improve oxygenation in unilateral lung disease
- Describe how various inflammatory processes injure the alveolar capillary membrane and produce severe shunting and hypoxemia in acute respiratory distress syndrome (ARDS)
- Explain how positive end expiratory pressure (PEEP) and continuous positive airway pressure (CPAP) improve oxygenation in ARDS
- Differentiate between PEEP and CPAP indications and mechanisms of action
- Describe how the interplay between alveolar and intrapleural pressures determines lung volume in both spontaneous and mechanically induced ventilation

- Explain why pressure and volume cannot function as independent variables in producing alveolar stretch injury
- Explain how to monitor alveolar pressure clinically and the rationale for its measurement
- Describe the mechanisms whereby alveolar overdistention, atelectrauma, and biotrauma are involved in ventilator-induced lung injury (VILI), and explain how they can be prevented during mechanical ventilation
- Explain why the accepted standard of care in mechanically ventilating patients with ARDS might require the development of hypercapnia and acidosis
- Describe the mechanisms whereby prone positioning of a mechanically ventilated patient with ARDS improves oxygenation and reduces VILI
- Differentiate both mechanically and functionally between volume-targeted and pressure-targeted mechanical ventilation
- Discuss which protective lung ventilation strategies have been conclusively shown to reduce mortality in ARDS

KEY TERMS

acute lung injury (ALI)
atelectrauma
biotrauma
cytokines
heterogeneous disease
homogeneous disease
multisystem organ dysfunction syndrome (MODS)

partial liquid ventilation (PLV)
permissive hypercapnia
prostaglandins
refractory hypoxemia
retinopathy of prematurity (ROP)
ventilator-induced lung injury (VILI)
volutrauma

TREATMENT OF HYPOXEMIA AND SEVERE SHUNTING

The reason for including a section on treating hypoxemia and shunting in this textbook is to establish the physiological basis for various treatment strategies. Rational therapy decisions and the proper evaluation of treatment effectiveness require clinicians to understand clearly the mechanisms whereby normal physiology becomes deranged; in addition, clinicians must have a clear understanding of the mechanisms by which they expect treatment strategies and mechanical devices to alter deranged physiology beneficially. The equipment used to treat patients is helpful only to the extent that it is applied in a physiologically appropriate way. The clinician's understanding of underlying physiological mechanisms is crucial for making wise treatment decisions and for recognizing the difference between harmful and desired effects.

Severe shunting impairs the lung's ability to transfer oxygen to the blood, resulting in hypoxemia that responds poorly to oxygen therapy, which is known as **refractory hypoxemia** (see Chapter 12). The primary defect in shunt-induced lung disease is the absence of ventilation in a large number of alveoli because they are either collapsed or filled with fluid. The first priority in treating this type of hypoxemia is to reestablish ventilation in these alveoli without injuring the lung or decreasing oxygen delivery to the tissues. The clinician must find a way to increase the arterial oxygen content while maintaining an adequate cardiac output. An important but less urgent priority is reversal of the underlying defect that caused hypoxemia.

Oxygen Therapy

Generally, oxygen therapy is used to maintain a PaO_2 of at least 60 mm Hg (which corresponds to an oxygen saturation in arterial blood [SaO_2] of approximately 90%).[1] However, in anemia, cardiac insufficiency, and coronary artery disease (hypoxic heart muscle), it is overly conservative to limit arterial oxygenation to these levels, especially if the F_IO_2 required to achieve a PaO_2 of 100 mm Hg ($SaO_2 = 98\%$) is 0.40 or less. The nearly 10% increase in arterial oxygen content accompanying a PaO_2 increase from 60 mm Hg to 100 mm Hg is clinically significant in such instances.

Oxygen therapy is effective in $\dot{V}_A/\dot{Q}_C$ mismatch but not if a large amount of absolute shunting is present (see Chapter 12). Oxygen therapy is also effective in diffusion defects and hypoventilation. However, oxygen therapy is not the appropriate way to treat hypoventilation because inadequate alveolar ventilation is the primary problem, not inability to oxygenate; that is, oxygen transfer across the alveolar capillary membrane is not impaired in pure uncomplicated hypoventilation.

Oxygen therapy must be closely monitored when treating patients who are chronically hypoxemic and hypercapnic (e.g., patients with severe chronic obstructive pulmonary disease [COPD]) because it can cause acute carbon dioxide retention and acidosis through mechanisms described in Chapter 11. However, oxygen should never be withheld from severely hypoxemic individuals, regardless of the cause. Hypercapnia and respiratory acidosis are of secondary importance if cerebral oxygenation is threatened. Oxygen should be administered to hypercapnic patients with COPD via devices that can produce relatively low, fixed, inspired oxygen concentrations not influenced by the patient's ventilatory pattern. In patients with severe hypoxemia, low inspired oxygen concentrations are effective because arterial hemoglobin saturation is located on the steep part of the oxygen-hemoglobin equilibrium curve. For example, a relatively large amount of oxygen is added to the blood when PaO_2 is increased from 30 to 60 mm Hg (see Chapter 8). A periodic $PaCO_2$ analysis is important in monitoring oxygen-induced hypercapnia.

CONCEPT QUESTION 14-1

Why is oxygen therapy less effective in absolute shunt than in $\dot{V}_A/\dot{Q}_C$ mismatch?

Excessively High F_IO_2

F_IO_2 values greater than 0.50 for prolonged periods may produce toxic damage to alveolar cells, known as pulmonary oxygen toxicity. High oxygen concentrations lead to the formation of free oxygen radicals, such as superoxide, hydrogen peroxide, and hydroxyl ions; the strong oxidizing effects of these ions damage the ultrastructure of the lung, causing effects similar to the effects seen in acute lung injury (ALI). Oxygen toxicity is marked by an inflammatory response of the lung that leads to alveolar capillary membrane injury and pulmonary edema, greatly impairing oxygen-transfer efficiency and lung compliance. Individual susceptibility to oxygen toxicity varies considerably; generally, F_IO_2 of 0.50 or less for 2 to 7 days does not produce significant lung impairment.[1] For this reason, the goal of oxygen therapy is to achieve a hemoglobin saturation of at least 90% (PaO_2 of at least 60 mm Hg) at F_IO_2 of 0.50 or less. This goal may not always be clinically feasible, and higher F_IO_2 values may be required. Such instances mark the presence of severe shunting and must be addressed by other therapeutic measures (discussed later in this chapter). Concerns about oxygen toxicity should never supersede concerns about tissue hypoxia.

Increased PaO_2, especially in premature infants, is also dangerous. A higher than normal PaO_2 may cause **retinopathy of prematurity (ROP)**, in which the retinal arteries of the infant's eyes constrict, possibly causing permanent blindness. PaO_2 is the critical factor in ROP, not F_IO_2 per se. In other words, PaO_2 may be at dangerous levels at F_IO_2 values well below 0.50; likewise, PaO_2 may be in a safe range at F_IO_2 values greater than 0.50.

Body Position

A simple change in body position may improve oxygenation by improving the match between ventilation and blood flow. Gravity affects the distribution of ventilation and perfusion, as discussed in Chapters 3 and 6. For example, cardiac output is greater in the supine than in the sitting position because venous blood does not have to be pumped "uphill," from the trunk and lower extremities up to the heart. The supine position improves venous return, pulmonary blood flow, and PaO_2 in patients with hypovolemic shock. The same position decreases PaO_2 in patients with congestive heart failure because increased venous return overwhelms the heart's pumping capacity, causing pulmonary edema (see Chapter 6).

The sitting or standing position usually improves PaO_2 over the supine position in obese patients and patients with obstructive lung disease. An upright position allows gravity to pull down on the diaphragm, expanding the lungs and increasing functional residual capacity (FRC). For this reason, it is common practice to get surgical patients out of bed, even on the same day of a major surgery, so that they can stand or walk; this improves overall ventilation and oxygenation because it improves lung mechanics.

Patients with unilateral lung disease (e.g., one lung with pneumonia) should be positioned in bed with the healthy lung down. Gravity causes blood to flow preferentially to the healthy lung, improving $\dot{V}_A/\dot{Q}_C$ and PaO_2.

Treatment of Shunting in Acute Lung Injury

Acute lung injury (ALI) is characterized by alveolar inflammation, alveolar-capillary membrane injury, high-permeability pulmonary edema, widespread atelectasis, and low lung compliance; the end result is severe shunting and refractory hypoxemia. Acute respiratory distress syndrome (ARDS) is the most severe form of ALI. According to the American-European Consensus Conference on ARDS, the PaO_2/F_IO_2 in ALI, regardless of applied positive end expiratory pressure (PEEP), is 300 mm Hg or less, whereas it is 200 mm Hg or less in ARDS.[2] ARDS is not a single disease entity; rather, it is a syndrome set in motion by any one of a wide variety of physiological insults to the lung (Table 14-1). The pathological feature common to each of these insults is injury to and increased permeability of the alveolar capillary membrane; the injury can be either direct (e.g., aspiration of gastric contents) or indirect (e.g., circulating bacterial endotoxins in sepsis).

Any of the risk factors listed in Table 14-1 can initiate the release of inflammatory mediators that attract and activate neutrophils (neutrophils are circulating white blood cells

TABLE 14-1

Conditions Associated with Acute Respiratory Distress Syndrome and Acute Lung Injury

Direct Injury	Indirect Injury
Pneumonia	Sepsis
Gastric content aspiration	Major nonpulmonary trauma
Pulmonary contusion	Multiple blood transfusions
Toxic gas/smoke inhalation	Pancreatitis
Near drowning	Heart-lung bypass machine
	Adverse drug effects
	Liver failure

essential for phagocytosis and destruction of bacteria and other pathological substances). Prostaglandins, endotoxins, and cytokines are examples of inflammatory mediators. **Prostaglandins** are substances that can change capillary permeability, cause platelet aggregation (which increases the risk for intravascular clotting), and change vascular smooth muscle tone. Endotoxins are contained in the cell walls of gram-negative bacteria and when released can injure the vascular endothelium and induce inappropriate synthesis of nitric oxide; the result is massive vasodilation (septic shock). **Cytokines** are any of several regulatory proteins released by immune system cells (e.g., T cells) in generating an inflammatory response. Interleukins are a subgroup of cytokines produced mainly by T cells (T cells are thymus-derived lymphocytes of the body's immune system that destroy or neutralize foreign substances); interleukins are signaling molecules that facilitate communication among neutrophils, causing them to migrate to the site of injury. Interleukins are thus important in mounting the inflammatory response.

Circulating neutrophils contain an array of toxic substances essential for destroying bacteria and other microorganisms. A hallmark of ARDS is the adherence of neutrophils to the pulmonary capillary endothelium (neutrophils become "sticky").[2] Toxic compounds released by neutrophils damage and increase the permeability of the capillary endothelium and alveolar epithelium as neutrophils transmigrate from the bloodstream into the alveoli. Among these compounds are reactive oxygen ions and proteolytic enzymes that degrade and destroy tissues (Figure 14-1). The end result is increased alveolar capillary membrane permeability and flooding of the alveolar airspaces with protein-rich fluids. These fluids interfere with surfactant function, increasing surface tension and inducing widespread atelectasis. Shunting is the result of both alveolar filling and alveolar collapsing processes. The loss of alveolar airspace greatly reduces FRC and lung compliance in ARDS.

CONCEPT QUESTION 14-2

Why would pulmonary edema fluid of ARDS be richer in proteins than edema fluid of congestive heart failure, and why would this make ARDS edema likely to be more severe?

The hypoxemic effect of shunt in ARDS is especially severe because the normal hypoxic pulmonary vasoconstriction (HPV) mechanism is severely blunted.[3,4] As noted in Chapter 6, the physiological function of HPV is to match blood flow and ventilation better. HPV normally reduces blood flow to nonventilated alveoli, lessening the hypoxemic effect they can exert on arterial blood. In ARDS, blood flows more freely through the capillaries of nonventilated alveoli, contributing to the profound refractory hypoxemia characteristic of ARDS.

ARDS does not affect the lung uniformly; computed tomography scans reveal that both normal-appearing lung and heavily consolidated lung coexist.[2] ARDS is often characterized as a **heterogeneous disease** (i.e., interspersed normal and abnormal regions) as opposed to a **homogeneous disease**. In effect, reduced open airspace creates a "small" lung in ARDS; in other words, one can think of the ARDS lung as a relatively small "normal" lung sharing the same major airways with an abnormal consolidated or atelectatic lung. This means the ARDS lung has marked regional differences in lung compliance, which presents an especially difficult challenge in mechanical ventilation of these patients. A mechanical positive pressure breath preferentially inflates the most compliant lung areas, potentially overdistending and damaging these "normal" regions. Thus, much attention has been given to the phenomenon of **ventilator-induced lung injury (VILI)** and to protective ventilation strategies. The remaining sections of this chapter address the physiological rationale for various therapeutic strategies designed to improve oxygenation and to protect the mechanically ventilated ARDS lung from further injury.

CONCEPT QUESTION 14-3

Considering that ARDS is more of an oxygenation problem than a ventilation problem, why are patients with ARDS likely to require mechanical ventilatory assistance?

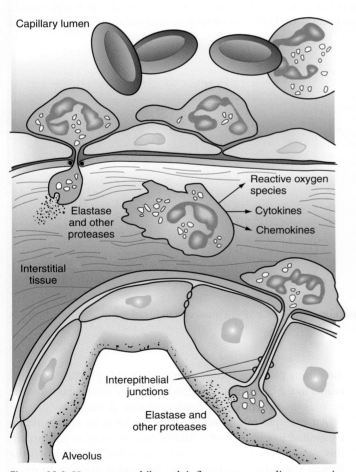

Figure 14-1 How neutrophils and inflammatory mediators are involved in ALI. Neutrophils in the blood migrate across the alveolar capillary membrane, releasing toxic compounds that are normally important in host defense against pathogens but that can damage tissues. (From Mason RJ, et al, editors: *Murray and Nadel's textbook of respiratory medicine,* ed 4, Philadelphia, 2005, Saunders.)

Positive End Expiratory Pressure

FRC in ARDS is greatly reduced because of widespread atelectasis and lung consolidation; it makes sense to use techniques that either reopen collapsed alveoli or prevent their collapse in the first place. Positive end expiratory pressure (PEEP) is aimed at accomplishing this effect. PEEP refers to airway pressure that remains above atmospheric levels at the end of expiration. PEEP is generally applied to the airway in conjunction with endotracheal intubation and positive pressure mechanical ventilation.

Mechanism of Action. In the atelectatic lung, PEEP increases FRC and lung compliance by increasing transpulmonary pressure ($P_A - P_{pl}$) at the end of expiration. This effect is beneficial only in people who already have abnormally low FRC and low lung compliance. In such individuals, PEEP may prevent alveolar collapse at the end of expiration and at sufficiently high levels may help to reopen collapsed alveoli.[5] The reopening of previously collapsed alveoli reduces intrapulmonary shunt and improves PaO_2. In addition, PEEP improves lung compliance (i.e., less pressure is required to inflate the lung to a given volume) by restoring the FRC of the diseased lung; that is, PEEP places the tidal volume on a steeper portion of the lung compliance curve (Figure 14-2), requiring less pressure to achieve a given tidal volume. As collapsed alveoli are reopened, the lung's compliance curve shifts back toward its normal position.

Continuous Positive Airway Pressure

A variation of PEEP that produces the same effect is continuous positive airway pressure (CPAP), which is applied to spontaneously breathing individuals. In CPAP, a relatively constant positive airway pressure is maintained throughout inspiration and expiration. CPAP can be applied through a facemask or an endotracheal tube. The beneficial effects of CPAP are similar to the effects of PEEP; alveolar collapse is prevented, and collapsed alveoli may be recruited. The improved lung compliance illustrated in Figure 14-2 decreases the patient's work of breathing. The major difference between CPAP and PEEP is that airway pressure does not increase during inspiration with CPAP as it does with PEEP. Therefore CPAP is associated with lower mean airway pressure than PEEP. Figure 14-3 illustrates PEEP and CPAP pressure waveforms.

How PEEP and CPAP Devices Work

It is beyond the scope of this chapter to review PEEP and CPAP devices in detail. However, a basic understanding of the mechanical principles involved helps one understand how PEEP and CPAP produce their physiological effects.

Modern mechanical ventilators use sophisticated microprocessor-controlled exhalation valves through which the patient exhales. As expiration proceeds, pressure in the ventilator tubing decreases until it reaches a preselected level, at which point the exhalation valve abruptly closes and traps positive pressure in the patient's lungs. In other words, the pressure in the patient's lungs is not allowed to decrease to atmospheric levels, which means the end expiratory volume of the lung (FRC) is increased, and alveolar collapse is presumably prevented. An ideal PEEP valve does not resist expiratory gas flow; instead, it establishes an end expiratory *threshold* pressure that abruptly stops exhalation

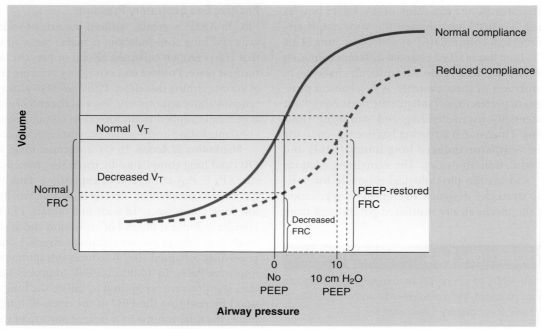

Figure 14-2 The reason PEEP improves lung compliance. With an increase in FRC in the abnormal lung, the same pressure change that produced a low tidal volume (V_T) at 0 cm H_2O PEEP produces a normal tidal volume at 10 cm H_2O PEEP. As PEEP reopens collapsed alveoli, lung compliance improves, shifting the curve back to the normal position.

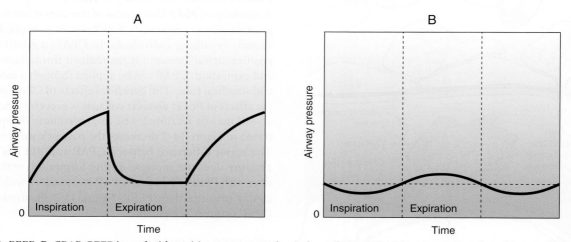

Figure 14-3 A, PEEP. **B,** CPAP. PEEP is used with positive pressure mechanical ventilation. CPAP is a spontaneous breathing mode. Both therapies increase FRC.

(i.e., PEEP does not resist expiratory flow above the preset threshold pressure). Sometimes PEEP is misunderstood to be a pressure that is forced into the lungs, but PEEP is not an inspiratory phenomenon; PEEP is applied at the end of expiration and simply prevents the patient from exhaling to his or her natural resting level.

A CPAP device may consist of a continuous flow apparatus or a demand valve system. In a continuous flow device, a source gas flows through a tube past the patient's airway (either through a mask or, as shown in Figure 14-4, through an adapter attached to an endotracheal tube) and out of a CPAP valve that can be adjusted to release gas at a given pressure threshold. A CPAP valve functions in a manner similar to a PEEP valve. For example, if the CPAP valve allows gas to escape only when

the tubing pressure exceeds 10 cm H_2O, this pressure is maintained in the breathing circuit as long as the source gas flow rate exceeds the patient's peak inspiratory flow demand.

An example of a demand valve device is an electronically controlled inspiratory valve that senses pressure in the circuit; this valve opens to allow gas to flow to the patient when the patient's inspiratory effort causes the circuit pressure to drop. In this way, gas flow meets the patient's inspiratory "demand." When the patient exhales, the inspiratory demand valve closes, and exhaled gas is directed through the expiratory valve, or CPAP valve. Thus, in a demand CPAP system, source gas flow is not continuous—it is present only during inspiration. A constant airway pressure is maintained in the breathing circuit as

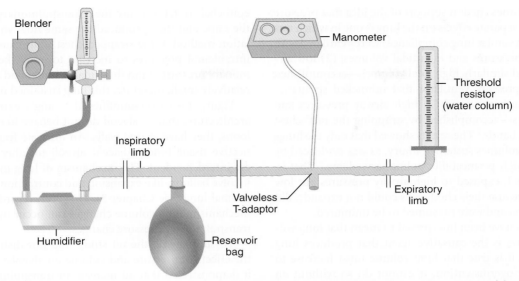

Figure 14-4 Diagram of a continuous flow CPAP circuit. The elastic reservoir bag helps keep inspiratory pressure constant if the patient's inspiratory flow demand momentarily exceeds the source gas flow rate. (Modified from Branson RD, Hurst JM, Dellayen CB: Mask CPAP: state of the art. Respir Care 30:846, 1985.)

long as the inspiratory flow of the source gas meets the patient's inspiratory flow demands.

Indications for PEEP and CPAP

The general indication for this type of airway pressure therapy is the presence of a significant amount of absolute shunting. Generally, if PaO_2 of at least 60 mm Hg with F_IO_2 of 0.5 or less cannot be achieved, PEEP or CPAP should be considered. Refractory hypoxemia combined with bilateral, uniform lung disease and uniformly low lung compliance are good indications for the use of PEEP or CPAP.[6] A classic indication for PEEP is diagnosed ARDS. As previously described, ARDS is associated with alveolar instability and collapse and extensive intrapulmonary shunting and refractory hypoxemia.

In addition to improving oxygen transfer across the lung, PEEP can have a protective effect on the lung in ARDS by preventing lung tissue stress caused by the repetitive opening and closing of alveoli during mechanical ventilation. This stabilizing effect of PEEP on the alveoli is discussed in more depth in a later section.

Poor candidates for PEEP and CPAP are patients with unilateral or localized lung disease (involving only one lung or one lobe) and patients with normally or highly compliant lungs.[6] In such individuals, PEEP preferentially affects the most compliant regions and may result in overdistention of normal alveoli. This overdistention leads to a high risk of pulmonary air leaks, lung rupture, and pneumothorax.

CPAP is reserved for patients who have adequate spontaneous ventilatory reserves, as confirmed by normal $PaCO_2$. CPAP does not mechanically ventilate the lungs; it is contraindicated in patients who cannot breathe on their own.

CONCEPT QUESTION 14-4

Why would CPAP or PEEP be less beneficial in $\dot{V}_A/\dot{Q}_C$ mismatch than in absolute shunt?

Concepts and Mechanisms of Ventilator-Induced Lung Injury

Over the past 20 years, it has become increasingly recognized that positive pressure mechanical ventilation in ALI can be as harmful, if not more so, than the pathological process itself. The extensive discussion of VILI in the medical literature has led to the coining of terms such as barotrauma and **volutrauma**, referring to the mechanical trauma produced by high pressures (barotrauma) and high volumes (volutrauma). These terms wrongly imply that pressure and volume are independent of one another and play separate roles in lung inflation.

Basic Concepts of Hyperinflation Injury. Few subjects have been made more complicated than the cause of hyperinflation lung injury. In thinking about what causes overdistention of the lung, during mechanical ventilation, one must keep in mind that changes in lung volume cannot be caused by any factor other than changes in alveolar distending pressure i.e., transpulmonary pressure (see Chapter 3). That is, if transpulmonary pressure does not change, volume cannot change. One must be clear about cause and effect: Pressure changes are the cause of lung volume changes; the lung cannot somehow gain volume independent of a pressure change. The separation of pressure changes from volume changes during ventilation, whether spontaneous or mechanical, is conceptually incorrect. Lung inflation, and thus stretch of the alveolar epithelium, can occur only when the transpulmonary pressure gradient ($P_A - P_{pl}$) increases. Several references in the medical literature erroneously imply that high volume produces alveolar trauma, not high pressure—as though pressure and volume changes are independent of one another.

CONCEPT QUESTION 14-5

Explain why a spontaneously taken breath of 1000 mL requires exactly the same transpulmonary pressure gradient and produces exactly the same alveolar epithelial stress as a 1000-mL breath induced by a mechanical positive pressure ventilator (in the same individual).

A study sometimes cited in support of the idea that pressure and volume have separate effects on the lung is one in which rats (presumably with similar lung compliance) were ventilated with (1) high airway pressures and high tidal volumes; (2) low airway pressures and similarly high tidal volumes—accomplished with a negative pressure ventilator that mimicked spontaneous breathing mechanics; and (3) high airway pressures and low tidal volumes—accomplished by strapping the rats' chest walls with rubber bands.[7] The results showed that only the lungs exposed to high volumes sustained injury, as was evidenced by the presence of high-permeability pulmonary edema.[8] That is, the rats in group 3, exposed to high airway pressures but low tidal volumes (because their chest walls could not expand), did not develop edema and were presumed to be uninjured.

These findings have been interpreted to mean that lung volume, not pressure, is the causative agent that produces lung injury. Although it is true that lung volume must increase to produce alveolar overdistention, it cannot do so without an increase in distending pressure, which should not be confused with the absolute alveolar pressure. The conclusion that volume is more important than pressure in producing lung injury is simplistic; it overlooks the inseparable relationship between transpulmonary pressures and lung volumes. The results of the rat study are not surprising when one realizes that transpulmonary pressure determined the alveolar volume and stretch in each ventilation method. As shown in Figure 14-5, ventilation with positive pressure (method 1) and with negative pressure (method 2) are the same with respect to their effects on alveolar epithelial stretch because their transpulmonary pressures were the same and thus produced the same tidal volumes. In ventilation method 3, the strapped chest walls caused alveolar and intrapleural pressures to increase together, keeping transpulmonary pressures (and thus tidal volumes and alveolar stretch) relatively small; therefore, this lung sustained no injury.

Figure 14-5 oversimplifies the lung's extremely complex architecture; that is, alveoli do not behave like individual balloons; they have shared walls. An intricate framework of connective tissue binds adjacent alveoli together such that they are interdependent. The mechanism of lung inflation does not involve balloon-like expansion and contraction of alveoli in the normal lung (see Chapter 3). However, regardless of inflation mechanism, lung volume changes can occur only as a result of transpulmonary pressure changes.

To summarize, the rat study[8] did not distinguish between the effects of pressure and volume on alveolar injury. Instead, it demonstrated that an increase in transpulmonary pressure, no matter how it is produced, generates an increase in lung volume, which, if great enough, injures the alveoli. It should be apparent that lung volume is a function of distending pressure and that volume and pressure cannot be separated in the roles they play in VILI. The idea that pressure and volume are independent of one another led to the suggestion that a mechanical ventilator can be engineered to guarantee delivery of a desired tidal volume without exceeding a preselected maximal pressure. In actuality, the microprocessor in such ventilators computes lung compliance and then determines whether or not the

---

CLINICAL FOCUS 14-1

Conservative vs. Aggressive Management

Mr. K, an alert, responsive, 80-kg man, sustained multiple injuries, including bone fractures and chest contusions, in an automobile accident. His current arterial blood gas values and vital signs, while spontaneously breathing supplemental oxygen at 12 L per minute from a nonrebreathing mask (F_IO_2 estimated at ≥0.80), are as follows:

Arterial Blood Gas Values
pH = 7.48
PCO_2 = 33 mm Hg
HCO_3^- = 24 mEq/L
PO_2 = 50 mm Hg
SO_2 (CO-oximeter) = 84%
Hemoglobin = 10 g/dL

Vital Signs
Blood pressure = 100/60 mm Hg
Temperature = 39.5° C
Respiratory rate = 28 breaths per minute
Heart rate = 136 beats per minute
The most recent chest x-ray shows bilateral infiltrates. Should this patient be intubated and placed on a mechanical ventilator, or is there reason to manage him more conservatively?

Discussion
This patient is at risk for developing ARDS (see Table 14-1). The $PaCO_2$ value rules out hypoventilation as the origin of hypoxemia, and the very poor response to the high inspired oxygen concentration indicates the presence of significant shunting. This situation and the chest x-ray are consistent with atelectasis and fluid-filled alveoli. The $PaCO_2$ and pH rule out ventilatory failure at this point; coupled with the patient's alert, responsive status, intubation and mechanical ventilation do not seem to be warranted. However, the current method of administering oxygen is inadequate. This situation calls for a trial of CPAP, which would be expected to increase FRC and facilitate alveolar recruitment and prevent alveolar recollapse. If CPAP accomplishes these beneficial effects, lung compliance would improve, work of breathing would decrease, and a lower concentration of oxygen would be necessary to maintain an acceptable PaO_2. CPAP does not actively ventilate an individual, but this patient's obvious ability to ventilate makes CPAP a reasonable option. In this situation, CPAP would be applied with a facemask with supplemental oxygen.

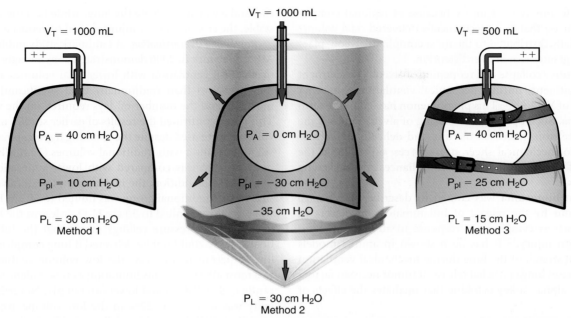

Figure 14-5 Conceptual illustration of three rat ventilation methods described in the text. *Method 1:* High airway pressure, high tidal volume; the pressure gradient responsible for the tidal volume (P_L) is $40 - 10 = 30$ cm H_2O. *Method 2:* Low airway pressure but the same tidal volume as in method 1, produced by decreasing the pressure around the chest wall below atmospheric levels; the pressure gradient responsible for the tidal volume (P_L) is exactly the same as in method 1, producing exactly the same degree of alveolar stretch. *Method 3:* High airway pressure, the same as in method 1, but low tidal volume because of a stiff chest wall that resists expansion; this compresses the intrapleural space more than in method 1. Intrapleural pressure (P_{pl}) increases more than in method 1, reducing the pressure gradient responsible for the tidal volume by half ($40 - 25 = 15$ cm H_2O), which reduces alveolar stretch.

selected volume can be delivered without exceeding the targeted pressure; if it cannot, the microprocessor simply adjusts the pressure target upward (within a factory preset limit) to deliver the desired volume. If still more inflation pressure is required to deliver the desired volume, the ventilator delivers only the volume that the lung can accept within the preset pressure limit (i.e., not all of the desired volume is delivered).

CONCEPT QUESTION 14-6

Explain why an alveolar pressure greater than 30 cm H_2O might nevertheless be safe with regard to alveolar injury if chest wall and diaphragm movement are abnormally restricted.

On the other hand, the rat study[8] points out the important fact that high alveolar pressure is not always associated with high lung volume. That is, high alveolar pressure does not always mean distention (transpulmonary) pressure is high, as demonstrated by the ventilation of rats with rubber-banded chest walls. Only when extrathoracic forces hinder chest wall expansion or hinder diaphragmatic displacement (e.g., rib cage deformities, severe abdominal distention, morbid obesity) is it possible for high alveolar pressures to be associated with a relatively low distention pressure. (Two other ordinary examples are the Valsalva maneuver, in which a person strains to exhale against a closed glottis, and the playing of a wind instrument such as an oboe, which presents high expiratory resistance; both situations increase the alveolar pressure without increasing transpulmonary pressure, as is evidenced by the lack of lung expansion.)

In mechanically ventilated patients, the correlate of alveolar pressure is plateau pressure, measured at the endotracheal tube at end-inspiration under zero airflow conditions (see Chapter 3). In all patients except patients with restricted chest wall and diaphragmatic movement, plateau pressure measurement is a reliable surrogate for assessing overdistention of the lung. It is generally accepted that the incidence of stretch-related lung injury is minimized if inspiratory plateau pressure is limited to less than 30 cm H_2O.[9,10]

This pressure may not be safe in highly compliant alveoli that are dispersed throughout the lungs, as seen in severe emphysema; such alveoli may sustain injury even if plateau pressure is less than 30 cm H_2O. That is, highly compliant alveoli may become overdistended at pressures much less than 30 cm H_2O.

Mechanisms of Lung Injury. Mechanisms of VILI fall into three general categories: (1) mechanical stretch injury from hyperinflation (barotrauma/volutrauma); (2) repetitive collapse and reinflation of alveoli (atelectrauma); and (3) toxic effects of inflammatory mediators on pulmonary tissues (biotrauma). As already indicated, mechanical overdistention of the alveoli disrupts the structural integrity of the lung, allowing air to dissect through lung tissues into the pleural space and mediastinum, producing pneumothorax and possibly dissection of air into subcutaneous tissues around the neck and upper chest (subcutaneous emphysema). In addition, overstretch of the alveoli disrupts the alveolar capillary membrane and induces the release of inflammatory mediators, both of which increase membrane permeability.[9-11] The heterogeneous distribution of diseased lung regions in ARDS makes the lung especially susceptible to this type of injury because of regional compliance differences; that is, a mechanically delivered tidal volume is preferentially distributed to the most compliant alveoli, placing them at greater risk of overdistension.

The repetitive collapse and reopening of alveoli (recruitment and derecruitment) during mechanical ventilation is another mechanism of VILI.[2,10,12] This phenomenon has led to the term **atelectrauma**. Such opening and closing of alveoli subjects the lung fibroskeleton, microvasculature, and delicate juxtaalveolar tissues to mechanical sheer stress forces, especially at the junctions of regions with differing compliances and anchoring attachments.[10]

The term **biotrauma** was coined to describe the damage brought about by the release of inflammatory mediators in the lung, such as cytokines, in response to atelectrauma and hyperinflation injury.[12] It has been shown in animal models that physical stretch of the lung during mechanical ventilation greatly increases lung epithelial release of tumor necrosis factor-alpha (TNF alpha), a key cytokine that mediates the effects of sepsis.[12]

CONCEPT QUESTION 14-7

Why is severe ARDS associated with the failure of other body organs besides the lungs?

Other cytokines, such as interleukins, may also be involved. Inflammatory mediators not only can affect the lung but also can affect other body organs; if alveolar disruption allows inflammatory mediators to translocate from the lung into the systemic circulation, it is possible that they can damage other body organs. It has been shown in adult patients with ARDS that a minimal stress mechanical ventilation strategy (low tidal volumes and the use of PEEP to prevent alveolar collapse) resulted in lower levels of cytokines in the systemic circulation than an injurious ventilation strategy (high tidal volumes with no PEEP).[12] Inflammatory mediators in the systemic circulation attract neutrophils and other inflammatory cells, potentially leading to injury of other organs, such as the kidneys and liver. This phenomenon may explain the increased incidence of **multisystem organ dysfunction syndrome (MODS)** seen in mechanically ventilated patients with severe ARDS.[12] A more recent study confirmed that a low tidal volume ventilation strategy coupled with adequate PEEP to prevent alveolar collapse during expiration reduces circulating cytokines.[13]

Physiological Rationale for Protective Ventilation Strategies

It stands to reason that if one can prevent lung overdistension, repetitive collapse and reopening of alveoli, and uneven distribution of the tidal volume, one can greatly reduce the incidence of VILI and its detrimental systemic effects. Although there is strong evidence that alveoli of normal lungs are very stable and do not change size during ventilation, alveoli do undergo large size changes in ALI, and alveolar recruitment and derecruitment is widespread.[14] It is reasonable to believe that if one

can find a way to ventilate the lungs while keeping alveolar size stable, the risk of alveolar injury should be reduced.

Preventing Overdistension. A landmark study published by the ARDS Network in 2000 demonstrated convincingly that in ALI, mechanical ventilation with lower tidal volumes and inspiratory pressures than traditionally used significantly decreases mortality and the number of days required on the ventilator.[11] This study confirmed the results of earlier studies in which low volumes were used despite the resulting hypercapnia and acidosis.[15] Ventilation with traditional volumes (12 mL/kg predicted body weight) was compared with lower ventilation volumes (6 mL/kg). In addition, the inspiratory plateau (alveolar) pressure in the traditional group was limited to 50 cm H_2O or less, whereas it was limited to 30 cm H_2O or less in the low-volume group. These pressure ceilings meant that the full calculated tidal volume could not be delivered if lung compliance was too low to permit its delivery; the low-volume ventilation group was most affected by this limitation as was evidenced by significantly higher $PaCO_2$ and lower arterial pH. Nevertheless, mortality was reduced by 22% in the low-volume group.[11] More recently, ARDS Network guidelines that limit plateau pressures to 30 cm H_2O or less were validated with regard to significant reduction in hospital mortality.[16] Ventilation with low volumes and the limitation of plateau pressures to 30 cm H_2O or less is considered the standard of care in the mechanical ventilation of patients with ARDS.[17]

If the low tidal volume ventilation strategy causes hypercapnia and acidosis, it is often referred to as **permissive hypercapnia**.[15] In other words, the adverse effects of hypercapnic acidosis that may result from low ventilation volumes are considered to be less detrimental to the patient than the alternative of overdistension lung injury. No safe upper limit for hypercapnia has been established, although some authorities believe the accompanying acidosis should not be allowed to fall below a pH of 7.20; infusion of sodium bicarbonate has been used to prevent arterial pH from falling below this level.[11,17] However, more recent evidence shows that hypercapnic acidosis may actually have a protective effect independent of lung volume.[18]

CONCEPT QUESTION 14-8

In what way might sodium bicarbonate infusion lead to higher $PaCO_2$?

Preventing Repetitive Collapse and Reopening of Alveoli (Atelectrauma). It stands to reason that a properly set PEEP level would prevent alveoli from collapsing at the end of expiration. Coupled with the low tidal volume strategy just outlined, the lung in ARDS would be protected from both overdistension and atelectrauma. That is, the lung would always be "open." This open-lung approach was first advocated in 1992[19]; an often cited study published in 1998 confirmed the protective effect of this ventilatory approach.[20] In this study, the investigator set PEEP just above the lower inflection point on the pressure-volume curve (see Chapter 3) to prevent repetitive alveolar collapse and reopening. The 28-day mortality rate was significantly lower in patients with ARDS ventilated with an open-lung approach

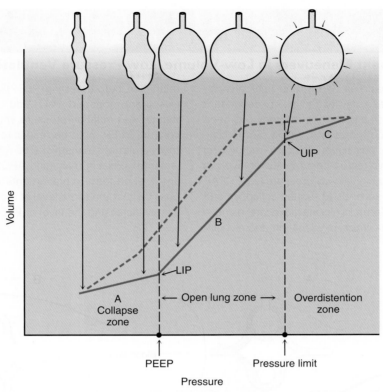

Figure 14-6 Pressure-volume waveform of a positive pressure breath (*solid line* = inspiration; *dotted line* = expiration). When the alveolus is collapsed, inflation pressure increases faster than volume (*line A*). The mass opening of many alveoli creates a lower inflection point (LIP), above which compliance dramatically improves (*line B*). When most alveoli reach their distention limit, an upper inflection point (UIP) is created, above which alveoli are dangerously overdistended (*line C*). If PEEP is set above the LIP and maximal inspiratory pressure is kept below the UIP, repetitive opening and closing injury and stretch-related injury are hypothetically avoided.

(38%) compared with a control group ventilated in the conventional manner (71%). The open-lung concept, or the use of enough PEEP to prevent alveolar collapse, and the limitation of plateau pressure to prevent overdistention—permitting hypercapnia if necessary—is now considered to be the standard of care against which all other strategies are measured in ventilating patients with ARDS (Figure 14-6).[21] As discussed in Chapter 3, it is now questioned whether the lower inflection point on the inspiratory pressure-volume curve is an appropriate criterion for setting PEEP at a level that prevents alveolar collapse; the hysteresis of the pressure-volume curve shows that lung volume is considerably greater at a given airway pressure on the expiratory limb of the curve than it is on the inspiratory limb. Nevertheless, the lower inflection point continues to be used by some practitioners as a criterion for setting PEEP in ALI,[22] although its use in this regard is controversial.

Prone Position: Improved $\dot{V}_A/\dot{Q}_C$ Match and Reduced Ventilator-Induced Lung Injury. Conventional mechanical ventilation is accomplished with the patient in the semisitting supine position. However, the prone position has been shown to improve oxygenation significantly and to delay VILI.[2,23-27]

Generally, the anterior (ventral) chest wall is more compliant and free to move than the posterior (dorsal) chest wall. The vertebral column limits dorsal rib cage movements much more than the sternum limits ventral rib cage movements. This condition is amplified in the supine position in which movements

of the rigid dorsal rib cage are further restricted by the body's weight against the bed's surface. For these reasons, ventral alveoli receive more ventilation than their dorsal counterparts (Figure 14-7, A). Moreover, in the supine position, the heart and the edematous ARDS lung weigh heavily on dorsal lung regions, possibly creating positive intrapleural pressure in this region. Consequently, dorsal alveoli tend to collapse. In mechanical ventilation, most of the tidal volume enters the more compliant ventral areas—both the lung and the rib cage are more compliant. Dorsal alveoli may open late in the inspiratory phase but then close again during expiration. Cyclical opening and closing of dorsal alveoli leads to lung injury, as previously described. For these reasons, VILI is most severe in dorsal lung regions of supine patients.[2]

In contrast to ventilation, pulmonary blood flow in the horizontal position (supine or prone) is relatively uniform from ventral to dorsal regions. Compared with the upright position, gravity has minimal effect on blood flow in the horizontal position because the ventral-to-dorsal lung distance is much less than the apex-to-base lung distance. Thus, dorsal lung units are very poorly ventilated with respect to their perfusion and are the site of the most significant shunting.

If the patient is turned to the prone position, the stiff dorsal component of the rib cage is freer to move than before, and the heart no longer compresses dorsal tissue (see Figure 14-7, B). The ventral rib cage is held against the bed surface,

CLINICAL FOCUS 14-2

Use of Lung Recruitment Maneuvers in Low-Volume, Low-Pressure Ventilation

Ventilation with low lung volumes, PEEP, and peak alveolar pressures of 30 cm H_2O or less may lead to gravity-dependent atelectasis, even though such a protective strategy has been shown conclusively to reduce mortality in ARDS. Some clinicians advocate the use of periodic hyperinflation to recruit lung volume. The most well-known recruitment maneuver involves the application of a sustained high airway pressure (e.g., CPAP of 30 to 50 cm H_2O) for 30 seconds to reopen collapsed and partly fluid-filled alveoli.[37] Some clinicians advocate using a recruitment maneuver to maximize oxygenation and alveolar reinflation before setting PEEP[10]; if a significant number of alveoli are reopened, PaO_2 and compliance should improve; that is, less inflation pressure should be required for a given volume. PEEP must be readjusted to sustain the benefits of the recruitment maneuver. The role of recruitment maneuvers is controversial in managing ARDS; studies have shown only small, short-term improvements in arterial oxygenation. It is possible that the same level of recruitment can be achieved by simply increasing the level of PEEP.

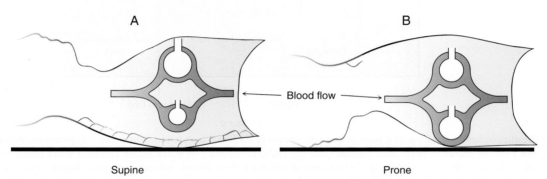

Figure 14-7 Theoretical mechanism whereby prone positioning improves oxygenation. Blood flow is similar in both dorsal and ventral lung regions regardless of position because of the small dorsal-ventral lung distance. This is not true for ventilation in the supine position. **A,** In the supine position, the ventral chest wall is freer to expand than the dorsal chest wall, which is restricted by the rigid vertebral column and the bed surface. Ventral alveoli receive more ventilation than dorsal alveoli. **B,** In the prone position, the bed surface reduces ventral chest wall compliance, resulting in approximately equal compliance in the ventral and dorsal chest wall. This equal compliance tends to distribute ventilation more uniformly, better matching it with blood flow distribution.

decreasing its compliance and freedom of movement. More of the mechanically delivered volume is directed toward dorsal regions than before. However, the natural stiffness of the dorsal rib cage limits how much ventilation can shift in its direction, forcing some of the volume into ventral units as well. The result is a fairly even tidal volume distribution in the lung and a better match between ventilation and blood flow; shunting is reduced, and oxygenation improves. To the extent that dorsal alveoli remain open, lung compliance improves, lowering the required inflation pressures. Because of less closing and reopening of alveoli in dorsal regions, the prone position is associated with less VILI.[25]

Prone positioning is generally combined with the other protective strategies already outlined, including low tidal volumes to prevent overdistention and PEEP adjusted to prevent alveolar recollapse. It is reasonable to believe that if prone ventilation is effective in improving oxygenation, it should also result in better carbon dioxide elimination, presumably through better ventilation of dorsal regions. It was found that a reduced $PaCO_2$ in response to prone ventilation was predictive of an improved survival rate; that is, patients in whom prone ventilation was associated with decreased $PaCO_2$ had a lower mortality rate

than patients in whom $PaCO_2$ remained the same.[28] Another predictor of response to prone positioning may be the distribution of disease in the ARDS lung.[29] ARDS is categorized as having one of three distribution patterns: (1) a lobar or segmental distribution; (2) a "patchy" distribution, in which lobar and segmental distribution coexist with areas not limited by anatomical boundaries; and (3) a "diffuse" distribution, in which disease is widespread and uniform throughout the lungs. Patients with lobar and patchy distributions are more likely to respond positively to prone positioning; that is, redistribution of densities is not as likely to occur in patients with diffuse, widespread patterns.[29]

CONCEPT QUESTION 14-9

Why might prone positioning be less effective in a diffuse, uniform pattern of ARDS than in ARDS with a patchy or lobar distribution?

A major meta-analysis of prone ventilation in ARDS did not show improved long-term patient survival, although oxygenation was significantly improved; however, there was a trend for lower mortality in the most severely ill patients when prone ventilation was used.[27] Longer duration in the prone position was associated with better outcomes; some authorities recommend maintaining the prone position for 12 to 20 hours per day.[10,27] Animal studies show reduced incidence of VILI with prone ventilation,[25] and it is thought that the prone position should be used sooner rather than later in the course of ARDS.[26,27] Generally, prone positioning is recommended for ARDS patients who require potentially harmful levels of F_IO_2 and plateau pressure, as long as positional changes do not place them at high risk, as might be the case in patients with spinal cord injuries.[10,17] Reversion to supine positioning at least once per day is recommended for patient washing and dressing changes; many patients with ARDS require almost continuous prone positioning for the first few days.[10] Of all lung protective ventilation strategies, volume-limiting and pressure-limiting strategies are the most universally accepted and most demonstrably effective in reducing mortality in ARDS.[30]

Pressure-Targeted versus Volume-Targeted Ventilation in Acute Respiratory Distress Syndrome. The realization that pressure-limiting ventilation strategies were associated with lower mortality in ARDS led manufacturers to develop ventilators that based the size of an inspiration on a preset pressure target rather than a preset volume target. Traditionally, intensive care ventilators were designed to cycle into expiration on delivery of a preselected volume at a preselected flow rate; in other words, these ventilators were "volume-targeted" machines. Inspiratory pressure depended on the elastic and resistive properties of the lung. If the lungs became less compliant over time, inspiratory pressure increased because the machine did not cycle into expiration until the preselected volume was delivered. In contrast, pressure-targeted machines were engineered to maintain a constant pressure at the endotracheal tube for the duration of inspiration (inspiratory pressure and inspiratory time were preselected by the clinician), regardless of lung compliance or airway resistance. Decreased lung compliance resulted in a reduced tidal volume; however, the lungs were never subjected to dangerously high pressures. Volume-targeted ventilators can be made to stop volume delivery if a pressure limit is preset; however, the ability to control pressure directly as a primary variable appealed to clinicians as a more intuitive way to protect the lung from excessive pressure.

CONCEPT QUESTION 14-10

Predict the nature of the inspiratory flow pattern produced by pressure-targeted mechanical ventilation.

Patients with ARDS can be effectively and safely ventilated by either type of ventilator. Low volumes can be used in volume-targeted machines, and high-pressure alarms can alert the clinician to dangerously high pressures. Likewise, desired pressure limits can be set in pressure-targeted ventilators, and low-volume alarms can alert the clinician of changing lung mechanics. However, one major difference between the two types of ventilators is the ventilator's flow rate response to the patient's spontaneous effort to breathe. In volume-targeted ventilators, the flow pattern is preset and does not change, whereas flow increases or decreases in response to patient demand in the pressure-targeted ventilator. By design, the pressure-targeted machine must maintain a constant pressure at the endotracheal tube for a specified time, which requires the ventilator to increase its flow output if the patient's inspiratory effort makes the circuit pressure drop. In the final analysis, the way in which inspiratory pressure is reduced (either by limiting the tidal volume in volume-targeted ventilation or by directly limiting inspiratory pressure in pressure-targeted ventilation) has no effect on mortality.[31] The important element influencing mortality is simply the use of low pressures and volumes.

Other Techniques for Treating Severe Oxygenation Failure

In addition to the ventilation strategies already outlined, pressure-limited mechanical ventilation and permissive hypercapnia, several other ventilation strategies have been described for severe ARDS. Airway pressure release ventilation (APRV) and bilevel positive airway pressure (BIPAP), nitric oxide inhalation, high-frequency oscillation ventilation, and liquid ventilation and their physiological rationales are briefly described in this section.

Airway Pressure Release Ventilation and Bilevel Positive Airway Pressure

APRV and BIPAP are mechanical ventilation modes that allow the patient to breathe spontaneously on top of the imposed mechanical ventilation pattern. Both modes supply the patient with alternating high and low levels of CPAP, which correspond to mechanical inspiration and expiration.[32] The term APRV traditionally refers to the mode in which the high CPAP level (inspiratory phase) lasts longer than the low CPAP level (expiratory phase), producing an inverse ratio pattern (i.e., inspiration lasts longer than expiration). The term BIPAP is used to describe the mode if high and low CPAP levels are applied for equal time periods or if low CPAP time is longer than high CPAP duration. However, these terms are not universally recognized; the numerous ventilator manufacturers tend to coin their own terms for these modes, each claiming some unique distinction that sets their ventilator's mode apart. For example, APRV is also known as Bi-Level Ventilation, Bi-Vent, and Duo-PAP.[32] Overall, APRV and BIPAP create higher mean airway pressures than the conventional low-volume, high-PEEP strategies mentioned earlier in this chapter.

The proposed mechanism of benefit for APRV and BIPAP is that these modes apply sustained levels of inspiratory pressure, which promote reopening of collapsed lung units, while still allowing the patient to breathe spontaneously at any time during the respiratory cycle. Enhanced alveolar recruitment should improve arterial oxygenation and decrease work of breathing by improving lung compliance. Spontaneous breathing efforts should provide a better distribution of ventilation than occurs with passive lung inflation through positive pressure ventilation; spontaneous breathing should also reduce mean intrathoracic pressure and lessen the adverse cardiovascular effects

CLINICAL FOCUS 14-3

ARDS Network Mechanical Ventilation Protocol for Acute Lung Injury and Acute Respiratory Distress Syndrome

In 1994, the National Institutes of Health and the National Heart, Lung, and Blood Institute initiated a clinical network (ARDS Network)[11] to find the best treatment strategies for ALI and ARDS through multicenter clinical trials. The network conducted a landmark randomized, controlled clinical trial that enrolled 861 subjects to compare lower tidal volume ventilation versus higher tidal volume in the treatment of patients with ALI early in their disease course. The study, published in the New England Journal of Medicine in 2000, conclusively showed for the first time that lower tidal volumes resulted in improved survival. The following mechanical ventilation protocol summary can be accessed on the Internet at www.ardsnet.org:

Ventilator Setup and Adjustment

- Calculate predicted body weight (PBW)
  Males: $50 + 2.3$ (height [inches]) $- 60$
  Females: $45.5 + 2.3$ (height [inches]) $- 60$
- Select assist/control mode
- Set initial V_T to 8 mL/kg PBW
- Reduce V_T by 1 mL/kg at intervals of 2 hours or less until $V_T = 6$ mL/kg
- Set initial respiratory rate (RR) to approximate baseline minute ventilation not greater than 35 breaths per minute
- Adjust V_T and RR to achieve pH and plateau pressure goals
- Set inspiratory flow to exceed patient demand (usually >80 L/min)

Oxygenation Goal: PaO_2 55 to 80 mm Hg or SpO_2 88% to 95%
- Use incremental F_IO_2/PEEP combinations to achieve goal:

F_IO_2	0.3	0.4	0.4	0.5	0.5	0.6	0.7	0.7
PEEP	5	5	8	8	10	10	10	12
F_IO_2	0.7	0.8	0.9	0.9	0.9	1.0	1.0	1.0
PEEP	14	14	14	16	18	20	22	24

Plateau Pressure (P_{plat}) Goal: 30 cm H_2O or Less
- Check P_{plat} (0.5 second inspiratory pause), SpO_2, RR, V_T, and pH at least every 4 hours and after each PEEP or V_T change
  If P_{plat} is greater than 30 cm H_2O: Decrease V_T by 1-mL/kg increments to minimum of 4 mL/kg
  If P_{plat} is less than 25 cm H_2O: If V_T is less than 6 mL/kg, increase V_T by 1-mL/kg increments until P_{plat} is greater than 25 cm H_2O, or $V_T = 6$ mL/kg
  If P_{plat} is less than 30 cm H_2O and breath stacking occurs: May increase V_T in 1-mL/kg increments to maximum of 8 mL/kg

pH Goal: 7.30 to 7.45
Acidosis Management (pH <7.30)
- **If pH is 7.15 to 7.30:** Increase RR until pH is greater than 7.30 or $PaCO_2$ is less than 25 mm Hg (maximum RR = 35)
  If RR = 35 and $PaCO_2$ is less than 25 mm Hg, may give sodium bicarbonate
- **If pH is less than 7.15:** Increase RR to 35
  If pH remains less than 7.15 and $NaHCO_3$ is considered or infused, V_T may be increased in 1-mL/kg steps until pH is greater than 7.15 (P_{plat} target may be exceeded)

Alkalosis Management (pH >7.45)
Decrease ventilator rate if possible

---

of these modes. In theory, APRV/BIPAP should make patients feel more comfortable because they can breathe spontaneously, and thus less sedation should be necessary; additionally, the patient's ability to use ventilatory muscles should improve muscle strength and endurance and shorten time spent on the ventilator.

At the time of this writing, none of the claims for the unique benefits of APRV and BIPAP have been subjected to rigorous scientific scrutiny; there is no strong evidence that these modes reduce the need for sedation, decrease the work of breathing, or reduce the time patients spend on mechanical ventilation.[32] Research efforts have been complicated by (1) disagreement among clinicians as to what constitutes APRV or BIPAP, (2) the lack of consistency among researchers in setting inspiratory/

expiratory timing ratios, and (3) the overlap of these modes with conventional pressure-targeted mechanical ventilation.[32]

Inhaled nitric oxide (iNO) may play a limited role in improving ventilation-perfusion relationships and PaO_2 in patients with severe ARDS.[33] As discussed in Chapter 6, nitric oxide is a potent pulmonary vasodilator and plays an important role in regulating pulmonary vascular resistance. In ARDS, hypoxic vasoconstriction (even though it is blunted in ARDS) reduces pulmonary blood flow in atelectatic regions of the lung. Inhalation of nitric oxide selectively dilates pulmonary vessels in well-ventilated regions where it is distributed; this diverts more blood flow to these regions and should improve their relationships. Studies have shown that iNO does improve $\dot{V}_A/\dot{Q}_C$, as evidenced by increased PaO_2; iNO also reduces pulmonary vascular resistance.[33] Such improved oxygenation may allow reductions in PEEP and F_IO_2, reducing the incidence of barotrauma and oxygen toxicity. However, iNO has not been shown to improve the survival rate in patients with ARDS; this is not surprising considering that most patients with ARDS die of multiorgan failure, not hypoxemia.[31] At the present time, evidence is insufficient to justify the routine use of iNO in patients with ARDS.[33,34]

High-Frequency Oscillatory Ventilation

In high-frequency oscillatory ventilation (HFOV), a continuous inspiratory flow (called bias flow) maintains a constant mean pressure in the airway. A rapidly oscillating (3 to 10 cycles per second) piston or diaphragm provides ventilation by creating small peak and trough pressures around the preset mean airway pressure. Gas exchange occurs essentially by diffusion; "tidal volumes" are less than the anatomical dead space volume. The constant mean oscillating airway pressure keeps the lung in a continuous partially inflated condition. Theoretically, HFOV is ideally suited for ARDS because alveoli are maintained in a continuously open state, avoiding atelectrauma and volutrauma because of the very small oscillating volumes. Nevertheless, clinical trials do not provide enough evidence to show improved mortality compared with conventional low-volume, low-pressure ventilation.[35]

Liquid Ventilation

Liquid ventilation uses an organic fluid that has a very high capacity for dissolving oxygen and carbon dioxide. The most widely used fluid is a perfluorocarbon compound known as perflubron.[2] The most common technique used is **partial liquid ventilation (PLV)**, in which the lung is filled with perflubron to the FRC level, and a conventional ventilator is used to deliver gas tidal volumes. Perflubron has a very low surface tension, which theoretically allows it to penetrate dependent lung regions and open collapsed alveoli.[2] Once filled with perflubron, alveoli cannot collapse again. The liquid also displaces secretions, making their removal more effective. PLV allows the use of lower pressures and volumes than conventional ventilation.[36] In theory, PLV should avoid the factors that produce VILI. However, there is not enough evidence at the present time to support its routine use in ARDS; clinical studies show no improvement in mortality over conventional low-volume, low-pressure ventilation.[36]

POINTS TO REMEMBER

- Oxygen therapy might cause hypercapnia in a patient with severe COPD.
- The nondiseased lung should be positioned in the down (gravity-dependent) position in unilateral lung disease to match blood flow better with normal lung tissue.
- The primary pathological feature of ALI and ARDS is lung inflammation that leads to alveolar capillary membrane injury and its increased permeability.
- Normal immune defense mechanisms are involved in producing ALI and ARDS.

- ARDS can be caused directly by external agents or indirectly by internal systemic agents.
- PEEP and CPAP work to recruit alveoli; prevent their collapse; and reduce shunt, increase FRC, and improve oxygenation.
- Any increase in lung volume and the resulting alveolar stretch must be instigated by an increase in pressure, whether the breath is spontaneously taken or mechanically induced.
- VILI is brought about by physical stress leading to ruptured alveoli, release of toxic inflammatory agents secondary to alveolar overdistention, and sheer forces of alveolar collapse and reopening.
- Adequate PEEP levels can prevent alveolar collapse and reopening injury.
- The prone position in mechanically ventilated patients with ARDS improves oxygenation and decreases physical lung trauma by distributing ventilation more evenly between dorsal and ventral lung regions and by preventing the repetitive collapse and reopening of dorsal alveoli.
- Mortality in ARDS is not differentially affected by volume-targeted versus pressure-targeted ventilation.
- The only protective ventilation strategy conclusively shown to decrease mortality in ARDS is the strategy employing low tidal volumes (≤6 mL/kg body weight) and low plateau pressures (≤30 cm H_2O).

References

1. American College of Chest Physicians–National Heart: Lung, and Blood Institute: National conference on O_2 therapy, *Respir Care* 29:922, 1984.
2. Lee WL, Slutsky AS: Hypoxemic respiratory failure, including acute respiratory distress syndrome. In Mason RJ, et al, editors: *Murray and Nadel's textbook of respiratory medicine*, ed 5, Philadelphia, 2010, Saunders.
3. Schuster DP, et al: Regional pulmonary perfusion in patients with acute pulmonary edema, *J Nucl Med* 43(7):863, 2002.
4. Patroniti N, et al: Measurement of pulmonary edema in patients with acute respiratory distress syndrome, *Crit Care Med* 33(11):2547, 2005.
5. Shapiro BA, Peruzzi WT, Templin R: *Clinical application of blood gases*, ed 5, St Louis, 1994, Mosby.
6. Marini JJ, Wheeler AP: *Critical care medicine: the essentials*, Baltimore, 1989, Williams & Wilkins.
7. Slutsky AS: Lung injury caused by mechanical ventilation, *Chest* 116(1):9S, 1999.
8. Dreyfuss D, et al: High inflation pressure pulmonary edema: respective effects of high airway pressure, high tidal volume, and positive end-expiratory pressure, *Am Rev Respir Dis* 137(5):1159, 1988.
9. Hess DR, Kacmarek RM: *Essentials of mechanical ventilation*, ed 2, New York, 2002, McGraw-Hill.
10. Marini JJ, Gattinoni L: Ventilatory management of acute respiratory stress syndrome: a consensus of two, *Crit Care Med* 32(1):250, 2004.
11. The Acute Respiratory Distress Syndrome Network: Ventilation with lower tidal volumes as compared with traditional tidal volumes for acute lung injury and the acute respiratory distress syndrome, *N Engl J Med* 342(18):1301, 2000.

12. Slutsky AS: Ventilator-induced lung injury: from barotrauma to biotrauma, *Respir Care* 50(5):646, 2005.

13. Reis Miranda D, et al: Ventilation according to the open lung concept attenuates inflammatory pulmonary inflammation response in cardiac surgery, *Eur J Cardiothorac Surg* 28(6):889, 2005.

14. Carney D, DiRocco J, Nieman G: Dynamic alveolar mechanics and ventilator-induced lung injury, *Crit Care Med* 33(Suppl 3):S122, 2005.

15. Hickling KG, Henderson SJ, Jackson R: Low mortality associated with low volume pressure limited ventilation with permissive hypercapnia in severe adult respiratory distress syndrome, *Intensive Care Med* 16(6):372, 1990.

16. Kallet RH, et al: Clinical implementation of the ARDS network protocol is associated with reduced hospital mortality compared with historical controls, *Crit Care Med* 33(5):925, 2005.

17. Sevransky JE, Levy MM, Marini JJ: Mechanical ventilation in sepsis-induced acute lung injury/acute respiratory distress syndrome: an evidence-based review, *Crit Care Med* 32(Suppl 11):S548, 2004.

18. Kregenow DA, et al: Hypercapnic acidosis and mortality in acute lung injury, *Crit Care Med* 34(1):1, 2006.

19. Lachmann B: Open up the lung and keep the lung open, *Intensive Care Med* 18(6):319, 1992.

20. Amato MB, et al: Effect of a protective-ventilation strategy on mortality in the acute respiratory distress syndrome, *N Engl J Med* 338(6):347, 1998.

21. Levy MM: Pathophysiology of oxygen delivery in respiratory failure, *Chest* 128(5 Suppl 2):547S, 2005.

22. Michaels AJ: Management of post traumatic respiratory failure, *Crit Care Clin* 20(1):83, 2004.

23. Gattinoni L, et al: Effect of prone positioning on the survival of patients with acute respiratory failure, *N Engl J Med* 345(8):568, 2001.

24. Slutsky AS: The acute respiratory distress syndrome, mechanical ventilation, and the prone position, *N Engl J Med* 345(8):610, 2001.

25. Valenza F, et al: Prone position delays the progression of ventilator-induced lung injury in rats: does lung strain distribution play a role? *Crit Care Med* 33(2):361, 2005.

26. Reignier J: Prone position: can we move from better oxygenation to better survival? *Crit Care Med* 33(2):453, 2005.

27. Alsaghir AH, Martin CM: Effect of prone positioning in patients with acute respiratory distress syndrome: a meta-analysis, *Crit Care Med* 36(2):603, 2008.

28. Gattinoni L, et al: Decrease in $PaCO_2$ with prone position is predictive of improved outcome in acute respiratory distress syndrome, *Crit Care Med* 31(12):2727, 2003.

29. Pelosi P, Brazzi L, Gattinoni L: Prone position in acute respiratory distress syndrome, *Eur Respir J* 20(4):1017, 2002.

30. Fan E, Needham DM, Stewart TE: Ventilatory management of acute lung injury and acute respiratory distress syndrome, *JAMA* 294(22):2889, 2005.

31. Esteban A, et al: Prospective randomized trial comparing pressure-controlled ventilation and volume-controlled ventilation in ARDS, *Chest* 117(6):1690, 2000.

32. Kallet RH: Patient-ventilator interaction during acute lung injury, and the role of spontaneous breathing: part 2: airway pressure release ventilation, *Respir Care* 56(2):190, 2011.

33. Fan E, Mehta S: High frequency oscillatory ventilation and adjunctive therapies: inhaled nitric oxide and prone positioning, *Crit Care Med* 33(Suppl 3):S182, 2005.

34. Sokol J, Jacobs SE, Bohn D: Inhaled nitric oxide for acute hypoxemic respiratory failure in children and adults, *Cochrane Database Syst Rev* (3), 2006. http://www.cochrane.org/reviews/en/ab002787.html.

35. Chan KPW, Stewart TE, Mehta S: High-frequency oscillatory ventilation for adult patients with ARDS, *Chest* 131(6):1907, 2007.

36. Davies MW, Sargent PH: Partial liquid ventilation for the prevention of mortality and morbidity in paediatric acute lung injury and acute respiratory distress syndrome, *Cochrane Database Syst Rev* (3), 2006. http://www.cochrane.org/reviews/en/ab003845.html.

37. Kacmarek RM, Kallet RH: Should recruitment maneuvers be used in the management of ALI and ARDS? *Respir Care* 52(5), 2007.

CHAPTER 15

Physiology of Sleep-Disordered Breathing

S. Gregory Marshall

OBJECTIVES

After reading this chapter, you will be able to:
- Explain how the brain regulates sleeping and waking cycles through neurocontrolled chemical mediators
- Explain why the upper airway anatomy plays such a major role in sleep-disordered breathing (SDB)
- Distinguish between the three stages of nonrapid eye movement sleep and rapid eye movement sleep
- Identify the six major categories of sleep disorders and the specific classification for SDB
- Differentiate between obstructive sleep apnea, central sleep apnea, mixed sleep apnea, childhood sleep apnea, and sudden infant death syndrome

- Explain the effects of SDB on the cardiovascular system
- Identify the mechanisms of central hemodynamic dysfunction secondary to SDB
- Classify SDB through the use of the polysomnogram
- Explain the physiological treatment of SDB using positive airway pressure, oral appliances, positional therapy, and airway enlargement treatment

KEY TERMS

alpha waves
apnea
apnea-hypopnea index (AHI)
bilevel positive airway pressure (BIPAP)
central sleep apnea (CSA)
circadian rhythm
congestive heart failure
continuous positive airway pressure (CPAP)
delta waves
durable medical equipment (DME)
dyssomnias
electroencephalogram (EEG)
electromyography (EMG)
excessive daytime somnolence
heart failure

hypersomnolence
hypopnea
hypothalamus
insomnia
macroglossia
Mallampati score
mandibular advancement device (MAD)
maxillomandibular advancement
micrognathia
mixed sleep apnea (MSA)
montage
nasal cycling
nonrapid eye movement (NREM)
obstructive sleep apnea (OSA)
polysomnogram (PSG)

KEY TERMS—cont'd

prescriptive pressure
radiofrequency tissue ablation
rapid eye movement (REM)
respiratory effort–related arousals (RERAs)
retrognathia
sleep architecture
sleep arousal
sleep-disordered breathing (SDB)

sleep histogram
sleep hygiene
sudden infant death syndrome (SIDS)
suprachiasmatic nucleus (SCN)
tongue retaining device (TRD)
uvulopalatopharyngoplasty (UPPP)
ventrolateral preoptic nucleus

FUNCTIONAL ANATOMY AND PHYSIOLOGY OF SLEEP

"To sleep: perchance to dream: ay, there's the rub."—William Shakespeare, *Hamlet* (III, I, 65-68)

The study of sleep has intrigued people through the ages. With more than one third of the human life span spent sleeping, the mystery of sleep and dreams is an experience common to everyone; yet, research has yielded few answers to the secrets of sleep. Although documentation of sleep disorders and dreaming can be found throughout recorded history, scientists have yet to discover the ultimate reason why humans need sleep, how it directly affects waking functionality, and the nature of physiological mechanisms associated with sleep. Certain anatomical and physiological disorders commonly associated with **sleep-disordered breathing (SDB)** are better understood; these include abnormal respiratory patterns and poor ventilation quality during sleep. Key to the understanding of SDB is a basic comprehension of the brain's role in controlling sleep and the anatomical and physiological features of the upper airways.

Neurocontrol of Sleep

Sleep has been described as "a reversible behavioral state of perceptual unresponsiveness to the environment with documentable, distinguishable physiological patterns of neural and muscle activity."[1] The diagnostic test performed to evaluate the quality of sleep is called a sleep study, or **polysomnogram (PSG)**. The PSG documents more than 20 individual physiological parameters during all phases of the sleep cycle. The term polysomnogram is derived from its prefix, root, and suffix definitions: "poly" means "many," "somno" means "sleep," and "gram" means "writing." This quantitative diagnostic study records physiological data during each second of sleep from wakefulness through the three sleep stages of **nonrapid eye movement (NREM)** to the **rapid eye movement (REM)** stage. Through the PSG, the sleep process can be classified in an objective, quantifiable way. However, the precise mechanisms responsible for sleep onset and waking from sleep continue to be the focus of intensive investigation. Although the brain plays a definitive role in sleep regulation, the specific anatomical region of the brain responsible for the sleep control is a subject

of controversy. It is now well established that the hypothalamus is the key regulator of sleep and wakefulness.[2] Since sleep research is now focused on the hypothalamus, new pharmaceutical and therapeutic breakthroughs for neurological sleep disorders have been developed.

The brain is composed of five major regions: the medulla oblongata, which is the most posterior portion of the brain that fuses with the spinal cord; the pons, located superiorly to the medulla oblongata; the midbrain or mesencephalon, located just above the pons; the telencephalon or cerebrum, which consists of five paired lobes within two convoluted hemispheres; and the diencephalon, which sits superior to the brainstem nestled between the two cerebral hemispheres. The diencephalon includes the thalamus, the **hypothalamus**, the optic chiasm, and the pineal gland (Figure 15-1). Sleep researchers have identified more than 70 distinct sleep disorders but have yet to identify the precise neurochemical mechanisms that "turn on and turn off" sleep and wakefulness. As mentioned, the central focus of study in sleep regulation is currently the hypothalamus.

Biomedical sleep research has definitively determined that the primary biological "sleep clock" resides in the **suprachiasmatic**

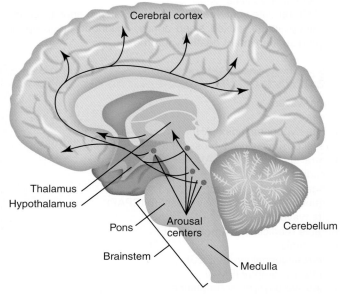

Figure 15-1 Illustration of the brain anatomy showing five component parts.

nucleus (**SCN**) of the hypothalamus where it controls the timing of the sleep cycle, or the **circadian rhythm**. When SCN function is disrupted, the circadian rhythm becomes random and sporadic. However, even though the onset of sleep may vary throughout a 24-hour period, the total sleep time remains the same. Located just above the optic chiasm, the SCN is believed to control certain neurologically secreted chemicals that regulate the sleep cycle. Light plays a very important role in the normal regulation of the SCN. Light is an environmental cue or stimulator known as the *zeitgeber*, or "time-giver," that regulates the sleep/wake cycle. The role that light plays as a circadian rhythm "cue" can be observed through the disrupted sleep habits of individuals living in geographical areas of prolonged winter darkness. A decrease in the amount of daylight exposure significantly alters the normal sleep/wake cycle during the winter seasons. The optic chiasm is thought to relay light/dark cues from the eye to the hypothalamus as a reference for the circadian rhythm. It is now understood that the SCN of the hypothalamus merely tracks day and night cycles, whereas the **ventrolateral preoptic nucleus (VLPO)** in the hypothalamus initiates sleep by inhibiting the brain's arousal centers in the brainstem (Figure 15-2).

The role of the hypothalamus in controlling the regulation of sleep/wake mechanisms has been confirmed. Various neurotransmitters released by the hypothalamus are believed to produce sleep by inhibiting the brain's arousal centers. The neurotransmitters that mediate arousal in the cortex include histamine, serotonin, norepinephrine, acetylcholine, and hypocretin (orexin) (Figure 15-3). Sleep research has shown that disruption of the VLPO and the lateral region of the hypothalamus results in arousal. The loss of the VLPO and the lateral hypothalamus structures have been associated with the symptoms of insomnia or narcolepsy respectively.[3]

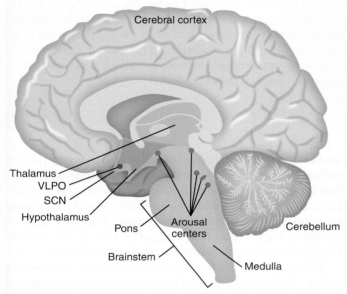

Figure 15-2 Suprachiasmatic nucleus (SCN) and ventrolateral preoptic nucleus (VLPO) inhibiting arousal centers.

CONCEPT QUESTION 15-1

What part of the brain has been shown to be the primary controller for sleep and wakefulness?

UPPER AIRWAY ANATOMY AND SLEEP

Human neonates have the remarkable ability to breathe, suck, and swallow simultaneously owing to the anatomical configuration of the upper airway at birth. Additionally, neonates are obligate nose breathers. During the first month of life, the neonatal upper airway grows and matures toward adult upper airway proportions; the infant's ability to breathe, suck, and swallow simultaneously wanes. Throughout infancy, adolescence, and

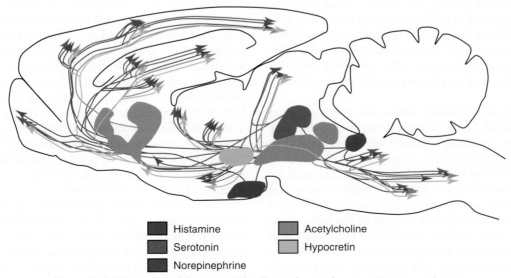

Figure 15-3 Illustration of the brain with release of arousal center neurotransmitters.

CLINICAL FOCUS 15-1

Effects of Nasal Cycling on Sleep-Disordered Breathing

Nasal cycling is an alternation of the degree of congestion between nares when the mucosa of one side of the nasal cavity becomes more swollen; this results in diminished airflow through the obstructed naris compared with the opposing naris. This autonomic nervous system response is believed to originate from the hypothalamus and was first described in 1895 by Kayser.[31] Nasal cycling is not to be confused with simple nasal congestion; nasal cycling is a normal event throughout the day and during sleep.

If a patient has a deviated septum resulting in diminished airflow through one nostril on a regular basis, what impact does nasal cycling have on the patient's sleep quality when nasal cycling decreases airflow through the more patent or open nostril? If the patient has SDB and is wearing a nasal mask, how does nasal cycling affect airway pressure? Could a decrease in airflow associated with nasal cycling prompt a RERA or sleep arousal? Would PAP devices compensate for the diminished flow through an obstructed naris?

Discussion

Nasal cycling is a frequently ignored issue that may play a significant role in regular patient use of PAP treatment of SDB. When an anatomical issue, such as a deviated septum, is present, special care should be taken in choosing the proper PAP patient adjunct or mask. Individual nasal pillows would not be the best choice because of the imbalance of pressure and nasal cycling events. The better choice for a patient with a deviated septum would be either a nasal mask or an oronasal mask. During nasal cycling, the decrease in patency of one naris obligates greater flow through the unobstructed naris. This sensation may disturb the sleep of the patient and trigger an arousal related to respiratory effort shifting the patient to a lighter stage of sleep or awakening the patient. Current PAP devices do not compensate for nasal cycling, but clinical trials are under way to address this issue.

---

adulthood, humans remain obligate nose breathers during sleep, which is often the source of significant problems for individuals with sleep disorders.

Oropharynx

The upper airways comprise three primary anatomical regions: the nose, pharynx, and larynx. As discussed in Chapter 1, normal pharyngeal muscle tone prevents the base of the tongue from falling backward in the oral cavity and obstructing the oropharyngeal airway. Sleep or unconscious states result in a loss of pharyngeal muscle tone and the relaxation of the soft tissue that constitutes the oropharynx and the tongue. Under the influence of gravity, the relaxed tongue falls into the oropharynx, partially or totally occluding the airway. Partial occlusions result in low-pitched snoring sounds, whereas complete occlusion results in apnea, characterized by ventilatory efforts without airflow. Several other soft tissue anatomical structures in the oropharynx may contribute to partial or total obstruction.

Obligate nose breathing during sleep causes problems when the nose is obstructed. Many individuals experience difficulty sleeping when nose breathing is limited because of nasal congestion that accompanies a cold or allergy. At the onset of sleep when obligate nose breathing begins, restricted nasal air passages usually cause sleepless or restless nights. Anatomical abnormalities such as a deviated septum create a permanent limitation of airflow through one or both of the nares. Poor quality of sleep is often a major complaint of individuals with nasal septum abnormalities. The assessment of a potential sleep disorder should always begin with inspection of each naris for patency and unrestricted airflow. If allergies are an issue,

medications that diminish nasal swelling or secretions to reduce airflow restriction should be considered. If anatomical obstruction is the primary cause of airflow limitations, corrective surgery may be the best remedy for the sleep disorder. If the nose is occluded during sleep, secondary mouth breathing becomes necessary. Regardless of nose or mouth breathing, the oropharyngeal airway must remain patent to allow ventilation.

Within the oral cavity, five specific structures can obstruct airflow. Mallampati was the first to categorize the amount of "open space" in the oropharynx by the visualization of five structures: the tongue, the soft palate, the hard palate, the uvula, and the tonsils.[4] Originally used to classify the difficulty level of oral endotracheal intubation, the **Mallampati score** is determined by direct visualization of the oropharynx through the open mouth. There are four categories of decreasing airway space (Figure 15-4). A class 1 score is considered normal, in which all five anatomical structures are visible. In class 2, all five structures can be identified, but only the upper portions of the tonsils and uvula are visible. Class 3 allows only the tongue, the soft and hard plate, and the base of the uvula to be seen. Class 4 allows visualization of only the hard palate and tongue. The higher the Mallampati classification number, the more anatomical crowding with less oropharyngeal room for airflow. Sleep research has shown a positive correlation between a high Mallampati score and the risk for obstructive sleep disorders when nasal obstruction is present.[5]

Because the mandible anatomically supports and positions the tongue and is part of the oropharyngeal structure, the size of the mandible may limit airflow during sleep. A small, recessed lower jaw, or **retrognathia**, results in a more retrograde or posteriorly positioned tongue. A posterior position of the tongue makes it easier for the tongue to fall back and

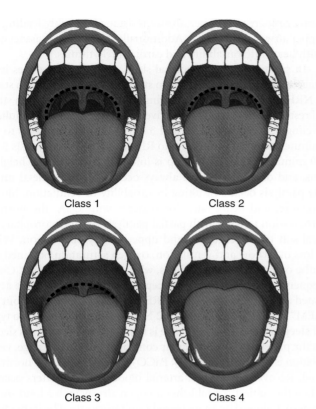

Figure 15-4 Mallampati scores. (Redrawn from Wilkins RL, et al: *Clinical assessment in respiratory care,* ed 6, St Louis, 2010, Mosby.)

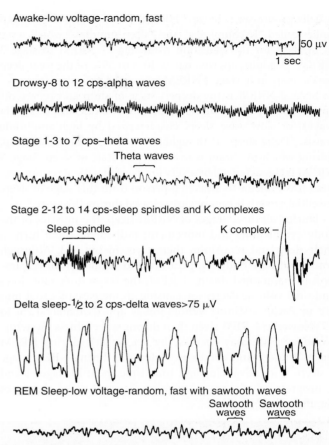

Figure 15-5 Electroencephalogram brain waves for wake and sleep stages. (From Wilkins RL, et al: *Clinical assessment in respiratory care,* ed 6, St Louis, 2010, Mosby.)

block the oropharynx as the pharyngeal muscles relax. An enlarged tongue, or **macroglossia**, as seen in individuals with Down syndrome, hypothyroidism, and acromegaly, can also crowd the oropharynx decreasing the size of the airway lumen. A shortened or widened neck may also crowd the anatomical structures, narrowing or obstructing the oropharyngeal lumen. A neck circumference greater than 17 inches in men or greater than 16 inches in women is highly correlated with the incidence of obstructive sleep apnea (OSA).[6,7]

CONCEPT QUESTION 15-2

During sleep, humans become obligate nose breathers. How does the oropharyngeal anatomy affect breathing during sleep?

CONCEPT QUESTION 15-3

How is the Mallampati score used to assess the possible presence of SDB?

STAGES OF SLEEP

Sleep is an active process in which specific regions of the brain show continuous electrical activity that can be physiologically monitored. An understanding of the normal stages of sleep is necessary for the clinician to evaluate sleep disorders. In adults

and children, the two major states of sleep are non-rapid eye movement (NREM) and rapid eye movement (REM). Sleep stages are categorized according to the absence or presence of eye movement.

The normal pattern of sleep stages involves the cycling back and forth between NREM and REM stages every 60 to 90 minutes for four to five cycles during an 8-hour sleep period. Sleep normally begins with the NREM stages and progresses to REM sleep. During the awake phase, the **electroencephalogram (EEG)**, or electrical waveform of brain activity, shows a pattern of small, fine waves oscillating at a high frequency, known as **alpha waves** (Figure 15-5). At the onset of sleep, alpha waveforms slow and change to waveforms characteristic of NREM sleep, suggesting a resting or restorative state of the brain.

Nonrapid Eye Movement

NREM sleep is composed of three stages with each progressive stage transitioning to a deeper state of sleep. Stage 1 NREM represents the onset of sleep for adults and children. During stage 1 NREM, the eyes roll gently and slowly while low-amplitude EEG brainwaves are noted during the sleep study. This change in EEG brain wave pattern is associated with the transition from awake to sleep. Only 5% to 10% of the entire sleep period is spent in stage 1 NREM, and within 2 to 10 minutes, sleep usually progresses to stage 2 NREM. EEG tracings show sharp spikes called "K-complexes" and "sleep spindles," which serve as markers for the transition from stage 1 NREM to stage 2 NREM. In adults, approximately 40% to 50% of the total sleep period is spent in stage 2 NREM.[8]

Stage 3 NREM is the deepest stage of sleep and represents approximately 25% of the sleep period. The EEG displays **delta waves**, or slow-wave sleep, characterized by high-amplitude waves. "Delta sleep" is thought to represent restorative sleep, during which the brain is in its deepest state of sleep. Stage 3 NREM is characterized by a very low level of patient responsiveness; it is difficult to awaken a person from this stage of sleep. Essential growth hormones are released during this stage.[8-10]

During all three stages of NREM sleep, the muscles of the body exhibit tone and movement; individuals often turn in their sleep and reposition themselves in the bed. Although control of core body temperature and regulation of respiration is maintained during NREM, the respiratory rate slows and tidal volume decreases, causing an increase of 2 to 4 mm Hg in $PaCO_2$. Minute ventilation is approximately 13% to 15% lower in NREM sleep than during wakefulness. Systemic blood pressure may decrease by 5% to 10% during NREM stages 1 and 2 and decrease 8% to 14% during NREM stage 3 sleep. With advancing age, total time spent in stages 1 and 2 progressively increases, whereas stage 3 sleep decreases significantly.[10,11]

> ### CONCEPT QUESTION 15-4
>
> *Explain the difference between NREM stages 1, 2, and 3 with regard to the sleep cycle.*

Rapid Eye Movement

REM sleep is associated with a loss of core body temperature regulation, whereas cerebral blood flow and cerebral temperature increase owing to increased brain activity. Systemic blood pressure becomes variable and elevated during REM. These normal physiological effects of REM place patients with preexisting pulmonary or cardiac disease at greater risk for exacerbations of their disease.

EEG tracings during REM strongly resemble the level of brain activity seen in the awake state (i.e. alpha-like, low-voltage, random, high-frequency waveforms) (see Figure 15-5). As sleep progresses, adults and children cycle back to NREM stages and return to the REM stage three to five times. The time spent in REM normally increases with each cycle for a total of approximately 25% of the sleep period. **Electromyography (EMG)** shows skeletal muscle tone at its lowest level during the REM stage, suggesting a paralyzed state. This partial paralysis results in a further decrease of the minute ventilation in healthy adults and children, producing a few associated episodes of hypoxemia and hypercapnia, which are normal during REM. Loss of skeletal muscle tone during REM affects pharyngeal muscles; upper airway resistance increases as pharyngeal tissues relax and narrow the upper airway lumen. As previously mentioned, relaxation of the tongue and soft tissues of the oropharynx are the primary cause of increased upper airway resistance, possibly leading to upper airway obstruction. Additionally, REM sleep is associated with heart rate variability and cardiac arrhythmias.[8-11]

In summary, during normal sleep, an individual dozes into stage 1 NREM and progresses to stage 2 NREM and then to stage 3 NREM as sleep deepens. During NREM, the brain is in a state of rest while the body is still active and can respond to stimuli. A cycling between stage 1, 2, and 3 NREM continues for 60 to 90 minutes before transitioning to REM, which normally lasts 5 to 30 minutes. Once REM sleep is initiated, brain activity heightens, and dreaming almost always occurs. Partial skeletal muscle paralysis occurs resulting in variability of ventilation, blood pressure, and heart rate. For patients with OSA, the normal progression to REM with partial paralysis results in oropharyngeal soft tissue relaxation and upper airway obstruction. With a loss of airflow and ventilation, oxygen saturation obtained by pulse oximeter (SpO_2) declines, whereas $PaCO_2$ increases. Consequently, medullary chemoreceptors sensitive to CO_2 are activated and disrupt the onset of REM, "pulling the patient out of REM" and back into stage 1 or 2 NREM sleep; this event is a type of **sleep arousal**. This sequence is repetitive and fragments sleep; as the patient regains muscular control in the NREM stage, ventilation is restored, and PaO_2, $PaCO_2$, and pH values are normalized. Recovery of normal arterial blood gas parameters occurs when the subject reestablishes an open airway with a loud snort or gasp, followed by an increased respiratory rate. The individual then slips back into the next NREM stage only to be disrupted from REM sleep repeatedly throughout the night. Patients with SDB commonly lack years of REM sleep; their histories often reveal that they have not dreamed for many years.

Sleep architecture refers to the pattern in which an individual moves back and forth between sleep stages throughout the night. Although the approximate percentage of sleep time spent in the three stages of NREM and the REM stage previously described represents normal sleep architecture, each person has a distinct pattern unique to his or her own sleep cycle. The graphic representation of a patient's sleep architecture is known as a **sleep histogram** and is a standard part of every sleep study; it depicts the summative time spent in each phase of sleep at a glance (Figure 15-6). When a patient's NREM and REM cycles become fragmented on a regular basis, the patient is said to have poor **sleep hygiene**. Poor sleep hygiene is often due to the lack of a sleep routine or the lack of appropriate sleep cues that signal the body to prepare for sleep, which is typical of the sleep habits of a night shift worker.[9-11]

> ### CONCEPT QUESTION 15-5
>
> *Describe the physiological changes that occur in the body during REM stage sleep.*

SLEEP DISORDERS

Approximately 1 in 6, or greater than 50 million, Americans have some form of sleep disorder. More than 84 sleep disorders have been identified and coded by the World Health Organization's *International Classification of Diseases and Related Health*

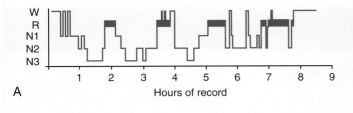

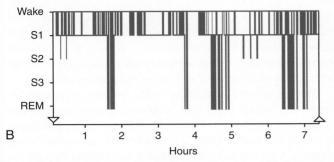

Figure 15-6 A, Represents a normal sleep histogram with time spent in Stages N1, N2, and N3 and increasing REM (R) sleep through the night. **B,** Represents an abnormal sleep histogram with sleep primarily restricted to Stage N1 and scattered irregular periods of REM sleep.

BOX 15-1

International Classification of Diseases and Related Health Problems, 10th Revision, Classification of Sleep Disorder Categories

Dyssomnias—sleep disorders characterized by hypersomnolence or insomnia
  Insomnia
  Narcolepsy
  Sleep apnea (adult and pediatric)
  Periodic limb movement disorders
  Hypersomnia
  Circadian rhythm sleep disorders
Parasomnias
  REM sleep behavior disorder
  Sleep terror
  Sleepwalking (somnambulism)
  Bruxism (teeth grinding)
  Bedwetting (nocturnal enuresis)
  Sleep talking (somniloquy)
  Sleep sex (sexsomnia)
  Exploding head syndrome (awaking hearing loud noises)
Medical or psychiatric conditions (producing sleep disorders)
  Psychoses (schizophrenia)
  Mood disorders
  Depression
  Anxiety
  Panic
  Alcoholism
Sleep sickness (parasitic disease caused by tsetse fly)
Snoring
Sudden infant death syndrome

Problems, 10th Revision (ICD-10), which assists health care providers in categorizing sleep disturbances. The ICD-10 coding system classifies diseases, signs and symptoms, abnormal findings, complaints, social circumstances, and external causes of injury or diseases.[12] In the latest edition of ICD-10, sleep disorders are classified under "Mental and Behavior Disorders" in a subcategory called "Behavior Syndromes Associated with Physiological Disturbances and Physical Factors." The physiology and comorbidities associated with sleep disturbances are complex; a growing number of patients with SDB complain of numerous chronic ailments, including hypertension, depression, heart failure, obesity, learning disorders, and posttraumatic stress syndrome.

There are six broad classifications of sleep disorders with multiple subcategories (Box 15-1). The six major categories include dyssomnias, parasomnias, medical or psychiatric conditions producing sleep disorders, sleep sickness, snoring, and sudden infant death syndrome (SIDS). The largest and most common category of sleep disorders is the dyssomnia group. **Dyssomnias** ("difficult sleep") are primarily characterized either as excessive daytime sleepiness (**hypersomnolence**) or as the inability to fall asleep (**insomnia**). SDBs in the dyssomnia category include **obstructive sleep apnea (OSA)**, **central sleep apnea (CSA)**, and **mixed sleep apnea (MSA)**.

Obstructive Sleep Apnea

In the United States, the most common SDB in adults is OSA, which affects an estimated 18 million Americans. The etiology of OSA is primarily anatomical, combining the complications of disordered REM physiology with a decreased oropharyngeal lumen. Contributing factors include macroglossia (large tongue), **micrognathia** (small mandible), deviated nasal septum, and retrognathia (recessed lower jaw). Depending on oropharyngeal anatomy, loss of muscle tone and muscle paralysis during REM sleep may partially or completely obstruct the airway lumen. Complete airway obstruction produces **apnea**, defined as the absence of ventilation lasting 10 seconds or more. Partial obstruction of the airway causes **hypopnea**, defined as a 50% reduction in the tidal volume. Apneic and hypopneic events are critical diagnostic markers documented in all sleep studies on the PSG.

During an apnea event, the patient with OSA continues to make ventilatory efforts despite complete airway obstruction. During inspiration, the diaphragms move downward, which generates greater negative intrapleural pressures as the patient tries to inhale. The chest and abdomen move paradoxically, or oppositely, producing a "seesaw" movement. When paradoxical breathing is matched with PSG tracings that document the absence of airflow for at least 10 seconds, an apneic event has occurred. The effect is similar to placing a hand over the nose and mouth of an individual and asking him or her to breathe in as deeply as possible. Full chest and abdominal efforts are apparent, but they produce no airflow. Patients with OSA commonly describe their regular sleeping experiences as episodes

CLINICAL FOCUS 15-2

Non–Sleep-Disordered Breathing Disorders

Although sleep apnea is the most common condition of the more than 84 sleep disorders currently identified, the remaining sleep disorders are not specifically characterized by difficult breathing during sleep. Box 15-1 details the ICD-10 Classifications of Sleep Disorder categories with SDB diagnoses such as OSA, CSA, and MSA falling under the general category of dyssomnia, or "difficulty sleeping." Generally, dyssomnias are characterized by hypersomnolence—excessive daytime sleepiness—or insomnia—the inability to sleep. Narcolepsy, the abrupt onset of REM sleep, is most often seen in young adults and can be quite dangerous for individuals suddenly falling into deep REM sleep with complete loss of consciousness for minutes to hours. Periodic limb movement disorders are persistent involuntary leg movements during sleep and routinely cause fragmented sleep because of multiple sleep arousals during the night. Hypersomnia is excessive sleepiness during the day and often a symptom of sleep fragmentation during sleep and the lack of delta, or slow-wave, sleep. Circadian rhythm sleep disorders represent a malfunction of the "internal sleep clock" signaling an individual to sleep or awaken during the day and night.

Parasomnias are associated with sleep fragmentation associated with abnormal activities performed during REM sleep. Because skeletal muscles are partially paralyzed during REM,

body movement is normally restricted during the REM phase. With parasomnia disorders, behaviors such as sleepwalking, teeth grinding, sleep talking, night terrors, sleep driving, sleep cooking, sleep sex, and multiple other activities occur while the patient remains in REM sleep. Patients wake up completely unaware of their behaviors or actions in a confused state. Bedwetting is also considered a parasomnia condition and may be accompanied with other REM sleep behaviors.

Sleep disorders associated with medical or psychiatric conditions include psychoses, depression, anxiety, panic disorders, and alcoholism. Treatment of the underlying problem is usually the best method for resolving the associated sleep disorder. Sleeping sickness, a disease transmitted through the bite of the tsetse fly, is a separate rare sleep disorder category. Similarly, SIDS is classified as a distinct category and represents specific criteria not associated with other sleep disorders. Finally, the category of snoring represents a specific classification associated with various contributing factors that produce a snoring sound. Although snoring is a symptom frequently associated with OSA and MSA, as a classification category, it suggests anatomical conditions that limit air movement during NREM and REM sleep. Disproportional anatomical size of the tongue, oropharynx, chin, jaw, and other structures contributes to the presence of snoring without apnea.

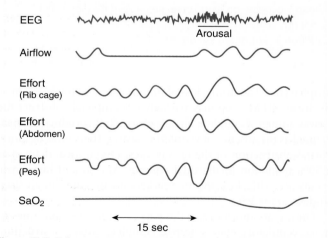

Figure 15-7 Polysomnogram representation of obstructive sleep apnea in the presence of apnea. (From Wilkins RL, et al: *Clinical assessment in respiratory care,* ed 6, St Louis, 2010, Mosby.)

of suffocation (Figure 15-7). The increase in $PaCO_2$ prompts arousal of the medullary chemoreceptors, which is documented by the EEG; the patient often gasps, is aroused from sleep, and sits up in bed to open the airway. Often the patient does not completely awaken; however, deep REM sleep is disrupted, bringing the patient into stage 1 or 2 NREM sleep. Most patients are unaware that they sit up in bed, gasp, or cough; they

simply lay down again, only to repeat the process throughout the night. As soon as the individual returns to REM sleep, the next obstruction begins. Because of anatomy and gravity, the most vulnerable sleeping position for the patient with OSA is supine. Turning to either side or the prone position may significantly decrease the degree of airway obstruction at REM onset.

If airway obstruction is partial, a hypopnea may occur, and the process just described is repeated except that ventilations are shallow rather than absent. Hypopneas frequently cause EEG arousals, and the patient may reposition in the bed before resuming sleep (Figure 15-8). Such arousals, as depicted on the PSG, are known as **respiratory effort–related arousals (RERAs)** (Figure 15-9). During RERAs, the thorax and abdomen move in a diminished, synchronous manner, although airflow does not appear to be reduced, and the SpO_2 remains stable. However, RERAs usually result in an EEG arousal, and sleep architecture may be disrupted.

OSA occurs most frequently in elderly obese men with a short neck greater than 17 inches in circumference. Heavy snoring that begins soon after falling asleep is the classic picture of a patient with OSA. Typically, the snoring becomes louder and is interrupted by a period of apnea followed by a loud snort or gasp. After reestablishing the airway, snoring returns, and the cycle repeats. The snoring and gasping events may drive the sleep partner from the bed to another room. Risk factors associated with worsening of OSA include a body mass index

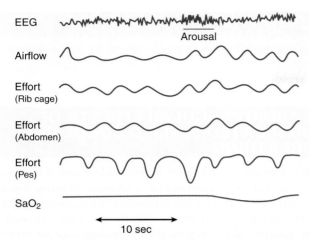

Figure 15-8 Polysomnogram representation of obstructive sleep apnea in the presence of hypopnea. (From Wilkins RL, et al: *Clinical assessment in respiratory care,* ed 6, St Louis, 2010, Mosby.)

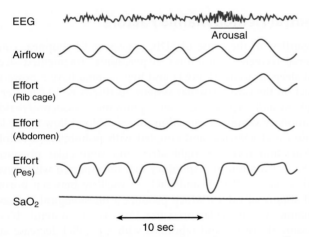

Figure 15-9 Polysomnogram representation of respiratory effort–related arousals. (From Wilkins RL, et al: *Clinical assessment in respiratory care,* ed 6, St Louis, 2010, Mosby.)

25 or greater, alcohol consumption before bedtime, smoking, nasal congestion at night, and large tonsils. The consequences of uncorrected OSA include decreased physical performance, decreased mental performance owing to a reduced ability to concentrate, psychosocial problems, impotence, decreased libido, hypertension, exacerbation of coronary artery disease, myocardial infarction, heart failure, and stroke.[9,10]

Central Sleep Apnea

The second frequently encountered classification of SDB is central sleep apnea (CSA). CSA is characterized by lack of airflow accompanied by the total absence of thoracoabdominal effort for at least 10 seconds. The cause of apnea is not obstruction of the airway but a lack of normal brain activity associated with the physiological drive to breathe. CSA is responsible for only about 10% of all adult SDB but is more common in children and infants. CSA is observed most often during stage 1 NREM or REM sleep. The cause of CSA is varied and complex. It is

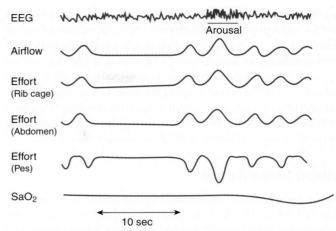

Figure 15-10 Polysomnogram representation of central sleep apnea. (From Wilkins RL, et al: *Clinical assessment in respiratory care,* ed 6, St Louis, 2010, Mosby.)

thought that CSA may be linked to a loss of the neurological control of breathing secondary to injury, stroke, brainstem lesion, encephalitis, neurodegeneration, radiation treatments to the cervical spine region, or congestive heart failure.[10,11,13]

Individuals with CSA are most often not obese and have a normal neck circumference. Snoring is not usually present; however, **excessive daytime somnolence**, or sleepiness, may occur because of frequent awakenings and lack of restorative sleep. Because CSA is closely associated with neurological issues, patients may report symptoms such as difficulty swallowing, a change in the ability to use their voices, or other body weakness or numbness. Any of these neurological symptoms should be immediately brought to the attention of a physician for complete assessment and diagnostic investigation. The most common sign of CSA is the presence of Cheyne-Stokes respirations (see Chapter 11).[9] Figure 15-10 shows a PSG study of a patient with CSA.

Children with Central Sleep Apnea

Although CSA is much less common in children than adults, it is often found in premature infants born before 37 weeks of gestation. CSA is associated with congenital cardiac disorders that cause an elevation of the $PaCO_2$. As with adults, hypercapnic drive centers in the brainstem may be insensitive or too immature to trigger corrective breathing stimuli to respiratory muscles. Multiple disorders may precipitate CSA in children and infants, including neuromuscular, neurological, metabolic, gastrointestinal, and hematological abnormalities and infections with an accompanying fever.[8,11]

Sudden infant death syndrome (SIDS) is thought by some experts to be associated with CSA, but there is no clinical evidence that the two are linked. The Centers for Disease Control and Prevention defines SIDS as "the sudden death of an infant less than one year of age that cannot be explained after a thorough investigation is conducted, including a complete autopsy, examination of the death scene and review of the clinical history."[14] Although the etiology is unknown, most reported SIDS cases occur in the first 6 months of life with a peak incidence between 2 and 4 months of age. Previously thought to be linked to CSA pathophysiology, SIDS is now believed to have a familial relationship to OSA and positional sleeping and to be associated with families that have a history of apparent life-threatening events.[14] Research during the last decade has linked SIDS to risk factors such as the prone sleeping position, bed sharing, maternal substance abuse, and maternal cigarette smoking. Despite a 38% decrease in SIDS incidence in the United States, it remains the leading cause of death in children younger than 1 year.

Mixed Sleep Apnea

As the name implies, mixed sleep apnea (MSA) is a combination of OSA and CSA in the same patient. A PSG study of the patient with MSA typically reveals an initial CSA event followed by an OSA phase (Figure 15-11). During the CSA portion of the MSA sequence, there is no thoracic wall or abdominal effort associated with loss of airflow and declining SpO_2. Following the CSA event, thoracic and abdominal efforts return, but the effort is met with an upper airway obstruction for the remainder of the MSA sequence. As is often the case, support of the collapsing airway through the use of CPAP may eliminate the OSA aspect of the sequence only to allow the CSA component and continued apnea to persist. Many times, as positive airway pressure (PAP) is titrated in the patient with OSA, an underlying CSA episode is discovered when the OSA issue is resolved. Without the PSG diagnostic/titration study, MSA is virtually impossible to confirm. When the OSA component is treated with PAP, the CSA component can be addressed by providing a backup respiratory rate controller on the PAP device. The use of rate controller PAP devices quickly resolves any CSA issues, and the patient can sleep without apneic episodes.[10,11]

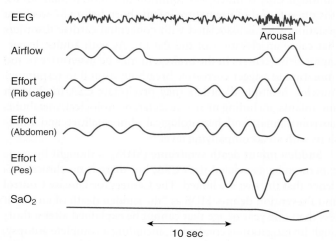

Figure 15-11 Polysomnogram representation of mixed sleep apnea. (From Wilkins RL, et al: *Clinical assessment in respiratory care,* ed 6, St Louis, 2010, Mosby.)

CARDIOVASCULAR EFFECTS OF UNTREATED SLEEP-DISORDERED BREATHING

SDB is a significant risk factor in the development of hypertension and multiple cardiovascular conditions. Effective therapy can eliminate or reverse the detrimental cardiovascular effects of SDB; nevertheless, cardiovascular disorders are increased in these patients either because SDB is undiagnosed or because patients fail to comply with prescribed PAP therapy. The simple act of "breathing while asleep" is key to the restoration of cardiovascular health and a decreased rate of morbidity and morality.[15]

Central Hemodynamic Factors

Regardless of the cause of SDB, apneas and hypopneas cause arterial oxygen desaturation, hypercapnia, fragmented sleep, and sleep arousals. Hypoxia and hypercapnia have a powerful effect on the cardiovascular system. As discussed in Chapter 6, hypoxia and hypercapnia cause pulmonary vasoconstriction. Pulmonary venous constriction impedes blood flow to the left atrium and ventricle and coupled with pulmonary arteriolar constriction increases right atrial and ventricular pressures. In SDB, variation in respiratory rate interspersed with apneic periods causes $PaCO_2$ and PaO_2 to vacillate between normal and abnormal values, which produce a physiological "seesaw" dynamic in ventricular pressures. As a result, systemic blood pressure decreases and rebounds with a parallel decrease and increase in heart rate. Cardiac pressures can increase and then decrease to the point that blood flow momentarily stops; the resulting blood stagnation and stasis clotting may lead to potential stroke or myocardial infarction.[15,16]

During periods of airway obstruction in OSA and MSA, thoracic inspiratory expansion creates large negative intrathoracic pressures, which decrease left ventricular stroke volume and cause a momentary decrease in systemic blood pressure. Blood flow through the already constricted pulmonary vasculature is decreased further, exacerbating cardiac function, as manifested by diminished cardiac output, stroke volume, and systemic blood pressure. When airway obstruction is resolved through sleep arousal or a change in position, stroke volume, heart rate, and blood pressure transiently increase. This physiological "seesaw" of hemodynamics in patients with SDB occurs during each cycle of apnea. Because episodes of apnea commonly result in some level of arousal, sleep is further fragmented as the patient swings between REM and NREM or is awakened by the event.[17,18]

Causal Role in Cardiovascular Disease

Studies have clearly documented the relationship between long-standing SDB and the predisposition for cardiovascular disease; sympathetic nervous system overactivity is thought to be a critical mechanism in the pathogenesis of hypertension. Repetitive airway occlusion, hypercapnia, and hypoxia, accompanied by vacillations in intrathoracic pressures elicit autonomic, neural, and humeral responses. A night of fragmented sleep may adversely affect cardiovascular function during waking hours the next day, although daytime breathing is normal.[18] Nocturnal hypoxemia results in endothelial cell dysfunction, producing vasoconstriction and elevated blood pressure during both sleeping and waking hours. Urinary catecholamine levels, an indicator of sympathetic stress and overstimulation, are elevated in patients with untreated SDB, manifesting the persistence of OSA-induced physiological stress throughout the day. Studies have also shown that when patients with OSA are treated with PAP, and sleep apnea is resolved, urinary catecholamine levels return to normal. Hypertension is frequently resolved or diminished through PAP treatment of OSA.[19]

Patients with untreated OSA have a higher risk of hypercoagulability (i.e., increased tendency to develop intravascular blood clots) and subsequent thrombosis than their PAP-treated counterparts. Hypercoagulability mechanisms are still under investigation, but current research suggests changes in clotting factors might be due to the increased number of neutrophils seen in patients with SDB, along with increased catecholamine levels and compromised blood flow.[17] Hypercoagulability increases the risk of coronary artery disease when it coexists with other conditions present in patients with OSA, including obesity, metabolic syndrome, insulin resistance, diabetes, and hyperlipidemia. Fluctuations in blood flow caused by repeated blood pressure surges in OSA result in additional myocardial work, which is associated with left ventricular hypertrophy, often a precursor of adverse cardiovascular events.

Heart failure, or systolic dysfunction (ejection fraction <40%), is asymptomatic in about 2% of the general population.[18] Additionally, diastolic dysfunction (failure of the ventricle to fill properly) is a major risk factor in the development of **congestive heart failure**, or left ventricular failure. Patients with OSA and CSA commonly have coexisting heart failure and its associated increase in mortality rate. Decreased blood flow leads to myocardial ischemia during periods of negative intrathoracic pressure, which may lead to an increased left ventricular afterload, a decreased left ventricular preload, and a subsequent reduction in stroke volume. The use of PAP produces immediate cardiovascular improvement by relieving hypoxia and hypercapnia; the associated improvement in myocardial oxygenation decreases left ventricular end-systolic volume and improves ejection fraction.[19]

SDB and cardiac arrhythmias are also significantly linked, although the association is not well understood. Atrial and ventricular premature ectopic beats are the most common arrhythmias in SDB. Separating cardiac arrhythmias that result from preexisting heart disease from the effects of SDB is difficult; however, successful treatment of SDB seems to decrease arrhythmias.[20] The role of SDB as an independent risk factor for cardiac arrhythmias is yet to be substantiated in the scientific literature.

CONCEPT QUESTION 15-8

Describe the physiological effects of hypoxia and hypercapnia on the cardiovascular system. What are the cardiovascular consequences of untreated SDB?

PHYSIOLOGICAL DIAGNOSIS OF SLEEP-DISORDERED BREATHING

Polysomnogram

The treatment of SBD begins with a definitive diagnosis based on a PSG sleep study, which is the "gold standard" diagnostic tool in determining the presence of a sleep disorder. The guidelines for conducting and evaluating sleep studies are established by the Association of Sleep Disorders Center and further defined by Medicare Practice Guidelines. The configuration of the various physiological tracings on the PSG display is called a **montage** (Figure 15-12). The montage for a typical sleep study includes a minimum of 17 channels of physiological tracings. Electrodes are strategically placed on the patient's head, face, chest, abdomen, and legs to collect the physiological data (Figure 15-13). All data are recorded continuously from "lights off" to "lights on" including four EEG channels to identify NREM or REM sleep stages, two channels recording right and left eye movement, one channel monitoring chin movement, two channels recording right and left leg movement, and nine more channels documenting snoring, nasal and oral airflow, thoracic and abdominal movement, SpO_2, heart rate, electrocardiogram (ECG), and body position.[8]

Sleep clinicians must adhere to strict criteria to conduct the PSG study properly and titrate the appropriate pressure needed to resolve apneas and hypopneas. Apneas and hypopneas must be counted during each hour of the sleep study and serve as the basis for certain calculations. The primary index defining the presence of apneas or hypopneas or both is the **apnea-hypopnea index (AHI)**, or the number of hypopneas and apneas per hour of sleep time. For adults, an AHI greater than 5 per hour with a 4% decrease in SpO_2 from baseline is considered abnormal and requires treatment. For infants and children, an AHI greater than 1 is considered abnormal when end-tidal PCO_2 is greater than 53 mm Hg or SpO_2 is less than 92%.[8-10] Whether SDB is anatomical or neurological, the AHI is the primary criterion on which the diagnosis of SDB is based. Ideally, the **prescriptive pressure** derived from a PSG study is the PAP in cm H_2O pressure required to keep the patient's airway patent. The goal in titrating PAP is to reduce AHI to 5 or less per hour while the patient is in the supine position. When PAP is correctly adjusted, the patient's apnea and hypopnea are immediately resolved. If the correct prescriptive PAP is applied, the patient is able to sleep through the night without sleep fragmentation.[10]

The classification of sleep disorder severity involves many factors, but sleep specialists generally agree that the AHI is a measure of sleep apnea severity. An AHI less than 5 is within normal limits. An AHI of 5 to 20 is termed "mild" sleep apnea. An AHI of 20 to 40 is "moderate" sleep apnea. An AHI greater

CLINICAL FOCUS 15-3

Sleep-Disordered Breathing and Comorbidities

The impact of untreated SDB is pervasive and significantly affects quality of life and longevity. SDB also exacerbates pre-existing disorders of the cardiovascular, pulmonary, and endocrine systems, accelerating the development of serious health issues.

Chronic Obstructive Pulmonary Disease

Patients with chronic obstructive pulmonary disease (COPD) experience progressive dyspnea with advancing lung disease accompanied by right heart failure, or cor pulmonale, secondary to pulmonary vascular hypertension. When these conditions exist in isolation, the impact on the quality of life is significant and debilitating. SDB superimposed on advanced COPD causes patients to develop persistent hypersomnolence, tiredness, loss of ability to concentrate, decreasing SaO_2 levels, and increasing $PaCO_2$ levels. Their inability to reach REM without upper airway obstruction (SDB), coupled with small airway obstruction leads to the development of respiratory failure and progressive right ventricular failure. The lack of restorative sleep accelerates muscle fatigue, which is critically detrimental to the ventilation of the hyperinflated COPD thorax.

Cardiovascular Disorders

Patients with concurrent SDB and cardiovascular conditions are at high risk for a rapid and progressive decline in cardiovascular function. OSA alone causes swings in central hemodynamic pressures; this occurs as left ventricular stroke volume decreases during inspiratory efforts against an obstructed upper airway followed by a surge in systemic arterial pressure when breathing is restored. Peripheral, cerebral, and pulmonary circulations are thus subjected to periods of hypertension and hypotension. SDB is highly correlated with congestive heart failure in the population at large. The large ventricular afterload produced by OSA events has been shown to depress cardiac function in patients with preexisting congestive heart failure. Additionally, untreated severe sleep apnea has been shown to be associated with stroke, coronary artery disease, cardiac arrhythmias, and pulmonary hypertension—which leads to right ventricular failure.

Insulin Resistance

Since 1993, studies have shown the relationship between glucose dysregulation and OSA. A growing body of evidence suggests OSA can independently impair insulin sensitivity resulting in insulin resistance. A newly described metabolic condition reaching near-epidemic proportions in Western society, "syndrome Z," has many features common to OSA, including obesity, hypertension, hyperlipidemia, and insulin resistance. Since PAP is the most common treatment for OSA, the question of the effect of PAP on insulin sensitivity is an unanswered question. In a group of 40 patients with OSA, Harsch et al.[32] showed that insulin sensitivity improved 18% after 2 days of PAP treatment and improved 31% after 3 months of treatment. It has been theorized that acute periods of hypoxic stress and sleep fragmentation may impair glucose homeostasis, leading to insulin resistance and type 2 diabetes.[33]

---

than 40 is "severe" sleep apnea in an adult. Other criteria and symptoms must also be considered in the evaluation of a sleep study. Patients with SDB and preexisting pulmonary or cardiac disease present a complicated clinical problem that requires additional assessment for treatment options.[11]

Following a sleep study, the clinician analyzes the EEG tracings and scores the study by identifying all the NREM and REM stages. Any abnormal breathing events such as apneas, hypopneas, arousals, and desaturations are noted, and calculations are made relative to each event. Ultimately, a physician trained in sleep medicine interprets the PSG and sends the findings to the patient's primary care physician, who informs the patient of the results. If the PSG study indicates the need for treatment, an additional night of study in the sleep laboratory is necessary to determine the PAP level needed.

PAP devices, such as **continuous positive airway pressure (CPAP)** and **bilevel positive airway pressure (BIPAP)** machines, provide the anatomical "cure" for the presence of OSA, CSA, or MSA. The "titration night" in the sleep laboratory is critically important to provide the correct mask fit for

the patient and to find the correct PAP required to resolve the obstruction. For CSA, BIPAP with a guaranteed back-up respiratory rate ensures that the patient remains appropriately ventilated during periods of CSA. Some physicians may prefer that the diagnostic and titration procedures be completed in one night, which is called a split-night sleep study. However, split-night studies are not recommended for optimal diagnosis and treatment of SDB because of time limitations. Many patients have a difficult time falling asleep soon enough to allow the sleep clinician to quantify the sleep disturbance and implement intervention protocols. Titration of the correct PAP and selection of a properly fitting mask can be difficult and time-consuming. The patient must fall asleep before a supine REM state can be documented with the level of PAP required to resolve the airway obstruction.[9,10]

CONCEPT QUESTION 15-9

Describe the diagnostic process of determining the presence of SDB.

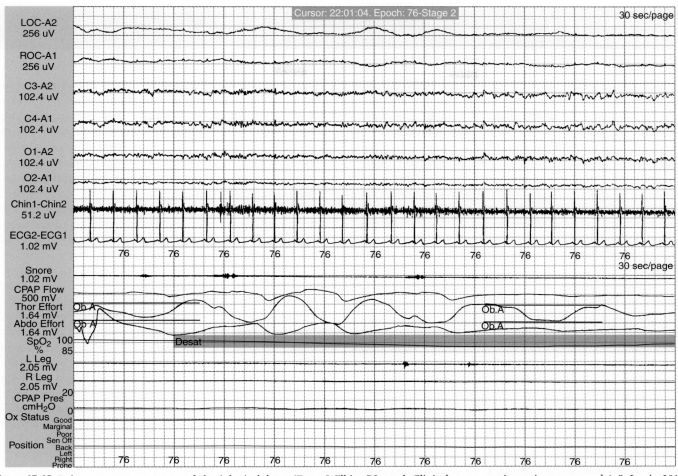

Figure 15-12 Polysomnogram montage of physiological data. (From Wilkins RL, et al: *Clinical assessment in respiratory care,* ed 6, St Louis, 2010, Mosby.)

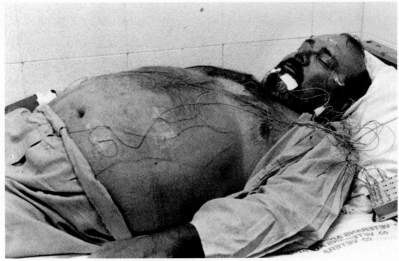

Figure 15-13 Patient with sleep-disordered breathing ready for a sleep study (From Wilkins RL, et al: *Clinical assessment in respiratory care,* ed 6, St Louis, 2010, Mosby.)

CLINICAL FOCUS 15-4

Pharmacology of Sleep-Disordered Breathing

Effective drug therapy for SDB is yet to be discovered. SDB refers to sleep disorders in which normal breathing is affected during sleep, and the specific pharmacology to relieve sleep apnea is lacking. Upper airway obstruction is the primary etiology of sleep apnea (OSA and MSA); a specific pharmaceutical agent that targets receptor sites, shrinks soft tissues, and reestablishes airway patency has not been found. Both serotoninergic and serotonin receptor antagonist drugs have been tested for effectiveness in reducing SDB, but none of these drugs have been shown conclusively to reduce sleep apnea. At best, sleep pharmacology may be helpful for some individuals as an adjunctive therapy when combined with PAP treatment.[34]

Ventilatory stimulants, including medroxyprogesterone, thyroxine, acetazolamide, and theophylline, have not been shown to benefit patients with moderate to severe OSA. In some cases, the induced ventilator efforts appear to increase chest wall work and airway collapse secondary to increased intrathoracic pressures.[35] Opioid antagonists and nicotine have also been used in attempts to stimulate ventilation in patients with OSA with minimal changes in the number of apneic events and an undesirable increase in sleep fragmentation. However, some studies have shown that ventilatory stimulation may be of some use for patients with CSA in the absence of upper airway obstruction.

Studies of psychotropic agents, such as protriptyline, serotonin precursors (L tryptophan), and benzodiazepines, have shown a varying impact on patients with SDB and a reduction in AHI and improved sleep in a small percentage of subjects but not to a statistically significant level. Antihypertensive agents, such as hydralazine, metoprolol, and cilazapril, have been used to decrease sympathetic tone to improve SDB. Although antihypertensive agents were found to decrease the number of apnea events, the mechanism is thought to be due to a REM-suppressing effect.[36]

Sleep pharmacology for non-SDB categories of sleep disorders is of significant importance. As popularly advertised, sleep medications address issues of insomnia rather than SDB. Insomnia often may be an accompanying symptom of excessive daytime sleepiness that results from OSA during the night. The patient becomes sleepy during the day, naps frequently, and has difficulty attaining sleep onset or experiences prolonged sleep onset at night, which is interpreted as insomnia. Agents such as modafinil (Provigil) taken once in the morning may reduce the excessive daytime sleepiness of OSA, narcolepsy, and shift work sleep disorder by maintaining alertness during the day. For other patients with SDB, the use of PAP treatment may lead to increased sleep efficiency, decreased excessive daytime sleepiness, and abatement of insomnia without adjunctive medication. Sleep pharmacology for primary sleep disorders is presented in Box 15-2.

BOX 15-2

Sleep Pharmacology for Primary Sleep Disorder Categories

Dyssomnias
Modafinil (Provigil)—excessive daytime sleepiness (EDS), narcolepsy, shift work sleep disorder
Medroxyprogesterone, acetazolamide—stimulate ventilation
Melatonin—alternative medicine
Bupropion—panic/mood disorders, idiopathic CSA
Ferritin—RLS
Dopamine agonists (levodopa)—RLS
Gabapentin—RLS and partial seizures
Low-dose opiates (tramadol, codeine)

Parasomnias
Benzodiazepines (flurazepam [Dalmane], temazepam [Restoril], triazolam [Halcion], estazolam [ProSom], clonazepam [Klonopin], diazepam [Valium])—may decrease periodic breathing
Tricyclic antidepressants (mirtazapine)
Anticonvulsants
Desmopressin—nocturnal enuresis
Imipramine (Tofranil)—chronic depression/pain
Barbiturates (secobarbital [Seconal], phenobarbital [Luminal], pentobarbital [Nembutal], butabarbital [Butisol])—insomnia
Nonbarbiturates (zolpidem [Ambien], zaleplon [Sonata], chloral hydrate [Noctec], eszopiclone [Lunesta])—insomnia

RLS, Restless legs syndrome.

Split-Night Polysomnogram Study

Patient Assessment

A 55-year-old man with complaints of snoring, apnea, daytime fatigue, restless legs, shortness of breath, nocturnal awakenings, and severe hypersomnia was referred to a sleep center for a diagnostic PSG and PAP titration, if indicated. Patient medical history includes hypertension, allergies, asthma, gastroesophageal reflux disease (GERD), tonsillectomy, and adenoidectomy. The patient's height of 69 inches and weight of 240 lb produces a calculated body mass index of 35.4. The patient is a former 20-pack-year smoker who quit approximately 10 years ago; he consumes 5 to 10 caffeinated beverages daily to maintain alertness, and consumes 3 to 4 alcoholic beverages each evening. He has no regular exercise routine. Neck circumference is 18.5 inches with a Mallampati classification of class III.

A complete PSG digital sleep system diagnostic was performed using the international 10- to 20-electrode placement for recording EEG, electrooculography near the eyes, EMG from the chin, ECG, respiratory effort, oximetry, body position, airflow, snoring monitor, pulse rate, and limb movement channels. Following full PSG hook-up, the patient was provided specific education regarding PAP titration should the diagnostic test meet standard guidelines for intervention.

Pretreatment Polysomnogram Summary

The patient's total sleep efficiency was 82.9% with 0.0% REM sleep, 22.9% stage 1 sleep, 76.6% stage 2 sleep, and 0.6% stage 3 sleep. There were 45 obstructive apneas, 0 central apneas, and 0 mixed apneas with 124 hypopneas with SpO_2 desaturations 3% or greater and 6 RERAs. The apnea index was 30.9, and the AHI was 115.9 with a respiratory disturbance index (RDI) of 118.6. The lowest SpO_2 recorded was 80% with 15.9 minutes of desaturations from 81% to 90%. The mean SpO_2 during sleep was 93%. There were 220 periodic limb movements, and no snoring was recorded during the pretreatment phase. The sleep architecture was severely fragmented during pretreatment owing to SDB. The respiratory arousal index was 117.9. The average heart rate associated with apnea or hypopnea was 74, and the ECG showed regular sinus rhythm without ectopic beats.

Post–Positive Airway Pressure Treatment Polysomnogram Summary

Within 87.5 minutes of sleep, the criteria for treatment with PAP titration were met. The patient was awakened and fitted with a CPAP mask and instructed to return to sleep. CPAP was initiated at 5 cm H_2O and increased incrementally to 12 cm H_2O, according to protocol. At 12 cm H_2O, no obstructions were noted, yielding an AHI of 0.0 and an RDI of 0.0 per hour. In the supine position, 18.5 minutes of REM was recorded with a low SpO_2 of 92%. With CPAP, sleep efficiency increased to 92% with 40.2% spent in REM sleep, 3.8% in stage 1 sleep, 42.8% in stage 2 sleep, and 13.1% in stage 3 sleep.

Discussion

Multiple symptoms relevant to OSA are present in the patient history, including snoring, apnea, daytime fatigue, restless legs, shortness of breath, nocturnal awakenings, and hypersomnia. Additionally, the presence of obesity, use of caffeinated beverages during the day to maintain alertness, use of alcohol before bedtime, a neck circumference greater than 17 inches, and a Mallampati classification of class III complete a scenario common to patients with OSA. The pretreatment PSG study shows no REM sleep with 22.9% stage 1 sleep, 76.6% stage 2 sleep, and 0.6% stage 3 sleep. This sleep architecture suggests very poor sleep quality with no REM and most of the sleep time spent in stage 2 sleep with negligible time spent in restorative stage 3 sleep. SpO_2 values indicate mild hypoxia during sleep with 220 leg movements during sleep that likely cause sleep arousals. The apnea index was 30.9 apneic events per hour; a normal apnea index is less than 5 events per hour. An apnea index of 30.9 equates to having an apnea episode of greater than 10 seconds every 30 seconds of sleep. Sleep fragmentation is quite severe.

After qualifying for PAP titration, the patient was fitted with a CPAP mask at a beginning pressure of 5 cm H_2O. After returning to sleep, the sleep technician began to titrate the CPAP incrementally while observing the number of apneic events. When a CPAP of 12 cm H_2O was reached, the sleep technician noted there were no apnea events and no hypopnea events. In the supine position, the likelihood of airway obstruction is greatest, but a CPAP of 12 cm H_2O held the upper airways open and prevented obstruction by the tongue or soft tissues. As a result, the patient experienced "REM rebound" spending 40.2% of the sleep time in REM sleep, 3.8% in stage 1 sleep, 42.8% in stage 2 sleep, and 13.1% in stage 3 sleep. Sleep efficiency was increased to 92%, and the prescription pressure of 12 cm H_2O was verified through an AHI of 0.0.

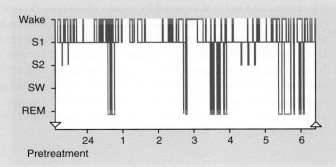

Pretreatment

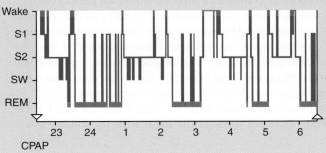

CPAP

ANATOMICAL TREATMENT OF SLEEP-DISORDERED BREATHING

In theory, the treatment for OSA is simply the maintenance of a patent airway during sleep. During REM, the relaxation of oropharyngeal muscles and the tongue partially or completely obstruct the airway. Options for treating SDB include PAP therapy, oral appliances, positional solutions, and airway enlargement procedures.

Positive Airway Pressure

SDB caused by soft tissue obstruction of the oropharynx can be immediately resolved without surgery or pharmaceuticals through the use of properly administered PAP therapy. Judicious titration of PAP is required to identify the precise pressure that alleviates sleep apnea, snoring, and hypopneas. Each titration sleep study is individually tailored to meet the specific needs of the patient, which are related to the degree of obstruction present. PAP treatment begins with a properly sized and fitted mask. With more than 50 brands and types of masks available, the sleep clinician must be an expert in finding the properly designed mask that accommodates each patient's particular facial features and anatomical structures. The clinician chooses a nasal or oronasal mask after assessing the patient's facial anatomy. If the patient requires high PAPs, nasal masks are not suitable, and an oronasal or full facial mask is needed to provide the appropriate pressure without leaking. Additionally, patient comfort is a critical factor affecting continued patient use or compliance with PAP therapy. Overtightening the mask can cause leaks or patient discomfort and is usually a sign of improper sizing. Without the proper mask fit, applied pressures do not reliably keep the airways patent (Figure 15-14).[21]

More than 50 models of PAP, CPAP, and BIPAP generators exist, and it is beyond the scope of this chapter to detail their differences. Various PAP modes and delivery systems are available to meet specific patient needs, including CPAP, BIPAP, average volume assured pressure support (AVAPS), auto-CPAP, BIPAP-autoSV (support ventilation), BIPAP S/T (spontaneous/timed), volume positive airway pressure (VPAP), Smart CPAP, and demand positive airway pressure (DPAP). Each mode has specific advantages that must be matched to the patient's specific SDB needs. For this reason, a titration sleep study must be completed in the sleep laboratory under direct supervision of a trained clinician to allow titration and adjustment of PAP equipment during the night. Some physicians and medical equipment companies attempt to provide treatment for documented SDB without a titration study, but patient compliance and continued use is threatened by this practice. Current manufacturers of PAP devices provide multiple-mode devices that are small, quiet, and efficient. Patients using PAP must be able to transport the device and all associated equipment safely when traveling away from home; the size of the device has a significant impact on patient compliance during travel.[8,11,21]

As previously mentioned, the length of the REM stage normally increases through the night with the longest phase of REM typically just before waking. Because the REM state represents skeletal muscle paralysis and decreased ventilation efforts, the PAP device must be adjusted to meet all ventilation needs and supply complete support of flaccid or collapsing soft tissue in the oropharyngeal cavity. With the CPAP or BIPAP adjunct in place with the appropriate PAP device, the PSG titration study documents the PAP setting required to stent open the airways while the patient transitions through each stage of sleep. PAPs are adjusted in each sleeping position until all sleep parameters are normalized and documented with an AHI less than 5. Because the supine sleeping position is the patient's most vulnerable position with regard to airway collapse, the therapist must ensure the PAP is titrated to the correct pressure during REM while the patient is supine. When this pressure is determined, all other stages of sleep and sleeping positions are likely to be supported with enough PAP for uninterrupted sleep.[10]

Following the titration sleep study in which PAP successfully normalizes the AHI, the prescription pressure and supporting documentation are reported back to the ordering physician, and the patient is referred to a **durable medical equipment (DME)** company to purchase a home PAP device. The respiratory therapist from the DME company properly fits the patient with a PAP adjunct, instructs the patient how to use the PAP equipment, and provides patient education relevant to the type of SDB present. PAPs are preset by the DME therapist according to the physician's order; the therapist instructs the patient on how to don the mask properly and activate the PAP device. The device should be set to pressurize to the prescriptive pressure automatically. Both the physician and the DME company are responsible to provide patient follow-up on PAP compliance and resolve any issues affecting treatment adherence.

Oral Appliances

Known also as dental appliances, oral appliances are acrylic devices that fit over the upper and lower teeth similar to a mouth guard. An oral appliance is designed to move the lower jaw, or mandible, slightly forward. Because the tongue is attached to the mandible, the tongue is also advanced forward to provide a larger oropharyngeal lumen. A dentist experienced in the treatment of snoring and sleep apnea must customize the oral appliance for each patient. Two of the oral appliances in current use are the **mandibular advancement device (MAD)** and the **tongue retaining device (TRD)**. The MAD device is designed with an adjustable mechanism that allows the patient to advance the mandible gradually daily, eventually increasing the oropharyngeal airway opening. The TRD fits around the tongue and holds it forward by means of suction; it is used most often by patients with lower dentures that are removed at night or by patients in whom the mandible cannot be effectively advanced. Both devices require the patient to be able to breathe through the nose adequately; otherwise, the oral appliance will not be tolerated (see Figure 15-15, *A* and *B*). Although oral appliances are an option for the treatment of OSA, results are marginally successful, and these appliances are effective only in patients diagnosed with mild OSA.[22,23]

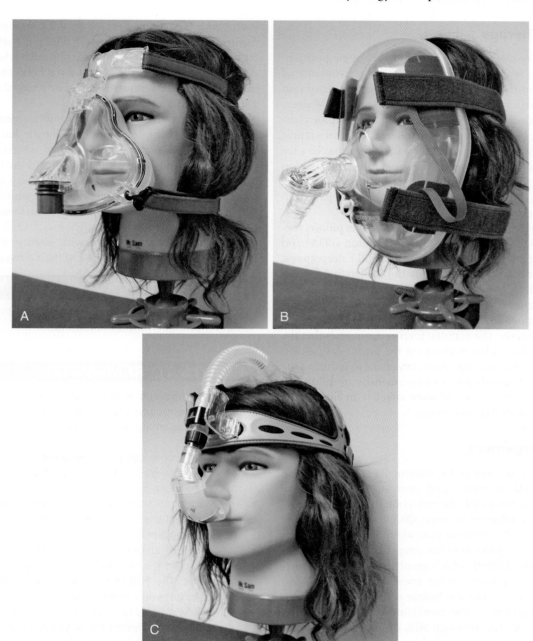

Figure 15-14 A-C, Continuous positive airway pressure and bilevel positive airway pressure masks.

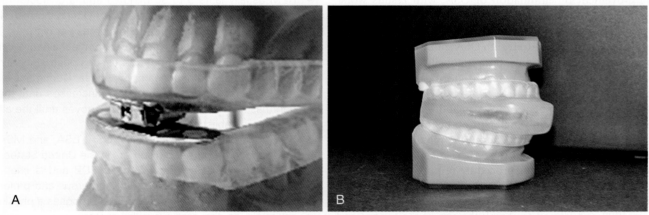

Figure 15-15 Mandibular advancement device (**A**) and tongue retaining device (**B**) oral appliances.

Positional Therapy

Given that gravity worsens sleep apnea in the supine position, one approach to reducing apneic episodes is the avoidance of the supine position. Individuals normally move and reposition themselves through the night during each cycle of NREM sleep. The goal of positional therapy is to maintain a nonsupine position. The "snore ball" is a hard plastic sphere the size of a tennis ball that is sewn into the middle of the back of pajamas or a tee shirt worn by the patient at night. The supine sleeping position is discouraged by the uncomfortable ball positioned over the spine. In theory, the discomfort prompts the sleeping patient to roll to either side and out of the supine position.

Another approach to positional therapy involves pillows registered by the U.S. Food and Drug Administration (FDA) and specifically designed to prevent snoring and mild sleep apnea. These pillows are designed to reposition the neck so that the oral airway is more likely to remain patent. The foam wedge-shaped pillows are designed at angles of various degrees and presumably reduce positional collapse of the airways and reduce apneas and snoring. However, the manufacturer recommends that the patient sleep in the supine position on the positional pillows. At best, positional therapy may prove beneficial in reducing the number of apneic periods and snoring intensity in mild sleep apnea, but it has not been found to be effective in eliminating moderate or severe obstructive apnea.[24]

Airway Enlargement

The treatment of last resort for obstructive SDB is surgical enlargement of the oropharyngeal cavity to provide a more patent airway. Surgery entails the reduction of soft tissue structures and may be effective in some OSA conditions, but the patient should be fully aware of potentially adverse outcomes. A common surgical procedure for sleep apnea is **uvulopala-topharyngoplasty (UPPP)**, which involves removal or shortening of the uvula, removal of the tonsils and adenoids, and excision of portions of the soft palate or roof of the mouth; the goal is enlargement of the airway lumen. The benefits of UPPP are controversial. Although 90% of patients experience symptomatic improvement from habitual snoring, studies have shown that only 41% to 66% of patients undergoing UPPP see improvement or elimination of OSA, with results worsening over time.[25] The efficacy of UPPP cannot be predicted, and nonsurgical options should be considered before resorting to the procedure. Children with OSA should be assessed for enlarged tonsils and adenoids. Simple tonsillectomy/adenoidectomy has been effective in relieving snoring and sleep apnea in children.[26,27]

Other surgical treatment of OSA includes midline glossectomy and lingualplasty, in which part of the tongue is removed to enlarge the oral cavity. In addition, **maxillomandibular advancement (MMA)**, which moves the mandible anteriorly, has been successful, but this procedure requires the jaw to be broken, extended, and wired shut until the mandible heals.[28] **Radiofrequency tissue ablation** (RFTA) was approved by the FDA in 1998 and is used to shrink the size of the tongue and palate with high-frequency waves; the procedure can be performed in the physician's office.[29] The most effective surgical treatment of OSA is a tracheotomy, although it is deemed unacceptable by most patients. When a tracheotomy is performed for this purpose, the stoma is closed or plugged during the day and unplugged during the night.

The least invasive method to promote airway enlargement is weight loss. Multiple studies have shown that when patients with OSA lose a significant amount of weight, the lumen of the oropharyngeal airway is increased, and the reduced weight on the chest, airways, and abdominal cavity decreases work of breathing during sleep. Obese patients who lose more than 100 lb may see a reduction in PAPs needed; in some cases, OSA may completely resolve with weight loss.[30] OSA is an anatomical issue not always associated with obesity; thin individuals may also experience OSA because of their airway anatomy.

CONCEPT QUESTION 15-10

Discuss the four major categories of SDB treatment, and identify the most common method of treatment.

■ POINTS TO REMEMBER

- The hypothalamus is responsible for the neurocontrol of sleep by controlling the timing of the sleep cycle through the suprachiasmatic nucleus and the ventrolateral preoptic nucleus.
- Humans become obligate nose breathers during sleep, and the upper airways must remain open to accommodate normal restful sleep.
- The Mallampati score can be used to assess whether the oropharyngeal anatomy is too crowded to allow proper ventilation during sleep.
- During NREM stages 1, 2, and 3, the brain enters a restful state while the skeletal muscles respond to stimuli with movement. The NREM cycle lasts 60 to 90 minutes with transitions between all three stages.
- In the REM stage, brain wave activity increases in intensity to a level that resembles the awake state. Skeletal muscles become partially paralyzed during REM, and the loss of muscle tone allows soft tissues to relax.
- REM usually lasts 5 to 30 minutes and is characterized by rapid eye movement and dreaming. During normal sleep, NREM and REM cycle three to five times per night.
- Relaxation of muscles in the oropharyngeal airways can result in the tongue and other soft tissues obstructing airflow producing a period of apnea or hypopnea. During this event, the PaO_2 decreases and the $PaCO_2$ increases until the patient has an EEG arousal, gasps, and moves until the airway can be reestablished.
- SDB is classified as dyssomnias; OSA, CSA, and MSA are the most common sleep disorders in the United States.
- OSA is the most common form of SDB and is characterized by snoring and gasping with numerous and prolonged periods of apnea and hypopnea. OSA imposes a physiological strain on the cardiovascular system with a significant

predisposition for hypertension, cardiac arrhythmias, heart failure, potential myocardial infarction, and stroke.

- CSA manifests with periods of apnea without respiratory effort or obstructed airways. A lack of neurocontrol of breathing is thought to be responsible; CSA is also seen in premature infants and children.
- The PSG is considered the "gold standard" diagnostic tool to determine the presence of a sleep disorder. Physiological data are collected and scored by the sleep technician or respiratory therapist before being interpreted by a qualified sleep physician.
- The goal of treatment for SDB is to establish open airways to allow breathing during sleep. Maintaining an open airway can be accomplished through PAP devices, oral appliances, positional therapy, and airway enlargement options.

References

1. Ranjbaran Z, et al: The relevance of sleep abnormalities to chronic inflammatory conditions, *Inflamm Res* 56(2):51, 2007.
2. Mignot E, Taheri S, Nishino S: Sleeping with the hypothalamus: emerging therapeutic targets for sleep disorders, *Neuroscience* 5(11):1071, 2002.
3. Szymusiak R, McGinty D: Hypothalamic regulation of sleep arousal, *Ann N Y Acad Sci* 1129(5):275, 2008.
4. Mallampati SR, et al: A clinical sign to predict difficult tracheal intubation: a prospective study, *Can Anaesth Soc J* 32(4):429, 1985.
5. Listro G, et al: High Mallampati score and nasal obstruction are associated risk factors for obstructive sleep apnea, *Eur Respir J* 21(2):248, 2003.
6. Davies RJ, Stradling JR: The relationship between neck circumference, radiographic pharyngeal anatomy, and the obstructive sleep apnea syndrome, *Eur Respir J* 3(5):509, 1990.
7. Katz I, et al: Do patients with obstructive sleep apnea have thick necks? *Am Rev Respir Dis* 141(5 pt 1):1228, 1990.
8. Spriggs WH: *Principles of polysomnography*, Salt Lake City, UT, 2002, Sleep Ed.
9. Wilkins RL, Dexter JR, Heuer AJ: *Clinical assessment in respiratory care*, ed 6, St Louis, 2010, Mosby.
10. Kryger HM, Roth T, Dement WC: *Principles and practice of sleep medicine*, ed 4, Philadelphia, 2005, Saunders.
11. Sprigg WH: *Essentials of polysomnography*, Carrollton, TX, 2008, Sleep Ed.
12. World Health Organization: *International statistical classification of diseases and related health problems, 10th revision*, Geneva, 2007, World Health Organization.
13. Quan SF, Gersh BJ: Cardiovascular consequences of sleep-disordered breathing: past, present and future, *Circulation* 109(8):951, 2004.
14. Centers for Disease Control and Prevention (CDC): Sudden infant death syndrome—United States, 1983-1994, *Morb Mortal Wkly Rep MMWR* 45(40):859, 1996.
15. Dempsey JA, et al: Pathophysiology of sleep apnea, *Physiol Rev* 90(1):47, 2010.
16. Somer VK, et al: Sympathetic neural mechanisms in obstructive sleep apnea, *J Clin Invest 96(4)*1995, 1897.
17. Arnult I, et al: Obstructive sleep apnea and venous thromboembolism, *JAMA* 287(20):2655, 2002.
18. Redfield MM, et al: Burden of systolic and diastolic ventricular dysfunction in the community: appreciating the scope of the heart failure epidemic, *JAMA* 289(2):194, 2003.
19. Kaneko Y, et al: Cardiovascular effects of continuous positive airway pressure in patients with heart failure and obstructive sleep apnea, *N Engl J Med* 349(13):1233, 2003.
20. Harbison J, O'Reilly P, McNicholas WT: Cardiac rhythm disturbances in the obstructive sleep apnea syndrome: effects of nasal continuous positive airway pressure therapy, *Chest* 188(3):591, 2000.
21. Wilkins RL, Stoller JK, Kacmarek RM: *Egan's fundamentals of respiratory care*, ed 9, St Louis, 2009, Mosby.
22. Chan ASL, Cistulli PA: Oral appliance treatment of obstructive sleep apnea: an update, *Curr Opin Pulm Med* 16(6):591, 2009.
23. Ferguson KA, et al: A short term controlled trial of an adjustable oral appliance for the treatment of mild to moderate obstructive sleep apnea, *Thorax* 52(4):362, 1997.
24. Permut I, et al: Comparison of positional therapy to CPAP in patients with positional obstructive sleep apnea, *J Clin Sleep Med* 6(3):238, 2010.
25. Pushkar M, Wolford LM: Surgical management of obstructive sleep apnea, *Baylor University Medical Center Proceedings* 13(4):338, 2000.
26. Littner M, et al: Practice parameters for the use of laser-assisted uvulopalatoplasty: an update for 2000, *Sleep* 24(5):603, 2000.
27. Kezirian EJ, et al: Risk factors for serious complication after uvulopalatopharyngoplasty, *Arch Otolaryngol Head Neck Surg* 132(10):1091, 2006.
28. Li KK: Maxillomandibular advancement for obstructive sleep apnea, *J Oral Maxillofac Surg* 69(3):687, 2011.
29. Steward DL: Effectiveness of multilevel (tongue and palate) radiofrequency tissue ablation for patients with obstructive sleep apnea syndrome, *Laryngoscope* 114(123):2073, 2004.
30. Tuomilehto HPI, et al: Lifestyle intervention with weight reduction: first-line treatment in mild obstructive sleep apnea, *Am J Respir Crit Care Med* 179(4):320, 2009.
31. Kayser R: Die exakte Messung der Luftdurchgängigkeit der Nase, *Arch Laryngol Rhinol* 8:101, 1895.
32. Harsch IA, et al: Continuous positive airway pressure treatment rapidly improves insulin sensitivity in patients with obstructive sleep apnea syndrome, *Am J Respir Crit Care Med* 169(2):156, 2004.
33. Dempsey JA, et al: Pathophysiology of sleep apnea, *Physiol Rev* 90(1):47, 2010.
34. Hudgel DW, Thanakitcharu S: Pharmacologic treatment of sleep-disordered breathing, *Am J Respir Crit Care Med* 158(3):691, 1998.
35. Hackett PH, et al: Respiratory stimulants and sleep periodic breathing at high altitude, *Am Rev Respir Dis* 135(4):896, 1987.
36. Issa FG: Effect of clonidine in obstructive sleep apnea, *Am Rev Respir Dis* 145(1):435, 1992.

CHAPTER 16

Fetal and Newborn Cardiopulmonary Physiology

Elizabeth A. Hughes
Christine K. Sperle

OBJECTIVES

After reading this chapter, you will be able to:
- Describe the events that occur during each of the five stages of fetal lung development
- Explain how prematurity might lead to respiratory failure in the newborn
- Explain how gas exchange occurs between fetal and maternal blood
- Describe how alterations in maternal-fetal physiology affect fetal development
- Identify the key anatomical differences between infant and adult airways
- Describe the physiological responses to heat loss in infants

- Explain how infants generate heat
- Explain how the fetal cardiovascular system forms and becomes functional early in gestation
- Identify the factors that determine whether a fetus is viable for postnatal life
- Describe the key anatomical and physiological differences between fetal and neonatal circulation
- Describe the key events that occur during transition from fetal to extrauterine life
- Differentiate acyanotic and cyanotic cardiac defects

KEY TERMS

abruptio placentae
acyanotic
alveolar period
amniocentesis
amniotic fluid

anomalous venous return
aortic stenosis
atrial septal defect (ASD)
atrioventricular septal defect (AVSD)
bulbus cordis

DEVELOPMENT OF THE RESPIRATORY SYSTEM

The development of the respiratory system progresses along a predetermined series of structural changes throughout gestation. Organs of the lower respiratory tract (larynx, trachea, bronchi, and lungs) begin to develop during the fourth week of gestation and continue to grow throughout early childhood. Development of the lung occurs in five overlapping stages: (1) the embryonic period, during which the trachea and major bronchi are formed; (2) the pseudoglandular period, during which the remaining conducting airways develop; (3) the canalicular period, in which the vascular bed and framework of the acinus are developed; (4) the saccular period, during which the terminal airways widen and form cylindrical structures known as saccules; and (5) the alveolar period, in which the alveoli are developed. Table 16-1 summarizes these events of development.

The embryo consists of three primary germ layers from which all tissues, organs, and organ systems arise (Figure 16-1). The endoderm is the innermost germ layer, the mesoderm is the middle layer, and the ectoderm is the outermost layer. Table 16-2 lists the structures that arise from each of the three germ layers. The epithelium of the respiratory tract originates from the endoderm, whereas supporting structures such as connective tissue and muscle arise from the mesoderm.

Embryonic Period

The **embryonic period** begins approximately 26 days after conception.[1-4] During this period, the lung begins to emerge as an outpouching of the primitive foregut (see Figure 16-1). This outpouching elongates and separates into two bronchial buds and the trachea. The right lung bud parallels the esophagus and branches further into three additional buds. The left lung bud is directed more laterally and divides into two additional buds. Thus, the asymmetry of the main bronchi present in the adult is

established. The right and left lung buds continue to grow and branch into segmental and subsegmental bronchi.

By the end of the embryonic period (near the sixth week of gestation), the major bronchi are formed, consisting of 10 right branches and 9 left branches (Figure 16-2).[1-4] During this time, the pulmonary arteries and veins emerge from the developing heart. The diaphragm also develops during this stage and is formed by about the seventh gestational week.[1-4] The diaphragm separates abdominal contents from the thorax. Failure of the diaphragm to form completely can result in **congenital diaphragmatic hernia**, allowing abdominal organs to enter the pleural cavity and compress the lungs and possibly lead to severe underdevelopment, or hypoplasia, of the lung.

The dorsal portion of the foregut evolves into the esophagus. The formation of the tracheoesophageal septum separates the esophagus from the trachea (Figure 16-3). **Teratogens** (agents that disturb fetal development, such as drugs, infection, or chemicals) can produce congenital anomalies and may cause injury to the embryo during this stage of development, such as **tracheoesophageal fistula** (an abnormal opening between the trachea and the esophagus), **choanal atresia** (occlusion of the passageway between the nose and the pharynx), and **pulmonary hypoplasia** (underdevelopment of the lung).

Pseudoglandular Period

The **pseudoglandular period** begins about the sixth week and continues into the sixteenth week of gestation.[1-3] The lung resembles a gland at this stage, giving rise to the name pseudoglandular. Branching and division of the tracheobronchial tree continue to occur asymmetrically and dichotomously (branching into two parts) forming the conducting airways. By the end of this period, the formation of respiratory bronchioles is nearly complete. Cilia, mucous glands, and goblet cells begin to appear in the epithelial lining at approximately 10 weeks' gestation.[1-4] Absence or dysfunction of cilia can impair mucous

TABLE 16-1
Summary of Pulmonary Development

Approximate Gestational Age	Development
Embryonic Period	
Day 26	Lung emerges as outpouching of primitive foregut
Week 4	Mainstem bronchi formed
Week 5	Lobar bronchi formed; pulmonary arteries and veins emerge
Week 6	Segmental bronchi formed
Pseudoglandular Period	
Week 7	Diaphragm complete
Week 8	Heart formation complete
Week 10	Cilia, mucous glands, and goblet cells appear
Week 12	Smooth muscle present in large bronchi
Week 16	Conducting airways completed; respiratory bronchiole near completion
Canalicular Period	
Week 17	Formation of terminal bronchioles
Week 22	Pulmonary capillary development begins
Week 23	Type I and type II cells and immature surfactant present
Weeks 24-26	Fetus potentially capable of gas exchange
Saccular Period	
Weeks 26-28	Development of saccules (primitive alveoli)
Week 35	Mature surfactant present
Week 36	Early alveoli development
Alveolar Period	
Weeks 36-40	Rapid alveolar development; efficient alveolar capillary membrane present
Birth–2 years	Alveoli continue to increase in number and size paralleled by arterial development

transport and lead to chronic respiratory infections (see Chapter 1). Smooth muscle, which originates from the mesoderm, also appears during this stage and is present in the large bronchi by the twelfth week. Any event that alters the development of smooth muscle, cartilage, or vascular structures during this stage can lead to pulmonary disorders in infancy. A fetus born prematurely during this period is unable to survive.

Canalicular Period

The third stage of development, or the **canalicular period**, begins at approximately 17 weeks and continues through 26 weeks' gestation.[1-4] During this stage, the terminal bronchioles subdivide further to form the basic structure of the acinus, or gas-exchanging unit.[1-4] Capillaries begin to establish a network around the alveoli allowing for limited gas exchange by 22 weeks.[1-4] At approximately 23 weeks' gestation, type I and type II alveolar cells begin to differentiate. Type I cells are important in the development of the alveolar capillary membrane, whereas type II cells are involved in surfactant production. By the end of the canalicular stage, some thin-walled primitive alveoli have developed, and the lung tissue is well vascularized. A fetus born prematurely at the end of this stage (approximately 24 to 26 weeks' gestation) is potentially capable of air breathing and may survive with intensive medical care. The immature respiratory system often requires mechanical ventilatory assistance or surfactant replacement therapy or both. (See Chapter 3 for further discussion of surfactant replacement therapy.)

CONCEPT QUESTION 16-1

What problems would you expect in a premature infant born at 24 weeks of gestation?

Saccular Period

The **saccular period** begins around 26 weeks of gestation.[1-4] During this stage of development, the terminal airways continue to widen and form cylindrical structures called saccules. These saccules subdivide to form subsaccules, which eventually develop into alveoli. By the end of this stage, the blood-air barrier is established allowing for adequate gas exchange for the fetus if it is born prematurely. Alveolar cells continue to differentiate into type I and type II cells, with type II cells synthesizing pulmonary surfactant. Surfactant is a complex mixture of phospholipids and proteins that lines the inner walls of the alveoli and offsets surface tension forces at the air-liquid interface of the alveoli (see Chapter 3). Surfactant production begins at approximately 20 weeks' gestation and is present in only small amounts in infants born prematurely. The production of surfactant increases during gestation and reaches adequate levels to support air breathing during the last two weeks of pregnancy. Mature surfactant contains the phospholipid phosphatidylglycerol (PG), which is required for normal surfactant function. PG first appears at about 35 weeks of gestation and increases to peak levels at term.[1-3] Immature surfactant has insufficient PG and is easily inhibited by hypoxia, hypothermia, and acidosis. Thus, premature infants, especially infants born before 35 weeks' gestation, are susceptible to developing **respiratory distress syndrome (RDS)** because of surfactant deficiency. Maternal administration of prenatal corticosteroids, which induce surfactant production, and the administration of exogenous surfactant directly into the newborn lungs after birth can decrease the severity of RDS and the need for mechanical ventilation.

Alveolar Period

The final period of lung development, the **alveolar period**, begins at approximately 36 weeks' gestation and extends

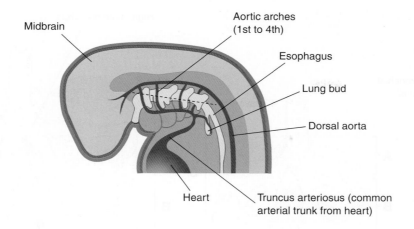

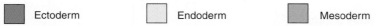

Germ-Layer Derivatives

Ectoderm   Endoderm   Mesoderm

Figure 16-1 Schematic drawing shows the lung bud that emerges as an outpouching of the primitive foregut eventually forming the lung. The three primary germ layers from which all tissues and organs originate are also illustrated. (From Moore KL, Persaud TVN: *The developing human: clinically oriented embryology,* ed 7, Philadelphia, 2003, Saunders.)

TABLE 16-2		
Structures Arising from the Three Embryonic Layers		
Ectoderm	**Mesoderm**	**Endoderm**
Central nervous system	Cardiovascular system	Epithelial tissue Respiratory,
Peripheral nervous system	Connective tissue	digestive, and urinary systems
Sensory epithelia	Bone, cartilage, muscle	Large glands: tonsils, thyroid, thymus
Glandular tissues	Kidney and spleen tissue	Auditory structures
Epidermal tissues	Reproductive tissues	
Teeth	Serous linings	

increased to about 300 million alveoli.[1-3] This explains why children who sustain lung injury during the neonatal period (birth to 28 days) can seemingly "outgrow" their lung disease. Alveolar development is usually complete by age 8; from this time on, alveoli increase in size until thoracic growth is complete.[1-4] Collateral pathways such as the canals of Lambert and pores of Kohn are poorly developed in young children. Consequently, children less than 10 years of age are more likely to develop airway obstruction and atelectasis than older children.[5]

FACTORS AFFECTING FETAL DEVELOPMENT

Fetal Lung Fluid

The fetal lung has no respiratory function before birth; it is a secretory organ that produces approximately 250 to 350 mL of fluid per day.[4] Fetal lung fluid is present by the sixth week of gestation and is derived from alveolar epithelium secretions. Most of the fluid produced remains in the lung; however, some is swallowed, and some is emitted into the amniotic fluid during periodic opening of the larynx when the fetus makes breathing movements. Lung fluid is constantly produced and plays a significant role in determining the size and shape of the developing air space. The composition of fetal lung fluid differs from the composition of amniotic fluid. Fetal lung fluid is higher in sodium and chloride concentrations; lower in pH; and lower in bicarbonate, potassium, and protein concentrations.[4] Lung fluid also contains components of pulmonary surfactant and other fluids from alveolar epithelial cells; its presence in amniotic fluid aids the clinician in determining the degree of lung maturity.

through infancy and childhood.[1-4] During this stage, alveoli continue to develop and mature at a rapid rate, and pulmonary surfactant production increases. The full-term fetus has developed numerous alveoli with mature surfactant, creating an efficient alveolar capillary gas-exchange membrane. Although the lungs are completely developed, they do not take on a respiratory function until the moment of birth.

The lung at birth is not a miniature adult lung; it continues to develop and grow well into childhood. During the first years of life, alveoli develop rapidly paralleled by the expansion of the pulmonary capillary bed. As body weight increases, alveolar development increases proportionally, matched by an increase in the lungs' oxygen uptake. At birth, approximately 50 million alveoli are present; by age 8 years, this number has

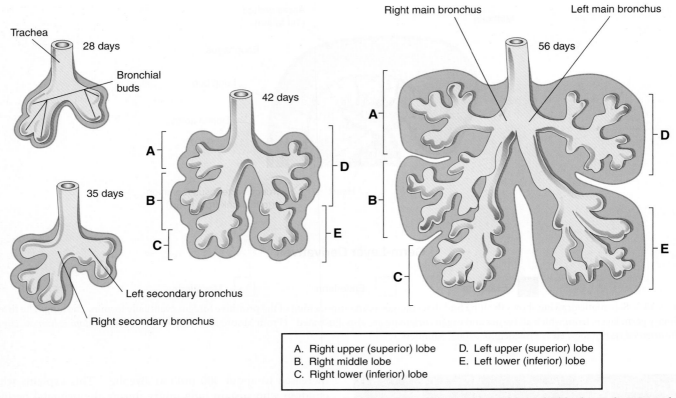

A. Right upper (superior) lobe   D. Left upper (superior) lobe
B. Right middle lobe   E. Left lower (inferior) lobe
C. Right lower (inferior) lobe

Figure 16-2 Stages of development of the bronchial buds and lung. *28 days,* Formation of the trachea and bronchial buds. *35 days,* Secondary bronchi that branch into segmental bronchi are formed. *42 days,* Beginning of pseudoglandular period; the lung takes on the appearance of a gland. *56 days,* Branching of the tracheobronchial tree that forms the conducting airways. (From Moore KL, Persaud TVN: *The developing human: clinically oriented embryology,* ed 7, Philadelphia, 2003, Saunders.)

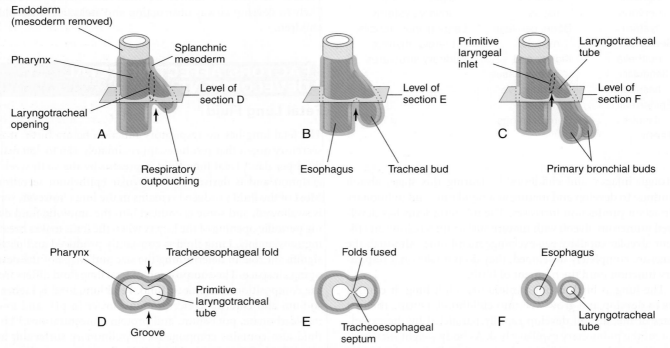

Figure 16-3 Developmental stages of the tracheoesophageal septum. **A-C,** Lateral views showing the outpouching of the foregut into the esophagus and laryngotracheal tube. **D-F,** The formation of the tracheoesophageal septum showing its separation into the laryngotracheal tube and esophagus. (From Moore KL, Persaud TVN: *The developing human: clinically oriented embryology,* ed 7, Philadelphia, 2003, Saunders.)

CLINICAL FOCUS 16-1

Respiratory Distress Syndrome and Surfactant Therapy

An infant girl with an estimated gestational age of 30 weeks was delivered with Apgar scores of 5 and 7 at 1 minute and 5 minutes (see Clinical Focus 16-4). Over the next hour, the infant's respiratory status began to deteriorate, with the infant exhibiting nasal flaring, expiratory grunting, and intercostal retractions. Arterial blood gas results on an F_IO_2 of 0.60 via oxygen hood results were as follows:

pH = 7.26
$PaCO_2$ = 50 mm Hg
PaO_2 = 40 mm Hg

A chest x-ray revealed findings consistent with RDS: bilateral ground-glass appearance and decreased lung volumes. The infant was intubated and placed on mechanical ventilation, and exogenous surfactant was delivered. Arterial blood gas results after surfactant administration were as follows:

pH = 7.36
$PaCO_2$ = 37 mm Hg
PaO_2 = 78 mm Hg on an F_IO_2 of 0.80

A few days later, the infant was extubated and placed on F_IO_2 of 0.30 via oxygen hood.

Discussion

RDS, a condition found primarily in premature infants, is characterized by respiratory failure after premature birth associated with severe atelectasis. The lack of adequate amounts of surfactant resulting in high surface tension is the major cause of alveolar collapse. To maintain alveolar ventilation, the infant must generate tremendous intrathoracic pressures with each breath, which results in increased work of breathing and eventually respiratory failure. A newborn with RDS presents with signs of respiratory distress at birth or within a few hours after birth. Diagnosis is made by clinical presentation (nasal flaring, expiratory grunting, and intercostal retraction), chest x-ray, and arterial blood gas results. The standard treatment for RDS is surfactant replacement therapy. (A premature infant born at 30 weeks is an automatic indication for prophylactic surfactant therapy.) Surfactant replacement therapy improves lung compliance by reducing surface tension, allowing alveoli to remain inflated. This improves arterial blood gas values and decreases the need for mechanical ventilation and oxygen delivery.

Although the presence of fetal lung fluid is essential for normal development of the lung, the switch from placental to pulmonary gas exchange at birth requires rapid removal of this fluid from the newborn lung. The production of lung fluid decreases shortly before term to approximately 65% of previous values. In addition, lung fluid is absorbed during labor so that only about 35% of the original lung fluid volume needs to be cleared during delivery.[4] At the time of birth, the infant's inspiratory effort generates an enormous amount of negative intrapulmonary pressure to fill the lungs with air. With the first few breaths, most fetal lung fluid is expelled; the remaining lung fluid is cleared by absorption through the pulmonary vasculature and lymphatic systems.

Fetal breathing movements begin at approximately 10 weeks of gestation and increase in strength and frequency as gestation progresses, increasing to a rate of 30 to 70 breathing efforts per minute during the last 10 weeks.[4] This early respiratory activity contributes to the regulation of lung fluid and aids in the stretch of lung tissue, which influences lung growth. Fetal breathing movements appear to originate from the diaphragm and are thought to be necessary for training and developing the respiratory muscles so that they can generate enough force to overcome the surface tension of airless alveoli during the initial breath. The absence of lung fluid and breathing movements during fetal development results in an underdeveloped lung.[2]

CONCEPT QUESTION 16-2

What abnormality might occur in the absence of adequate amounts of fetal lung fluid?

Maternal-Fetal Gas Exchange

The **placenta** is a highly vascular gas-exchange organ, providing a circulatory link between mother and embryo; it is required for survival of the fetus. The fetus relies on maternal blood flow through the placenta for the exchange of nutrients and wastes, including oxygen delivery and carbon dioxide removal. The placenta separates the fetus from the **endometrium** (mucous membrane lining) of the uterus and consists of two compartments: (1) the fetal compartment, arising from the embryonic sac, and (2) the maternal compartment, derived from the endometrium. The placenta transports nutrients and wastes between mother and fetus through the umbilical cord. **Abruptio placentae**, or premature detachment of the placenta from the uterine wall, is a medical emergency and may result in life-threatening maternal hemorrhage and fetal asphyxia.

Shortly after the fertilized egg implants in the uterine wall, the placenta begins to develop with small finger-like projections invading the endometrial lining of the uterus. These projections, called **chorionic villi**, continue to branch further into the endometrium, creating irregular pockets around the villi called intervillous spaces (Figure 16-4). Maternal blood fills these spaces supplying oxygen and nutrients to the fetus. As the fetus matures, villi increase in number, expanding the surface area for gas exchange.

Maternal blood enters the intervillous space through the spiral arteries (see Figure 16-4). At this point, the diffusion of oxygen, carbon dioxide, and metabolic products occurs between maternal and fetal blood. After this exchange, maternal blood exits the intervillous spaces through venous channels.

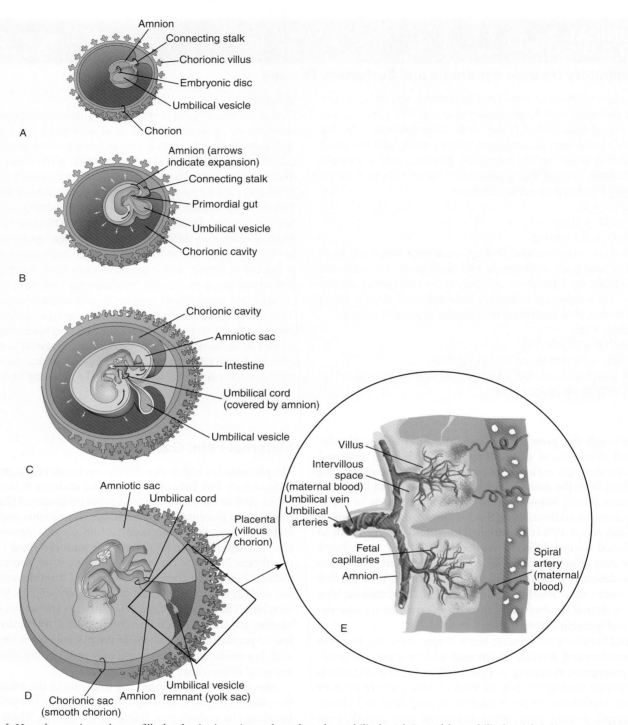

Figure 16-4   How the amnion enlarges, fills the chorionic cavity, and envelops the umbilical cord. Part of the umbilical vesicle is incorporated into the embryo as the primordial gut. **A,** At 3 weeks. **B,** At 4 weeks. **C,** At 10 weeks. **D,** At 20 weeks. **E,** Cutaway view of the placenta showing spiral arteries that supply maternal blood to the intervillous space and villus capillaries that supply oxygenated blood to the fetus through the umbilical vein (*red*). The umbilical arteries (*blue*) return deoxygenated blood from the fetus to the placenta.   (**A-D,** From Moore KL: The developing human: clinically oriented embryology, ed 8, Philadelphia, 2008, Saunders; **E,** From Wilkins RL, et al, editors: *Fundamentals of respiratory care,* ed 8, St Louis, 2003, Mosby.)

Oxygenated fetal blood leaves the chorionic villi via capillaries that merge into a single umbilical vein.

The placenta is not a very efficient gas-exchange organ. The PO_2 of maternal blood in the intervillous spaces is about 50 mm Hg, but blood leaving the placenta through the umbilical vein to oxygenate the fetus has a PO_2 value of only about 30 mm Hg. Fetal blood returning through the umbilical arteries to the placenta for reoxygenation has a PO_2 of only about 19 mm Hg.[2] The maximum PO_2 experienced by the fetus is about 30 mm Hg. The primary factor limiting oxygen

TABLE 16-3

Normal Blood Gas Values in a Term Fetus

	PO$_2$ (mm Hg)	PCO$_2$ (mm Hg)	pH
Umbilical artery	19	47	7.36
Umbilical vein	30	43	7.39

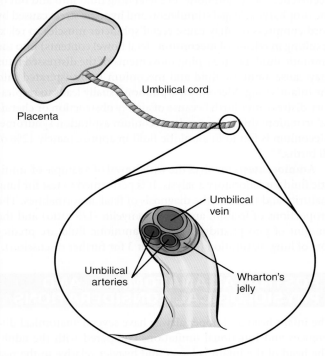

Figure 16-5 Cross-section view of the umbilical cord showing the umbilical vein, arteries, and Wharton's jelly.

transport to the fetus is blood flow. Any factor diminishing uterine or fetal blood flow results in fetal hypoxia and intrauterine growth retardation (IUGR). Severe reduction in fetal blood flow may result in fetal asphyxia and death. Table 16-3 shows normal blood gas values of the umbilical arteries and veins in a full-term fetus.

The umbilical cord connecting the placenta to the fetus contains one vein that delivers oxygenated blood to the fetus and two arteries that carry deoxygenated blood from the fetus back to the placenta. Placental circulation can be compared with the pulmonary circulation in postnatal life: The placenta functions similar to the lungs. The umbilical vein carries oxygenated blood from the placenta to the fetus just as the pulmonary veins carry oxygenated blood from the lungs to the left atrium. Umbilical arteries carry deoxygenated fetal blood back to the placenta for reoxygenation, just as the pulmonary artery carries deoxygenated blood from the body back to the lungs. See the section on fetal circulation later in this chapter for a complete description of fetal circulation.

A tough gelatinous material called Wharton's jelly surrounds the umbilical vessels, which prevents the cord from kinking and occluding blood flow to the fetus (Figure 16-5). After birth, the

umbilical vessels remain open for a short time, allowing vascular access for fluid infusion and blood sampling.

CONCEPT QUESTION 16-3

What maternal factors could adversely affect gas exchange in the fetus?

Fetal Hemoglobin

Fetal blood oxygen tension is low compared with values seen after birth. As stated previously, the most oxygenated fetal blood is found in the umbilical vein with a PO$_2$ of approximately 30 mm Hg. Nevertheless, fetal tissues are adequately oxygenated for the following reasons: (1) the unique blood flow through fetal circulation results in increased blood flow to vital organs (liver, heart, and brain); (2) the fetus has an increased number of red blood cells and hemoglobin compared with the adult; (3) and fetal hemoglobin (HbF) has an increased affinity for oxygen compared with adult hemoglobin.[6]

HbF is the predominant form of hemoglobin in the fetus at approximately eight weeks of gestation; HbF continues to increase until the third trimester when its concentration begins to decline gradually. At 24 weeks of gestation, HbF constitutes about 90% of the total hemoglobin, whereas at birth, HbF represents approximately 70% of the total hemoglobin.[4] The production of HbF decreases rapidly after birth, and by 6 to 12 months of age, HbF has been replaced by adult hemoglobin (HbA).[4]

HbF has a greater affinity for oxygen than HbA. This increase in oxygen affinity is associated with a left shift of the fetal oxyhemoglobin dissociation curve (Figure 16-6), which means that oxygen binds more readily to HbF. The placental transfer of oxygen from maternal blood to fetal blood is thus facilitated, allowing the fetus to survive in a relatively hypoxic environment. Therefore, a PO$_2$ of 30 mm Hg in the fetus corresponds to a hemoglobin saturation of 75% to 80% (see Chapter 8 for further discussion of the oxyhemoglobin equilibrium curve). Maternal hypoxia or hyperventilation can have profound effects on fetal oxygenation; in the case of maternal hyperventilation, the resulting alkalosis shifts the maternal oxygen-hemoglobin equilibrium curve to the left (greater hemoglobin affinity for oxygen), decreasing oxygen availability to the fetus and potentially causing fetal distress.[4]

CONCEPT QUESTION 16-4

Why can a fetus tolerate and thrive on a PaO$_2$ of 30 mm Hg?

Amniotic Fluid

Amniotic fluid, a clear liquid produced by the fetal membranes and the fetus, appears early and surrounds the fetus throughout pregnancy. Amniotic fluid is composed mainly of water; however, its composition changes throughout gestation. During the first half of gestation, amniotic fluid is similar to maternal and fetal serum; in the second half, it is similar to dilute fetal urine with added phospholipids from the fetal lung.[4] Amniotic fluid

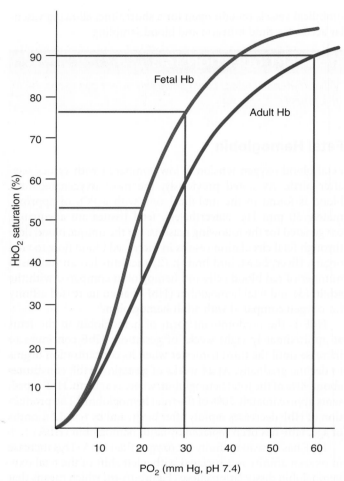

Figure 16-6 Left shift of the fetal oxyhemoglobin dissociation curve illustrating the greater affinity of fetal hemoglobin for oxygen. The fetus' normal PO_2 of 30 mm Hg produces a saturation of about 78%. (From Wilkins RL, et al, editors: *Fundamentals of respiratory care*, ed 8, St Louis, 2003, Mosby.)

is continuously secreted and reabsorbed throughout gestation with a volume reaching approximately 1000 mL at full term. The fetus swallows this fluid, which is absorbed by the digestive tract and excreted as urine. Amniotic fluid serves many important functions. It protects the fetus from trauma by cushioning any blows or impacts to the maternal abdomen, and it allows the fetus to move freely, permitting fetal growth and development. In addition, amniotic fluid helps control the temperature of the fetus by maintaining a relatively constant thermal environment.

Polyhydramnios—an excessive amount of amniotic fluid—occurs when the fetus does not swallow and absorb the usual amount of amniotic fluid. The most common cause of polyhydramnios is a birth defect of the central nervous system or gastrointestinal tract resulting in a fetal swallowing dysfunction. A complication associated with polyhydramnios is premature rupture of amniotic membranes, which may lead to premature delivery.

Oligohydramnios—too little amniotic fluid—results from prematurely ruptured membranes, placental dysfunction, or

fetal abnormalities such as renal agenesis (failure of the kidneys to form). The absence of fetal urine as a component of amniotic fluid is the most common cause of oligohydramnios. Complications for the fetus with oligohydramnios include asphyxia secondary to umbilical cord compression and skeletal deformities caused by uterine wall compression of the fetus.

As stated previously, the fetus periodically exhibits shallow respiratory chest movements or "fetal breathing." This normal occurrence moves amniotic and fetal lung fluid into and out of the oropharynx. Vagal stimulation and hypoxic stress caused by cord compression may cause rectal sphincter muscles to relax, resulting in release of **meconium** (fetal bowel contents) into the amniotic fluid. Deep gasping movements of the distressed fetus may cause amniotic fluid and meconium to be aspirated into the infant's lung. Meconium aspiration usually leads to respiratory distress after birth because of airway obstruction or chemical irritation; this is known as meconium aspiration syndrome. Meconium is found in amniotic fluid in approximately 12% of all births.[4]

Amniocentesis involves the withdrawal of a sample of amniotic fluid for laboratory analysis. It is performed to test for lung maturity and to aid in the diagnosis of fetal abnormalities. The proportions of lecithin and sphingomyelin (L/S ratio) and the amount of phosphatidylglycerol in amniotic fluid are predictors of lung maturation (see Chapter 3 for further discussion).

POSTNATAL ANATOMICAL AND PHYSIOLOGICAL CONSIDERATIONS

The infant head and upper airway have several anatomical differences and functional limitations compared with the adult. The head of the infant is larger and heavier relative to the rest of the body. In addition, the head is poorly supported on a relatively small neck, making the neck mechanically more susceptible to injury with abrupt movement. The mouth and nose of an infant are smaller and more easily obstructed. The relatively large tongue and small oral cavity make mouth breathing more difficult and is probably one reason infants tend to be preferential nose breathers when they are not crying.

All infant airway structures are smaller and narrower than in the adult; the infant's upper airway mucosa is thinner and more easily traumatized. The infant larynx is positioned higher in the neck and is more cone-shaped than it is in the adult; the cricoid ring is the narrowest portion of the upper airway in the infant (Figure 16-7). The newborn trachea is shorter, narrower, softer, and more collapsible than the trachea of the adult (Figure 16-8). Because of the small diameter of the infant airway, a minor degree of mucosal edema can very quickly produce significant airway narrowing and increased airflow resistance.

Croup, the most common cause of upper airway obstruction in children, is a viral infection that causes subglottal mucosal edema of the larynx and trachea. The illness begins with an upper respiratory tract infection, progressing to an inspiratory stridor and a "barky" cough after several days. Stridor is a harsh sound caused by the vibration of air through a narrowed upper airway. The obstruction is occasionally severe enough to require an artificial airway.

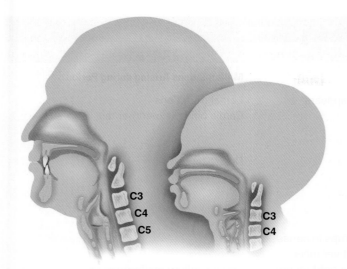

Figure 16-7 Location of the larynx in an infant compared with an adult. Note the narrow cone-shaped infant airway. (From Wilkins RL, et al, editors: *Fundamentals of respiratory care*, ed 8, St Louis, 2003, Mosby.)

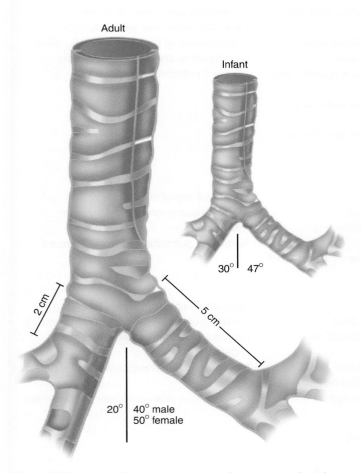

Figure 16-8 Size of the trachea in an infant compared with an adult. (From Wilkins RL, et al, editors: *Fundamentals of respiratory care*, ed 8, St Louis, 2003, Mosby.)

Epiglottitis is a life-threatening bacterial infection primarily affecting the soft tissue of the epiglottis. The epiglottis can rapidly swell and severely obstruct or totally occlude the glottis, causing respiratory arrest. The onset of epiglottitis is abrupt and associated with a high fever. Symptoms include a severe sore throat, drooling (inability to swallow), and a muffled cough, which progress rapidly to stridor and inability to speak. Complete airway obstruction can occur within hours, requiring immediate endotracheal intubation or tracheostomy.

The chest wall of the infant is very compliant with the ribs positioned more horizontally than in the adult. The infant's ribs and sternum are mostly cartilage offering little support to the chest wall, and intercostal muscles are immature and fatigue easily causing the infant to rely more heavily on the diaphragm for respiration; this can cause the chest and abdomen to move in opposite directions (paradoxical breathing) during respiratory distress. Signs of respiratory distress and high airway resistance in the infant include inspiratory nasal flaring, expiratory grunting, inspiratory intercostal retractions, and paradoxical breathing. Table 16-4 shows normal vital signs of full-term neonates at birth.

In utero, the fetus lives in an environment that maintains a stable fetal body temperature. However, at the time of delivery, the infant's body temperature may decrease rapidly as it passes from the warm protected fluid environment to the cooler air environment of the delivery room where heat can be lost rapidly through convection. Delayed warming can lead to cold stress, which may have serious consequences for all newborns, especially premature infants or infants who are small for gestational age. The thermal environment of the newborn infant must be carefully maintained to prevent heat loss and cold stress.

The infant is capable of heat production through both physical and chemical mechanisms. Physical mechanisms produce heat by increased activity such as restlessness, hyperactivity, crying, and shivering. As mentioned previously, the musculature of newborns, especially premature infants, is underdeveloped and weak; therefore, the ability to produce heat via physical mechanisms is limited. Chemical mechanisms of heat production in the infant include an increase in metabolic rate and the metabolism of brown adipose tissue, or brown fat.

Brown fat metabolism is the most important means of heat production in the newborn infant. This special fat is located between the scapulae; around the muscles and blood vessels of the neck, axillae, and mediastinum; and around the kidneys and adrenal glands. Brown fat begins to appear at approximately 26 weeks' gestation and continues to develop until 3 to 5 weeks after birth, accounting for one tenth of the adipose tissue in term infants.[4] Brown fat stores are much lower in preterm infants and almost nonexistent in infants of very low birth weight.

The physiological response to heat loss in the neonate includes (1) peripheral vasoconstriction to prevent blood from reaching the skin, where heat loss occurs; (2) movement and flexion of the extremities to generate heat and decrease the surface area for heat loss; and (3) brown fat metabolism to warm adjacent blood circulation. On exposure to cold, thermal receptors located on the face of the infant signal the sympathetic nervous system to release norepinephrine. Norepinephrine

TABLE 16-4

Timelines in Normal and Abnormal Cardiac Development

Normal Time	Developmental Events	Malformations Arising during Period
18 days	Horseshoe-shaped cardiac primordium appears	Lethal mutations
20 days	Bilateral cardia primordial fuse	Cardia bifida (experimental)
	Cardiac jelly appears	
	Aortic arch is forming	
22 days	Heart is looping into S shape	Dextrocardia
	Heart begins to beat	
	Dorsal mesocardium is breaking down	
	Aortic arches I and II are forming	
24 days	Atria are beginning to bulge	
	Right and left ventricles act like two pumps in series	
	Outflow tract is distinguished from right ventricle	
Late in week 4	Sinus venosus is being incorporated into right atrium	Venous inflow malformations
	Endocardial cushions appear	Persistent atrioventricular canal
	Septum primum appears between right and left atria	Common atrium
	Muscular interventricular septum is forming	Common ventricle
	Truncoconal ridges are forming	Persistent truncus arteriosus
	Aortic arch I is regressing	
	Aortic arch III is forming	
	Aortic arch IV is forming	
Early in week 5	Endocardial cushions are coming together, forming right and left atrioventricular canals	Persistent atrioventricular canal
	Further growth of interatrial septum primum and muscular interventricular septum occurs	Muscular ventricular septal defects
		Transposition of the great vessels; aortic and pulmonary stenosis or atresia
	Truncus arteriosus is dividing into aorta and pulmonary artery	Aberrant pulmonary drainage
	Atrioventricular bundle is forming; there is possible neurogenic control of heartbeat	
	Pulmonary veins are being incorporated into atrium	
	Aortic arches I and II have regressed	
	Aortic arches III and IV have formed	
	Aortic arch VI is forming	
Late in week 5–early week 6	Endocardial cushions fuse	Low atrial septal defects
	Interatrial foramen secundum is forming	Membranous interventricular septal defects
	Interatrial septum primum is almost contacting endocardial cushions	Aortic and pulmonary vascular stenosis
	Membranous part of interventricular septum starts to form	
	Semilunar valves begin to form	
Late in week 6	Interatrial foramen secundum is large	High atrial septal defects
	Interatrial septum secundum starts to form	Tricuspid or mitral valve stenosis or atresia
	Atrioventricular valves and papillary muscles are forming	Membranous interventricular septal defects
	Interventricular septum is almost complete	Membranous interventricular septal defect
	Coronary circulation is becoming established	
8-9 weeks	Membranous part of interventricular septum is complete	Membranous interventricular septal defect

From Carlson BM: *Human embryology and developmental biology,* ed 3, St Louis, 2004, Mosby.

stimulates the breakdown of brown fat. The rapid metabolism of brown fat produces heat and warms the blood perfusing the surrounding tissues. Heat is transferred to the rest of the body via the systemic circulation. The production of heat from the metabolism of brown fat involves the breakdown of triglycerides into glycerol and fatty acids. This process depends on the availability of oxygen, glucose, and production of adenosine triphosphate (ATP). Therefore, the ability to generate heat is severely diminished in infants with hypoxia, acidosis, and hypoglycemia.

Several factors lead to increased heat loss in the newborn infant. Infants have a very large surface area-to-body mass ratio, they have little subcutaneous fat, and they have a relatively large head. For these reasons, heat loss is proportionally greater in infants than in adults. The infant's thin skin with blood vessels near the surface provides poor insulation, leading to further heat loss. In addition, shivering, which is a major method of heat gain in adults, is not well developed in newborns. Hypothermia, or cold stress, is a serious condition that can be fatal if not detected and treated early. Hypothermia occurs when heat is lost at a greater rate than it can be replaced. Clinical manifestations of cold stress include tachypnea, peripheral vasoconstriction, pallor, skin mottling, and metabolic acidosis. Cold stress may occur when the infant's core body temperature decreases to less than 36° C.[7] Therefore, the clinician should ensure that the infant is placed in a **neutral thermal environment** and is kept warm and dry; this minimizes heat loss, improves survival, and decreases metabolic demands (see Clinical Focus 16-3).

CONCEPT QUESTION 16-5

Why are infants more prone to airway obstruction than adults?

FETAL AND NEONATAL CARDIOVASCULAR DEVELOPMENT AND PHYSIOLOGY

The cardiovascular system is the first organ system to develop and function in the fetus, appearing at about 18 or 19 days of gestation. The rapidly growing embryo requires an efficient method to transport oxygen and nutrients; cardiac contractions begin by day 22, and blood flow can be observed by Doppler ultrasonography by gestational week 4.[3] The primitive heart and its relationship to the fetal cardiovascular system is shown in Figure 16-9. Understanding this development is of value to students when studying the various cardiac anomalies discussed later in this chapter.

The cardiovascular system arises from the mesoderm layer of the embryo (see Table 16-2). The first identifiable features are cell clusters that can induce blood vessel formation (angiogenic cells) arranged on both sides of the embryo's central axis.[8] Late in gestational week 3, a pair of cardiac tubes forms from the combination of these cell clusters. Fusion of these heart tubes creates a single, three-layer endocardial heart tube (Figure 16-10). The inner layer of the heart tube becomes the internal endothelial lining of the heart—the **endocardium**—whereas the primitive **myocardium** becomes the muscular, myocardial layer of the heart.[4] These layers are separated by a middle

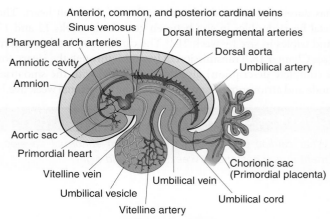

Figure 16-9 The fetal cardiovascular system (approximately 26 days) showing vessels on the left side only. The umbilical vein carries well-oxygenated blood and nutrients from the chorionic sac to the fetus. The umbilical arteries carry poorly oxygenated blood and waste products from the fetus to the chorionic sac. The umbilical vesicle (yolk sac) provides for the transfer of nutrients during weeks 2 and 3 of gestation when uteroplacental circulation is being established. During the fourth week, the endoderm of the umbilical vesicle is incorporated into the embryo as the primordial gut (see Figure 16-4). (From Moore KL: *The developing human: clinically oriented embryology,* ed 8, Philadelphia, 2008, Saunders.)

layer of gelatinous connective tissue referred to as **cardiac jelly**, which participates later in the separation of the heart chambers and formation of the atrioventricular valves.[9] The **epicardium**, also known as the visceral pericardium, is part of the outer layer of the heart and develops from mesothelial cells that arise from the area of the sinus venosus.[3]

The developing heart lengthens and bends, giving rise to three recognizable structures—the **bulbus cordis**, the ventricle, and the primordial (primitive) atrium—from which the right ventricle, the left ventricle, and the atria arise respectively (Figure 16-11, *A*). The truncus arteriosus is identifiable shortly thereafter, and it divides into the pulmonary artery and aorta sometime during gestational week six (Figure 16-11, *B*). The fetal heart continues to bend in an S-shaped pattern, pushing the atrial bulge in a superior direction (Figure 16-12). If this process of bending and looping (sometimes referred to as cardiac looping) progresses abnormally, cardiac malformation can occur (Table 16-4 describes malformations that may arise during cardiac development). By the end of the fourth gestational week, the external appearance of the fetal heart is similar to the appearance of a mature heart; however, internal structures are incomplete. Development of the atrial and ventricular septa and the atrioventricular (tricuspid and bicuspid) and semilunar (pulmonary and aortic) valves begins between days 25 and 30 and continues through weeks 7 and 8 (Figure 16-13), during which time blood begins to flow through the fetal circulation pathway (explained later).

A heart rate of approximately 100 beats per minute may be detected by gestational week five and increases to an average rate of 140 beats per minute before term delivery.[4,10] By gestational week 12, the fetal heart is positioned normally in the chest and has developed into a miniature version of the adult heart. The fetal heart doubles in size between gestational weeks 12 and 17 and triples in size by week 21.[11] The cardiac conduction system (see Chapter 18, Transmission of Impulses through the Heart, for a complete description) also develops early, with the sinoatrial node and atrioventricular node evident by gestational week five.[12]

CONCEPT QUESTION 16-6

What cardiac defects could result from abnormal development during gestational weeks seven and eight?

FETAL CIRCULATION

The design of the fetal cardiovascular system meets the needs of the developing fetus and allows for the transition to neonatal circulation that occurs after birth. Figure 16-14 illustrates fetal blood flow, including the three fetal shunts that must close after birth. As mentioned earlier, the placenta, a highly vascular, low-resistance organ, supplies oxygen-rich blood to the fetus via the umbilical vein. Blood from the umbilical vein flows first to the liver where 18% to 30% of oxygenated blood is shunted around the liver, through the **ductus venosus** (the first shunt) into

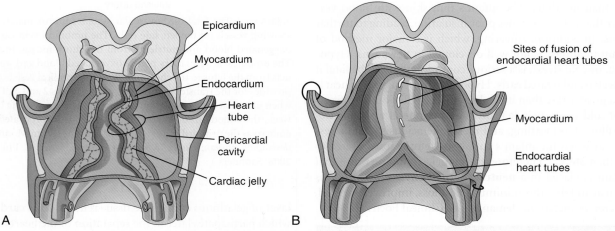

Figure 16-10 The developing heart (end of week 3 of gestation). The heart tubes fuse (**A**) to form a single tube (**B**). The fusion begins at the cranial end of the tubes and extends downward until a single heart tube is formed. (From Moore KL: *The developing human: clinically oriented embryology,* ed 8, Philadelphia, 2008, Saunders.)

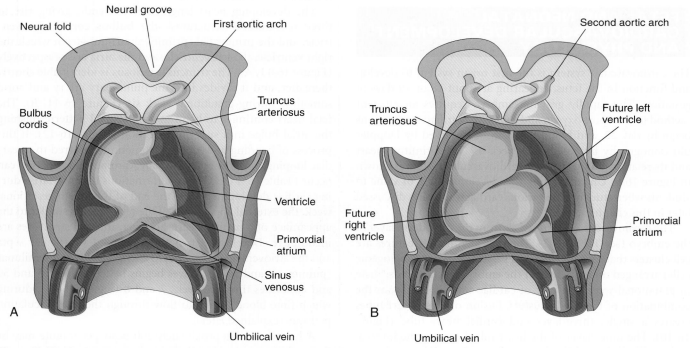

Figure 16-11 The developing heart (days 22 to 25 of gestation). As the heart elongates, it loops to the right and bends (**A**), forming regional segments from which the future atria and ventricles will arise (**B**). (From Moore KL: *The developing human: clinically oriented embryology,* ed 7, Philadelphia, 2003, Saunders.)

the inferior vena cava (IVC). Blood flow through the ductus venosus increases in response to fetal distress; flow through this shunt normally decreases in the near-term infant, which helps to supply the liver with additional nutrients.[4] Because of the angle at which the IVC enters the right atrium, most of the oxygenated blood supply is directed through the opening between the right and left atrium, the **foramen ovale** (the second shunt) to the left atrium, where it mixes with a small amount of poorly oxygenated blood returning from the lungs through the pulmonary veins. This partially oxygenated blood mixture flows down into the left ventricle and out of the ascending aorta to perfuse myocardial and cerebral circulations. Blood with poor oxygen content coming from the superior vena cava (SVC) mixes with oxygenated blood from the IVC and because of the anatomical orientation of the SVC, blood from it tends to preferentially flow through the tricuspid valve into the right ventricle. This moderately oxygenated blood is pumped through the pulmonary valve into the pulmonary artery where only about 13% to 25% of the blood enters the pulmonary circulation to perfuse the developing lungs; the remaining 75% to 90% bypasses the lungs through the third shunt, the **ductus arteriosus**, which connects the pulmonary artery with the descending aorta.[13]

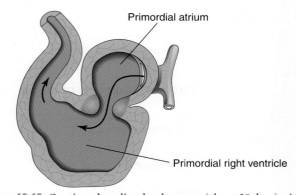

Figure 16-12 Continued cardiac development (about 28 days) with the common atrium moving into a superior position. (From Moore KL: *The developing human: clinically oriented embryology*, ed 7, Philadelphia, 2003, Saunders.)

The fetal lung requires little blood flow because it does not participate in gas exchange. Fetal pulmonary vascular resistance (PVR) is increased because the fluid-filled lungs have a very low PO_2, leading to hypoxic pulmonary vasoconstriction and consequently, an increase in the medial muscle layer of pulmonary arteries.[14] The high PVR explains why 75% to 90% of the pulmonary artery blood flows preferentially through the ductus arterious, a path of much less resistance. The ductal blood mingles with descending aortic blood that supplies the lower extremities. Two umbilical arteries, branching from the iliac arteries, carry blood back to the placenta for reoxygenation and carbon dioxide removal (see Figure 16-14). The three fetal shunts are necessary for fetal cardiovascular function, but it is equally necessary that they close after birth.

TRANSITION TO EXTRAUTERINE LIFE

The transition from fetal life to neonatal life is defined by a complex series of events. The fluid in the lungs must be replaced with air, diffusion of oxygen and carbon dioxide across the alveolar-capillary membranes must begin, and blood flow through the heart and lungs must change course.

Respiratory Transition

As stated previously, the production of fetal lung fluid decreases shortly before term delivery, leaving approximately 35% of the original lung volume to be removed by the squeeze effect on the chest during vaginal delivery and by absorption via pulmonary capillaries and the lymphatic system after birth. Before delivery, the fetal lung contains 10 to 30 mL/kg of fluid, which is comparable to newborn functional residual capacity (FRC).[4] Infants born by cesarean section and infants born after a precipitous (rapid) delivery do not benefit from vaginal chest compression and may experience retention of fetal lung fluid. Such fluid retention can result in short-term respiratory distress known as **transient tachypnea of the newborn**.[4]

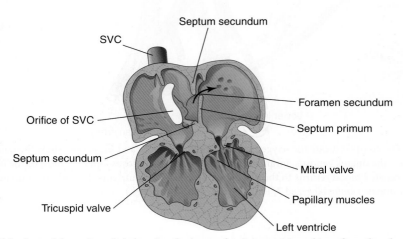

Figure 16-13 Frontal section of the heart (about 8 weeks) showing the heart after it is partitioned into four chambers. The *arrow* indicates the flow of well-oxygenated blood (from the placenta) moving from the right to the left atrium. *SVC,* Superior vena cava. (From Moore KL: *The developing human: clinically oriented embryology,* ed 7, Philadelphia, 2003, Saunders.)

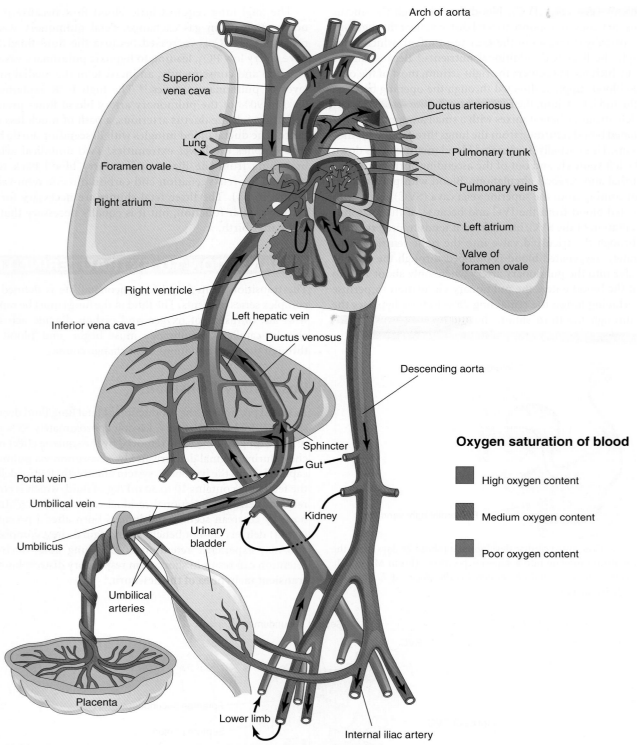

Figure 16-14 Fetal circulation. The colors indicate the oxygen saturation of the blood, and the *arrows* show the course of the blood from the placenta to the heart. Three shunts—the ductus venosus, foramen ovale, and ductus arteriosus—permit most of the oxygenated blood to bypass the liver and lungs. The poorly oxygenated blood returns to the placenta for oxygen and nutrients through the umbilical arteries. (From Moore KL: *The developing human: clinically oriented embryology,* ed 7, Philadelphia, 2003, Saunders.)

CONCEPT QUESTION 16-7

What is the purpose of fetal lung fluid?

After vaginal delivery, the thorax is decompressed and expands, creating a negative intrathoracic pressure that facilitates air entry into the lungs. With the first breaths, a newborn must generate pressures of −20 to −70 cm H_2O to overcome the surface tension of airless alveoli and the viscosity of residual lung fluid.[15] As additional alveoli inflate with subsequent breaths, surface tension is reduced and transpulmonary pressures decrease, allowing the FRC to be established within a few hours of birth. A premature infant born with underdeveloped pulmonary surfactant has great difficulty establishing the FRC because of the continued need for high transpulmonary pressures to overcome the surface tension of collapsed alveoli; this predisposes the premature infant to the development of respiratory distress syndrome (see Clinical Focus 16-1).

CONCEPT QUESTION 16-8

What clinical signs and symptoms would be evident in an infant experiencing retention of fetal lung fluid?

A transient period of asphyxia occurs after the umbilical cord is clamped and placental blood flow ceases; this lack of oxygen helps activate chemoreceptors that stimulate breathing efforts. The sensory stimulation experienced by the neonate when transitioning from the warm, moist intrauterine environment to the cooler, drier delivery room, coupled with handling and drying further stimulate breathing. Approximately 10% of newborns require some assistance to begin breathing at birth, usually in the form of oxygen administration or positive pressure ventilation, or both.[7] Box 16-1 summarizes conditions that may necessitate these interventions, known as neonatal resuscitation.

CLINICAL FOCUS 16-2

Maternal Steroid Therapy to Enhance Fetal Lung Development

Infants born prematurely have a significant risk for developing RDS. A significant decrease in the incidence of RDS has been shown in infants born to mothers who received prenatal steroid therapy to enhance lung maturity by accelerating the production of fetal surfactant. The National Institutes of Health recommends that all pregnant women at risk of delivering between 24 and 34 weeks' gestation are candidates for prenatal steroid therapy.[22] Treatment consists of two 12-mg doses of betamethasone given intramuscularly 24 hours apart or four 6-mg doses of dexamethasone given intramuscularly 12 hours apart. The guidelines suggest a complete course of prenatal steroids starting at 24 hours to 7 days before delivery for the most benefit.

CLINICAL FOCUS 16-3

Effects of Cold Stress on a Newborn

A respiratory therapist is called to a small rural hospital to transport a 29-week gestational age newborn boy to a regional medical center. On arrival, the infant is found lying in an open radiant warmer loosely covered with a wet blanket. The infant is intubated and placed on mechanical ventilation; vital signs are stable except for temperature, which is recorded as 89° F, and blood pressure, which is unattainable. On arrival to the regional medical center, the infant's heart rate decreases to 60 beats per minute. Chest compressions are initiated, and blood gases are drawn with the following results:

pH = 7.00
PCO_2 = 80.5 mm Hg
PO_2 = 11.5 mm Hg
HCO_3^- = 19.9 mEq/L

Despite aggressive resuscitation maneuvers, the neonate dies soon thereafter. How did this infant's low temperature affect the outcome?

Discussion

The initial response of the neonate to cold is peripheral vasoconstriction. Neonates also have a large skin surface area in relation to body mass and lose core body heat to the atmosphere much more rapidly than adults. Newborn infants rely on a special fat called brown fat for heat production. Brown fat first appears around 26 weeks' gestation and increases as pregnancy advances. A neonate metabolizes brown fat in response to cold, which increases oxygen consumption. The combination of immature lungs and insufficient brown fat stores in this infant caused additional hypoxic vasoconstriction, respiratory and metabolic acidosis, and ultimately death. It is important to provide all newborns with a neutral thermal environment by providing an environment that is in equilibrium with the infant's body temperature allowing the infant to maintain a normal internal temperature without increasing oxygen consumption.

Circulatory Transition

The transition from fetal to neonatal circulation is characterized by a series of dramatic cardiovascular changes. The fetus prepares for this transition by increasing the expression of pulmonary vasodilators, nitric oxide synthase, and soluble guanylate cyclase (see Chapter 6, Humoral Agents and Nitric Oxide) late in gestational life.[16] Figure 16-15 illustrates neonatal circulation. Shortly after delivery, the umbilical cord is clamped, eliminating the low-resistance placenta from the circulation; this decreases blood flow to the right atrium from the umbilical vein, resulting in a decrease in pressure on the right side of the heart. Clamping of the cord also stops blood flow from the descending aorta into the placenta, increasing left-sided pressures and systemic vascular resistance (SVR). As a result,

CLINICAL FOCUS 16-4

Use of Apgar Scoring in Newborn Assessment

Following a 10-hour period of intense labor, a 2000-g girl is born by vaginal delivery. At 1 minute after delivery, the infant has a heart rate of 120 beats per minute, exerts little respiratory effort, and has good color except for some cyanosis in her extremities. The infant cries when a suction catheter is passed into her nasal passages and has good muscle tone. How will these findings help you in your assessment and treatment of this newborn?

The Apgar score was introduced by Virginia Apgar in 1952 as a rapid method of newborn assessment. Five physical signs are evaluated and given a rating of 0, 1, or 2 points, depending on the severity of the findings. The scores are totaled and become the infant's Apgar score (see chart). Apgar assessment is done at 1 minute and 5 minutes after birth, with additional scoring every 5 minutes for 20 minutes for infants who score less than 7 initially. Infants with low scores (0 to 2) require immediate resuscitation efforts. Infants with a score of 3 to 6 may need oxygen and additional stimulation, whereas infants with scores of 7 or more are considered stable. Resuscitation efforts should not be delayed until after 1 minute in severely depressed infants. This newborn's Apgar score is 8, suggesting no additional intervention is necessary. The acronym APGAR may be used to help remember the five areas of assessment (see chart).

Apgar Score

Sign	0	1	2
Appearance (color)	Pale, blue	Pink body, blue extremities	Completely pink
Pulse	None	<100 beats/min	>100 beats/min
Grimace (reflex irritability, catheter in nares, tactile stimulation)	No response	Grimace	Cough, cry, sneeze
Activity (muscle tone)	Limp	Some flexion	Active motion, good flexion
Respirations	None	Slow, irregular	Good, crying

left-sided heart pressures become greater than right-sided heart pressures. This reversal in pressure gradients physically pushes and closes the flaplike valve between the atria, functionally closing the foramen ovale. Anatomical closure of the foramen ovale occurs as tissue grows around the opening; this process may not be complete for weeks to months. Occasionally, the foramen remains patent into adulthood.[17]

Elimination of blood flow through the umbilical circulation also results in closure of the ductus venosus within one week of delivery. The ductus venosus becomes the ligamentum

BOX 16-1

Risk Factors Associated with the Need for Neonatal Resuscitation

Risk Factors before Labor and Delivery

Maternal infection
Pregnancy-induced hypertension
Chronic hypertension
Anemia
Maternal diabetes
Polyhydramnios
Premature rupture of membranes
Diminished fetal activity
Maternal bleeding
Previous fetal or neonatal death
Postterm status
Multiple gestation
Small-for-dates fetus
Substance abuse
Congenital abnormalities
Oligohydramnios
No prenatal care
Maternal age (<16 or >35)
Chronic maternal illness (e.g., cardiopulmonary, neurological)
Drug therapy (e.g., adrenergic blockers, lithium, magnesium)
Fetal hydrops

Risk Factors during Labor and Delivery

Emergency cesarean section
Forceps or vacuum-assisted delivery
Fetal distress (e.g., abnormal heart rate)
Breech or other abnormal presentation
Meconium-stained amniotic fluid
Prolonged labor
Premature labor
Prolonged rupture of membranes (>18 hours before delivery)
Macrosomia
Uterine hyperstimulation
Postterm gestation
Use of general anesthesia
Chorioamnionitis
Prolapsed cord
Precipitous delivery
Abruptio placentae
Placenta previa
Breech or abnormal presentation
Significant intrapartum bleeding
Narcotics administered to mother within 4 hours of delivery

Adapted from Kattwinkel J, editor: *Neonatal resuscitation textbook*, ed 5, Elk Grove Village, IL, 2006, American Academy of Pediatrics and the American Heart Association.

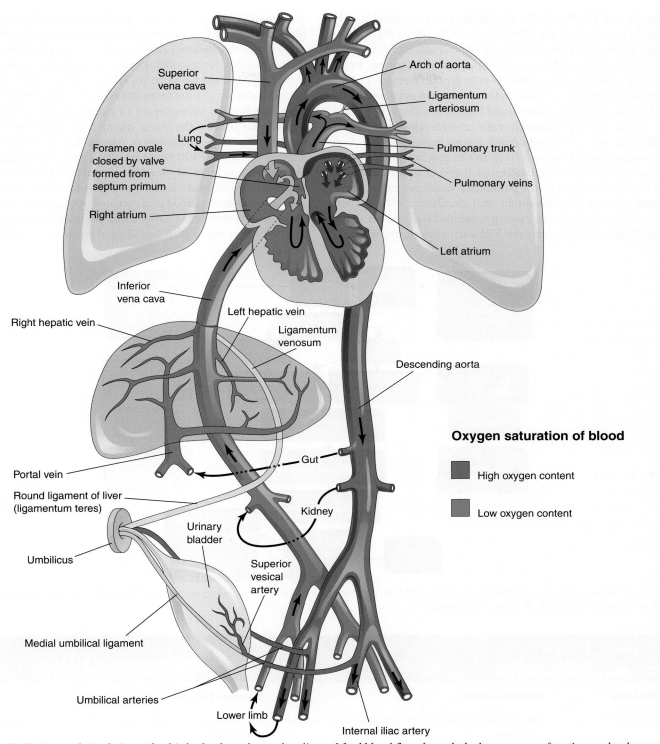

Figure 16-15 Neonatal circulation. After birth, the three shunts that directed fetal blood flow through the heart cease to function, and pulmonary and systemic circulation become separated. The *arrows* indicate the direction of blood flow in the infant. The adult versions of the fetal vessels and structures that become nonfunctional at birth are shown (foramen ovale, ligamentum arteriosum, ligamentum venosum, medial umbilical ligament, and ligamentum teres). (From Moore KL: *The developing human: clinically oriented embryology,* ed 7, Philadelphia, 2003, Saunders.)

venosum. As shown in Figure 16-16, PVR decreases after birth because of pulmonary vessel dilation associated with the ever increasing PO_2 and decreasing PCO_2 caused by ventilation—that is, ventilation removes the stimulus for hypoxic pulmonary vasoconstriction. Consequently, more blood flows to the lungs from the right ventricle, decreasing blood flow through the

ductus arteriosus. Anatomical closure of the ductus arteriosus begins before birth, when endothelial tissue (known as *intimal mounds*) forms in the ductal lumen.[13] At birth, smooth muscle surrounding the ductus arteriosus begins to constrict because ventilation elevates blood oxygen levels, which in turn inhibits the synthesis of prostaglandins responsible for ductal patency during fetal life. Normally, the ductus arteriosus anatomically closes two to four weeks after delivery and becomes the *ligamentum arteriosum* by the twelfth week of postnatal life.[3,13] Hypoxia and acidosis may delay closure of the ductus arteriosus, maintaining a pathway that allows blood to flow between the pulmonary artery and aorta. This condition is known as patent ductus arteriosus (PDA) and is discussed later in this chapter.

Infants born prematurely with underdeveloped surfactant (RDS) or with cardiopulmonary compromise (e.g., infection, meconium aspiration) may be unable to generate the high pressures required to expand collapsed alveoli at birth; this results in low PaO_2 and persistent pulmonary vasoconstriction, sometimes referred to as persistent fetal circulation. PVR remains elevated in these infants, causing continued right-to-left shunting through the foramen ovale and ductus arteriosus, similar to

conditions in fetal life. Unoxygenated venous blood bypasses the lungs through the fetal anatomical shunts and flows directly into the systemic circulation, causing significant arterial hypoxemia. This condition, commonly known as persistent pulmonary hypertension of the newborn (PPHN), manifests in the first 12 hours after birth, causing respiratory distress and arterial hypoxemia that is often unresponsive to oxygen therapy (refractory hypoxemia) because the blood supply does not come in contact with the lungs. Nevertheless, oxygen therapy is used in an attempt to reduce PVR. Some infants require more aggressive therapy, such as **extracorporeal life support** (ECLS), also known as extracorporeal membrane oxygenation (ECMO), which is a process whereby the blood is oxygenated outside of the body via a mechanical membrane oxygenator. Nitric oxide therapy may also be used to reduce PVR (see Clinical Focus 16-5). Table 16-5

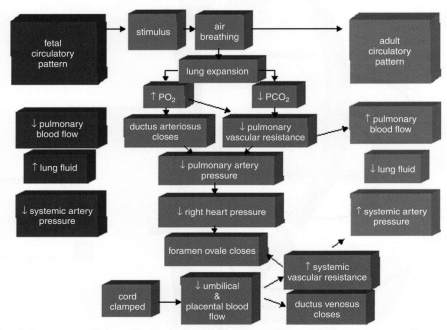

Figure 16-16 Sequence of cardiopulmonary changes after birth. (From Hicks GH: The respiratory system. In Wilkins RL, et al, editors: *Fundamentals of respiratory care,* ed 9. St Louis, 2009, Mosby.)

TABLE 16-5

Circulatory Transition at Birth

Structure	Fetal Circulation	Newborn Circulation
Placenta	Site of gas exchange between fetal and maternal vessels	Placental oxygenation ceases when umbilical cord is clamped
Foramen ovale	Allows blood to be shunted from right to left	Closes against intraatrial septum–atrium, bypassing the right ventricle and fetal lungs shortly after birth
Ductus arteriosus	Provides shunt for blood from pulmonary artery to descending aorta, bypassing fetal lungs	Constricts soon after birth in most infants in response to ↑ PO_2 levels
Aorta	Mixes oxygenated blood and unoxygenated blood and directs it to the rest of the body	Delivers oxygenated blood from left ventricle to the rest of the body
Lungs	No gas exchange; receive minimal flow owing to high PVR	Gas exchange

PVR, Pulmonary vascular resistance.

CLINICAL FOCUS 16-5

Nitric Oxide in the Treatment of Persistent Pulmonary Hypertension of the Neonate

Numerous factors have been associated with the development of PPHN, including birth asphyxia caused by meconium aspiration or prematurity, infection, pulmonary hypoplasia (underdevelopment of fetal lungs) associated with congenital diaphragmatic hernia, and in 10% to 20% of cases of PPHN, remodeling of the pulmonary vasculature owing to unknown (idiopathic) causes.[16]

The primary problem in PPHN is pulmonary artery pressures that remain higher than systemic arterial pressures, impeding blood flow to the lungs and causing hypoxemia and acidosis. Pulmonary arterioles constrict in response to acidosis, further increasing PVR. Blood is shunted through the path of least resistance, from the right atrium into the left atrium through the foramen ovale and from the pulmonary artery into the aorta through the ductus arteriosus (both are examples of right-to-left shunting). The primary goal in treatment of PPHN is a reduction of PVR.

Discussion

Conventional therapy for PPHN includes the use of oxygen and hyperventilation to aid in pulmonary vasodilation. Tolazoline hydrochloride (Priscoline), a potent systemic vasodilator drug, has been used in the past to decrease PVR; however, because of systemic hypotension associated with its use, it is rarely used now. Inhaled nitric oxide (iNO) has proven to be a promising therapy for treatment of PPHN. Nitric oxide is produced in the body and acts through cyclic guanosine monophosphate to cause smooth muscle relaxation, resulting in vasodilation (see Chapter 6). iNO is delivered to pulmonary vessels in contact with functioning alveoli, selectively dilating these blood vessels, enhancing ventilation-perfusion relationships, and improving oxygenation. PVR decreases as oxygenation improves. Areas of poorly ventilated lung do not receive iNO; infants with severe lung disease may benefit from ventilation strategies (i.e., high-frequency ventilation) that optimize lung expansion. Not all infants with PPHN respond or sustain a response to nitric oxide therapy, particularly infants with cardiac disease secondary to left ventricular dysfunction.[16] The benefits of using iNO include selective vasodilation of the pulmonary circulation and a short half-life. The U.S. Food and Drug Administration approved the use of iNO for PPHN in 2000. Concerns surrounding the use of iNO include optimum dosage, the formation of methemoglobin, and the potential for the formation of NO_2, a toxic gas.

---

summarizes the major cardiovascular changes that occur during transition to extrauterine life. Many congenital cardiac defects require a PDA for survival, in which case prostaglandin therapy may be initiated to keep the ductus open. These conditions are described in the next section.

CONCEPT QUESTION 16-9

Would a blood PO_2 value obtained from a right radial artery differ from a blood PO_2 value obtained from an umbilical artery catheter in an infant with right-to-left shunt? Why?

CONGENITAL CARDIAC DEFECTS

Congenital cardiac defects are present at birth and are usually caused by developmental abnormalities occurring during gestational weeks three through eight.[18] Approximately 1% of infants are born with some congenital heart defect, with a higher incidence in premature infants.[18] Defects described in this section account for most cardiac anomalies and fall into three major categories: **acyanotic** (nonhypoxemic) disorders, **cyanotic** (hypoxemic) disorders, and obstructive disorders. Acyanotic disorders shunt already oxygenated blood from the left side of the heart to the right side of the heart, increasing pulmonary blood flow. This additional blood flow overloads the pulmonary circulation, increasing the workload of the right ventricle. Cyanotic disorders shunt deoxygenated blood from the right side of the heart to the left side of the heart, causing serious arterial hypoxemia and possible cyanosis. Acyanotic disorders may progress to cyanotic disorders if they are severe and uncorrected. Obstructive disorders create blood flow limitation within the vessels or at the level of the heart valves. A complete discussion of congenital cardiac defects is beyond the scope of this chapter, but important characteristics of the most common defects are listed subsequently.

ACYANOTIC DISORDERS

Atrial Septal Defect

An **atrial septal defect (ASD)** is an abnormal opening in the atrial septum that allows blood to flow between the left atria and right atria (Figure 16-17). Atrial septal defect is one of the most common congenital cardiac anomalies but is usually asymptomatic and undetected until adulthood, when increased left-to-right blood flow can result in right atrial and ventricular hypertrophy. Surgical or catheter-based closure is an option in severe cases.

Ventricular Septal Defect

Failure of the septum between the right and left ventricles to close is known as a **ventricular septal defect (VSD)** and is the most common type of congenital heart defect (Figure 16-18).[18] VSD may occur as an isolated defect or in association with other defects, such as tetralogy of Fallot. Symptoms depend on the

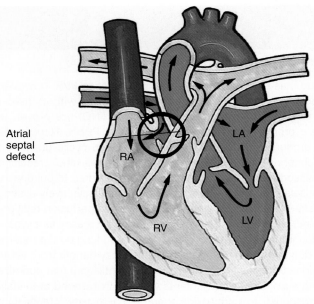

Figure 16-17 Atrial septal defect. Blood flows from the higher pressure left atrium (LA) into the lower pressure right atrium (RA) through the defect in the atrial septum. *LV,* Left ventricle; *RV,* right ventricle. (Modified from Hockenberry MJ, et al: *Wong's essentials of pediatric nursing,* ed 8, St Louis, 2009, Mosby.)

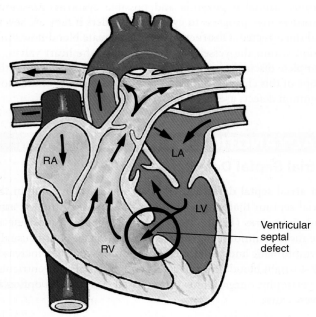

Figure 16-18 Ventricular septal defect. Blood flows from the higher pressure left ventricle (LV) into the lower pressure right ventricle (RV) through an abnormal opening between the ventricles. If pulmonary vascular resistance exceeds systemic vascular resistance, blood flows from the right ventricle into the left ventricle across the ventricular septal defect. *LA,* Left atrium; *RA,* right atrium. (Modified from Hockenberry MJ, et al: *Wong's essentials of pediatric nursing,* ed 8, St Louis, 2009, Mosby.)

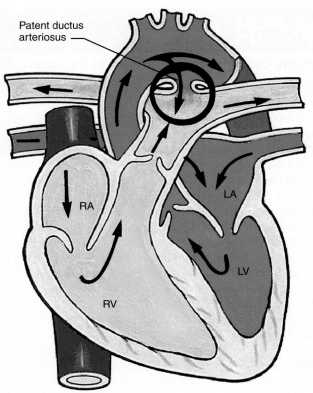

Figure 16-19 Patent ductus arteriosus. Blood flows from the higher pressure aorta through the patent ductus arteriosus into the pulmonary artery. If pulmonary vascular resistance exceeds systemic vascular resistance, blood flow reverses and flows from the pulmonary artery across the ductus arteriosus into the aorta. *LA,* Left atrium; *RA,* right atrium; *LV,* left ventricle; *RV,* right ventricle. (Modified from Hockenberry MJ, et al: *Wong's essentials of pediatric nursing,* ed 8, St Louis, 2009, Mosby.)

size of the defect, which shunts blood from the left ventricle (higher pressure) to the right ventricle (lower pressure), causing right ventricular hypertrophy and pulmonary hypertension. Left untreated, a VSD may result in right-sided heart pressures exceeding left-sided heart pressures, reversing the direction of the shunt and causing cyanosis. Small VSDs may close on their own, whereas larger defects require surgical or catheter-based closure.

Patent Ductus Arteriosus

Patent ductus arteriosus (PDA) occurs when the ductus arteriosus, the fetal shunt between the pulmonary artery and the aorta, does not close after birth (Figure 16-19). The size of the PDA determines how much blood is shunted from the aorta into the pulmonary artery or, in reverse, from the pulmonary artery into the aorta. The latter occurs when PVR exceeds SVR (often seen in hypoxic premature infants), creating a cyanosis-producing defect. A large PDA shunts significant volumes of blood into the pulmonary circulation, causing pulmonary hypertension. Infants requiring treatment have two options: (1) administration of indomethacin (Indocin) or ibuprofen lysine (NeoProfen) to block the production of ductal prostaglandin

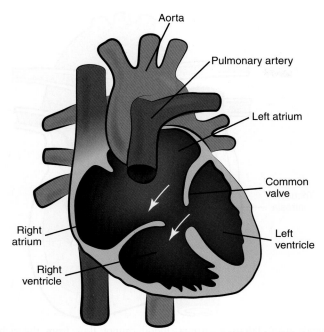

Figure 16-20 Atrioventricular septal defect. Blood flows freely between all heart chambers, owing to incomplete development of atrial and ventricular septa and malformation of tricuspid and mitral valves.

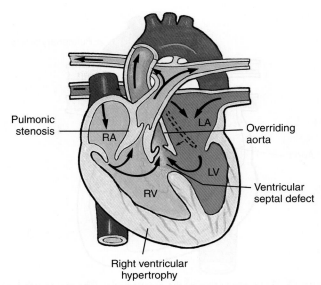

Figure 16-21 Tetralogy of Fallot. The four defects associated with this defect are (1) pulmonary stenosis, (2) ventricular septal defect, (3) overriding aorta, and (4) right ventricular hypertrophy. (Modified from Hockenberry MJ, et al: *Wong's essentials of pediatric nursing,* ed 8, St Louis, 2009, Mosby.)

(allowing ductal smooth muscle constriction) or (2) surgical intervention, either with a percutaneous transcatheter ductal closure (PTDC) device or by surgical closure.[19,20]

Atrioventricular Septal Defect

Atrioventricular septal defect (AVSD), also called atrioventricular canal (AV canal) defect, results from failure of the septa between the atria and ventricles to develop (Figure 16-20). Varying degrees of tricuspid and mitral valve malformation are also present, resulting in one large chamber or "hole" that allows blood to mix freely between all four chambers. The resultant left-to-right shunt increases pulmonary blood flow and causes volume hypertrophy of all chambers. The scooped-out appearance of the heart gives rise to the term AV canal defect, which is one of the most common types of heart defect present in patients with Down syndrome. Surgical repair is possible.[21]

CYANOTIC DISORDERS

Tetralogy of Fallot

Tetralogy of Fallot is the most common cyanotic congenital heart defect.[18] The four defects that characterize this anomaly are (1) pulmonary stenosis (narrowing), (2) VSD, (3) right ventricular hypertrophy, and (4) overriding or dextroposition of the aorta (Figure 16-21). The amount of blood flow to the lungs depends on the severity of obstruction to flow through the pulmonary artery. With mild narrowing, enough blood may flow through the pulmonary artery to keep right-sided pressures lower than left-sided pressures, and the shunt will be left-to-right through the VSD (no cyanosis). Severe narrowing creates high resistance

to pulmonary blood flow, increasing PVR over SVR, causing right-to-left shunting across the VSD and into the overriding aorta. Infants with tetralogy of Fallot may exhibit a "boot-shaped" heart on chest x-ray secondary to right ventricular hypertrophy caused by high PVR. Periods of cyanosis may be mild or severe, depending on the degree of pulmonary stenosis. Surgical repair is recommended, with the type of repair and timing of the surgery determined by the specific details of the defect. Infants with severe pulmonary stenosis require prostaglandin therapy to maintain adequate pulmonary blood flow through a PDA.

Transposition of the Great Arteries

Transposition of the great arteries (TGA) causes severe cyanosis that is usually evident shortly after birth. In TGA, the aorta arises from the right ventricle, and the pulmonary artery arises from the left ventricle, creating two parallel circulations (Figure 16-22). Deoxygenated blood flows from the right atrium, through the right ventricle to the aorta, out into the systemic circulation and then back to the right atrium. Oxygenated blood returning to the left atrium through the pulmonary veins travels through the left ventricle, into the pulmonary circulation, and back to the left atrium.

Some form of communication (e.g., PDA, VSD, ASD) must exist between the two circulations for mixing of blood to occur and to allow some oxygenated blood to be delivered to the tissues. Prostaglandin therapy may be initiated to ensure patency of the ductus arteriosus while the infant awaits corrective surgery.

Anomalous Venous Return

In **anomalous venous return**, oxygenated blood returning from the lungs is carried by the pulmonary veins abnormally

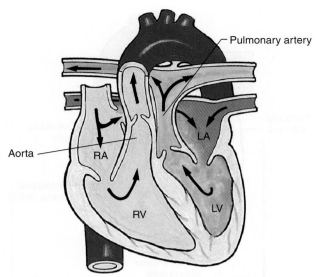

Figure 16-22 Transposition of the great arteries. The major arteries of the heart are reversed. The aorta comes off the right ventricle (RV), and the pulmonary artery arises from the left ventricle (LV). A communication channel must exist between the two circulations (atrial septal defect or patent ductus arteriosus) to sustain life. (Modified from Hockenberry MJ, et al: *Wong's essentials of pediatric nursing,* ed 8, St Louis, 2009, Mosby.)

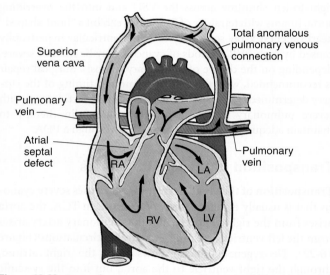

Figure 16-23 Anomalous venous return. Oxygenated blood is carried abnormally to the right atrium (RA) instead of the left atrium (LA). An atrial septal defect is essential for life, allowing oxygenated blood to reach the left atrium. (Modified from Hockenberry MJ, et al: *Wong's essentials of pediatric nursing,* ed 8, St Louis, 2009, Mosby.)

to the right atrium instead of the left atrium (Figure 16-23). The result is mixing of pulmonary and systemic blood in the right atrium, increasing pressures on the right side of the heart. An ASD must be present for oxygenated blood to move across to the left side of the heart and into systemic circulation. These infants are usually cyanotic and must have early surgical intervention.

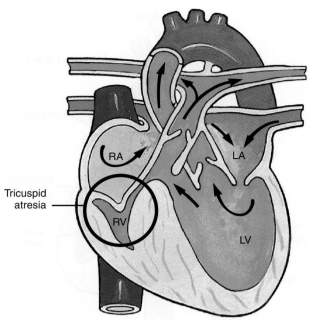

Figure 16-24 Tricuspid atresia. Blood cannot flow from the right atrium (RA) into the right ventricle (RV), requiring an atrial septal defect, ventricular septal defect, or patent ductus arteriosus for survival. (Modified from Hockenberry MJ, et al: *Wong's essentials of pediatric nursing,* ed 8, St Louis, 2009, Mosby.)

Tricuspid Atresia

Complete occlusion of the tricuspid valve and hypoplastic (underdeveloped) right ventricle characterizes **tricuspid atresia** (Figure 16-24). Blood cannot flow from the right atrium into the right ventricle, so circulation is maintained by a right-to-left shunt through either an ASD or patent foramen ovale. A VSD is also present, allowing small amounts of blood to be directed to the right ventricle and pulmonary circulation. With this disorder, cyanosis is usually present at birth. Numerous surgical options are available for treatment. Preoperative management includes prostaglandin administration to maintain ductal patency and enhance pulmonary blood flow.

Truncus Arteriosus

Truncus arteriosus is a defect resulting from failure of the embryonic truncus arteriosus to separate into the aorta and pulmonary artery (Figure 16-25). A single great artery overlies the left and right ventricles, receiving blood through a large VSD. Pulmonary and systemic blood mix and circulate throughout the body, resulting in cyanosis. Surgical treatment involves separating the common vessel into two separate vessels and closing the VSD.

OBSTRUCTIVE CONGENITAL ANOMALIES

Coarctation of the Aorta

A constricted area of the aortic lumen is known as **coarctation of the aorta** (Figure 16-26). Narrowing may occur at any point

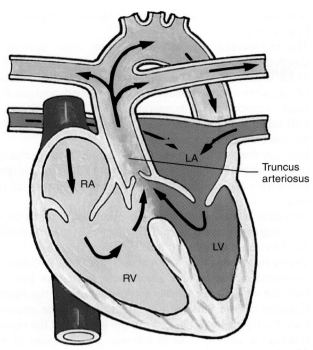

Figure 16-25 Truncus arteriosus. An overriding aorta receives blood from both ventricles through a ventricular septal defect. (Modified from Hockenberry MJ, et al: *Wong's essentials of pediatric nursing,* ed 8, St Louis, 2009, Mosby.)

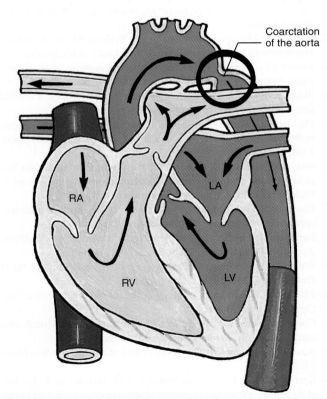

Figure 16-26 Coarctation of the aorta. Vessels supplying the head and upper extremities occur before the area of narrowing (coarctation). This accounts for the upper and lower extremity blood pressure differences. (Modified from Hockenberry MJ, et al: *Wong's essentials of pediatric nursing,* ed 8, St Louis, 2009, Mosby.)

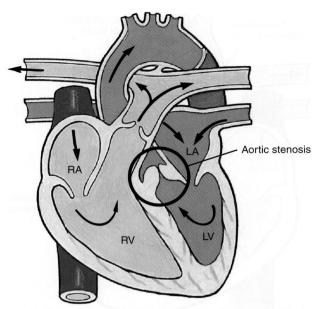

Figure 16-27 Aortic stenosis. Blood flow into the aorta is obstructed by a narrowed lumen. (Modified from Hockenberry MJ, et al: *Wong's essentials of pediatric nursing,* ed 8, St Louis, 2009, Mosby.)

along the aorta; however, in 90% of the cases, the constriction is found directly opposite the ductal entrance into the aorta.[3] Clinical manifestations depend on the severity of obstruction. Blood pressure is higher in the upper extremities than in the lower extremities; heart murmurs (fluttering sound heard with a stethoscope, associated with blood moving through a narrowed lumen) can be heard; and cardiomegaly (enlarged heart) may be seen on chest x-ray. Cardiomegaly occurs because of an increased workload caused by high blood flow resistance through the narrowed aorta. Coarctation of the aorta may occur in association with other cardiac defects such as PDA, VSD, ASD, or mitral regurgitation. Treatment is usually surgical repair or sometimes balloon dilation of the constricted area (balloon angioplasty).

Aortic Stenosis

Narrowing found above, below, or at the level of the aortic valve obstructs flow out of the left ventricle and is the cause of the congenital heart defect known as **aortic stenosis** (Figure 16-27). Clinical manifestations depend on the degree of stenosis. Resistance to blood flow through the aorta results in increased left ventricular work and eventual hypertrophy. Left ventricular pressures may become high enough to cause elevation of pulmonary venous and pulmonary capillary pressures, causing pulmonary edema and congestive heart failure. Numerous options exist for surgical repair, including balloon dilation of the stenotic aortic valve, removal of the stenotic area of the aortic valve, and repair of the area above the valve with a patch to widen the narrowed area.

Hypoplastic Left Heart Syndrome

Hypoplastic left heart syndrome includes (1) hypoplastic left ventricle, (2) aortic and mitral valve stenosis or atresia, and

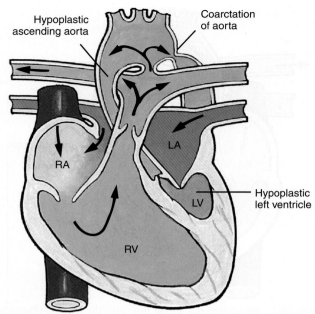

Figure 16-28 Hypoplastic left heart syndrome. A patent ductus arteriosus is necessary to supply the systemic circulation. (Modified from Hockenberry MJ, et al: *Wong's essentials of pediatric nursing,* ed 8, St Louis, 2009, Mosby.)

often (3) hypoplasia of the ascending aorta (Figure 16-28). Blood flow through the left ventricle is severely compromised, necessitating a PDA to supply the systemic circulation and an ASD to allow pulmonary venous blood to flow into the right atrium. Infants born with hypoplastic left heart syndrome appear gray and hypotensive shortly after birth and die without surgical intervention or heart transplantation.

CONCEPT QUESTION 16-10

Why could oxygen delivery to an infant born with hypoplastic left heart syndrome be detrimental?

POINTS TO REMEMBER

- Lung development occurs in five stages, beginning 26 days after conception and continuing through childhood.
- The fetal lung is capable of supporting limited gas exchange by 24 to 26 weeks of gestation.
- Premature birth frequently results in respiratory distress secondary to underdeveloped surfactant.
- The placenta functions as the organ of respiration in the fetus, exchanging nutrients and waste products between maternal and fetal blood.
- Fetal lung fluid plays a significant role in determining the size and shape of the developing air space.
- Fetal hemoglobin has a greater affinity for oxygen than adult hemoglobin facilitating placental transfer of oxygen from maternal blood to fetal blood.
- Infants are much more susceptible to upper airway obstruction than adults because the diameter of an infant's airway is smaller.

- A newborn infant relies on a special fat called brown fat for heat production.
- The cardiovascular system is the first organ system to develop and function in the fetus.
- In the fetus, right-sided heart pressures are elevated because of hypoxic pulmonary vasoconstriction secondary to low PO_2 values associated with nonaerated lungs.
- Left-sided heart pressures are low in the fetus because of low resistance from the placenta.
- Because the fetal lung does not participate in gas exchange, three anatomical shunts are necessary to carry oxygenated blood from the placenta to the systemic circulation of the fetus.
- Transition to neonatal circulation occurs as a result of (1) clamping of the umbilical cord, (2) initiation of the first breath, and (3) closure of fetal shunts.
- Severe hypoxemia may result in persistent fetal circulation.
- Acyanotic cardiac defects are defects that cause shunting from the left side of the heart to the right side of the heart.
- Cyanotic cardiac defects are defects that cause shunting from the right side of the heart to the left side of the heart.
- Obstructive cardiac defects increase the workload of the heart.

References

1. Schnapf B, Kirley S: Fetal lung development. In Walsh BK, et al, editors: *Perinatal and pediatric respiratory care,* ed 3, St Louis, 2010, Saunders.
2. Hicks GH: The respiratory system. In Wilkins RL, et al, editors: *Fundamentals of respiratory care,* ed 9, St Louis, 2009, Mosby.
3. Moore KL, Persaud TVN: *The developing human: clinically oriented embryology,* ed 8, Philadelphia, 2008, Saunders.
4. Blackburn ST: *Maternal, fetal, and neonatal physiology: a clinical perspective,* ed 3, St Louis, 2007, Saunders.
5. Haddad GG, Fontan JJP: Development of the respiratory system. In Berham RE, et al, editors: *Textbook of pediatrics,* ed 17, St Louis, 2004, Saunders.
6. Ross MG, Ervin MG, Novak D: Fetal physiology. In Gabbe SG, et al, editors: *Obstetrics: normal and problem pregnancies,* ed 5, Philadelphia, 2007, Churchill Livingstone.
7. Bissinger RL: *Neonatal resuscitation,* 2011, http://emedicine.medscape.com/article/977002-overview.
8. Bernstein D: Cardiac development. In Behrman RE, et al, editors: *Textbook of pediatrics,* ed 19, St Louis, 2011, Saunders.
9. Sedmera D, McQuinn T: Embryogenesis of heart muscle, *Heart Fail Clin* 4(3):235, 2008.
10. Phoon C: Circulatory physiology in the developing embryo, *Curr Opin Pediatr* 13(5):456, 2001.
11. Cook AC, Yates RW, Anderson RH: Normal and abnormal fetal cardiac anatomy, *Prenat Diagn* 24(13):1032, 2004.
12. Boulinn J, Morgan JM: The development of cardiac rhythm, *Heart* 91(7):874, 2005.
13. Czervinske MP: Fetal gas exchange and circulation. In Walsh BK, et al, editors: *Perinatal and pediatric respiratory care,* ed 3, St Louis, 2010, Saunders.
14. Rosenberg AA: The neonate. In Gabbe SG, et al, editors: *Normal and problem pregnancies,* ed 4, New York, 2002, Churchill Livingstone.

15. Niermeyer S, Clarke SB: Delivery room care. In Merenstein GB, Gardner SL, editors: *Handbook of neonatal intensive care*, ed 5, St Louis, 2006, Mosby.

16. Steinhorn RH: Neonatal pulmonary hypertension, *Pediatr Crit Care Med* 11(Suppl 2):S79, 2010.

17. Keane JF, Geva T, Fyler DC: Atrial septal defect. In Keane JF, et al, editors: *Nadas' pediatric cardiology*, ed 2, Philadelphia, 2006, Saunders.

18. Schoen FJ, Mitchell RN: The heart. In Kumar V, et al, editors: *Robbins and Cotran pathologic basis of disease*, ed 8, St Louis, 2009, Saunders.

19. Katakam LI, et al: Safety and effectiveness of indomethacin versus ibuprofen for treatment of patent ductus arteriosus, *Am J Perinatol* 27(5):425, 2010.

20. Giroud JM, Jacobs JP: Evolution of strategies for management of the patent arterial ductus, *Cardiol Young* 17(Suppl 2):68–74, 2007.

21. Sayler J, Butiu TD, Crotwell DN: Congenital cardiac defects. In Walsh BK, et al, editors: *Perinatal and pediatric respiratory care*, ed 3, St Louis, 2010, Saunders.

22. Antenatal corticosteroids revisited: repeat courses, *NIH Consensus Statement Online* 17(2):1, 2000.

THE CARDIOVASCULAR SYSTEM

CHAPTER 17

Functional Anatomy of the Cardiovascular System

OBJECTIVES

After reading this chapter, you will be able to:
- Describe the gross anatomy and function of each structure of the heart
- Explain how the atria, ventricles, and heart valves work together to pump blood through the pulmonary and systemic circulations
- Explain why the heart muscle is more blood flow dependent for oxygenation than other muscles in the body
- Explain why extremely high heart rates can result in low cardiac stroke volumes and coronary artery blood flow
- Explain how the specialized cardiac conduction system coordinates the synchronized contraction and relaxation of the atria and ventricles
- Explain how cellular mechanisms, calcium ions, and adenosine triphosphate work together to bring about myocardial contraction and relaxation

- Describe how the Frank-Starling mechanism helps the heart adjust to pump-varying amounts of blood
- Discuss the timing and sequence of all mechanical events in the cardiac cycle
- Explain how pumping action and arterial elasticity work together to produce continuous blood flow
- Explain how different mechanisms work to control the distribution of blood flow through systemic capillary beds
- Explain why high diastolic pressure is more indicative of increased vascular resistance than high systolic pressure
- Explain why independent right ventricular pumping failure produces a different type of circulatory derangement than left ventricular failure
- Describe how local, central, and humoral mechanisms regulate blood pressure

KEY TERMS

actin
afterload
angina pectoris
angiotensin-converting enzyme (ACE)
aortic semilunar valve
atherosclerosis
atrioventricular (AV) node
atrioventricular (AV) valves
atrium
autoregulation
AV bundle (bundle of His)
bicuspid (mitral) valve
B-type natriuretic peptide (BNP)
bundle branches
cardiac tamponade
chordae tendineae
cross-bridges
dicrotic notch
ejection fraction
endocardium
epicardium
Frank-Starling mechanism
hematocrit

interatrial septum
interventricular septum
mean arterial pressure (MAP)
myocardial infarction (MI)
myocardium
myosin
papillary muscles
pericardium
point of maximal impact (PMI)
prolapse
pulmonary semilunar valve
pulse pressure
Purkinje fibers
renin-angiotensin-aldosterone system (RAAS)
sarcomere
sinoatrial (SA) node
stroke volume
titin
tricuspid valve
tropomyosin
troponin
vasopressin mechanism
ventricle

The lungs could not accomplish their purpose without the cardiovascular system. The heart and blood vessels link gas exchange at the lungs with gas exchange at the tissues. Cardiovascular function is as vital as lung function in oxygenating tissues. In this sense, the heart and lungs are a single, integrated cardiopulmonary system, dedicated to tissue oxygenation.

HEART

Gross Anatomy

The human heart is a hollow muscular pump about the size of its owner's closed fist. It lies in the mediastinum of the thorax just behind the sternum (Figure 17-1). About two thirds of its mass is left of the sternal midline.

The heart resembles an inverted cone, its lower apex pointing to the left such that one side lies on the diaphragm at the level of the fifth intercostal space at the midclavicular line. Its upper base is just below the second rib at the midsternal line. The apical beat or the **point of maximal impact** (**PMI**) is created by the repeated impact of the beating heart on the inner chest wall. The PMI can be felt and sometimes seen at the intersection of the fifth intercostal space and the midclavicular line. A shift in the PMI indicates a change in the anatomical position of the heart, which could occur in a pneumothorax when the mediastinum is pushed to one side.

CONCEPT QUESTION 17-1

A tension pneumothorax of the left lung shifts the PMI in which direction?

From a posterior perspective, the heart rests against the fifth through eighth thoracic vertebrae. Its position between the sternum and vertebral column allows the heart to be compressed when pressure is applied to the sternum. This is the basis for external cardiac compression, applied during cardiopulmonary resuscitation (CPR), in which the heel of the hand compresses the sternum. Rhythmic compression of the valved, hollow muscular heart during cardiac arrest can produce enough blood

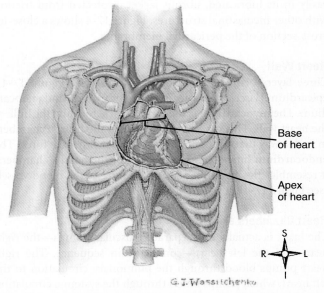

Figure 17-1 Location of the heart in the chest. (From Thibodeau GA, Patton KT: *Anatomy & physiology,* ed 3, St Louis, 1996, Mosby.)

flow to sustain life briefly if combined with effective artificial ventilation.

Knowledge of the heart's anatomical position and boundaries is clinically important; palpation and percussion of the external chest wall helps the clinician determine where these boundaries lie. Heart size also can be assessed with chest x-ray films. The heart may be enlarged in certain conditions, such as congestive heart failure, in which the heart becomes engorged or congested with blood. Knowledge of the heart's normal position helps the clinician position a stethoscope properly to hear heart valve sounds.

External Features

Figure 17-2 shows anterior and posterior views of the external heart surfaces. The right ventricle constitutes most of the anterior portion of the heart; the left ventricle is located more posteriorly. (Notice the small size of the atria compared with the ventricles.)

Pericardium

The heart is covered with a loose-fitting membranous sac called the **pericardium** (Figure 17-3). The pericardium consists of a tough, fibrous outer portion continuous with the connective tissue covering the great vessels. Inferiorly, it attaches to the surface of the diaphragm. The fibrous pericardium limits overexpansion of the heart, holding it in place in the mediastinum. Inside the fibrous pericardium is a thin transparent membrane called the serous pericardium. The serous pericardium is a closed envelope containing a small amount of pericardial fluid. The part of the membrane that lines the inner surface of the fibrous pericardium is the parietal pericardium. The visceral pericardium, also known as the **epicardium**, is the part of the serous pericardium that is fused to the heart's surface. The space between the parietal and visceral pericardium is the pericardial space. The fluid in this space lubricates the membranes, allowing smooth, frictionless movement. As the heart beats, it moves easily in its lubricated, fibrous jacket, protected from friction with other mediastinal structures. Figure 17-4 shows a close-up cross-section of the pericardial membranes.

Heart Wall

Three layers of tissue form the heart wall (see Figure 17-4): epicardium (visceral pericardium), myocardium, and endocardium. The **myocardium** is the heart muscle forming the bulk of the heart wall. This muscle wraps around the heart's chambers in such a way that contraction ejects blood with great force. The **endocardium** lines the inner surfaces of the heart's chambers; it resembles the smooth endothelial lining of the blood vessels (see Figure 17-4).

Heart Chambers and Valves

The heart is actually two separate muscular pumps—the right heart and the left heart—connected in sequence. The right heart pumps blood through the pulmonary circulation to the left heart, which pumps blood through the systemic circulation back to the right heart. Each heart consists of two chambers: an **atrium** located superiorly to a **ventricle** (Figure 17-5). The atria

are weak pumps that prime the more powerful ventricles; they passively funnel blood into the ventricles except when they contract at the last instant to complete the filling process actively.

The atria are thin-walled collecting chambers, whereas the ventricles are heavily muscled pumping chambers; the inner surfaces of the ventricles are muscle bundles undercut by open spaces called trabeculae carneae (see Figure 17-4). These irregular surfaces may prevent endocardial wrinkling and damage during ventricular contraction.[1] The muscle mass of the left ventricle is greater than the muscle mass of the right ventricle (see Figure 17-5) because the left ventricle pumps against a much greater resistance (systemic vascular resistance [SVR]) than the right ventricle (pulmonary vascular resistance [PVR]). The left ventricle is more spherical in cross-section than the right ventricle (Figure 17-6). The thinner walled right ventricle is crescent-shaped, appearing to wrap partly around and "hug" the left ventricle. This arrangement tends to flatten the right ventricle during left ventricular contraction, aiding ejection of blood by the right ventricle.

The right atrium receives deoxygenated systemic venous blood from the superior and inferior vena cava and coronary venous blood from the coronary sinus. The left atrium receives oxygenated pulmonary venous blood from four pulmonary veins, two from each lung. Both atria channel their blood into the ventricles through one-way **atrioventricular (AV) valves**. These valves prevent backflow of blood into the atria during ventricular contraction. The right AV valve is the **tricuspid valve** (three cusps or leaflets); the left AV valve is the **bicuspid (mitral) valve** (two cusps). The two atria are separated by the **interatrial septum**, which prevents mixing of oxygenated and deoxygenated blood. A small depression in this septum marks the former location of the foramen ovale, an opening between the left and right atria during fetal life (see Chapter 16).

CONCEPT QUESTION 17-2

What are the consequences of a mitral valve that leaks or allows backflow of blood during ventricular systole?

Each ventricle has a large outflow tract located superiorly near the AV valves. The right ventricle pumps blood through the **pulmonary semilunar valve** into the pulmonary trunk, whereas the left ventricle pumps blood through the **aortic semilunar valve** into the aorta (see Figure 17-5). These valves prevent backflow of blood into the ventricles during ventricular relaxation. The **interventricular septum** separates right and left ventricles, preventing mixing of oxygenated and unoxygenated blood.

Each ventricle contains cone-shaped pillars called **papillary muscles** from which thin, strong connective tissue strings (**chordae tendineae**) attach to tricuspid and mitral valve cusps (see Figure 17-5). The chordae tendineae tether the AV valve leaflets, preventing them from bulging up into the atria and opening during ventricular contraction (called regurgitation). When the ventricles relax, these valves open again, allowing blood to fill the ventricles. Most of the ventricular filling is a passive process; the atria do not contract until very near the end of ventricular relaxation (diastolic) time.

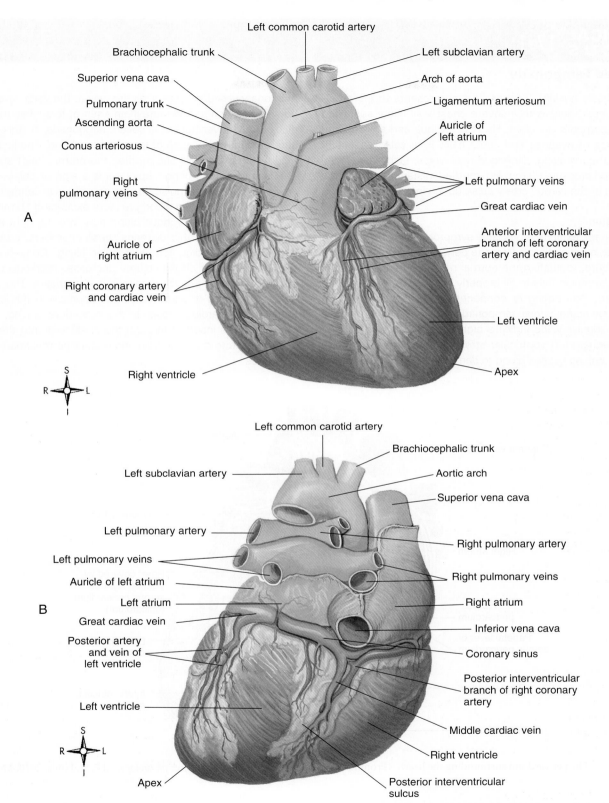

Figure 17-2 The heart and coronary arteries. **A,** Anterior view. **B,** Posterior view. (From Thibodeau GA, Patton KT: *Anatomy & physiology,* ed 3, St Louis, 1996, Mosby.)

CLINICAL FOCUS 17-1

Cardiac Tamponade

A previously healthy, 32-year-old man presents to the emergency department with a severe chest wall injury sustained in an automobile accident. He is conscious and anxious and complains of dyspnea and chest pain. Physical examination reveals the following: distended neck veins; tachycardia; systolic blood pressure 90 mm Hg; muffled, distant heart sounds; and loss of the carotid artery pulse during inspiration.

Discussion

This patient exhibits signs and symptoms of **cardiac tamponade**, in which fluid enters the pericardial space and builds up pressure, restricting the normal movements of the heart. The left ventricle fails to fill properly because its expansion is restricted. Penetrating or nonpenetrating chest wall trauma may cause acute cardiac tamponade. This patient's distended neck or jugular veins indicate high venous pressure caused by inadequate left ventricular stroke volume—that is, inadequate pumping causes blood to dam up throughout the entire pulmonary vascular system, all the way to the vena cava. The body increases the heart rate in an attempt to sustain the cardiac output; nevertheless, in severe tamponade, systolic pressure decreases because of low stroke volume. The jacket of fluid in the pericardial sac muffles the normal heart sounds. The loss of pulse during inspiration is a sign of pulsus paradoxus, or paradoxical pulse. Pulsus paradoxus is defined as an inspiratory reduction in blood pressure exceeding 10 mm Hg. Inspiration increases venous blood flow into the right atrium and right ventricle; this distends these chambers, crowding and further impeding left ventricular filling. Consequently, the left ventricular stroke volume decreases markedly during inspiration, and the pulse weakens or disappears. The emergency treatment of acute cardiac tamponade in this clinical setting is pericardiocentesis. In this procedure, a long, large-bore needle is inserted through the chest wall into the pericardial space to drain the fluid and restore normal heart-filling pressures.

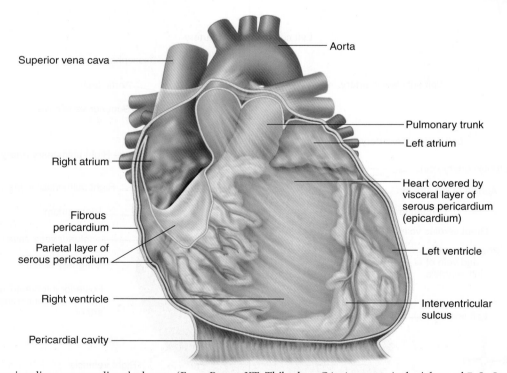

Figure 17-3 The pericardium surrounding the heart. (From Patton KT, Thibodeau GA: *Anatomy & physiology*, ed 7, St. Louis, 2010, Mosby.)

Cardiac Skeleton and Valvular Function

A tough set of connected rings (fibrous annuli) form a semirigid framework to which the heart valves and cardiac muscle are attached (Figure 17-7, *A*). This framework forms a fibrous skeleton, which is an electrical insulator and a physical barrier between atrial and ventricular muscle masses. The only electrical connection between atrial and ventricular muscle is a single bundle of specialized conductive tissue that penetrates the fibrous skeleton (discussed in a later section).

The spiral arrangement of ventricular muscle fibers (see Figure 17-7, *A*) propels blood upward into the aorta and pulmonary artery during contraction. This action "wrings" blood

CLINICAL FOCUS 17-2

Effects of a Ventricular Septal Defect

Ventricular septal defect (VSD) is the most common congenital malformation of the heart reported in children. In VSD, a defect in the septum dividing the right and left ventricles allows blood to flow directly from one chamber to the other. The functional disturbance caused by a VSD depends mainly on its size and the pulmonary vascular resistance. Normally, left ventricular pressure greatly exceeds right ventricular pressure, causing a left-to-right shunt through the VSD. That is, some oxygenated blood mixes with deoxygenated blood and is pumped back into the pulmonary circulation. A small, high-resistance VSD permits only a small left-to-right shunt. A large VSD is more likely to allow some mixing of right ventricular deoxygenated blood with oxygenated left ventricular blood (i.e., right-to-left shunt). This is especially true if pulmonary vascular resistance is elevated or if the pulmonic valve is narrowed; in these circumstances, right ventricular pressure rises, increasing right-to-left shunting. In very large defects, both ventricles act as a single pumping chamber with two outlets, equalizing the pulmonary and systemic pressures. In any case, only right-to-left shunting causes systemic arterial hypoxemia. Left-to-right shunting merely returns already oxygenated blood to the pulmonary circulation for reoxygenation. Left-to-right shunting increases right ventricular work. The treatment for a large, symptomatic VSD is surgical correction.

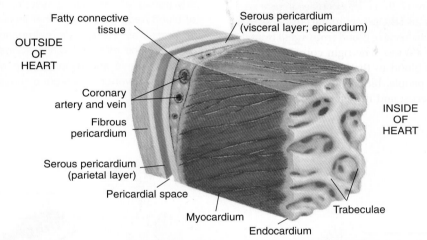

Figure 17-4 Cross-section of the wall of the heart. (From Thibodeau GA, Patton KT: *Anatomy & physiology,* ed 3, St Louis, 1996, Mosby.)

out of ventricles from apex to base. As the heart contracts, it rotates to the right, swinging the left ventricle to the front of the chest; this creates the PMI.

The fibrous rings supporting the tricuspid and mitral valves are more compliant than the rings supporting the semilunar valves. For this reason, mitral and tricuspid rings are compressed to smaller sizes during ventricular systole; consequently, their valve cusps are larger than the area to be covered; this ensures a complete seal during contraction.[1] If the size disproportion is too great, the valve cusps balloon upward into the atrium during ventricular contraction (**prolapse**). Heart valve function during ventricular diastole is illustrated in Figure 17-7, *B*; Figure 17-7, *C*, illustrates valvular function during ventricular systole. These illustrations correspond with ventricular filling (diastole) and ejection (systole) shown in Figure 17-8, *A* and *B*.

The crescent-shaped (semilunar) pulmonic and aortic valve cusps permit them to open fully during ventricular ejection and seal perfectly during ventricular diastole. The aortic diameter is slightly enlarged at the base just above the semilunar valves. This provides a space behind the valve cusps when they open during ventricular ejection, preventing them from occluding the coronary artery orifices.[1] Coronary arteries branch off from the aorta immediately above the semilunar valve. The enlarged aortic base also keeps the valve cusps away from the aortic wall. As the ventricles relax, the backflow of blood immediately catches the valve cusps and sharply closes them, preventing blood from flowing back into the ventricles.

Coronary Circulation

Coronary Arteries

The heart muscle itself receives its blood supply from the right and left coronary arteries, which arise from the aorta immediately above the aortic semilunar valve. These arteries and their branches lie on the heart's surface (see Figure 17-2); smaller arteries penetrate into the cardiac muscle mass. Figure 17-9, *A*, illustrates the coronary arterial circulation. The heart relies almost exclusively on the two main coronary arteries for its oxygen supply. The endocardial surface obtains a very small amount of oxygen directly from the blood in the heart chambers.[2]

Very few connections exist between the major coronary arteries; blood flow can take few detours if its main route becomes obstructed. This lack of collateral circulation explains why sudden coronary artery occlusion, such as occurs with a blood clot, is life threatening. The heart muscle supplied by the occluded artery becomes hypoxic (ischemic), which can lead to myocardial tissue death, or **myocardial infarction (MI)**. If the narrowing of coronary arteries progresses gradually over a long time, some collateral circulation develops to supply ischemic areas; this lessens the chances that a blocked coronary artery will cause an MI.[2]

Ischemia produced by coronary artery occlusion stimulates myocardial nociceptive (pain-eliciting) fibers, producing the characteristic pain known as **angina pectoris**.[3] This pain is often felt beneath the sternum, in the left arm, and in the neck. Frequent attacks of angina are associated with a greatly increased risk of coronary artery occlusion. About 35% of all deaths in the United States are caused by coronary artery disease.[2]

The left anterior descending and circumflex branches of the left coronary artery supply the anterior and lateral portions of the left ventricle (see Figure 17-9, *A*). The right coronary artery supplies the right ventricle and the posterior part of the left ventricle. The left and right atria receive blood from small branches of left and right coronary arteries. The right coronary artery is the dominant supplier of blood to the heart in about 50% of people; in about 30% of people, blood flow is equal through right and left coronary arteries; and the left artery predominates in about 20% of people.[2]

CLINICAL FOCUS 17-3

Pulmonary Effects of Mitral Valve Regurgitation and Stenosis

A patient with diagnosed severe mitral valve stenosis is in the cardiac intensive care unit. This patient requires oxygen and shows signs and symptoms of pulmonary edema on physical examination and chest x-ray film. What is the connection between this patient's cardiac and pulmonary problems?

Discussion

Mitral valve stenosis is a condition characterized by a narrowed, stiff mitral valve. The narrowed valve creates high resistance to blood flow, increasing pulmonary venous and capillary pressures. A stenosed valve is likely to seal improperly during left ventricular systole, allowing some backflow of blood (regurgitation), further increasing pulmonary vascular pressures. Hydrostatic pulmonary edema is a common consequence of mitral valve stenosis, which accounts for the hypoxemia and dyspnea that often accompany mitral stenosis. Severe cases require surgical correction.

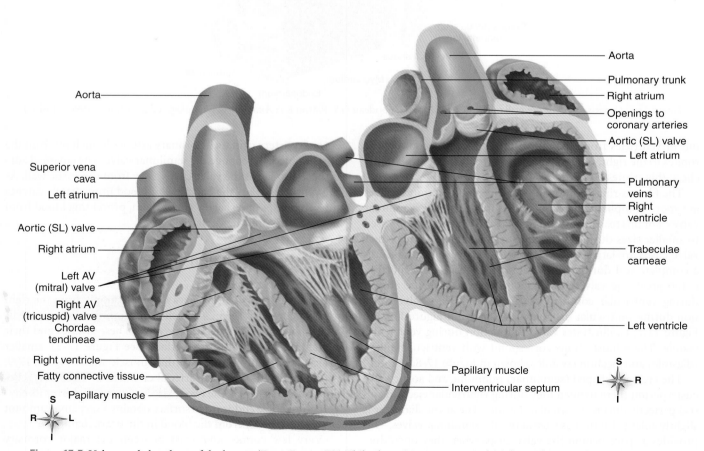

Figure 17-5 Valves and chambers of the heart. (From Patton KT, Thibodeau GA: *Anatomy & physiology*, ed 7, St. Louis, 2010, Mosby.)

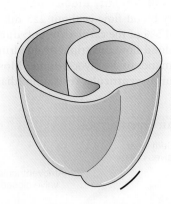

Figure 17-6 Cross-section of the ventricles.

Coronary Veins

The coronary venous drainage (see Figure 17-9, *B*) follows a path generally parallel to the path of the coronary arteries. The cardiac veins converge to empty into a large venous cavity within the right atrium, the coronary sinus. In addition, the thebesian veins (not shown) empty directly into all heart chambers; this venous drainage into the left heart contributes to the normal anatomical shunt that prevents arterial blood from being fully saturated with oxygen. About 75% of coronary venous flow is through the coronary sinus.[2]

Oxygen Requirements and Coronary Blood Flow

Even at rest, the myocardium extracts about 70% of the oxygen from its arterial blood flow compared with a 25% extraction rate for the whole body.[2] During exercise, this extraction rate is higher still. Because heart muscle cannot extract much additional oxygen from the blood, the only way it can receive more

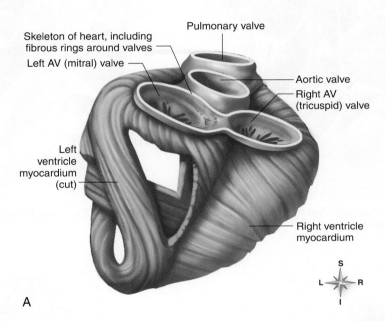

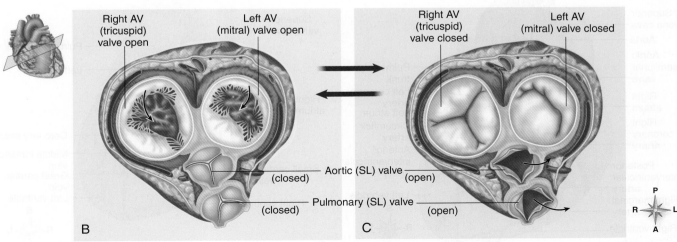

Figure 17-7 The cardiac skeleton and heart valves. **A,** Posterior view. Note the muscle fiber arrangement. **B,** View from above. The ventricles are relaxing—the atrioventricular (AV) valves are open. **C,** The ventricles are contracting—the semilunar (SL) valves are open, and the AV valves are closed. (From Patton KT, Thibodeau GA: *Anatomy & physiology,* ed 7, St. Louis, 2010, Mosby.)

oxygen is through increased coronary blood flow. Myocardial oxygenation is highly dependent on blood flow.

Myocardial oxygen need is the major factor governing coronary blood flow. Increased metabolic activity and myocardial hypoxia cause the release of a potent coronary vasodilator called adenosine.[3]

Diastolic Time and Coronary Blood Flow

At rest, coronary blood flow is about 225 mL per minute, or between 4% and 5% of the cardiac output; during heavy exercise, coronary blood flow can triple or quadruple to meet the extra oxygen demands of the myocardium.[2] Most coronary perfusion occurs during ventricular relaxation (diastole), opposite

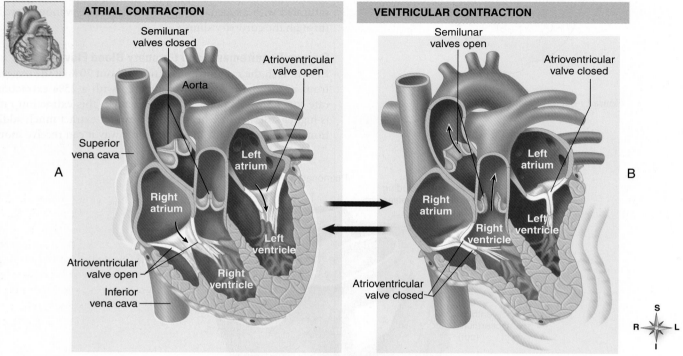

Figure 17-8 Action of valves and chambers when the ventricles are in diastole (**A**) and systole (**B**). (From Patton KT, Thibodeau GA: *Anatomy & physiology*, ed 7, St. Louis, 2010, Mosby.)

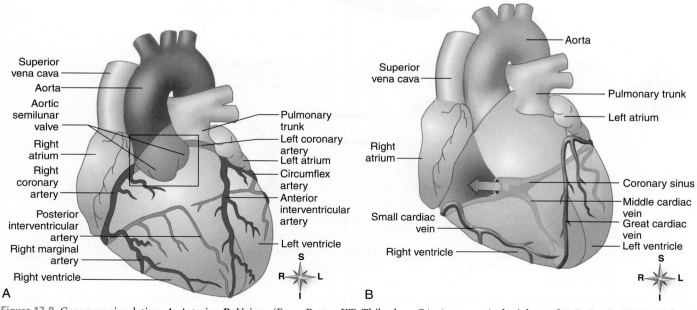

Figure 17-9 Coronary circulation. **A,** Arteries. **B,** Veins. (From Patton KT, Thibodeau GA: *Anatomy & physiology,* ed 7, St. Louis, 2010, Mosby.)

to flow through other vascular beds of the body. The powerful contractile force of the ventricles during systole compresses the coronary vessels, momentarily stopping or reversing the direction of their blood flow.[3] Thus, sufficient diastolic time (normally about two times as long as systolic time) is important for adequate coronary blood flow. Extreme tachycardia, especially in persons with narrowed coronary arteries, may shorten diastolic time so much that coronary blood flow becomes inadequate. In healthy people, the effect of this shortened diastolic time is overridden by the coronary vasodilation that occurs with increased myocardial oxygen demand.

Cardiac Conduction System

A specialized system of modified cardiac muscle tissue (distinct from nerve tissue) conducts regular electrical impulses that stimulate rhythmic, synchronized heart muscle contractions. This conduction system also transmits the impulses rapidly and uniformly throughout the heart, much more rapidly than over regular myocardial fibers. Rapid and uniform conduction of electrical impulses is important to ensure effective, properly timed pumping action of the heart. With normal impulse conduction, the atria contract to complete the ventricular filling process about one sixth of a second before the ventricles contract.[2] Figure 17-10 illustrates the electrical conduction system of the heart.

The **sinoatrial (SA) node**, embedded in the right atrial muscle near the superior vena cava, is responsible for initiating the electrical impulses that produce sequential atrial and ventricular contraction. The impulses of the SA node travel over specialized internodal pathways to the **atrioventricular (AV) node** at a velocity of about 1 m per second (regular atrial muscle conducts impulses at about 0.3 m per second). The AV node and the AV bundle slow the impulse velocity considerably before transmitting it into the ventricles. It takes the SA node impulse about 0.03 second to reach the AV node, which along with the AV bundle delays the impulse another 0.13 second before conducting it on to the ventricles; thus, about 0.16 second elapses from the time the SA node generates its impulse until the ventricles receive the signal.[2] This transmission delay prevents impulses from arriving at the ventricles too rapidly in succession; in this way, the ventricles have enough time to fill between contractions.

> ### CONCEPT QUESTION 17-3
>
> *What is the effect of a very high heart rate on ventricular stroke volume?*

The only electrical connection between atrial and ventricular muscle is the **AV bundle** (also known as the **bundle of His**). This bundle conducts impulses to the right and left **bundle branches** in the forward direction only (toward the ventricles). This one-way transmission prevents impulses from traveling backward from ventricles to atria. The bundle branches travel downward through the ventricular septum and subdivide many times to form the **Purkinje fibers**. Purkinje fibers spread out diffusely from the apex throughout the ventricles, transmitting

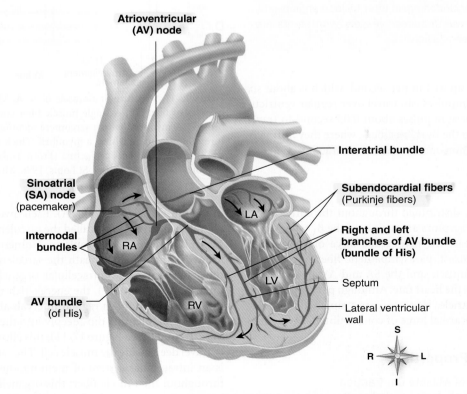

Figure 17-10 Conduction system of the heart. *Arrows* show direction of electrical current flow. (From Patton KT, Thibodeau GA: *Anatomy & physiology,* ed 7, St. Louis, 2010, Mosby.)

Surgical Treatment Options for Blocked Coronary Arteries

When blockage of the major coronary arteries is severe and life threatening, coronary artery bypass graft (CABG) surgery and coronary angioplasty are common treatment options. In CABG surgery, a vein taken from another part of the patient's body (often the saphenous vein of the leg) is grafted such that it provides a channel around the vessel obstruction, allowing the hypoxic myocardium to be resupplied with blood. In an aortocoronary bypass graft, the grafted vein connects the aorta to the coronary artery distal to the obstruction site. Veins can be grafted from other nearby arteries as well. If more than one coronary artery is blocked, multiple bypass grafts are done.

In coronary angioplasty, a small stainless steel mesh sleeve called a stent is positioned over a small, balloon-tipped catheter about 1 mm in diameter; the catheter is usually introduced into a femoral artery and advanced through the abdominal and thoracic aorta and into the coronary artery until the deflated balloon and stent lie in the partially occluded part of the vessel. The balloon is abruptly inflated with high pressure, permanently dilating the stent, which keeps the artery propped open; the balloon is then deflated, and the catheter is withdrawn. After this procedure, blood flow through the vessel is often restored to normal, reoxygenating the myocardium. Before the advent of stents, vessels often became occluded again after balloon angioplasty, and CABG surgery was required; vessels with stents are less susceptible to reocclusion.

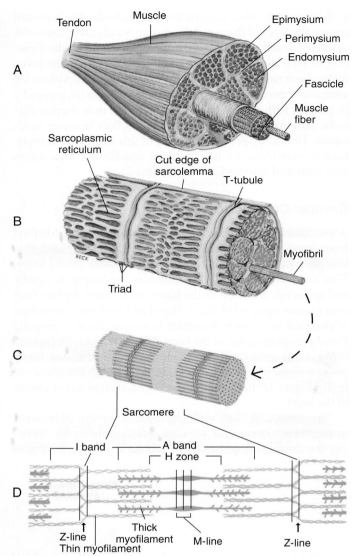

Figure 17-11 Structure of a muscle fiber. **A,** Muscle organ containing bundles of fibers. **B,** A single muscle fiber containing smaller myofibrils. **C,** A myofibril with a sarcomere identified. **D,** Molecular structure of a sarcomere within a myofibril. Thick myofilaments are myosin; thin myofilaments are actin. (From Thibodeau GA, Patton KT: *Anatomy & physiology,* ed 3, St Louis, 1996, Mosby.)

impulses at a velocity up to 4 m per second, which is about six times faster than the impulses can travel over regular ventricular muscle. It takes these impulses about 0.03 second to travel from the AV bundle to the Purkinje fibers, where they normally stimulate rapid, simultaneous ventricular contractions.[2]

Innervation

Sympathetic fibers are distributed throughout the entire heart. Cardiac sympathetic receptors are mainly of the β_1 type. When stimulated, they increase the myocardial force of contraction and heart rate. In contrast, parasympathetic fibers are distributed mostly to atrial muscle and the SA and AV nodes where their stimulation slows the heart rate. Although parasympathetic innervation of the ventricles is sparse, parasympathetic stimulation can decrease myocardial force of contraction by 30%.[2]

Cardiac Muscle Properties

General Mechanism of Muscle Contraction

Gross muscle is composed of muscle bundles, which contain numerous muscle fibers or cells (myocytes) extending the length of the muscle (Figure 17-11, *A*). Each myocyte is bounded by a complex cell membrane called the sarcolemma; the cell's protoplasm is known as the cytoplasm. Numerous mitochondria are located immediately beneath the sarcolemma and throughout the cytoplasm; these intracellular organelles generate adenosine triphosphate (ATP), the energy-rich molecules that power muscle contraction. At regular intervals along the length of the fiber, the sarcolemma dips deeply into the cell's interior, forming a T-tubule (see Figure 17-11); this allows electrical impulses to travel deep inside the muscle cell. The sarcoplasmic reticulum is an intracellular system of membranous tubules that spread throughout the muscle fiber; this organelle forms an extensive interconnected network of canals that converge to form a single tube alongside the T-tubules. The sarcoplasmic reticulum is a

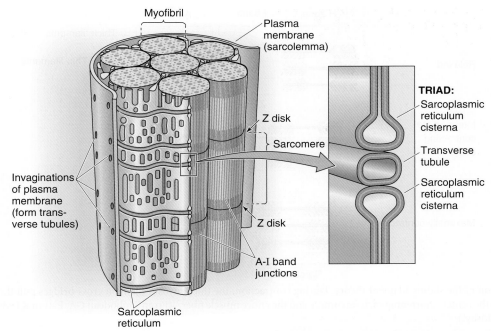

Figure 17-12 Illustration of the sarcolemma's formation of transverse tubules as it dips deeply into the sarcoplasmic reticulum, forming the triad (*inset*). (From Boron WF, Boulpaep EL, editors: *Medical physiology,* ed 2, Philadelphia, 2009, Saunders.)

storehouse for calcium ions. As shown in Figure 17-12 (*inset*), the T-tubule is sandwiched tightly between two sarcoplasmic reticulum tubules or cisterna, forming a so-called triad. Electrical impulses within the T-tubule stimulate the adjacent sarcoplasmic reticulum tubules, causing them to release calcium ions into the cell's cytoplasm through specialized calcium release channels. Calcium ions are essential for muscle contraction, as explained later.

Each muscle fiber consists of numerous myofibrils (see Figures 17-11, *B* and *C*, and 17-12), which are composed of numerous myofilaments. Myofilaments are mainly composed of the contractile proteins **myosin** and **actin**. The configuration of the thick myosin and thin actin myofilaments give the myofibrils a banded or striated appearance. As shown in Figure 17-11, *D*, the thin actin filaments are anchored to protein disklike structures, which form the Z-line. The basic contractile unit, the **sarcomere**, extends from Z-line to Z-line. The thick myosin filaments in the center of the sarcomere extend between the actin filaments on both sides toward the Z-lines (see Figure 17-11, *D*). **Titin**, a giant elastic protein molecule, tethers the myosin filament to the Z-line (Figure 17-13). The titin molecule is composed of an inflexible anchoring segment and a flexible elastic segment that stretches as the sarcomere elongates during cardiac diastole. The more the titin molecule stretches as the heart fills with blood, the more vigorously it recoils when the heart contracts; this helps explain the Frank-Starling mechanism (discussed later).[4] During muscle contraction, the actin myofilaments slide toward each other over the myosin filaments, bringing the Z-lines closer together and shortening the sarcomere (Figure 17-14); neither actin nor myosin filaments actually shorten. As numerous sarcomeres shorten, the muscle fiber as a whole shortens.

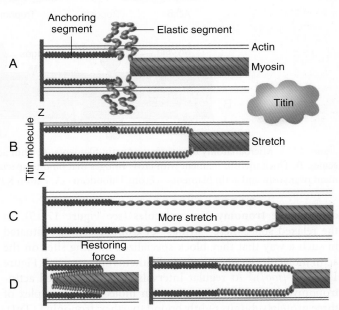

Figure 17-13 Titin, a large elastic protein molecule, anchors myosin filaments to the Z-line; it consists of an anchoring segment and an elastic segment, which acts as a spring when the muscle fiber is stretched (**A–C**). Titin's recoil during muscle shortening (contraction) may help explain the Frank-Starling mechanism. At short sarcomere lengths, the elastic segment is folded in on itself, generating a restoring force (**D**). (From Zipes DP, et al, editors: *Braunwald's heart disease: a textbook of cardiovascular medicine,* ed 7, St Louis, 2005, Saunders.)

Excitation-Contraction Coupling

Figure 17-15 shows the microanatomy of the thin actin and thick myosin filaments. Thin filaments are composed of two beadlike actin strands twisted in a helical fashion around a "backbone"

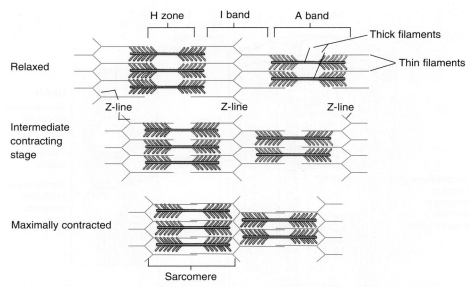

Figure 17-14 Illustration of the sliding filament theory. During contraction, the thick myosin filament cross-bridges pull the thin actin filaments from each side toward the center, shortening each sarcomere and the entire muscle fiber. (From Thibodeau GA, Patton KT: *Anatomy & physiology,* ed 3, St Louis, 1996, Mosby.)

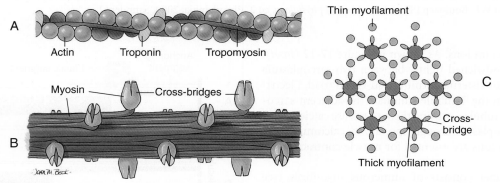

Figure 17-15 Microanatomy of myosin and actin filaments. **A,** Thin actin filament with a tropomyosin molecule held in place by troponin molecules. **B,** Thick myosin filament with cross-bridges that bind to special sites on the actin filament. **C,** Cross-section showing the spatial arrangement of myosin and actin filaments. (From Thibodeau GA, Patton KT: *Anatomy & physiology,* ed 3, St Louis, 1996, Mosby.)

of stringlike **tropomyosin** molecules (see Figure 17-15). In the relaxed state, these "strings" of tropomyosin are situated in such a way that they block specialized binding sites on the actin molecules to which myosin filaments are attracted (Figure 17-16, *A [top]*).[4] At regular intervals along the twisted actin-tropomyosin structure are **troponin** molecules, a complex of three protein subunits tightly bound together: troponin I (TnI), troponin T (TnT), and troponin C (TnC) (Figure 17-16, *A [top]* and *B*). TnC binds calcium ions, TnI binds to actin, and TnT binds to tropomyosin; the entire troponin complex is attached to the actin filament. The TnI subunit is responsible for inhibiting actin-myosin interaction when the myocardial fiber is in the relaxed state (see Figure 17-16, *B*); that is, TnI interacts with TnT to hold the tropomyosin molecule in a position that blocks the binding sites of the actin molecule.[4]

The thick myosin filaments (see Figure 17-15, *B*) consist of numerous individual myosin molecules shaped like golf clubs. Their "shafts" form the length of the myosin bundle with club-like "heads" sticking outward, attracted to the covered binding sites of adjacent actin molecules. The myosin heads are known as **cross-bridges**.

Contraction occurs when a nerve impulse causes acetylcholine to stimulate the muscle cell sarcolemma. The impulse travels deep into the T-tubules causing the sarcoplasmic reticulum to release Ca^{++} ions, which bind with and activate TnC. Activated TnC initiates a complex interaction among all three troponin subunits that removes the inhibitory effect of TnI; this repositions the tropomyosin molecule to expose the binding sites of the actin molecule (see Figure 17-16, *A [bottom]* and *C*).

Figure 17-17 illustrates the sequence of events that occur in actin and myosin filament cross-bridge formation; at the top of the figure, the myosin head is still attached to binding sites on the actin filament from the previous cross-bridge cycle. In *(1)*, ATP binds with the myosin head, which reduces its affinity for actin and causes it to detach. In *(2)*, ATP is broken down (hydrolyzed) into adenosine diphosphate (ADP) and inorganic phosphate (P) on the myosin head, causing it to swivel on its hinge so that it is positioned immediately across from a new

CLINICAL FOCUS 17-5

Blood Biomarkers of Myocardial Infarction

In MI, cardiac muscle cells die (become necrotic) from a lack of blood flow and oxygen. This cell necrosis disrupts the integrity of the sarcolemma, the muscle cell membrane, allowing intracellular macromolecules (serum cardiac biomarkers) to leak out into the interstitial spaces and eventually the systemic circulation. Sensitive laboratory tests (assays) can detect the presence of these cardiac biomarkers. Cardiac-specific troponins are the preferred biomarkers for diagnosing MI, in particular, TnI and TnT.[8] Most of the TnT and TnI is incorporated into the troponin complex, but small amounts also are dissolved in the cytoplasm. After the sarcolemmal membrane disintegrates, the troponin dissolved in the cytoplasm is released first, followed by a more drawn-out release from the disintegrating actin filaments.

In acute MI, blood levels of these troponins increase within 3 to 12 hours to about 20 to 50 times their baseline reference limit, peaking in 12 hours to 2 days (TnT) or 24 hours (TnI).[8] Although troponin is present in skeletal muscle, it is encoded by different genes and has a different amino acid sequence in cardiac muscle; this allows development of specific laboratory assays for cardiac troponins. Another less specific cardiac biomarker is an isoenzyme of creatine kinase (CK) known as CK-MB; however, small quantities of CK-MB are present in various other body tissues. Strenuous exercise in trained long-distance runners or professional athletes can increase blood levels of CK-MB; for this reason, the cardiac-specific troponins are the preferred biomarker for diagnosing MI.[8]

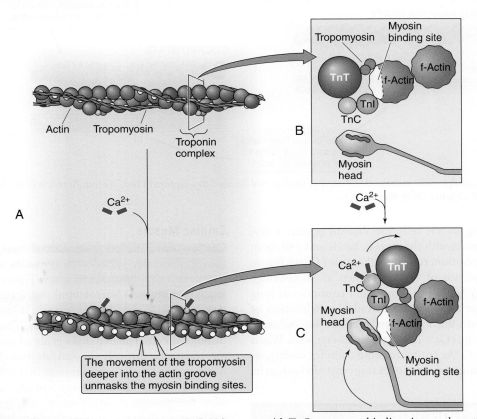

Figure 17-16 Detailed view of myocardial microanatomy: **A–C,** Ca^{++} interacts with TnC to uncover binding sites on the actin myofilament. **C,** The myosin head moves to bind with the actin filament (f-Actin) after the binding site is uncovered. (From Boron WF, Boulpaep EL, editors: *Medical physiology,* ed 2, Philadelphia, 2009, Saunders.)

binding site farther along on the actin filament. In *(3)*, the myosin head binds to its new position on the actin filament, forming a cross-bridge. This action causes the inorganic phosphate molecule to dissociate from ADP, which causes the myosin head (still attached to the actin filament) to flex on its hinge, pulling the actin filament toward the myosin filament's tail (the "power stroke"). This action causes ADP to dissociate from the myosin head *(5)*, leaving the actin-myosin complex in a rigid state (*top figure*). In the absence of ATP, the strong binding state between myosin and actin persists, which would potentially prevent the contractile proteins from relaxing (this occurs soon after death because ATP cannot be generated, creating a state known as

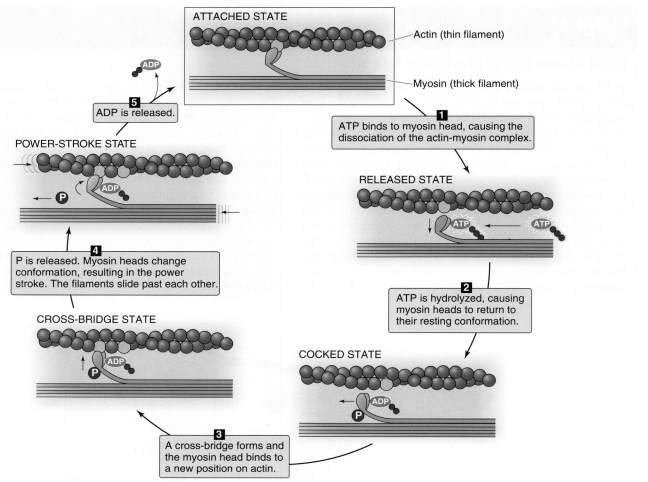

Figure 17-17 The cross-bridge cycle in skeletal and cardiac muscle. See detailed description in text. (From Boron WF, Boulpaep EL, editors: *Medical physiology,* ed 2, Philadelphia, 2009, Saunders.)

rigor mortis). In living muscle cells, metabolism generates new ATP molecules that react with the myosin heads and pull them back to their resting position, restarting the cycle *(1)* (see Figure 17-15, *A*). This sequence of events, known as cross-bridge cycling, repeats many times per second and continues as long as ATP molecules are produced and available. Relaxation of the muscle occurs when the nerve impulse ceases; sarcoplasmic reticulum rapidly pumps Ca^{++} back into its storage sites. When calcium ions leave TnC, the entire troponin complex undergoes a conformational change, which moves tropomyosin back to its blocking position.

CONCEPT QUESTION 17-4

What would be the effect of a drug that blocks Ca^{++} entry into the muscle fiber?

Increased cytoplasm Ca^{++} concentration increases the heart's force of contraction. The opposite occurs with decreased Ca^{++} concentration or with drugs that block calcium ion entry into the muscle cell. This explains why calcium chloride ($CaCl_2$) is sometimes given to patients to improve the heart's force of contraction.

Cardiac Muscle

Cardiac muscle differs from skeletal muscle in that individual muscle fibers are joined end-to-end to other fibers through junctions called intercalated disks (Figure 17-18). These disks are cell membranes (sarcolemma) separating individual cardiac muscle cells. That is, cardiac muscle is made up of many individual cells joined together in series. The electrical resistance through the intercalated disks is about one four-hundredth of the resistance through the outside muscle fiber membrane.[2] A reason for this low resistance is that cell membranes fuse at places along the disks, forming so-called gap junctions, which allow free passage of ions between cells. Functionally, the entire cardiac muscle mass acts as a single muscle fiber; for this reason, the myocardium is known as a syncytium.[2] If one fiber in the syncytium contracts, all fibers contract ("all-or-none" principle). The heart consists of two distinctly separate syncytia: the atrial syncytium and the ventricular syncytium. These two syncytia are electrically connected only by the AV bundle.

Frank-Starling Mechanism: Sarcomere Length–Dependent Activation

The inherent ability of the heart to increase its force of contraction as increasing amounts of blood flow into it is known as the

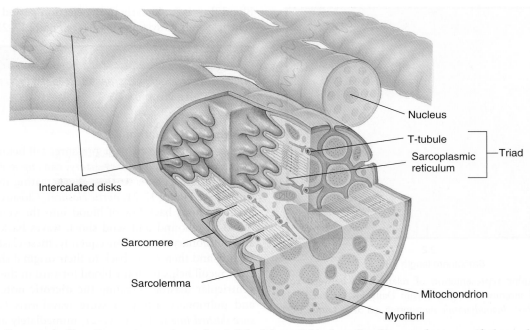

Figure 17-18 Cardiac muscle fiber. Low-resistance intercalated disks join individual cardiac fibers to form a unified muscle mass or syncytium. (From Thibodeau GA, Patton KT: *Anatomy & physiology,* ed 3, St Louis, 1996, Mosby.)

Frank-Starling mechanism, named after two physiologists of the late nineteenth and early twentieth centuries.[2] Frank and Starling observed that the greater the diastolic volume of the heart, the greater the force of contraction. This phenomenon occurs in hearts removed from the body and is thus independent of neural mechanisms. The force of myocardial contraction is proportional to the rate of cross-bridge formation between actin and myosin filaments, which is influenced by the sarcomere's length (length-dependent activation).[4] The exact mechanism is incompletely understood. The traditional explanation is that myocardial stretch brings actin and myosin filaments into a more optimal degree of overlap for cross-bridge formation. Figure 17-19 shows that too much stretch disengages some cross-bridges, whereas extremely foreshortened fibers cause actin filaments to bypass one another and overlap. A more current view is that an increase in sarcomere length increases the sensitivity of TnC to calcium, which increases the rate of cross-bridge cycling.[4] In addition, the passive recoil of stretched titin molecules also may contribute to increased contractile force; a combination of mechanisms is probably at work.[4] Whatever the mechanism, a precontraction sarcomere length of about 2.2 μ is associated with the greatest force of contraction.[4]

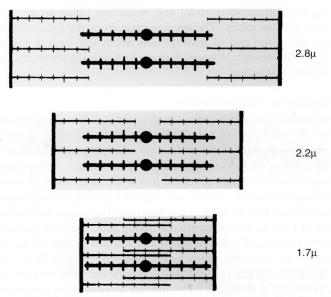

Figure 17-19 Sarcomere length and actin-myosin cross-bridge formation. Too much stretch (*top*) or too much fiber shortening (*bottom*) decreases the number of cross-bridges that can form, weakening contractile strength. (From Daily EK, Schroeder JS: *Techniques in bedside hemodynamic monitoring,* ed 5, St Louis, 1994, Mosby.)

CONCEPT QUESTION 17-5

In congestive heart failure, the left ventricle may become overdistended. Why may this decrease the heart's force of contraction?

The precontraction length of the cardiac muscle fiber is known as the heart's preload. The clinician can measure ventricular preload by measuring ventricular filling pressure just before contraction (end-diastolic pressure). The assumption is that greater end-diastolic pressures stretch the muscle fibers to greater lengths. In clinical terms, the Frank-Starling mechanism states, "the greater the preload, the greater the force of contraction." This statement is true only to a point because too much fiber stretch decreases the force of contraction (Figure 17-20).

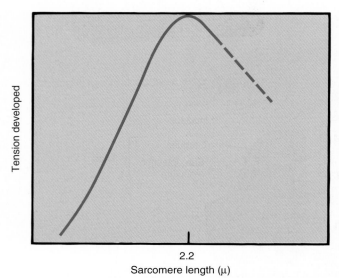

Figure 17-20 Graphic representation of relationship between contractile force and sarcomere length. (From Daily EK, Schroeder JS: *Techniques in bedside hemodynamic monitoring*, ed 5, St Louis, 1994, Mosby.)

Cardiac Cycle

The cardiac cycle refers to a complete pumping cycle, consisting of contraction (systole) and relaxation (diastole) of both atria and ventricles. The average cycle from the beginning of systole to the end of diastole lasts about 0.8 second. Figure 17-21, known as a Wiggers diagram,[4] graphically illustrates the sequence of events.

Ventricular Filling (Preload)

As soon as the ventricles relax, the pressure that accumulated in the atria during ventricular contraction pushes the AV valves open, and blood rushes into the ventricles, creating a rapid filling phase (see Figure 17-21, *f*) and a slow filling phase (see Figure 17-21, *g*). As blood leaves the atria, atrial pressure decreases abruptly and is only slightly higher than ventricular pressure as blood continues to drain into the ventricles. During the last 0.1 second of ventricular filling time, the atria contract (atrial kick) and force an additional amount of blood into the ventricles, distending their walls slightly (see Figure 17-21, *a*). About 80% of ventricular filling is passive; the remaining 20% is caused by the atrial kick.[2] The atria are mere priming pumps for the ventricles, completing the "preloading" process.

Ventricular Emptying

Contraction of the ventricles rapidly builds up pressure, forcefully snapping the AV valves closed; this creates the first heart sound (see Figure 17-21, *M₁* and *b*). A fraction of a second passes before the ventricular pressure increases enough to push the aortic and pulmonary semilunar valves open against the opposing aortic and pulmonary artery pressures. During this brief time, no blood leaves the ventricles (see *isovolumetric contraction*, Figure 17-21, *b*). The ejection period occurs immediately after aortic and pulmonary semilunar valves open (see Figure 17-21, *AO*); the resistance to this ejection is called **afterload**.

Blood flow is rapid early in the ejection period, slowing as the ventricle ends its systolic phase (see Figure 17-21, *c* and *d*).

Ventricular Relaxation

As the ventricles relax, their pressures fall below the pressures of the aorta and pulmonary artery, causing aortic and pulmonary semilunar valves to snap shut, creating the second heart sound (see Figure 17-21, *aortic closure*). Closure of these valves abruptly stops backflow of blood into the ventricles, causing blood to rebound and send shock waves back into the aorta and pulmonary artery. Consequently, these elastic vessels dilate slightly and then recoil back to their original shapes. This vascular recoil helps push the blood forward in the arteries during ventricular diastole, creating the **dicrotic notch** in the aortic and pulmonary artery pressure waveforms (see *aortic pressure dashed line* in Figure 17-21, immediately after *aortic valve closure*).

A fraction of a second passes before ventricular pressures decrease enough to allow AV valves to open again. This time period is called isovolumetric relaxation (see Figure 17-21, *e*). Passive ventricular filling then begins, and the cycle is repeated.

The end-diastolic volume of each ventricle is about 110 to 120 mL.[2] Contraction ejects about 70 mL of blood (**stroke volume**), leaving behind about 40 to 50 mL (end-systolic volume). The filled ventricles normally eject about 60% of their volume (**ejection fraction**). A low ejection fraction (<50%) indicates poor contractility and pumping failure. Very powerful contractions during exercise can increase the ejection fraction to about 90%.[2]

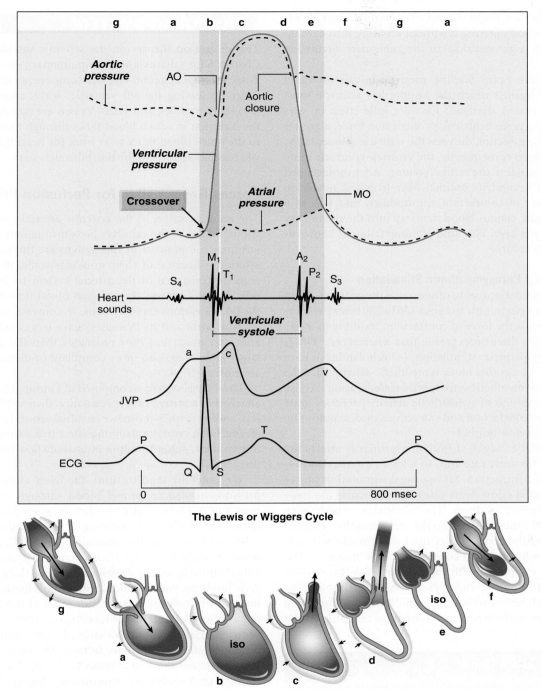

The Lewis or Wiggers Cycle

Figure 17-21 Composite graphic representation of cardiac function. A cycle length of 0.8 second produces a heart rate of 75 beats per minute. *AO,* Aortic valve opening; *MO,* mitral valve opening; M_1 and T_1, mitral valve and tricuspid valve closure component of first heart sound; A_2 and P_2, aortic and pulmonic valve closure components of second heart sound; S_3 and S_4, third and fourth heart sounds; *JVP,* jugular venous pressure (*a,* right atrial contraction; *c,* carotid artery artifact during rapid ventricular ejection; *v,* venous return wave causing atrial pressure rise when tricuspid valve is closed); *ECG,* electrocardiogram. See text for explanation of figures *g* through *a.* (From Zipes DP, et al, editors: *Braunwald's heart disease: a textbook of cardiovascular medicine,* ed 7, St Louis, 2005, Saunders.)

Regulation of Heart Pumping Activity

Frank-Starling Mechanism
The amount of blood flowing into the heart from the vena cava determines how much blood the heart pumps each minute; that is, venous blood return to the right atrium determines the cardiac output. The heart automatically adjusts to the incoming blood flow, pumping it out at the same rate that it enters. This ability to adapt to changing inflow of blood is known as the Frank-Starling mechanism (explained previously). The greater the inflow of blood, the greater is the ventricular volume and fiber length, and the greater is the force of contraction. The

result is an increased stroke volume. The normal heart always pumps all the blood entering it without allowing it to dam up in the vena cava (right ventricle) or the pulmonary circulation (left ventricle).

Because of the Frank-Starling mechanism, an increased aortic pressure against which the healthy left ventricle must pump (i.e., increased afterload) has very little effect on cardiac output. At a given ventricular contraction force, a greater pressure-opposing ejection distends the ventricle momentarily, stretching its fibers; consequently, the ventricle contracts more forcefully and sustains the stroke volume. An overdistended heart stretched beyond its optimal fiber length is unable to increase its force of contraction appropriately and fails as a pump. As a result, venous blood dams up into the pulmonary veins and the vena cava. This kind of pump failure is known as congestive heart failure.

Sympathetic and Parasympathetic Stimulation

Strong sympathetic stimulation can increase the heart rate from a normal 70 beats per minute to about 180 to 200 beats per minute and can double the force of contraction, resulting in a cardiac output two or three times greater than when at rest.[2] Drugs that mimic sympathetic stimulation (catecholamines) have the same effect. Drugs that block sympathetic activity have the opposite effect. Sympathetic activity is increased during exercise and anxiety. Inhibition of sympathetic activity decreases heart rate and force of contraction and can reduce cardiac output by as much as 30% below normal.[2]

Parasympathetic (vagal) stimulation primarily affects the atria, slowing the heart rate and, to a lesser extent, decreasing the force of contraction. Strong vagal stimulation causes severe bradycardia (slow heart rate) and can cause momentary cardiac arrest; however, the ventricles, which have much less vagal innervation than the atria, usually "escape" the influence of the atria and set up a rhythm of their own at a rate of about 20 to 40 contractions per minute.[2] The trachea is richly supplied with vagal nerves. For this reason, the common respiratory care practice of inserting a catheter into the trachea to remove accumulated secretions may stimulate severe bradycardia or momentary cessation of the heartbeat.

CONCEPT QUESTION 17-7

What is the cardiac effect of a drug that blocks parasympathetic activity?

Effect of Heart Rate

An increased heart rate generally increases cardiac output, but this effect is limited when heart rate exceeds 170 to 220 beats per minute.[2] Above this critical range, diastolic time becomes so short that blood flow from the atria does not have enough time to fill the ventricles completely. The volume of blood the ventricles can eject with each stroke is reduced, offsetting the increase in cardiac output that normally accompanies increased heart rate.

VASCULAR SYSTEM

This discussion focuses on the systemic vascular system; see Chapter 6 for a discussion of the pulmonary vasculature. Blood flows through systemic vascular components in the following order on leaving the left ventricle: aorta, arteries, arterioles, capillaries, venules, and veins. Vessels are named according to the direction in which blood flows through them with respect to the heart: Blood flows away from the heart through arteries, whereas blood flows to the heart through veins.

Forces Responsible for Perfusion Pressure

The main function of the systemic arterial system is to distribute blood to the capillary beds throughout the body. The terminal components of this system are the small, muscular arterioles. Because of their muscular walls, they are able to regulate resistance of the arterial system by constricting or dilating. In so doing, they control blood flow distribution to the body's various capillary beds. In contrast, the larger arteries (the aorta and its branches) have less constricting ability and offer much less flow resistance than the arterioles. The larger arteries are also more compliant or distensible than the arterioles.

The arterial system is composed of a pump (the left ventricle) attached to a system of low-resistance, distensible tubes (arteries), ending in high-resistance terminal vessels (arterioles). This arrangement creates a damping effect that converts the heart's intermittent, pulsatile output into steady flow through the capillary beds.[2]

We generally tend to think the heart alone provides the pressure needed to propel blood through tissue capillary beds, but this is not entirely true. Perfusion pressure is maintained by the heart's pumping action combined with the elastic recoil force of the arteries. Figure 17-22 illustrates this point. A single ventricular contraction discharges the stroke volume into the arteries, lasting about one third of the cardiac cycle duration. Much of the contraction's force propels blood forward through the arteries, but some of the force distends the arteries to larger diameters (Figure 17-22, *A*). When the ventricle relaxes, its outflow stops, but the recoil force of the distended arteries continues to move the blood forward during ventricular diastole (Figure 17-22, *B*). Thus, blood flow through the capillaries is continuous. Hypothetically, if arterial walls were perfectly rigid, the entire stroke volume would flow through the capillaries in a single contraction; because arterial walls could not recoil, blood flow would cease during diastole (Figure 17-22, *C* and *D*). Although this extreme situation does not occur in the body, vascular diseases that reduce vessel wall compliance (arteriosclerosis) have a similar effect, creating a wide difference between systolic and diastolic pressures.

CONCEPT QUESTION 17-8

Why do rigid arterial walls increase the difference between systolic and diastolic blood pressures?

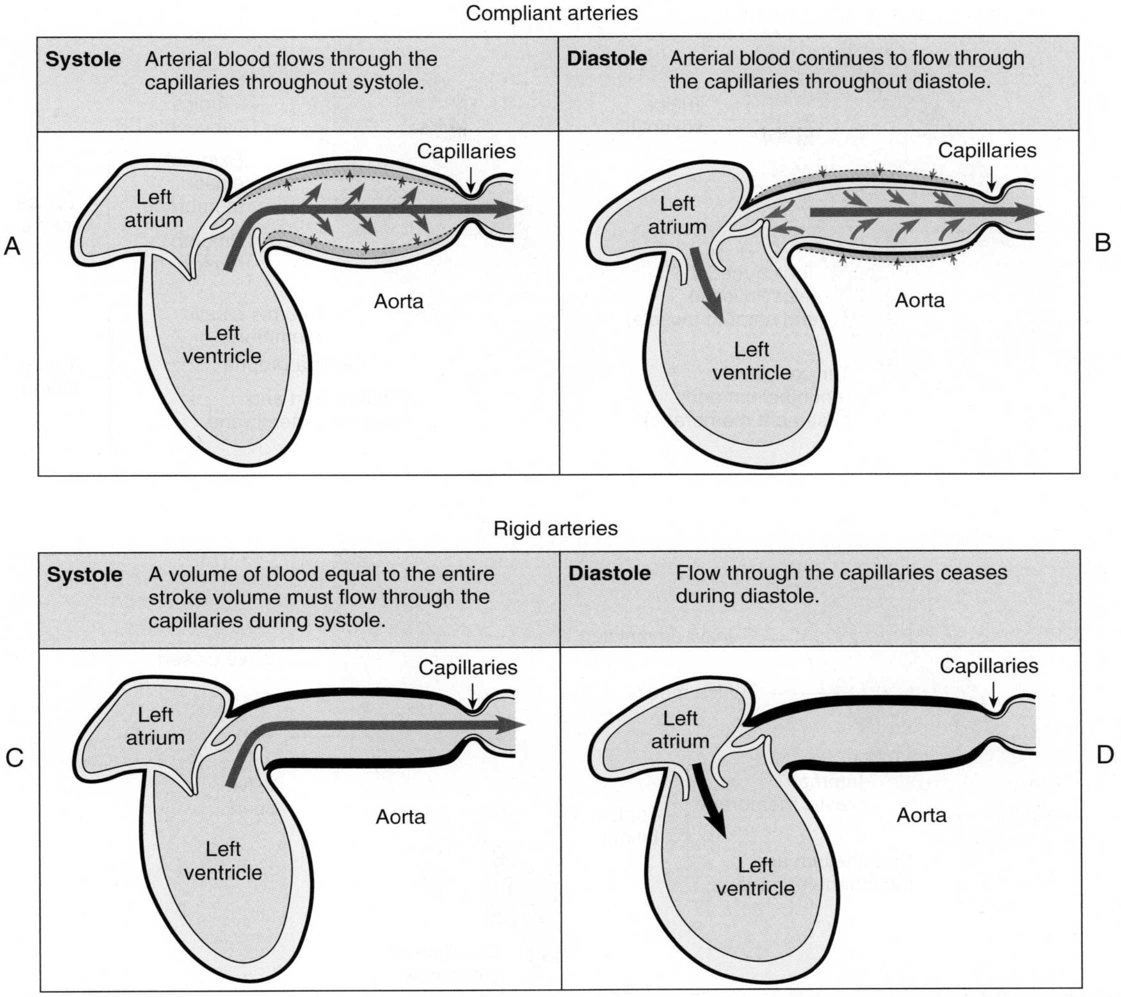

Compliant arteries

Rigid arteries

Figure 17-22 Pumping action and elastic recoil both provide the force for blood flow. Pulsatile flow is converted to steady flow. **A,** In normal, compliant arteries, systole propels blood forward through capillaries. **B,** Recoil of stretched arteries continues to propel blood after contraction ends. **C,** If the arteries were rigid pipes, the entire stroke volume would flow through the capillaries during ventricular contraction. **D,** During diastole, blood flow would cease because arteries have no recoil. (From Berne RM, Levy MN: *Principles of physiology,* ed 2, St Louis, 1996, Mosby.)

Vascular Structure

Figure 17-23 compares the structures of arteries and veins. All have similar general features. However, arterial muscular layers are generally thicker than their venous counterparts; thus, arteries have greater constricting ability. The largest arteries (see Figure 17-23, *A*), often called conducting arteries, have more elastic tissue and less smooth muscle than smaller arteries and arterioles. Pressures are relatively high in them, fluctuating markedly between systolic and diastolic phases of the heartbeat.

Smaller arteries and arterioles have thick walls compared with their diameters because of their thick muscle layers. The arterioles are known as resistance vessels because of their powerful constricting ability. Through vasoconstriction and vasodilation, arterioles exert a major influence on systemic blood pressure and flow.

Near the point at which capillaries originate, smooth muscle in the arterioles forms precapillary sphincters (Figure 17-24). These circular bands of muscle control blood flow through local capillary beds. Hypoxia dilates precapillary sphincters, increasing blood flow. At rest, some of the sphincters are constricted,

reducing blood flow to tissues with low metabolic activity. During strenuous activity, precapillary sphincters dilate, opening (recruiting) more capillaries to meet local tissue blood flow needs.

The capillary circulation is often called the microcirculation (see Figure 17-24). Capillary walls consist of a single layer of endothelial cells with no muscle tissue whatsoever; they have no intrinsic ability to constrict or dilate. Capillary diameters are determined passively, solely by the volume and pressure of blood within them, which is controlled by the precapillary sphincters. Besides oxygen and carbon dioxide exchange between blood and tissues, nutrient and waste product exchange also occur across the capillary cell walls.

CONCEPT QUESTION 17-9

When respiratory mucous membrane capillaries are engorged with blood, they may leak, resulting in mucosal edema. Drugs that constrict arterioles are called decongestants because they relieve mucosal edema. Explain how such a drug relieves mucosal swelling.

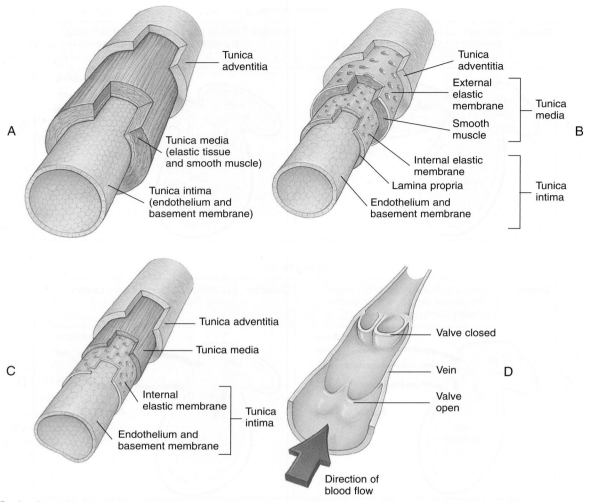

Figure 17-23 Blood vessel types. **A,** Large elastic artery. **B,** Smaller muscular arteriole. **C,** Small venule. **D,** Large distensible vein with unidirectional valves. (From Seeley RR, Stephens TD, Tate P: *Anatomy & physiology,* ed 3, New York, 1995, McGraw-Hill.)

Capillaries converge to form venules. A relatively direct connection between arterioles and venules is called an arteriovenous anastomosis, or thoroughfare channel (see Figure 17-24). In this way, blood can shunt past tissue capillary beds directly to the venous circulation, especially when local tissue metabolic needs are low. This kind of shunting is thought to be present in critically ill patients with septic shock. Septic shock is characterized by profound vasodilation and altered oxygen-extraction capabilities of the tissue cells. For example, venous oxygen saturation could be normal or elevated in patients with septic shock even though severe tissue hypoxia is present.[5] This occurs because blood is shunted past tissue capillary beds through thoroughfare channels and fails to release adequate oxygen. For this reason, mixed venous oxygen content is an unreliable indicator of cardiac output changes in patients with septic shock (see Chapter 8 discussion of the Fick cardiac output equation).

Venules converge to form veins (see Figure 17-23, *C* and *D*). Veins contain much less smooth muscle and are generally much more distensible than arteries. Larger veins contain one-way valves (see Figure 17-23, *D*) to aid venous blood flow toward the heart against gravitational force. Many such veins exist in the legs where the muscles squeeze them, producing a "milking" action, propelling blood upward to the heart. For this reason, muscular activity in the lower extremities is important to prevent venous "pooling" and impaired venous circulation. This venous "pooling" explains the uncomfortable feeling one has in the legs after long periods of standing still or sitting.

Venous Reservoir

Because of their distensibility, the veins contain by far the greatest proportion of the blood volume at any given time (Table 17-1). Veins are an important blood reservoir, containing about 64% of the total blood volume. When large amounts of blood are lost from the body, reflex sympathetic venous constriction shifts blood into the arterial system. This compensatory venous constriction allows essentially normal circulatory function, even after 20% of the total blood volume is lost.[2]

The veins manage to return blood to the heart against the force of gravity through four basic mechanisms: (1) muscular "milking" of leg veins containing one-way valves; (2) sympathetic venous constriction; (3) cardiac pumping action, creating

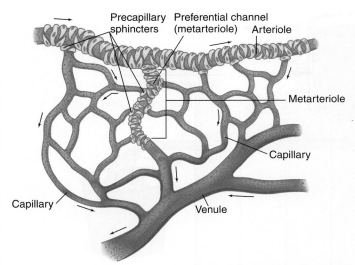

Figure 17-24 The microcirculation or capillary network. Precapillary sphincters control blood flow through the capillary bed. (From McCance KL, et al: *Pathophysiology: The biologic basis for disease in adults and children,* ed 6, 2010, Mosby.)

TABLE 17-1
Distribution of Blood Volume in Blood Vessels

Vessels	Total Blood Volume (%)
Systemic veins	64
Large veins (39%)	
Small veins (25%)	
Arteries	15
Large arteries (8%)	
Small arteries (5%)	
Arterioles (2%)	
Capillaries	5
Total in systemic vessels	*84*
Pulmonary vessels	9
Heart	7
Total blood volume	*100*

From Seeley RR, Stephens TD, Tate P: *Anatomy & physiology,* ed 3, New York, 1995, McGraw-Hill.

a "cardiac suction"; and (4) subatmospheric intrathoracic pressures during breathing. The normal subatmospheric pressure within the chest cavity aids venous return because abdominal venous pressure is positive.

Arterial Blood Pressure, Velocity, Flow Rate, and Resistance

Blood Pressure
Blood flows out of the left ventricle and returns to the right atrium of the heart because a pressure gradient exists between these two structures. The basic principle of circulation is simply that blood flows from areas of high pressure to areas of low pressure; blood does not flow between two structures if the pressure is the same in both places.

Blood pressure in large and medium-sized arteries varies considerably between systolic and diastolic pressures. The difference between these two pressures (**pulse pressure**) diminishes as blood flows farther away from the heart. The pulse pressure is influenced by stroke volume and arterial compliance. Increased stroke volume increases systolic pressure and thus increases pulse pressure. Decreased arterial compliance, as occurs with age or vascular disease, causes aortic pressure to rise higher and more sharply during systole and to fall more abruptly during diastole (see earlier discussion). For a given stroke volume, systolic pressure and pulse pressure are higher if arterial compliance is low. Figure 17-25 illustrates blood pressures in various parts of the systemic vascular system. Notice the progressive decline in pressure from aorta to vena cava and the lack of a pulsatile pressure waveform in the capillaries and venous system. This occurs because systolic and diastolic pressure fluctuations are dampened by the high-resistance arterioles.

Mean Arterial Pressure
Mean arterial pressure (MAP) is not simply the average of systolic and diastolic pressures as implied in Figure 17-25. The heart remains in systole for about one third of the cardiac cycle duration; thus, the arteries are exposed to the systolic pressure one third of the time and the diastolic pressure two thirds of the time. MAP is roughly estimated by the following equation:

MAP = (Systolic pressure + 2[diastolic pressure])/3

An arterial systolic blood pressure of 120 mm Hg and diastolic pressure of 80 mm Hg (i.e., 120/80) yields an MAP of:

MAP = 120 + 2(80)/3

MAP = 93.3 mm Hg

The MAP is simply the average driving pressure that propels blood from the left ventricle to right atrium. MAP is closely related to overall adequacy of tissue perfusion in the body. The previous calculation is an estimate only; accurate measurement of MAP requires integration of the arterial pressure waveform.

The greatest fall in MAP occurs across the high-resistance arterioles: blood pressure is 85 mm Hg on entering the arterioles and 35 mm Hg on exiting them (see Figure 17-25). The reason for this large fall in MAP is that the arterioles offer the greatest resistance of any circulatory component. Flow across a resistance always produces a drop in pressure; the greater the resistance, the greater the pressure drop downstream from the site of resistance.

Systemic Vascular Resistance
Vascular resistance is measured as units of pressure required to produce a flow of 1 L per minute (mm Hg/L/min) through the vessels. To calculate SVR, one must measure the pressure gradient across the systemic circulation and the blood flow rate (cardiac output). The pressure across the systemic vasculature is equal to the MAP minus the right atrial pressure (RAP); after measuring cardiac output (CO), we calculate SVR as follows:

SVR = (MAP−RAP)/CO

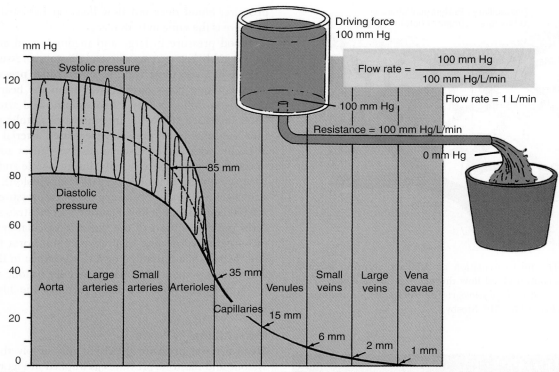

Figure 17-25 Blood pressure in various parts of the systemic circulation. High-resistance arterioles dampen systolic-diastolic pressure fluctuations in the capillaries and veins. (From Thibodeau GA, Patton KT: *Anatomy & physiology,* ed 3, St Louis, 1996, Mosby.)

Assuming MAP of 100 mm Hg, RAP of 0 mm Hg, and CO of 5 L/min, SVR is:

$$SVR = (100-0)/5$$
$$SVR = 20 \text{ mm Hg/L/min}$$

The SVR is a measure of the average resistance against which the left ventricle must work to eject the stroke volume; thus, SVR is an indicator of left ventricular afterload. (See Chapter 20 for a more thorough discussion of SVR measurement and its conversion to centimeter-gram-second or CGS units.)

The **hematocrit** (percentage of the blood volume composed of cells) also affects vascular resistance. The greater the number of cells, the greater is the friction between successive layers of blood (i.e., the greater is the blood's viscosity). As blood hematocrit or viscosity increases, the heart must pump more forcefully to maintain the blood flow rate; that is, a higher pressure gradient is required to produce the same blood flow. This increases the numerator of the SVR equation, yielding a greater SVR value.

Blood Flow Rate and Velocity

Blood flow rate is determined by two factors: (1) driving pressure (pressure difference between two ends of a vessel) and (2) vascular resistance. This is simply a rearrangement of the SVR equation:

Blood flow = Driving pressure/resistance
CO = (MAP−RAP)/SVR

For a given driving pressure, an increased resistance decreases blood flow.

An increased peripheral or arteriolar resistance does not always decrease the blood flow (cardiac output) however.

Arteriole constriction does decrease arteriole outflow or "arteriole runoff" into the capillaries, but it also increases pressure in the larger arteries and aorta. Increased arterial pressure offsets the increased vascular resistance, and blood flow may remain constant (see the previous equation). This kind of an increase in arterial blood pressure increases blood flow to organs not affected by arteriolar constriction. This is an important protective mechanism in shock caused by acute blood loss; reflex sympathetic stimulation causes peripheral vasoconstriction, maintaining arterial blood pressure and redirecting blood flow to vital central ("core") organs, such as the heart, kidneys, lungs, liver, and brain. However, if the heart fails to increase its contractile force in the face of increased vascular resistance, blood flow decreases.

Although total blood flow rate throughout the vasculature is fairly constant under steady-state conditions, blood velocity is not constant. Velocity refers to the speed with which blood flows, or distance traveled per minute. Velocity is distinct from flow rate; flow rate is volume moved per minute. Given a constant blood flow rate, velocity is determined by the summative cross-sectional area of the vascular components. For example, the aorta's cross-sectional area is about 5 cm², and the millions of capillaries have a combined cross-sectional area of about 2500 cm². For a cardiac output of 5 L per minute, blood velocity in the aorta is very high, but blood velocity in capillaries is very low (Figure 17-26). For this reason, aortic blood flow is normally turbulent, whereas capillary blood flow is laminar.

Turbulent flow vibrates the vessel walls, transmitting sound to the surface of the body. Abnormal vessel narrowing causes turbulent flow, which may be detected by a stethoscope.

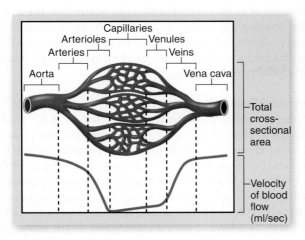

Figure 17-26 Blood flow velocity related to vascular cross-sectional area. (From Patton KT, Thibodeau GA: *Anatomy & physiology*, ed 7, St. Louis, 2010, Mosby.)

The swirling eddy currents of turbulent blood flow in partly obstructed arteries (e.g., arteries partially blocked by arteriosclerotic plaque) increase the probability of blood clot formation.

Determinants of Systolic and Diastolic Blood Pressure

For a given circulating blood volume, mean blood pressure is determined by (1) stroke volume, (2) arterial compliance, and (3) arterial resistance. For any given resistance and stroke volume, a "stiffer" aorta causes a higher systolic pressure. Likewise, at any given compliance and resistance, an increased stroke volume mainly increases the systolic pressure. The higher systolic pressure increases peripheral blood runoff during systole, and thus, diastolic pressure is affected to a lesser extent.

On the other hand, for a given heart rate, stroke volume, and arterial compliance, diastolic pressure depends purely on the peripheral vascular resistance.[6] If peripheral resistance decreases, blood runoff rate from the arterioles is greater, decreasing the diastolic pressure. Increased peripheral resistance slows arteriole runoff rate, increasing the diastolic pressure. In other words, if peripheral vascular resistance is high, the vascular pressure falls so slowly during the diastolic time interval that systole occurs before the pressure can fall to its normal diastolic level. That is, how rapidly and how far vascular pressure falls from its systolic peak depends on arteriole runoff rate.

CONCEPT QUESTION 17-10

Two patients have the same heart rate. Patient A's blood pressure is 170/80 mm Hg; patient B's blood pressure is 150/100 mm Hg. Which patient has the greatest degree of peripheral vascular resistance?

An increased heart rate also may increase diastolic pressure for a given peripheral vascular resistance. The mechanism is

TABLE 17-2

Effect of a Given Factor on Systolic and Diastolic Pressures When Other Factors Are Constant

Factor	Systolic Pressure	Diastolic Pressure
Stroke Volume		
Increased	++	+
Decreased	−−	−
Peripheral Resistance		
Increased	+	++
Decreased	−	−−
Arterial Compliance		
Increased	−	+
Decreased	+	−
Heart Rate		
Increased	+	++
Decreased	−	−−

Modified from Little RC: *Physiology of the heart and circulation*, ed 4, Chicago, 1989, Year Book Medical Publishers.

similar to that just described; the shortened diastolic time interval does not allow vascular pressure to fall to its normal diastolic level. Table 17-2 summarizes the isolated effects of various factors on systolic and diastolic pressures.

Hypertension

Hypertension, or high blood pressure, usually refers to a MAP greater than 110 mm Hg at rest; this coincides with a diastolic pressure of about 90 mm Hg and a systolic pressure of about 135 to 140 mm Hg.[2] The detrimental effects of hypertension occur in three major ways:[2] (1) excessive workload on the heart, leading to heart failure; (2) rupture of a major blood vessel in the brain, known as a stroke or cerebrovascular accident (CVA); and (3) multiple kidney hemorrhages leading to extensive renal tissue destruction.

Chronically high systolic pressures are associated with a stiffening, noncompliant arterial system, as occurs with old age and **atherosclerosis** (commonly known as "hardening of the arteries," secondary to endothelial inflammation and buildup of fatty substances under the endothelium in the vessel wall). A high systolic pressure per se is not always abnormal. Systolic pressure naturally increases during exercise as stroke volume increases and more blood flow is needed. A high systolic pressure with a normal diastolic pressure means that peripheral vascular resistance is normal. That is, normally vascular resistance is low enough so that the peak pressures during systole fall to normal values during diastole.

An elevated diastolic pressure is a more serious sign of high SVR. As explained in the previous section, high peripheral resistance decreases the arteriole runoff rate—the rate at which blood

CLINICAL FOCUS 17-7

Measurement of Arterial Blood Pressure with a Blood Pressure Cuff

Blood pressure is measured with an instrument called a sphygmomanometer. This instrument consists of a hollow balloon-like rubber cuff with two tubes. One tube is attached to a compressible bulb, and the other tube is attached to a pressure gauge. The cuff is wrapped around the arm above the elbow. By squeezing the bulb, one can inflate the cuff until it compresses the arm's brachial artery, stopping blood flow. A stethoscope is placed over the brachial artery at the inner bend of the elbow.

No pulse can be heard when the artery is occluded. Air is then slowly released from the cuff while the clinician closely watches the pressure gauge and listens to the stethoscope. When the cuff pressure decreases to a level just below the systolic pressure of the brachial artery, a small amount of blood spurts through the artery during systole. These spurts of blood flow sound like sharp, tapping sounds through the stethoscope; this identifies the systolic pressure. As the cuff pressure continues to decrease, the pulse sounds become muffled and faint and then disappear. This point identifies the diastolic pressure because blood now flows unrestricted through the artery and creates no sound. The sounds heard through the stethoscope are called Korotkoff sounds.

flows from the arterioles into the capillary beds. High arteriolar resistance slows the rate at which the peak pressure achieved during systole falls during diastole; this causes diastolic pressure to be higher than normal when the next ventricular contraction occurs. In the end, systolic pressure and MAP also increase.

About 90% of all people with hypertension have essential hypertension, or hypertension of unknown origin.[2] The peripheral vascular resistance in these individuals is about 40% to 60% above normal, about the same amount that MAP is increased.

Venous Pressures

Right Atrial Pressure

Blood pressure in the right atrium is often called central venous pressure (CVP) because blood from all systemic veins flows into the right atrium. Therefore, anything that affects right atrial pressure (RAP) affects all venous pressures in the body.

Pressure in the right atrium is determined by the heart's ability to pump blood out of it and the rate at which blood flows back into it from the vena cava. Powerful pumping action decreases RAP, whereas ineffective, weak pumping allows blood to dam up and increase RAP. Rapid return of venous blood to the right atrium tends to increase RAP. Venous blood flow increases if (1) there is an increased blood volume (e.g., intravenous fluid infusion); (2) venous tone increases, elevating venous pressures; and (3) arteriolar dilation occurs, causing more rapid blood flow into the venous system.[2] RAP can

be thought of as the preload of the right ventricle—that is, RAP is the "loading" or "filling" pressure of the right ventricle just before it contracts. In this way, RAP helps determine stroke volume and cardiac output (Frank-Starling mechanism). Normal RAP is about 0 to 5 mm Hg.

Peripheral Venous Pressure

Peripheral venous pressure is not affected by RAP until it increases to about 6 mm Hg.[2] At that pressure, the veins are distended enough that their pressures rise with further RAP increases. Pumping failure of the heart—congestive heart failure—is a major reason for the elevation of venous pressure. If systemic venous pressure rises high enough, it may be transmitted back into the capillary beds and force fluid out into interstitial spaces. This kind of fluid accumulation on the venous side of systemic capillary beds is known as peripheral edema and is a sign of right ventricular failure. In such cases, structures upstream from the right atrium (jugular veins, liver, abdominal viscera, leg veins) become engorged with dammed-up blood and swell. These events result in jugular venous distention (JVD), hepatomegaly (enlarged liver), ascites (fluid accumulation in the abdominal cavity), and pedal edema (edema of the ankles and feet).

Normal peripheral venous pressures are affected by gravitational forces. Beginning at the right atrium, where pressure is about 0 mm Hg, venous pressure increases to about 22 mm Hg in the lower abdominal cavity, to 40 mm Hg in the femoral veins, and to 90 mm Hg in the feet.[2] (These pressures apply to an adult standing perfectly still.) Thus, a gradient normally exists for venous blood return to the heart.

CONCEPT QUESTION 17-11

Explain how positive pressure mechanical ventilation may improve rather than hinder cardiac function in congestive heart failure.

Vascular System Regulation

The vasculature is controlled by both local and central control mechanisms. Local or intrinsic mechanisms do not need input from the central nervous system. These mechanisms respond to local metabolic needs of the tissues. Central, or extrinsic, mechanisms involve the central nervous system and circulating hormones (humoral agents). These mechanisms function to maintain a baseline level of vascular muscle tone. Vascular tone refers to a small degree of continuous vascular smooth muscle contraction. Only when a basal level of tone is maintained can vessels dilate further to increase blood flow or constrict either to decrease blood flow or to increase arterial pressure.

Local Control

Blood flow varies widely from organ to organ depending on the organ's metabolic needs or its functional purpose. Table 17-3 summarizes the blood flow to different organs. Generally, the higher the metabolic rate of the tissue, the greater its blood flow. Per gram of tissue weight, glandular structures receive a very

TABLE 17-3

Blood Flow to Different Organs and Tissues under Basal Conditions

Organ	%	mL/min	mL/min/100 g
Brain	14	700	50
Heart	4	200	70
Bronchi	2	100	25
Kidneys	22	1100	360
Liver	27	1350	95
Portal	(21)	(1050)	
Arterial	(6)	(300)	
Muscle (inactive state)	15	750	4
Bone	5	250	3
Skin (cool weather)	6	300	3
Thyroid gland	1	50	160
Adrenal glands	0.5	25	300
Other tissues	3.5	175	1.3
Total	100.0	5000	—

From Guyton AC: *Textbook of medical physiology,* ed 8, Philadelphia, 1991, Saunders. Based on data compiled by LA Sapirstein.

high blood flow (see Table 17-3); likewise, the kidneys receive a high blood flow relative to their mass. High renal flow is necessary to cleanse the blood of waste products.

Two theories for the local regulation of blood flow are the vasodilator theory and the oxygen demand theory.[2] According to the vasodilator theory, as tissues become more metabolically active, they produce a vasodilator substance that dilates precapillary sphincters and arterioles. Various substances, including carbon dioxide, adenosine, lactic acid, nitric oxide, potassium ions, hydrogen ions, and phosphate compounds, cause vasodilation; the concentrations of these substances increase with increases in metabolic rate. Adenosine has been suggested as the most important of these local vasodilators; this substance is especially important in dilating coronary arteries in response to increased myocardial oxygen demand.[2] Endothelial nitric oxide is also an important substance in regulating local vascular resistance. Controlled release of nitric oxide from the vascular endothelium is responsible for maintaining a continuous state of vasodilation.[7,8] In the presence of hypoxemia, endothelial cells release more nitric oxide, promoting vasodilation.[8]

The oxygen demand theory is not much different than the vasodilator theory; it states that a lack of oxygen and other nutrients dilates precapillary sphincters and arterioles, causing local blood flow to increase. When adequate amounts of oxygen and nutrients are restored to the tissues, precapillary sphincters close again. For this reason, blood flow through capillaries is not continuous; rather, it is cyclic, fluctuating because precapillary sphincters periodically relax and contract. The duration of the open phases of the cycle is proportional to oxygen requirements of the tissues. This cyclic opening and closing of precapillary sphincters is called vasomotion.[2]

The same mechanisms responsible for vasomotion are responsible for **autoregulation** of blood flow. Arterial blood

pressure can range from 75 to 175 mm Hg, but blood flow through tissues remains fairly constant. Even at minimum blood pressures, tissue perfusion can be maintained by local vasodilator mechanisms.

Central Control

Central neural control of the vascular system is mediated mainly through the autonomic nervous system, especially the sympathetic division. Sympathetic stimulation may cause either vasoconstriction or vasodilation, depending on which adrenergic receptor is stimulated. Adrenergic receptors respond to the sympathetic fiber's release of norepinephrine (noradrenaline). The β_2-adrenergic receptors mediate vasodilation, and the α-adrenergic receptors mediate vasoconstriction.

CONCEPT QUESTION 17-12

Which kinds of drugs would benefit a patient with high SVR: (1) alpha-receptor stimulator, (2) beta-receptor stimulator, (3) alpha-receptor blocker, or (4) beta-receptor blocker?

Nervous control is responsible for shifting blood flow from one large area of the peripheral circulation to another. In severe blood loss, neural mechanisms induce peripheral vasoconstriction, increasing the blood pressure in central vessels sufficiently to maintain perfusion of the brain and heart. This response is rapid, occurring within seconds.

The vasomotor center of the lower pons and upper medulla in the brain discharges a continuous low level of impulses to sympathetic vasoconstrictor fibers. This continuous low-level state of constriction is counterbalanced by vasodilator substances, which produces a resting vasomotor tone.[2] Sympathetic impulses also cause the adrenal gland (the adrenal medulla) to release epinephrine and norepinephrine into the blood. These hormones are carried by the circulation to various parts of the body where they exert influences on vessel diameter similar to direct sympathetic nervous stimulation.

Baroreceptor Reflex

Baroreceptors (also known as pressoreceptors) are special sensory fibers in the walls of large systemic arteries that are responsive to stretch. They are most numerous at the fork of the internal and external carotid arteries and in the aortic arch. When stretched by high blood pressures, carotid and aortic baroreceptors transmit impulses through the glossopharyngeal and vagus nerves to the brain's vasomotor and cardioregulatory centers. In response, the vasomotor center causes vasodilation, and the cardioregulatory center slows the heart rate. Consequently, arterial blood pressure decreases. A sudden reduction in blood pressure decreases the normal baseline impulse frequency transmitted by the baroreceptors to the brain; this causes vasoconstriction and increased heart rate. Through these mechanisms, the baroreceptors maintain blood pressure in a narrow range on a minute-to-minute basis.[2] The baroreceptors are responsible for maintaining a fairly constant blood pressure in the head and upper body when a person abruptly changes body posture (e.g., standing up after lying down).

Renin-Angiotensin-Aldosterone, Antidiuretic Hormone, and B-Natriuretic Peptide Systems

Baroreceptors do not control blood pressure on a long-term basis; they reset to any new blood pressure within 1 to 2 days.[2] Mechanisms that play important roles in long-term blood pressure regulation involve the kidney and include the **renin-angiotensin-aldosterone system (RAAS)**, the vasopressin mechanism, and a natriuretic peptide produced by ventricular walls.[2]

In the **RAAS**, low blood pressure stimulates specialized tubular cells in the kidneys to produce the enzyme, renin. Renin acts on a plasma protein to produce angiotensin I. Angiotensin I circulates through the body to the lungs; there, the pulmonary vascular endothelium produces **angiotensin-converting enzyme (ACE)**, which acts on angiotensin I to produce angiotensin II. Angiotensin II is a powerful vasoconstrictor that increases blood pressure significantly. Angiotensin II also increases blood pressure in another way; it causes the adrenal cortex to secrete aldosterone, which acts on the kidney tubules to increase their reabsorption of sodium ions and consequently water. The overall effect is an increased circulating blood volume and pressure. The RAAS is important in maintaining blood pressure in cases of circulatory shock.

In the **vasopressin mechanism**, a fall in blood pressure stimulates hypothalamic neurons in the brain to transmit impulses to the pituitary gland, stimulating the production of vasopressin, also known as antidiuretic hormone (ADH). ADH acts directly on blood vessels as a vasoconstrictor, but more importantly, it increases the kidney's reabsorption of water by increasing the permeability of the distal tubules in the kidney. These mechanisms increase blood volume and blood pressure.

Ventricular cells of the heart release a hormone, **B-type natriuretic peptide (BNP)**, in response to high blood pressure and stretch of ventricular walls.[9] This hormone inhibits aldosterone and promotes sodium loss (diuresis) by the kidney and subsequently water loss, reducing blood volume and blood pressure. In this way, BNP inhibits the RAAS; it is an aldosterone antagonist. In congestive heart failure (pumping failure), the ventricles become distended, and their walls are stretched, increasing blood levels of BNP. (For this reason, increased blood levels of BNP are a diagnostic marker for heart failure and help differentiate cardiac and pulmonary causes of dyspnea.[10]) Increased blood BNP levels inhibit aldosterone, blocking sodium reabsorption and subsequently water reabsorption. In this way, diuresis occurs, and blood volume is reduced. However, when the heart fails to pump adequately, the body's priority is to maintain the arterial blood pressure, and the fluid-retaining effects of the RAAS easily overwhelm the counteracting effects of increased BNP levels. The RAAS often causes too much fluid retention, which makes matters worse because it stresses the already failing heart even more. This harmful effect is only mildly lessened by increased blood levels of BNP.

CONCEPT QUESTION 17-13

In what kind of condition may an ACE inhibitor drug be beneficial?

POINTS TO REMEMBER

- The atria of the heart are mainly priming chambers for the ventricles, which are the pumping chambers.
- Tricuspid and mitral valves prevent backflow of blood from ventricles into atria during ventricular systole; likewise, pulmonary and aortic semilunar valves prevent backflow into the ventricles during ventricular diastole.
- The atrial and ventricular muscle masses are physically separated from each other by the fibrous cardiac skeleton, which consists of the structure that supports the heart valves.
- Forceful closure of the heart valves produces the major heart sounds.
- Coronary vessel perfusion occurs during the ventricular diastolic interval; factors that reduce diastolic time, such as a greatly increased heart rate, decrease coronary vessel perfusion.
- Very high heart rates reduce ventricular filling time and thus reduce ventricular stroke volume.
- The specialized conducting fibers in the AV node slow impulse transmission from atria to ventricles, preventing dangerously high ventricular rates.
- Heart muscle oxygenation is very blood flow dependent because of the heart's high oxygen extraction ratio and because the heart has very little collateral circulation.
- Calcium ions and ATP are essential for the formation of cross-bridges between actin and myosin filaments and subsequent muscle contraction.
- Heart muscle intercellular membranes pose almost no electrical resistance; thus, the stimulation of one muscle fiber causes all heart muscle fibers to contract as one ("all-or-none" principle).
- Preload refers to the ventricle's priming pressure, and afterload refers to the resistance to ventricular ejection.
- Stretching heart muscle fibers increases their force of contraction, which is called the Frank-Starling mechanism.
- The Frank-Starling mechanism is a basic way the heart adjusts stroke volume from minute to minute.
- Diastole lasts about twice as long as systole; MAP is therefore estimated by: (2[diastolic pressure] + systolic pressure)/3.
- High diastolic pressure is more indicative of high peripheral vascular resistance than high systolic pressure.
- Capillary diameters are dependent on the volume and pressure of blood within them; capillaries have no intrinsic ability to constrict or dilate.
- Flow through capillaries is controlled by precapillary sphincters, which respond to local tissue metabolic needs.
- The venous system is much more distensible and contains much less pressure than the arterial system; most of the blood volume at any given moment is in the venous system.
- During shock, peripheral vasoconstriction diverts blood flow and pressure to the vital central core organs.
- Compensatory mechanisms that maintain blood pressure in heart failure often result in too much fluid retention and further stress the heart.

- The RAAS often causes too much fluid retention during cardiac failure, stressing the already failing heart even more.
- BNP released by overstretched atrial muscle promotes blood volume reduction by increasing renal sodium loss and subsequent water loss.

References

1. Little RC: *Physiology of the heart and circulation*, ed 3, Chicago, 1985, Year Book Medical Publishers.
2. Hall JE: *Guyton and Hall textbook of medical physiology*, ed 12, Philadelphia, 2011, Saunders.
3. Segal S: Special circulations. In Boron WF, Boulpaep EL, editors: *Medical physiology*, ed 2, Philadelphia, 2009, Saunders.
4. Opie LH: Mechanisms of cardiac contraction and relaxation. In Zipes DP, et al, editors: *Braunwald's heart disease: a textbook of cardiovascular medicine*, ed 7, Philadelphia, 2005, Saunders.
5. Silance PG, Simon C, Vincent JL: The relations between cardiac index and oxygen extraction in acutely ill patients, *Chest* 105(4):1190, 1994.
6. Green JF: *Fundamental cardiovascular and pulmonary physiology*, Philadelphia, 1987, Lea & Febiger.
7. Anggard E: Nitric oxide: mediator, murderer, and medicine, *Lancet* 343(8907):1199, 1994.
8. Kam PC, Govender G: Nitric oxide: basic science and clinical applications, *Anaesthesia* 49(8):515, 1994.
9. Antman EM: ST-elevation myocardial infarction: pathology, pathophysiology, and clinical features. In Bonow RO, et al, editors: *Braunwald's heart disease: a textbook of cardiovascular medicine*, ed 9, Philadelphia, 2011, Saunders.
10. Greenberg B, Kahn AM: Clinical assessment of heart failure. In Bonow RO, et al, editors: *Braunwald's heart disease: a textbook of cardiovascular medicine*, ed 9, Philadelphia, 2011, Saunders.

Cardiac Electrophysiology

OBJECTIVES

After reading this chapter, you will be able to:
- Explain the physiological significance of the resting membrane potential (RMP) of the cardiac fiber and how it is established
- Describe how the relationship between the RMP of the cardiac fiber and threshold potential affects the fiber's tendency to depolarize
- Explain why depolarization of the cardiac fiber causes the fiber to contract
- Explain the nature of the electrochemical events that cause the cardiac muscle fiber to depolarize spontaneously
- Describe the mechanism whereby electrical charge differences across the cardiac cell membrane affect its permeability to Na^+, K^+, and Ca^{++} ions
- Explain why abnormalities in blood Ca^{++} and K^+ concentrations affect cardiac muscle depolarization
- Correlate the activity of ion channels and gates with the graphical voltage versus time representation (action potential) of depolarization and repolarization of a single cardiac fiber

- Explain why catecholamine drugs increase cardiac contractility
- Explain why calcium channel–blocking drugs affect heart muscle contractility
- Describe the mechanisms whereby various drugs affect cardiac contractility and excitability
- Explain how ectopic foci arising from increased tissue excitability and the sinoatrial (SA) nodal block differ from each other
- Describe the purpose of the impulse transmission delay between the SA node and ventricles
- Describe the consequences of blocked atrial impulses that fail to enter the ventricles
- Explain how sympathetic and parasympathetic stimulation affects heart muscle automaticity, rhythmicity, and excitability

action potential
automaticity
Bachmann's bundle
calcium ion channels
contractility
depolarization
ectopic beats
ectopic focus
electrocardiograph
excitability
internodal pathways
membrane potential

pacemaker
premature beat
refractory
repolarization
resting membrane potential (RMP)
rhythmicity
sinus rhythm
Stokes-Adams syndrome
threshold potential (TP)
transitional (junctional) fibers
ventricular escape

MEMBRANE POTENTIALS

All living cells maintain a difference in ion concentrations across their membranes. Specifically, cardiac muscle cells (fibers) maintain high concentrations of positive ions just outside their membranes and high concentrations of negative ions just inside their membranes. This difference in ion concentrations creates an electrical charge across the membrane of the fiber, called the **membrane potential**. The term membrane potential comes from the fact that oppositely charged ions have the potential to move together across the membrane because of their electrostatic attraction. At rest, when heart muscle fibers are relaxed, their membranes are almost impermeable to these ions. The potential energy the electrical charge difference generates across the membrane reflects the strength of ionic electrostatic forces. This charge difference polarizes the membrane; the fiber's interior is the negative pole, and its exterior is the positive pole.

The difference in positive and negative charges on either side of the cell membrane involves only a few ions in the immediate vicinity of the membrane. Overall, intracellular and extracellular fluids contain equal numbers of positively charged and negatively charged ions.

If the permeability of the cardiac fiber membrane suddenly increases, ions explosively rush in and out of the cell similar to water bursting through a dam, depolarizing the membrane. Cardiac cell permeability changes cyclically, alternating between almost complete impermeability and complete permeability. This cyclical change in permeability (explained in greater detail later) is the basis for rhythmic contraction and relaxation of the ventricles. Membrane depolarization initiates a series of electrochemical events responsible for heart muscle contraction.

Generation of Resting Membrane Potential

The electrical charge difference between two sides of a polarized myocardial cell membrane is called the **resting membrane potential (RMP)**. The strength of RMP is measured in millivolts. Myocardial cell RMP is about −85 to −90 mV.[1] The outside of the cell is assumed to have 0 (ground) potential. The RMP is therefore the difference between the cell's inside potential and zero. The negative sign in front of the cardiac cell RMP (−90 mV) indicates the polarity of the cell's interior.

Figure 18-1 illustrates the measurement of the RMP through the placement of one microelectrode inside the cell and another

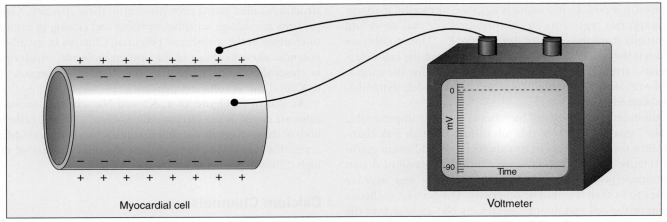

Figure 18-1 Measurement of the RMP. The recording electrode is inside and the reference electrode is outside of the cell, measuring a potential difference (voltage) of −90 mV.

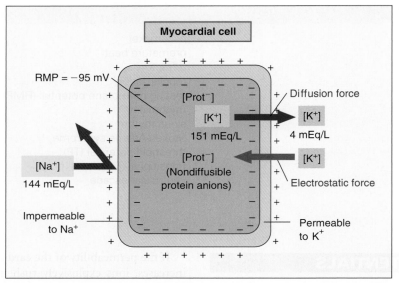

Figure 18-2 Potassium equilibrium potential. The outward diffusion force of potassium is in equilibrium with the inward electrostatic attraction exerted by nondiffusible protein anions.

outside the cell. A wire from each microelectrode is connected to a voltmeter, which measures the electrical potential difference across the membrane at about −90 mV.

The main ions involved in generating the RMP are sodium (Na⁺), potassium (K⁺), calcium (Ca⁺⁺), and large protein anions (negatively charged ions). As with all other cells in the body, K⁺ ion concentration inside the cardiac cell is much greater than outside the cell (about 151 mEq/L vs. 4 mEq/L).[2] The opposite is true for Na⁺ and Ca⁺⁺ ions; [Na⁺] is about 144 mEq/L outside the cell and about 7 mEq/L inside the cell, and [Ca⁺⁺] is 5 mEq/L outside the cell and less than 1 mEq/L inside the cell.

The resting cardiac cell membrane is fairly permeable to K⁺ ions but only slightly permeable to Na⁺ and Ca⁺⁺ ions. The permeability of the membrane to K⁺ allows potassium to diffuse out of the cell, down its high concentration gradient (Figure 18-2). Large, negatively charged protein ions and molecules cannot diffuse outward with K⁺ because the cell membrane is completely impermeable to them. Thus, as potassium leaves, an increasingly negative intracellular charge develops; this represents an electrostatic force that slows and eventually stops the outward diffusion of K⁺. The equilibrium between the outward diffusion force of K⁺ and the cell's electrostatic attractive force is largely responsible for the cardiac cell RMP, altered only slightly by Na⁺ ion diffusion dynamics, as explained next.

Although the cardiac cell membrane is highly impermeable to Na⁺, small amounts of this ion diffuse through leak channels into the cell because of its extremely high diffusion gradient (Figure 18-3).[1] This diffusion alters the potassium-driven membrane potential, causing it to be slightly less negative (closer to 0) than it would be otherwise. The Na⁺-K⁺ exchange pump in the cell membrane counteracts Na⁺ leakage into the cell by actively pumping it out while pumping potassium back in. Three Na⁺ ions are pumped out of the cell for every two

K⁺ ions pumped back in, adding to the electronegativity of the intracellular environment (see Figure 18-3). In the end, the RMP is the result of the complex interactions between (1) chemical diffusion forces, (2) electrostatic attractive forces, and (3) the Na⁺-K⁺ exchange pump.

CONCEPT QUESTION 18-1

Explain how high extracellular K⁺ concentration affects the RMP and heart muscle excitability.

ION CHANNELS AND GATES

Sodium and Potassium Channels

The permeability of the myocardial cell membrane to Na⁺ and K⁺ ions is mainly controlled by voltage-gated ion channels in the membrane (Figure 18-4). These channels are formed by large protein molecules and are specific for each ion. Gatelike structures called gating proteins control these channels. Gating proteins are voltage sensitive, opening and closing in response to changes in the membrane potential. Changes in membrane potential alter the shape of the protein molecule, which opens or closes the channel gates[2] (i.e., the membrane's permeability to K⁺ and Na⁺ is voltage dependent).

As shown in Figure 18-4, K⁺ and Na⁺ channel activation gates are closed at the cardiac cell's RMP of −90 mV. Although both of these channels are closed, some K⁺ and Na⁺ ions diffuse across the membrane through leak channels because of their high diffusion gradients.

Calcium Channels

In addition to the Na⁺ and K⁺ channels, cardiac fibers have numerous **calcium ion channels**. These channels are similar

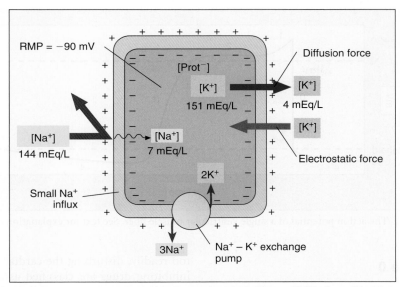

Figure 18-3 Generation of the RMP. The potassium equilibrium potential is altered by a small influx of Na$^+$ ions through leak channels and the unequal pumping of Na$^+$ and K$^+$ ions.

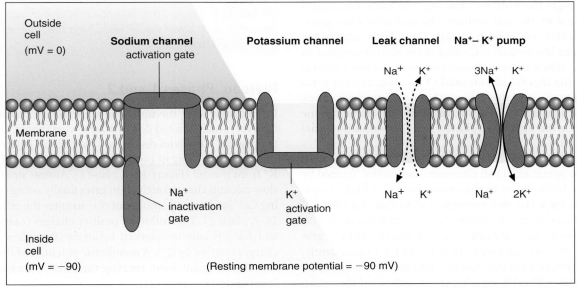

Figure 18-4 Selective sodium and potassium channels and voltage-sensitive gates. At rest, when the RMP equals −90 mV, Na$^+$ and K$^+$ gates are closed. The leak channel is about 100 times more permeable to K$^+$ than Na$^+$. The RMP of −90 mV is maintained by the balance between the outward diffusion force of the K$^+$ ion and intracellular electrostatic attractive forces plus the Na$^+$-K$^+$ pump activity.

to Na$^+$ channels in that they have activation and inactivation gates. However, calcium channel gates respond 10 to 20 times more slowly than sodium channel gates to changes in membrane potential.[1] Calcium channels are therefore called slow channels, whereas sodium channels are called fast channels. Although they mainly transmit Ca^{++} ions, calcium channels also permit the passage of some Na$^+$ ions. The responses of sodium, potassium, and calcium channels to changes in their membrane potentials bring about an event known as the **action potential**. The action potential is an electrical event ultimately leading to the mechanical event of muscle fiber contraction.

ACTION POTENTIAL

Cardiac muscle fiber **depolarization** occurs when the fiber RMP of −90 mV abruptly changes to 0 mV. **Repolarization** occurs when the RMP is again established at −90 mV. The action potential is a real-time recording of the moment-to-moment changes in the membrane potential as the cardiac fiber depolarizes and repolarizes. This recording plots voltage against time on specially designed graph paper or a monitoring screen. Figure 18-5 illustrates the action potential of a single ventricular muscle fiber. The different phases of the action potential (0 to 4) are created by Na$^+$, K$^+$, and Ca^{++} movement in and out of the cell.

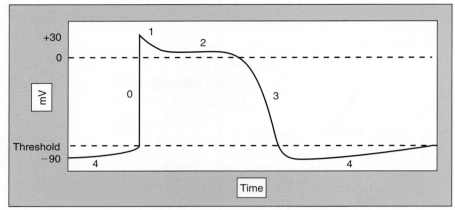

Figure 18-5 The action potential of a single ventricular muscle fiber. See text for explanation of phases.

Depolarization: Phase 0

The action potential of a ventricular muscle fiber (see Figure 18-5) is normally initiated by an electrical impulse originating from the sinoatrial (SA) node in the right atrium. The impulse changes the RMP to a less negative value that begins to open some of the fast sodium channel activation gates. Increased influx of sodium makes the fiber's membrane potential even less negative, causing more activation gates to swing open. When the membrane potential reaches a critical level called the **threshold potential (TP)**, all activation gates open instantaneously; this brings about an explosive influx of Na[+], which instantaneously depolarizes the cell membrane and generates the upstroke (phase 0) of the action potential (see Figure 18-5).

Two forces cause Na[+] ions to enter the cell during phase 0 of the action potential: (1) an electrostatic attraction created by the negative intracellular environment and (2) a high chemical diffusion force favoring movement of sodium into the cell (Figure 18-6, *A*). When the membrane potential reaches 0 mV, Na[+] continues to enter the cell because a strong diffusion gradient is still present (see Figure 18-6, *B* and *C*). Consequently, the cell membrane's polarity reverses (the membrane potential peaks at about +30 mV), creating the overshoot of the action potential (see Figures 18-5 and 18-6, *D*).

The rapid change in membrane potential from −90 mV to +30 mV causes the voltage-sensitive inactivation gates of the sodium channel to swing closed rapidly, stopping the influx of sodium (see Figure 18-6, *E*). These inactivation gates close only a few ten-thousandths of a second after the activation gates open—about the time the upstroke of the action potential reaches 0 mV, on its way to +30 mV.[1] The inactivation gates do not reopen until the original RMP is restored; thus, the heart muscle fiber first must repolarize before it can respond to another depolarizing stimulus. That is, the heart muscle fiber is **refractory** to depolarizing stimuli from phase 0 through the end of phase 3 of the action potential (see Figure 18-5).

Some cardiac drugs inhibit the opening of fast sodium channels, decreasing the membrane's susceptibility to depolarization. Such drugs are used when the membrane depolarizes too readily, disturbing the cardiac rhythm. Sodium channel–inhibiting drugs are classified as antiarrhythmic drugs (e.g., quinidine, amiodarone, and lidocaine).

CONCEPT QUESTION 18-2

Referring to Figure 18-5, do antiarrhythmic drugs raise (bring closer to 0) or lower the TP (assuming the RMP remains constant at −90 mV)?

Plateau: Phases 1 and 2

Immediately after the upstroke of the action potential (phase 0), a very small, limited downstroke occurs (phase 1) just before the plateau. This brief decline in intracellular positivity reflects the sudden opening of potassium channel gates and outflow of K[+] from the cell (Figure 18-7, *phase 1*). Almost simultaneously, slow calcium channel activation gates finally swing open, allowing Ca[++] and a small amount of Na[+] to enter the cell (see Figure 18-7, *phase 2*). This inflow of positive charges (carried by Ca[++] and Na[+]) is counterbalanced by an equal outflow of positive charges (carried by K[+]). A membrane potential of about 0 mV is thus briefly maintained, creating the action potential's plateau (see Figure 18-7, *phase 2*).

Compared with the depolarization phase (see Figure 18-7, *phase 0*), which lasts only a few ten-thousandths of a second, the plateau phase lasts for about 0.2 to 0.3 second.[1] Therefore, cardiac muscle contraction also lasts for this relatively long time, a property of cardiac muscle that enhances its pumping effectiveness.

Ca[++] ions entering the myocardial fiber during the plateau phase participate in the excitation-contraction coupling between actin and myosin fibers, as described in Chapter 17. Some drugs, such as digitalis, increase the intracellular level of Ca[++], which enhances myocardial contractility during this phase of the action potential. Drugs that increase contractility are called inotropic drugs.

The equilibrium between Ca[++] inflow and K[+] outflow during the plateau occurs in ventricular but not in atrial myocardial fibers. K[+] outflow exceeds Ca[++] inflow in atrial fibers, preventing the development of a plateau.[1]

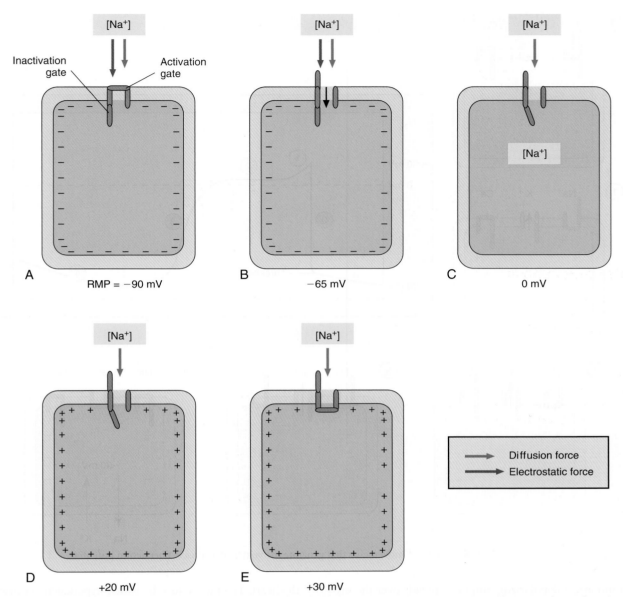

Figure 18-6 **A-E,** Sodium channel gating activity generating the upstroke (phase 0) of the action potential. See text for explanation.

Repolarization: Phase 3

The outflow of K+ ions gradually increases throughout the action potential plateau. The plateau phase ends when Ca++ inactivation gates close, stopping Ca++ inflow (see Figure 18-7, *phase 3*). The membrane is now highly permeable to only K+ ions. Intracellular negativity is rapidly restored to the resting level as K+ explosively rushes out of the cell, down its high diffusion gradient. After repolarization is complete and the RMP is restored, excess Na+ that entered the cell during phases 0 and 2 is pumped out by the Na+-K+ exchange pump. At the same time, K+ that exited the cell during phases 2 and 3 is pumped back into the cell, restoring the original Na+ and K+ concentrations inside and outside the cell (see Figure 18-7, *phase 4*). The muscle fiber is then ready to accept another depolarizing stimulus. Box 18-1 summarizes the events causing the action potential.

Action Potential Propagation

Depolarization of a specific point on a cardiac fiber membrane opens sodium channels at that point. Positive electrical charges carried by the inflow of Na+ ions decrease the intracellular negativity immediately adjacent to the point of entry, bringing these areas to their threshold potentials. Sodium channels in these areas immediately open, allowing more Na+ to rush in. This new incoming Na+ brings areas farther along the fiber to their threshold potentials, and so on, instantaneously spreading the action potential along the fiber. The inflow of positively charged Na+ ions leaves a relatively negative charge on the outside fiber surface. Thus, the action potential spreads as a wave of electronegativity across the surface of the depolarizing fiber membrane (Figure 18-8). This electronegative wave is called an electrical impulse, which can be detected on the body's surface with a special instrument called an **electrocardiograph**.

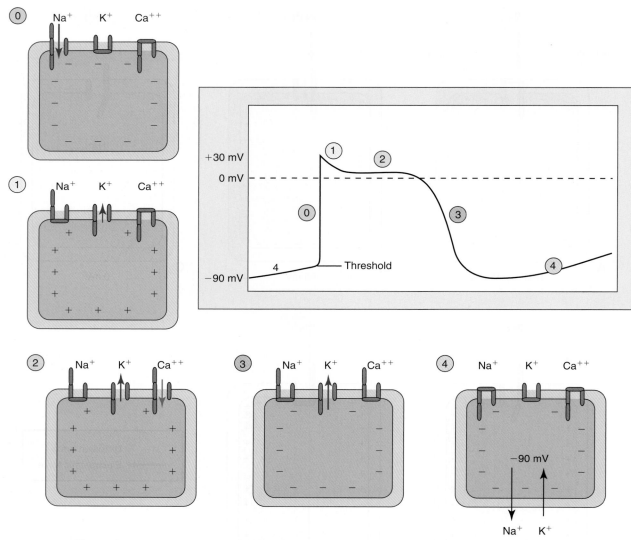

Figure 18-7 Na$^+$, K$^+$, and Ca^{++} movements that generate the ventricular muscle fiber action potential.

In summary, a depolarizing impulse spreads over the myocardial surface and deep into the fiber through the T-tubules (see Chapter 17). This impulse ultimately opens calcium channels, allowing Ca^{++} to enter the fiber and catalyze the excitation-contraction coupling of actin and myosin myofibrils. The mechanical muscle contraction event occurs only a few milliseconds after muscle fiber depolarization.

EFFECTS OF DRUGS AND EXTRACELLULAR ION CONCENTRATION ON THE ACTION POTENTIAL

Extracellular Ions

Potassium

An excess of potassium ions (hyperkalemia) in the extracellular fluid surrounding cardiac fibers decreases the heart rate and stroke volume. Severe hyperkalemia causes heart block, or the inability of cardiac fibers to conduct action potentials through the heart. The mechanism by which hyperkalemia causes these effects is illustrated in Figure 18-9.

As mentioned previously, K$^+$ diffusion out of the cell down its concentration gradient is primarily responsible for generating RMP (see Figure 18-2). High extracellular [K$^+$] diminishes the outward diffusion gradient of K$^+$. As a result, a smaller degree of intracellular electronegativity develops when potassium diffuses out of the cell. This means that the RMP across the cell membrane is less negative (closer to 0) and closer to the TP (see Figure 18-9). Hyperkalemia thus has a depolarizing influence on the membrane, making it more excitable (easier to depolarize). Excitability is defined as the difference between the RMP and the TP; the less the difference, the more excitable the membrane.[3]

Besides making the RMP less electronegative, hyperkalemia reduces the amplitude (strength) of the action potential, decreasing its rate of conduction along muscle fibers, which explains why hyperkalemia decreases the heart rate. The decreased action potential amplitude also reduces the amount of Ca^{++} that enters the muscle fiber during depolarization,

Generation of the Ventricular Fiber Action Potential

1. The SA nodal impulse changes the RMP to a less negative value.
2. Some fast Na⁺ channel gates respond by opening.
3. Na⁺ moves into the cell, bringing the RMP to the threshold.
4. At the threshold, all Na⁺ channels open; Na⁺ explosively rushes into the cell, depolarizing the membrane.

Repolarization

1. K⁺ and Ca⁺⁺ channel gates respond to depolarization by opening.
2. Ca⁺⁺ inflow equals K⁺ outflow, maintaining a plateau membrane potential of about 0 mV for 0.2 to 0.3 second.
3. Ca⁺⁺ channel inactivation gates close, stopping Ca⁺⁺ inflow.
4. Explosive outflow of K⁺ rapidly repolarizes the membrane.
5. Na⁺-K⁺ exchange pump restores prepotential ionic distribution.
6. Fiber is now ready to accept another depolarizing stimulus.

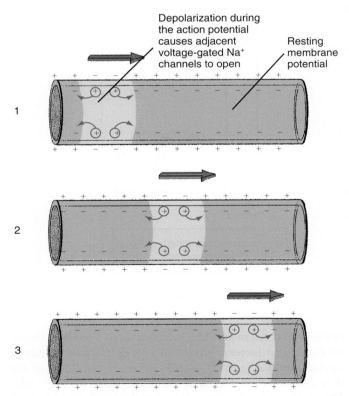

Figure 18-8 Propagation of the action potential along the cardiac fiber. (From Thibodeau GA, Patton KT: *Anatomy & physiology*, ed 3, St Louis, 1996, Mosby.)

which decreases ventricular contraction force and stroke volume. Severe hyperkalemia may depolarize the membrane to the extent that its resting potential is less (closer to 0) than its TP.[3] In this case, the muscle fiber is unable to repolarize after a single action potential and is no longer excitable (i.e., the fiber is in a continual state of depolarization). This leads to cardiac muscle paralysis and is why hyperkalemia may cause heart block.

Conversely, hypokalemia increases the diffusion gradient for K⁺ movement out of the cell, creating a greater intracellular electronegativity than normal. As a result, the RMP is lower than normal, hyperpolarizing the membrane (see Figure 18-9); this makes the membrane less excitable or less sensitive to depolarizing stimuli. In severe hypokalemia, the heart muscle may fail to depolarize, resulting in flaccid paralysis (cardiac arrest).[3] Hypokalemia may decrease the heart rate because a longer time is required for the membrane to depolarize to its threshold level. The muscle contraction force is not affected in this instance because adequate amounts of Ca⁺⁺ enter the cell during the action potential.

Calcium

Ca⁺⁺ entry into cardiac fibers during the plateau phase of the action potential is essential for muscle contraction (see Chapter 17). Generally, the heart muscle contractile force is directly related to extracellular [Ca⁺⁺].

Calcium ions affect membrane excitability by changing the TP rather than the RMP. This phenomenon is explained by the effect of Ca⁺⁺ on sodium channel activation. When extracellular [Ca⁺⁺] is low (hypocalcemia), an extremely small amount of membrane depolarization above the resting potential opens the sodium channels. In other words, hypocalcemia brings the threshold at which Na⁺ activation gates open closer to the RMP. For example, rather than opening at a normal TP of −65 mV, Na⁺ gates open at −75 mV, a value much closer to the −90-mV RMP (Figure 18-10). Thus, hypocalcemia increases heart muscle excitability, causing an effect similar to hyperkalemia. Apparently, Ca⁺⁺ ions bind to sodium channel protein molecules, increasing the amount of membrane depolarization that must occur to open the gate. Therefore, low extracellular [Ca⁺⁺] allows the gate to open with an extremely small degree of membrane depolarization.[1]

Conversely, hypercalcemia decreases membrane excitability because it raises the TP, requiring a greater amount of membrane depolarization to open the Na⁺ gates (see Figure 18-10). Because of its direct effect on the muscle contractile process, extremely high [Ca⁺⁺] can cause the heart to develop repetitive, spastic contractions. Because blood [Ca⁺⁺] is regulated within extremely narrow ranges, calcium-induced cardiac abnormalities are rarely a clinical concern.[1] However, administering Ca⁺⁺ to treat severe hyperkalemia may be clinically beneficial because doing so counteracts the effect of hyperkalemia on membrane excitability.[3]

Sodium

Changes in extracellular [Na⁺] have little effect on the RMP of cardiac muscle because the membrane is highly impermeable to Na⁺. Therefore, abnormal depolarization is rarely related to abnormal extracellular [Na⁺].

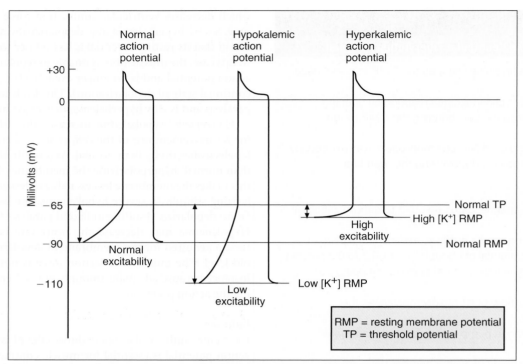

Figure 18-9 Effect of extracellular potassium concentration on RMP and excitability. The closer the RMP is to the TP, the more excitable is the muscle fiber membrane.

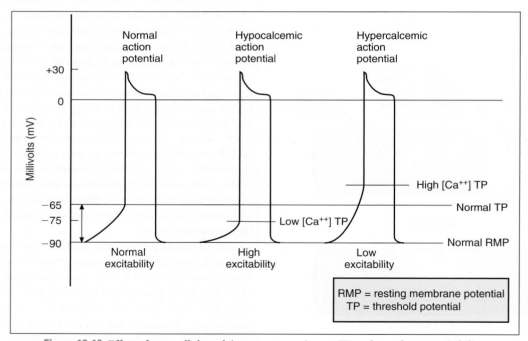

Figure 18-10 Effect of extracellular calcium concentration on TP and membrane excitability.

Drugs Affecting the Action Potential

Catecholamines

Catecholamines are compounds with chemical structures similar to epinephrine and norepinephrine. Such drugs increase the influx of Ca^{++} into the myocardial cell during the plateau phase of the action potential. Catecholamines activate beta receptors in the cardiac cell membrane, bringing about a series of chemical events that increase intracellular levels of cyclic adenosine monophosphate (cAMP). cAMP enhances activation of the slow calcium channels, augmenting the influx of Ca^{++} ions. This is the main mechanism by which catecholamine drugs increase cardiac muscle contractility.[2] Sympathetic nervous activity raises heart muscle contractility by the same mechanism because it raises adrenal secretion of epinephrine into the circulation.

Beta-blocking drugs such as propranolol compete with catecholamines for beta-receptor sites and thus reduce cardiac contractility and the heart rate. These drugs are sometimes given to control abnormally high heart rates or to reduce cardiac work and oxygen consumption. Beta blockers also decrease vascular smooth muscle tone and are sometimes used to treat high blood pressure.

As mentioned previously, digitalis increases contractility by increasing calcium stores in the cardiac fiber. Digitalis is sometimes given to patients with congestive heart failure to improve contractility and pumping effectiveness.

Calcium Channel Blockers

As the name implies, calcium channel–blocking drugs block the calcium channel, decreasing the entry of Ca^{++} into the cell during muscle contraction (plateau phase of the action potential). These drugs are also known as slow channel blockers or calcium antagonists. As expected, their main effect is to decrease the muscle's contractile force, reducing the heart's stroke volume. This effect may be beneficial in coronary artery disease, in which the blood and oxygen supply to the myocardium is impaired. Decreased contractility requires less oxygen consumption by the heart muscle. Calcium antagonists also decrease smooth vascular muscle contraction and are widely used as coronary vasodilators to improve coronary circulation. They are also used to treat systemic hypertension. Examples of these drugs include verapamil, nifedipine, diltiazem, and nicardipine.

RHYTHMIC EXCITATION OF THE HEART

Automatic Rhythmicity of the Cardiac Fibers

Although sympathetic and parasympathetic nerves innervate the heart, cardiac function does not require intact nervous pathways. A clinical example is a patient with a cardiac transplant whose heart is completely denervated but functions normally and adapts to stress appropriately. The heart can continue to beat even when removed from the body if it is appropriately nourished by artificial means. All cardiac tissue has properties of (1) **automaticity** (the ability to depolarize spontaneously), (2) **rhythmicity** (the ability to depolarize spontaneously in a repetitive manner), (3) **excitability** (the inclination to depolarize spontaneously), and (4) **contractility** (the ability to shorten muscle fibers).

Pacemaker Function of the Sinus Node

The cardiac tissue that generates the greatest frequency of impulses is the SA node in the right atrium because it is the most excitable tissue; this makes the SA node the heart's natural **pacemaker**. Although every other cardiac cell is a potential pacemaker, none can initiate depolarization because the SA node impulse depolarizes them first before they can reach their threshold potentials.

CONCEPT QUESTION 18-3

What happens if the SA node fails to generate any impulses in an otherwise healthy heart?

The RMP of sinus node fibers is only about −55 mV compared with −90 mV of ventricular fibers (Figure 18-11).[1] Sinus node tissue is naturally leakier than ventricular fibers to sodium ions; hence, its intracellular environment is less negative. In addition, the RMP of the SA node is closer to its TP than other heart muscle; its threshold is about −40 mV, creating an RMP-TP difference of about 15 mV. In contrast, ventricular muscle RMP and TP are about −90 mV and −65 mV, for an RMP-TP difference of about 25 mV. Thus, the ventricles require more time than the SA node to reach the TP (see Figure 18-11). Hence, the SA node sets the pace and suppresses all other cardiac cell pacemaker tendencies.

Sinus Node Self-Excitation

Figure 18-11 illustrates the sinus node's gradually rising RMP caused by the slow leak of Na^+ into the cell. When its threshold of −40 mV is reached, the SA node fires (depolarizes), initiating an impulse that spreads to all heart muscle over the specialized conduction system. As soon as repolarization is achieved, RMP immediately begins to decay again toward the TP, causing the cycle to repeat itself at regular intervals. The heart rate pattern established by the SA node is known as **sinus rhythm** and is normally about 70 to 80 beats per minute.[1]

Ectopic Beats

If the sinus node fails to discharge its impulses, the next most excitable myocardial cell spontaneously depolarizes and initiates the heartbeat at a lower rate. Alternatively, if the sinus node is functioning properly but another area in the heart muscle becomes irritated (e.g., hypoxic) and develops an abnormal RMP, it may depolarize sooner than the sinus node and initiate a premature heartbeat. Both of these situations represent **ectopic beats**. The term ectopic means the impulse originated from an area outside of the sinus node. The point from which such an impulse originates is known as an **ectopic focus**. Ectopic foci may become ectopic pacemakers if (1) they become more excitable or irritable than the SA fibers, (2) the SA node fails to initiate the impulse, or (3) conduction pathways between ectopic foci and the SA node become blocked.

Premature Beat

A **premature beat** occurs early between otherwise evenly spaced, sinus-generated beats. A premature beat is evidence that an ectopic focus has fired. In other words, an ectopic focus can initiate a beat prematurely only if it depolarizes more rapidly than the SA node. Factors that may produce such premature beats include (1) local areas of tissue hypoxia (ischemia); (2) mechanical irritation produced by calcified plaque in a diseased heart; and (3) toxic irritation caused by nicotine,

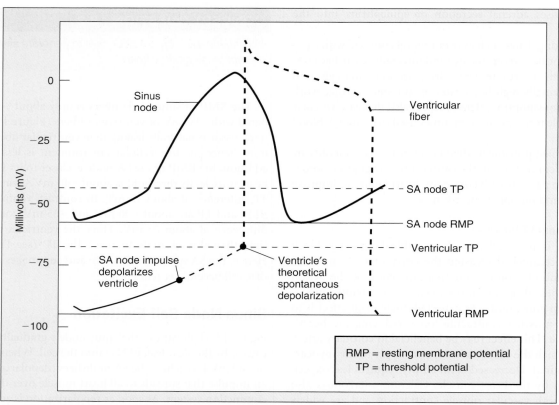

Figure 18-11 Pacemaker function of the SA node. Because the RMP of the SA node is closer to its TP, its fibers depolarize sooner than ventricular fibers. The SA node is the dominant pacemaker because its impulses depolarize other pacemaker cells before they can reach their thresholds.

caffeine, or other drugs.[1] All of these factors cause the heart muscle to become more excitable and more susceptible to depolarization.

CONCEPT QUESTION 18-4

Does an atrial ectopic focus acting as the heart's pacemaker have a greater firing rate than the SA node?

Downward Displacement of the Pacemaker

All cells in the cardiac conduction system are potential pacemakers, but not all have the same spontaneous depolarization rate. Lower order pacemakers (pacemakers with spontaneous depolarization rates lower than the SA node) normally cannot pace the heartbeat because the rapidly firing SA node suppresses them. If the SA node suddenly stops firing, lower order pacemaker cells begin to fire after a few seconds' pause. This brief pause is known as overdrive suppression. When lower order pacemaker cells are driven at high frequencies, their automaticity is temporarily depressed. These pacemaker cells remain inactive for a few seconds after the SA node stops firing and then establish a new, lower firing rate. The takeover of pacemaking activity by lower order pacemakers is known as downward displacement of the pacemaker.

After the SA node, the atrioventricular (AV) nodal fibers have the next highest spontaneous depolarization rate. If not stimulated from some outside source, AV fibers fire at a rate of 40 to 60 times per minute. If AV impulses fail to reach the ventricles after several seconds, the Purkinje fibers begin to fire at a rate of 15 to 40 times per minute.[1] These rates contrast with the intrinsic SA nodal rate of 70 to 80 beats per minute.

Lower order pacemakers not only fire at lower rates, they also tend to be more unreliable than the SA node. Ventricular pacemakers are especially unstable in this regard. If impulses from atria are totally blocked, the Purkinje cells may pause for 30 seconds before establishing a rate of 15 to 40 beats per minute. During this pause, there is no cardiac output, and the person may faint from lack of blood flow to the brain. This delayed ventricular takeover of the heartbeat is known as **Stokes-Adams syndrome**.[1]

TRANSMISSION OF IMPULSES THROUGH THE HEART

Atrial Transmission

The cardiac conduction system anatomy is discussed in Chapter 17. From the SA node, the depolarizing impulse spreads rapidly over atrial muscle to the AV node. The impulse is preferentially conducted along three specialized **internodal pathways** that eventually converge at the AV node.[1] One of these pathways, **Bachmann's bundle**, conducts SA nodal impulses directly to the left atrium (Figure 18-12). The impulse velocity over these specialized conductive pathways is about 1 m per second compared with 0.3 m per second over other atrial muscle.[1]

CLINICAL FOCUS 18-1

Clinical Benefits of Using Drugs to Alter Electrophysiological Events

Drugs that alter electrophysiological events in the heart often benefit patients with atherosclerotic heart disease. In this disease, abnormal fatty substances (atheroma) build up under the endothelium of coronary arteries, partially occluding them. As a result, blood flow may not meet the heart's oxygen requirements, creating myocardial ischemia and its associated pain, angina pectoris. Lack of oxygen causes myocardial irritability, increasing the chances that tachycardia and dangerous ectopic rhythms may develop. Complete lack of oxygen for a sustained period may cause a myocardial infarction (MI), an area of dead heart tissue, especially if myocardial work increases. Antianginal and antiarrhythmic drugs are beneficial in these patients.

Antiarrhythmic drugs decrease the irritability of ectopic foci, allowing normal SA nodal pacing. In this group of drugs, lidocaine (Xylocaine) and amiodarone (Cordarone) block Na^+ channels, decreasing the membrane's tendency to depolarize. Beta-receptor blockers such as carvedilol (Coreg) and bisoprolol (Zebeta) depress the myocardium's automaticity,

decreasing tachycardia and myocardial work. Calcium channel blockers such as amlodipine (Norvasc) and diltiazem (Cardizem) inhibit slow channel influx of Ca^{++} in the SA node and other myocardial cells. This inhibition depresses atrial automaticity, slows AV conduction velocity, and decreases myocardial contractility.

Calcium channel blockers also inhibit Ca^{++} entry into vascular smooth muscle, dilating coronary and systemic vessels. Systemic vascular resistance is lowered, allowing the heart to sustain an adequate cardiac output despite its reduced contractility. By decreasing myocardial contractility, Ca^{++} channel blockers reduce the heart's oxygen requirements, decreasing the chances for developing an MI. Because of their coronary vasodilating properties, these drugs improve blood and oxygen supply to the myocardium, further decreasing the potential for MI. Calcium channel blockers are thus also classified as antiarrhythmic and antianginal drugs. Other antianginal drugs include nitrates, such as nitroglycerin. These drugs dilate coronary arteries by releasing nitric oxide in vascular smooth muscle.

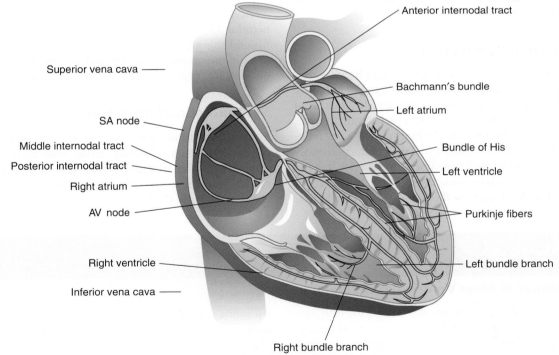

Figure 18-12 The heart's specialized conductive tissues.

CONCEPT QUESTION 18-5

Extremely rapid heart rates decrease the ventricular filling time. Besides being more rapid, how does this change the character of the pulse palpated at the radial artery?

Atrioventricular Conduction

If the SA nodal impulse was immediately conducted into the ventricles, ventricular contraction would begin before the atria have time to fill them with blood. The AV node delays impulse conduction enough to allow adequate ventricular filling time.

The AV node is located in the septal wall of the right atrium, just behind the tricuspid valve. The SA node impulse travels across atrial muscle to the AV node in about 0.03 second; however, the impulse does not emerge from the AV node for another 0.13 second.[1] About one fourth of the total delay occurs in the **transitional (junctional) fibers** (extremely small fibers connecting atrial muscle to nodal fibers). The conduction velocity in junctional fibers is about one twelfth of the velocity in normal cardiac muscle.[1] Nodal resistance to conduction is not quite as high as junctional resistance but is still greater than that for other heart muscle.

The AV bundle, also known as the bundle of His (see Figure 18-12), is the penetrating portion of the AV nodal system. It penetrates the fibrous cardiac skeleton and is the only electrically conductive connection between atrial and ventricular muscle masses. This penetrating portion of the bundle also has greater electrical resistance than regular cardiac muscle. A unique feature of the AV bundle is its one-way conduction from atria to ventricles. Ventricular impulses cannot be conducted backward through the bundle to the atria; this prevents reentry of the cardiac impulse back to the atria.

In summary, the AV nodal system consists of (1) junctional (transitional) fibers, (2) the node proper, and (3) the AV bundle (bundle of His). After they are depolarized, AV nodal fibers require a longer time to repolarize than any other cardiac fiber. The AV node is refractory to depolarizing stimuli longer than any other cardiac fiber.

Purkinje System Conduction

After it penetrates the fibrous cardiac skeleton, the AV bundle enters the intraventricular septum and divides into left and right bundle branches (see Figure 18-12). At the heart's apex, smaller branches of each bundle spread throughout the ventricles back toward the base. These Purkinje fibers penetrate into the heart muscle a few millimeters and fuse with other ventricular muscle. Conduction velocity is greatly accelerated through these fibers (about 1.5 to 4 m per second). Ventricular muscle is almost instantly depolarized; about 0.03 second elapses from the time the impulse enters the bundle branches until it reaches the terminal Purkinje fibers. Conduction velocity through other ventricular muscle is only about one sixth the conduction velocity of the Purkinje fibers (0.3 to 0.5 m per second); only about 0.06 second is required for impulse transmission from bundle branches to the last ventricular muscle fiber. The total time required for impulse transmission from the SA node to the last ventricular fiber is normally about 0.22 second.[1]

This uniform and rapid ventricular conduction is physiologically important for coordinated, synchronized contraction and relaxation. Synchronized ventricular action is necessary for normal cardiac output and ventricular filling.

ROLE OF SYMPATHETIC AND PARASYMPATHETIC NERVOUS CONTROL

Parasympathetic stimulation releases acetylcholine from postganglionic nerve endings. This decreases (1) SA nodal firing rate and (2) AV nodal fiber excitability, reducing the heart rate and slowing the conduction of atrial impulses to the ventricles. Strong vagal stimulation can totally block AV conduction or completely stop SA nodal firing.[1] However, if this state persists, the ventricular Purkinje system takes over the pacemaker function, producing a slow rate of 15 to 40 beats per minute. Such ventricular takeover is called **ventricular escape** (i.e., the ventricles escape the dominance of the SA node).

Acetylcholine (from vagal stimulation) greatly increases K^+ permeability of the cardiac fiber, allowing rapid outward K^+ diffusion;[1] this greatly increases intracellular negativity, hyperpolarizing the cardiac membrane and making depolarization more difficult. This explains why vagal stimulation causes AV heart block.

Sympathetic Stimulation

Sympathetic stimulation increases the SA nodal firing rate, conduction rate, and overall cardiac fiber excitability. This is explained by the fact that sympathetic postganglionic fibers release norepinephrine, which increases cardiac fiber permeability to Na^+ and Ca^{++}.[1]

CLINICAL FOCUS 18-2

Clinical Danger of Slow Ventricular Conduction Time

In normal ventricular depolarization, the cardiac impulse dies out after it travels through the ventricles because all ventricular muscle fibers are refractory and cannot conduct the impulse further. When the ventricular conduction time is abnormally slow, this normal dying out of the impulse may not occur. Heart muscle fibers tend to be arranged in a circular fashion as they wrap around their chambers. An impulse initiated at one point may travel in a circular path and end up in the vicinity of its origin. When the conduction velocity is abnormally slow, the impulse may reenter its point of origin if that area of the heart has already repolarized. In such instances, impulses are propagated through the same pathways repeatedly in a pattern described as circus movement. This circus reentry phenomenon is one of the causes of ventricular fibrillation, a pattern of uncoordinated, ineffective ventricular twitching. When they fibrillate, the ventricles have no effective pumping action, and cardiac output ceases, causing death in minutes. Besides slow conduction time, a lengthened conduction pathway (dilated, enlarged heart) or a shortened refractory time (various drug effects) also may create the circus reentry phenomenon. (See Chapter 19 for a detailed discussion of this lethal arrhythmia.)

POINTS TO REMEMBER

- Differences in ion concentrations immediately inside and outside the cardiac cell membrane create an electrical charge difference called the resting membrane potential (RMP).
- Because the cell membrane is impermeable to negatively charged intracellular protein ions, the outward diffusion of potassium down its concentration gradient creates a negatively charged cell interior, a polarized membrane, and a negative RMP.
- The slow leak of Na^+ ions into the cardiac cell changes the transmembrane voltage, which opens Na^+ channel gates and rapidly depolarizes the cell membrane.
- The closer the RMP of a cardiac cell is to its TP, the greater is its tendency to depolarize (the greater is its excitability).
- Ca^{++} channels open and Ca^{++} ions enter the cell immediately after the Na^+ ion influx depolarizes the cell membrane; Ca^{++} ions catalyze actin-myosin interaction and bring about muscle contraction.
- The depolarization of a single cardiac fiber depolarizes all cardiac fibers ("all-or-none" principle).
- Depolarization of the heart muscle is associated with contraction; repolarization is associated with relaxation.
- Cardiac drugs bring about their effects by blocking ion channels, by blocking or stimulating autonomic neural receptors, or by changing the RMP or the TP.
- Extracellular potassium and calcium ion concentrations affect the RMP and TP and depolarization characteristics of the cardiac fiber.
- The SA node of the heart depolarizes spontaneously and cyclically faster than any other cardiac fibers; thus the SA node is the heart's normal pacemaker.
- Any pacemaker other than the SA node is an ectopic pacemaker.
- Ectopic pacemakers may arise if the SA node is suppressed or other foci become more excitable than the SA node.
- Premature atrial or ventricular contractions are the result of ectopic foci.
- The slight delay of the cardiac impulse at the AV node normally allows adequate ventricular filling time.
- Parasympathetic stimulation slows the heart rate and contraction force, whereas sympathetic stimulation has the opposite effect.

References

1. Hall JE: *Guyton and Hall textbook of medical physiology*, ed 12, Philadelphia, 2011, Saunders.
2. Rubart M, Zipes DP: Genesis of cardiac arrhythmias: electrophysiological considerations. In Bonow RO, et al, editors: *Braunwald's heart disease: a textbook of cardiovascular medicine*, ed 9, Philadelphia, 2011, Saunders.
3. Rose BD, Post T, Rose B: *Clinical physiology of acid-base and electrolyte disorders*, ed 5, New York, 2001, McGraw-Hill.

CHAPTER 19

The Electrocardiogram and Cardiac Arrhythmias in Adults

CHAPTER OUTLINE

I. Normal Electrocardiogram
- A. Electrocardiogram Components
  - 1. Waves and Complexes
  - 2. Intervals and Segments
- B. Positive and Negative Electrocardiogram Deflections
  - 1. Lead Axis and Current Flow
- C. Electrocardiogram Graph Paper

II. Electrocardiogram Leads
- A. Standard Bipolar Limb Leads: Einthoven's Triangle
- B. Standard Unipolar Limb Leads
- C. Precordial (Chest) Leads
- D. Hexaxial Reference Figure

III. Locating the Heart's Electrical Axis
- A. Determinants of the Electrical Axis
- B. Easy Method for Determining the Electrical Axis
  - 1. Using Leads I and aV_F to Determine the Cardiac Axis

IV. Identifying Common Cardiac Arrhythmias
- A. Systematic Electrocardiogram Analysis
  - 1. Step One
  - 2. Step Two
  - 3. Step Three
  - 4. Step Four
- B. Normal Sinus Rhythm
- C. Abnormal Sinus Rhythms
  - 1. Tachycardia
  - 2. Bradycardia
  - 3. Sinus Arrhythmia
- D. Premature Atrial Contraction
- E. Supraventricular Arrhythmias
  - 1. Atrial Flutter
  - 2. Atrial Fibrillation
- F. Junctional Arrhythmias
- G. Ventricular Arrhythmias
  - 1. Premature Ventricular Contractions
  - 2. Ventricular Tachycardia
  - 3. Ventricular Fibrillation
  - 4. Circus Reentry in Ventricular Fibrillation
- H. Atrioventricular Conduction Blocks

V. Points to Remember

OBJECTIVES

After reading this chapter you will be able to:
- Explain how the components of the electrocardiogram (ECG) relate to the electrical and mechanical activity of the heart
- Explain how heart muscle mass affects ECG amplitude
- Identify factors that determine the QRS complex polarity (positivity or negativity)
- Describe how each of the 12 ECG leads is configured with respect to the heart and the hexaxial reference system
- Explain how the QRS complex recorded in different ECG leads is used to determine the mean direction of current flow (electrical axis) in the heart
- Explain why cardiac electrical axis abnormalities are correlated with certain physiological abnormalities
- Calculate the heart rate from an ECG recording
- Identify ECG characteristics of common cardiac arrhythmias
- Describe the physiological basis for common cardiac arrhythmias
- Discuss the treatment focus for various cardiac arrhythmias

KEY TERMS

atrial fibrillation
atrial flutter
axis deviation
bigeminy
bipolar leads
circus movement (circus reentry)
defibrillation
Einthoven's triangle

NORMAL ELECTROCARDIOGRAM

The action potentials conducted through myocardial fibers during depolarization produce small electrical currents that can be detected at the body's surface with the aid of proper equipment. As the heart depolarizes, the current flows from depolarized to polarized regions.[1] Because a depolarized membrane is negatively charged on the outside with respect to the inside, the depolarization impulse sweeps over the surface of myocardial fibers as a wave of electronegativity. Figure 19-1 illustrates the depolarization wave and current flow of a depolarizing, contracting fiber. (The current flows from negatively to positively charged regions.)

Electrodes placed on the skin and attached to a specialized voltmeter, known as an electrocardiograph, can detect small voltage changes as the heart depolarizes and repolarizes. This device reflects the summation of all action potentials conducted through millions of myocardial fibers during the cardiac cycle. This summated recording is called the **electrocardiogram (ECG)**, which is simply a graphic recording of voltage plotted against time during myocardial depolarization and repolarization (Figure 19-2). The ECG may be traced on specialized graph paper or displayed on an LCD monitoring screen.

The electrodes used to record the ECG are called leads. ECG leads may be placed directly on the chest surface or attached to the arms and legs—hence the terms chest leads and limb leads. The placement of leads in different positions allows the heart's electrical activity to be monitored from several different vantage points. The ECG reflects only electrical events; it does not reflect mechanical events or contraction force, although contractions are initiated by electrical events in the heart. The ECG is an extremely valuable diagnostic tool for detecting cardiac abnormalities. From the ECG, it is possible to detect abnormal

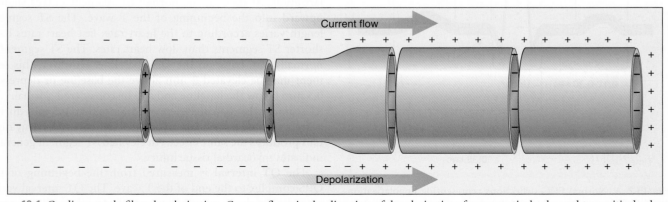

Figure 19-1 Cardiac muscle fiber depolarization. Current flows in the direction of depolarization, from negatively charged to positively charged areas.

heart rhythms, conduction problems, and the location of damaged heart muscle.

Electrocardiogram Components

Waves and Complexes

The ECG consists of waves and complexes plotted as voltage on the vertical axis and time on the horizontal axis (see Figure 19-2).

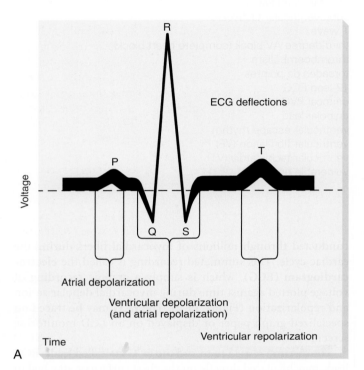

A

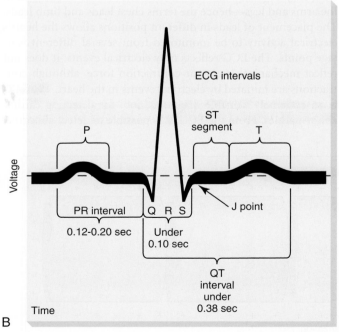

B

Figure 19-2 **A,** Normal ECG deflections representing depolarization and repolarization. **B,** Normal ECG time intervals. (From Thibodeau GA, Patton KT: *Anatomy & physiology,* ed 3, St Louis, 1996, Mosby.)

The spaces between waves and complexes are called intervals and segments. The **P wave** (see Figure 19-2, *A*) is produced as a result of atrial depolarization. The mechanical event of atrial contraction normally follows a fraction of a second after the P wave appears.

The **QRS complex**, produced by ventricular depolarization, is composed of three separate waves: the Q, R, and S waves. The first small downward (negative) deflection from the baseline that occurs after the P wave is called the Q wave, the next tall upward (positive) deflection is the R wave, and the following small negative deflection is called the S wave. The QRS complex may not always possess Q or S waves, depending on the lead from which it is recorded. The QRS complex represents the electrical events associated with ventricular contraction (systole).

The **T wave** is produced by ventricular repolarization and is associated with ventricular relaxation (diastole). The atria also have a repolarization wave, but it is hidden by the QRS complex.

Height, or amplitude, on the ECG represents voltage. Because the ventricular muscle mass is much greater than the atrial muscle mass, ventricles generate a much greater voltage when they depolarize. (Notice the difference in height between the P wave and QRS complex.) The amplitude of waves and complexes is related to the muscle mass involved.

Intervals and Segments

Figure 19-2, *B*, illustrates various ECG time intervals and segments. The **PR interval** is the time required for the sinus node impulse to reach the ventricles. It is measured from the beginning of the P wave to the next deflection, whether it is a Q or an R wave. The average adult PR interval is between 0.12 second and 0.20 second; a PR interval greater than 0.20 second indicates abnormally slowed impulse conduction from atria to ventricles. The PR interval is normally shorter in fast heart rates than in slow heart rates.

The adult QRS complex lasts on average about 0.08 to 0.10 second. QRS width represents ventricular depolarization time and is measured from the point at which the tracing leaves the baseline to the point at which it returns to baseline (see Figure 19-2, *B*). This point of return is called the **J point**.

The ST segment extends from the J point to the beginning of the T wave and represents the early phase of ventricular repolarization. At its end, the normal ST segment curves slightly upward into the beginning of the T wave. The ST segment length varies according to the heart rate; fast heart rates have shorter ST segments than slow heart rates. The ST segment is normally flat, lying on the ECG baseline. However, this segment may be elevated 2 mm above the baseline or depressed 0.5 mm below the baseline and still be considered normal.[2] An ST segment that becomes depressed more than 0.5 mm during a stress exercise test signals myocardial ischemia. The drug digitalis produces the same effect. An elevated ST segment generally indicates myocardial tissue injury.[3]

The **QT interval** is measured from the beginning of the QRS complex to the end of the T wave. The QT interval varies according to the heart rate but is usually less than 0.40 second.[1] It represents the general refractory period of the ventricles.

During this time, the ventricles generally cannot accept another depolarizing stimulus. However, as repolarization progresses, some of the ventricular muscle fibers are repolarized, while other fibers are still depolarized. This represents a **vulnerable period** during which part of the heart can respond to an additional stimulus and part of it cannot. The most vulnerable period is located at about the peak of the T wave and is sometimes called the **relative refractory period** of the heart. A depolarizing stimulus during this vulnerable time can create electrical chaos in the heart, rendering it quivering (fibrillating) and unable to pump blood. A prolonged QT interval is associated with life-threatening fibrillation because it is associated with a longer vulnerable period.[2]

CONCEPT QUESTION 19-1

What does a high-amplitude P wave indicate about atrial muscle mass, and what condition might be the cause of this abnormality?

Positive and Negative Electrocardiogram Deflections

ECG leads consist either of two opposite polarity electrodes (one positive and the other negative) or one positive electrode and a reference (ground) electrode. Leads composed of two opposite polarity electrodes are known as **bipolar leads**. A single positive electrode and its reference point are known as a **unipolar lead**.

The heart depolarizes in a base-to-apex direction (i.e., from atria to ventricles); the electrical current generated by depolarization flows in the same direction. Current flowing toward a lead's positive electrode generates a positive, or upward, deflection on the ECG. Conversely, current flowing away from a positive electrode generates a negative, or downward, deflection.

Lead Axis and Current Flow

An imaginary straight line between the positive and negative electrodes of a bipolar lead is defined as the lead axis. Similarly, an imaginary line between a unipolar lead's positive electrode and the center of the heart is the unipolar lead's axis. In Figure 19-3, a myocardial depolarization current flowing at right angles to a lead's axis generates an equiphasic or isoelectric deflection on the ECG monitored by the unipolar lead. Current flowing parallel to a lead's axis generates a strongly negative or positive ECG deflection, depending on whether the current flows toward or away from the positive electrode; this is illustrated by the bipolar lead in Figure 19-3. Figure 19-4 illustrates the range of ECG deflection possibilities, depending on the direction of current flow relative to the lead's axis.

The heart's **electrical axis** refers to the average direction of current flow in the heart. The heavy arrow in the heart in Figure 19-3 is the heart's electrical axis. The length of this arrow is proportional to the current's intensity and is called a vector because it has direction and magnitude. For this reason, the average direction of current flow in the heart is commonly called the **mean cardiac vector** (**MCV**).

CONCEPT QUESTION 19-2

In what way would you expect an increased right ventricular muscle mass to affect the MCV?

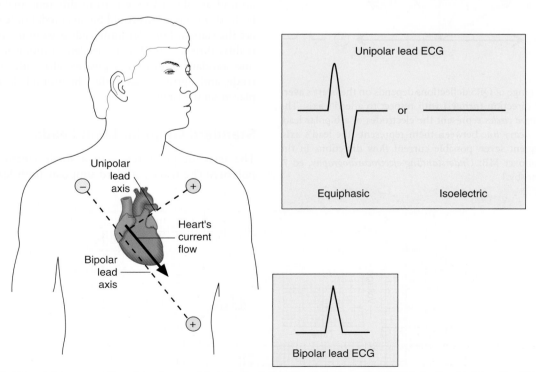

Figure 19-3 Lead axis and the average direction of current flow in the heart. The polarity of the QRS deflection is determined by the direction of current flow relative to the recording lead's axis.

Electrocardiogram Graph Paper

ECG graph paper is a grid, permitting time measurement along the horizontal lines and voltage measurement along the vertical lines (Figure 19-5). Dark and light intersecting lines form large and small squares. The light vertical lines that help form the small squares are 1 mm apart and represent 0.04 second at a standard sweep speed of 25 mm per second. The heavy vertical lines are 5 mm apart and represent 0.20 second at standard recording speed. (The large squares have five small squares on each side [see Figure 19-5]).

Vertically, each small square represents 0.1 mV, which means each large square represents 0.5 mV (see Figure 19-5). By convention, ECG machines are adjusted, or standardized, so that a 1-mV electrical signal produces a 10-mm (two large squares) deflection. The amplitude of the ECG is discussed in terms of millivolts.

The hard copy (paper) ECG grid is convenient for determining the heart rate and uniformity of spacing between QRS complexes. Because each large square represents 0.2 second, five large squares represent 1.0 second. Five large squares are 25 mm, or 2.5 cm, long; thus, 1 inch of horizontal distance equals 1 second on ECG graph paper.

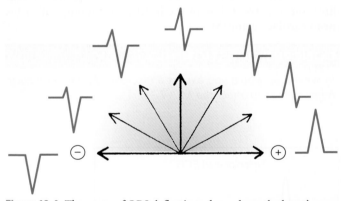

Figure 19-4 The range of QRS deflections depends on the heart's average current flow direction (*arrows*) with respect to a lead's axis. The *positive and negative circles* represent the electrodes of a bipolar lead, and the *straight, heavy line* between them represents the lead's axis. The *arrows* represent seven possible current flow directions in the heart. (From Conover MB: *Understanding electrocardiography,* ed 7, St Louis, 1996, Mosby.)

Short vertical markers spaced 3 seconds apart (15 large squares or 75 small squares) are usually placed at the upper edge of the ECG paper. These markers allow a 3-second or 6-second time interval to be easily selected for analysis. The 6-second "strip" is a common ECG paper length used for electrocardiographic analysis and interpretation. These strips may be placed in the hard copy medical records of patients undergoing cardiac evaluations.

ELECTROCARDIOGRAM LEADS

Standard Bipolar Limb Leads: Einthoven's Triangle

At the turn of the twentieth century, Einthoven invented the ECG machine and introduced the three bipolar limb leads.[3] Figure 19-6 illustrates these three **standard limb leads**. In lead I, the negative electrode is placed on the right arm, and the positive electrode is placed on the left arm. The axis of lead I is a horizontal line running from shoulder to shoulder. In lead II, the negative electrode is on the right arm, and the positive electrode is on the left leg; the axis of lead II runs from the right arm to the left leg (see Figure 19-6). Lead III has a negative electrode on the left arm and a positive electrode on the left leg. The lead III axis runs from the left arm to the left leg.

The axes of these three leads form an equilateral triangle around the heart, called **Einthoven's triangle**. Einthoven discovered that the voltage (amplitude) of the QRS complex recorded in lead II is always equal to the sum of the voltages in leads I and III (Einthoven's law).

The ECG recorded from three different leads gives three different views of the heart's electrical activity—similar to walking around an object to see it from different angles. Other bipolar lead combinations could be invented, but leads I, II, and III are the standard bipolar limb leads used in medical practice. In reality, three electrodes are needed to monitor the ECG from one standard limb lead: a positive electrode, a negative electrode, and a ground electrode. The ground electrode is usually placed on the right leg.

Standard Unipolar Limb Leads

The term unipolar refers to a single electrode of positive polarity. The three standard unipolar limb leads use similar

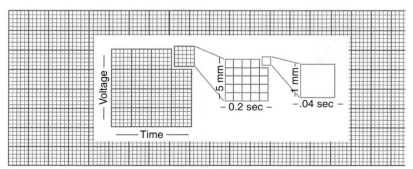

Figure 19-5 ECG graph paper. The horizontal axis represents time, and the vertical axis represents amplitude or voltage. (From Aehlert B: *ECGs made easy,* ed 4, St Louis, 2011, Mosby.)

CLINICAL FOCUS 19-1

Methods for Assessing Heart Rate on the Electrocardiogram

At least two different ways exist to determine the heart rate from the ECG recording. One method works well for regular heart rhythms, and the other method is better for irregular rhythms.

Method 1

Look at Figure 19-5. Notice that five large squares equal 1 second (0.2 sec × 5 = 1.0 sec). Because 1 minute contains 60 seconds, 1 minute is represented by 300 large squares (5 squares/sec × 60 sec = 300 squares). If the heart rate is 300 beats per minute, the interval between two QRS complexes is one large square (i.e., a heartbeat [QRS complex] occurs every 0.2 second). When the heart rate is 150 beats per minute, the interval between two QRS complexes is two large squares. For determining the heart rate, the number 300 is divided by the number of large squares between two QRS complexes. This is summarized as follows:

Number of Large Squares between Two QRS Complexes	Rate (beats/min)
1	300 (300 ÷ 1)
2	150 (300 ÷ 2)
3	100 (300 ÷ 3)
4	75 (300 ÷ 4)
5	60 (300 ÷ 5)
6	50 (300 ÷ 6)

Memorization of the numbers in the right column ("300, 150, 100, then 75, 60, 50") allows quick identification of the heart rate at the patient's bedside. This method is appropriate only for regular heart rhythms in which QRS complexes are uniformly spaced.

Method 2

In Figure 19-5, markers identify 3-second intervals on the ECG paper. First, a 6-second interval is identified by using these markers (two 3-second intervals). Next, within this 6-second strip, the number of QRS complexes is counted. Because 1 minute contains 10 6-second intervals, the number of QRS complexes that were counted is multiplied by 10. For example, if eight QRS complexes are counted in a 6-second strip, the heart rate is 8 × 10 or 80 beats per minute. This method is best for averaging the heart rate when the rhythm is irregular (i.e., when the interval between QRS complexes varies).

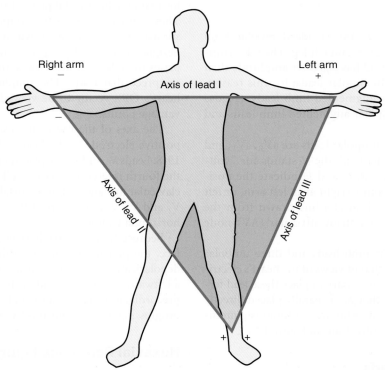

Figure 19-6 The axes of leads I, II, and III form Einthoven's triangle. (From Seidel JC, editor: *Basic electrocardiography: a modular approach,* St Louis, 1986, Mosby.)

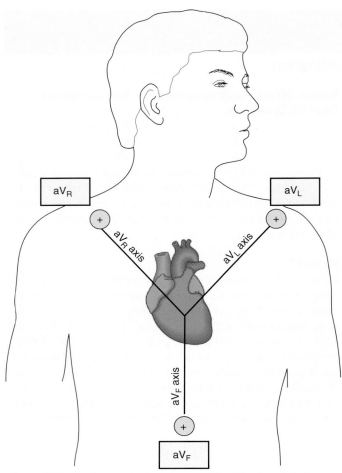

Figure 19-7 The three unipolar augmented limb leads and their axes.

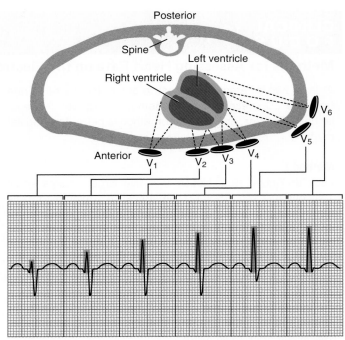

Figure 19-8 The electrocardiographic tracing from the chest leads (V_1 to V_6), showing the gradual changes that occur in the polarity of the QRS complex. (From Hillegrass E: *Essentials of cardiopulmonary physical therapy,* ed 3, St. Louis, 2011, Saunders.)

electrode attachment points as the standard bipolar limb leads—that is, right arm, left arm, and left leg. The QRS complex recorded by a unipolar lead has a greater amplitude than the QRS complex recorded by bipolar leads; for this reason, unipolar leads are known as augmented limb leads. (Figure 19-7 illustrates the three unipolar augmented limb leads and their axes.)

The symbols for the three unipolar leads are aV_R, aV_L, and aV_F. The *a* stands for "augmented," the *V* stands for "voltage," and the subscript letters *R*, *L*, and *F* indicate the positive electrode's attachment points (right arm, left arm, or left foot). The axis of a unipolar lead is a line drawn from the positive electrode to the heart's atrioventricular (AV) node (see Figure 19-7).

The three standard bipolar limb leads and three unipolar leads combined provide six different views of the heart's electrical activity. In practice, it is unnecessary to place these lead terminals on the limbs; instead, they are generally placed directly on the anterior chest in patients who are continuously monitored (as shown for the augmented leads in Figure 19-7).

Precordial (Chest) Leads

The six ECG leads discussed up to this point are categorized as frontal plane leads because their axes lie in the frontal or vertical plane of the chest. From these leads, information can be obtained about current flowing right, left, up, or down but not about current flowing from the front of the chest toward the back, or vice versa. The axes of the **precordial leads** are located on a horizontal plane through the chest (Figure 19-8). They consist of six positive unipolar electrodes placed on the surface of the chest, as shown in Figure 19-9. These leads are designated V_1, V_2, V_3, V_4, V_5, and V_6. The **12-lead ECG** comprises three bipolar limb leads, three unipolar limb leads, and six precordial leads. The standard 12-lead ECG allows the heart's QRS vector to be viewed from 12 different electrical vantage points.

The axes of the precordial leads are lines drawn from the positive electrode to the heart's AV node, as shown in Figure 19-8. Leads V_1 and V_2 are placed on either side of the sternum at the fourth intercostal space (see Figure 19-9). V_4 is at the midclavicular line and fifth intercostal space. V_3 is equidistant from V_1 and V_4. V_5 and V_6 are at the anterior and midaxillary lines, horizontal with V_4.

Because they lie directly over the heart on the chest's surface, the precordial leads are valuable in localizing abnormal depolarization of the myocardium. The ventricles depolarize in a leftward, downward, and posterior direction.[2] Therefore, the precordial leads record a strongly negative QRS complex in V_1, progressing to a strongly positive QRS in V_6.

Hexaxial Reference Figure

If the axes of the six frontal plane leads are superimposed on one another such that all six lead axes have the same midpoint, the **hexaxial reference figure** is formed (Figure 19-10);

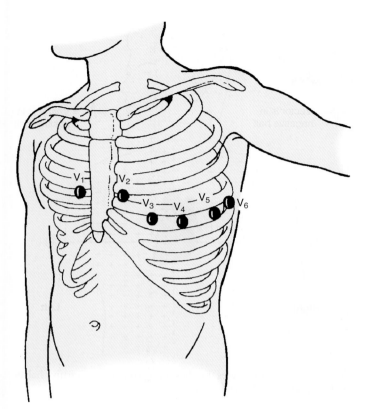

Figure 19-9 Electrode sites for the precordial leads. (From Conover MB: *Understanding electrocardiography,* ed 7, St Louis, 1996, Mosby.)

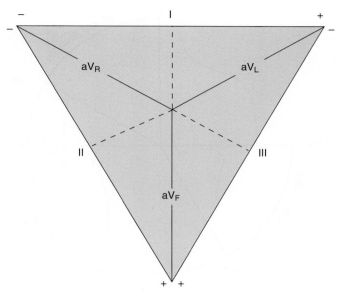

Figure 19-10 Axes of the three unipolar and three bipolar limb leads combined. Each unipolar lead axis is perpendicular to a bipolar lead axis. (From Conover MB: *Understanding electrocardiography,* ed 7, St Louis, 1996, Mosby.)

the three unipolar limb lead axes are plotted inside the triangle formed by the axes of leads I through III. In Figure 19-10, the axis of each unipolar lead is extended through the heart (*dotted lines*) and is perpendicular to the opposite side's bipolar lead axis. For example, the aV_R axis is perpendicular to the lead III axis. Imagine pushing each side of the triangle in Figure 19-10 to the center (keeping the angles of the sides constant) so that all six axes of unipolar and bipolar leads intersect each other at a single point in the heart's center. This forms the hexaxial reference figure (Figure 19-11), which allows the direction of the MCV to be determined precisely.

The six axes of the hexaxial figure form 12 "spokes," spaced 30 degrees apart (see Figure 19-11). By standard convention, the zero-degree point is placed at the 3-o'clock position. Negative values are assigned to degrees moving counterclockwise from 0 degrees; positive values are assigned to degrees moving clockwise from 0 degrees. Figure 19-3 shows that the normal MCV points toward +60 degrees. This direction is parallel to the standard limb lead II axis and points toward the lead II positive electrode. Lead II is thus expected to record a strongly positive QRS complex (see Figure 19-3).

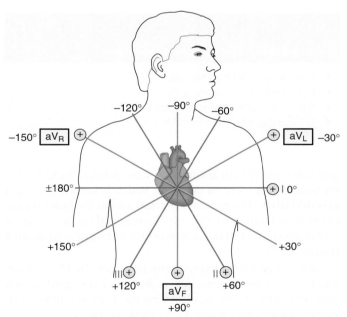

Figure 19-11 The hexaxial reference system formed by the unipolar and bipolar limb leads.

LOCATING THE HEART'S ELECTRICAL AXIS

Determinants of the Electrical Axis

The normal QRS vector points slightly to the left side of the chest toward +60 degrees. The larger left ventricular muscle mass generates most of the heart's electrical activity, explaining why the QRS vector points to the left. Relative ventricular muscle mass is a major determinant of the MCV direction. For example, if high pulmonary vascular resistance overworks the right ventricle, it may gain mass (hypertrophy) and

CONCEPT QUESTION 19-3

Assuming the MCV points at +60 degrees (see Figure 19-11), is the QRS complex recorded from lead aV_R positive or negative?

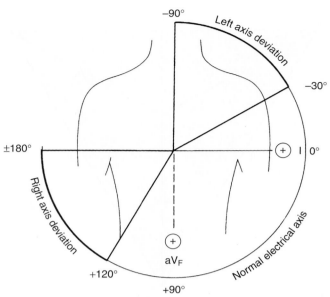

Figure 19-12 The range for the normal electrical axis of the heart is −30 to +120 degrees. (From Conover MB: *Understanding electrocardiography,* ed 7, St Louis, 1996, Mosby.)

BOX 19-1

Factors Causing Electrical Axis Deviations

- Change in heart position (obesity)
- Hypertrophy of one ventricle
- Bundle branch conduction block
- Myocardial infarction (dead heart tissue)

---

generate more electrical current. Consequently, the QRS vector would shift more to the right, which is known as a right **axis deviation**. The normal electrical axis of the heart is usually between 0 degrees and +90 degrees, although a range of −30 degrees to +120 degrees may still be considered normal (Figure 19-12).[2]

Factors other than hypertrophy influence the QRS vector. These factors are summarized in Box 19-1. Extreme obesity pushes the diaphragm up, displacing the heart to a more horizontal position and causing a left axis deviation.

If a major bundle branch is blocked, the cardiac impulse depolarizes the unblocked ventricle first before it depolarizes the blocked ventricle. The depolarized ventricle is momentarily electronegative, while the blocked ventricle is still electropositive. This polarity difference causes a strong electrical current to flow from the depolarized ventricle to the polarized ventricle, creating a marked axis deviation toward the blocked side.[4]

Myocardial infarction produces a dead (necrotic) area in the heart that cannot conduct electrical impulses. Because this area generates no electrical current, the QRS vector deviates from the infarcted area toward normal, current-generating tissue.[3]

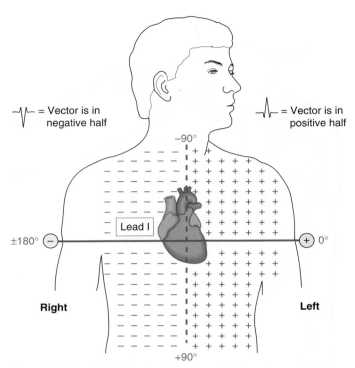

Figure 19-13 Lead I divides the chest into positive and negative halves with respect to the QRS it records.

Easy Method for Determining the Electrical Axis

A positive QRS complex is recorded from leads in which the heart's depolarizing current flows toward the positive electrode. Lead II generates a positive QRS recording because the MCV normally points directly at the lead II positive electrode. If lead II records a totally negative QRS, this means (1) the lead's electrode placement is reversed or (2) the heart's current actually flows in the opposite direction from normal (i.e., toward −120 degrees [see Figure 19-11]).

Use of Leads I and aV_F to Determine the Cardiac Axis

Figure 19-13 shows that standard limb lead I separates the chest into positive and negative halves (*dashed vertical line*). That is, any cardiac vector pointing to the right of the chest produces a negative QRS in lead I. Any cardiac vector pointing to the left of the chest produces a positive QRS in lead I. The QRS recorded from lead I merely reveals whether the cardiac vector points toward the right or left half of the patient's chest. If the QRS is more positive than negative, the vector points to the left half; if it is more negative than positive, the vector points to the right half.

Figure 19-14 shows that the QRS from lead aV_F similarly separates the chest into upper negative and lower positive halves (*dashed line*). Lead aV_F records a positive QRS if the MCV points below the dashed line. Likewise, lead aV_F records a negative QRS for vectors pointing above the dashed line. The use of aV_F alone or lead I alone does not allow the cardiac vector to be pinpointed with any degree of precision.

The comparison of QRS configurations from both leads I and aV_F allows the cardiac vector to be located within a

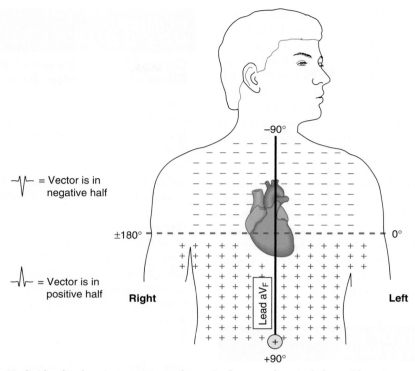

Figure 19-14 Lead aV$_F$ divides the chest into positive and negative lower and upper halves with respect to the QRS it records.

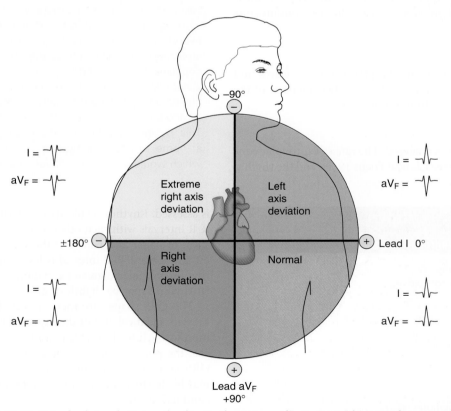

Figure 19-15 Using leads I and aV$_F$ together locates the mean cardiac vector within a 90-degree quadrant.

90-degree quadrant (Figure 19-15). A positive QRS complex recorded by both leads means the cardiac vector is located in the left lower quadrant, or the normal range (-0 degrees to $+90$ degrees). Conversely, a positive QRS in lead I and a negative QRS in aV_F means the cardiac vector points to the left upper quadrant (0 degrees to -90 degrees), which indicates a left axis deviation. A negative QRS in lead I and positive QRS in aV_F means the vector lies in the right lower quadrant ($+90$ degrees to $+180$ degrees), or a right axis deviation (see Figure 19-15).

After locating the quadrant in which the MCV lies, one can pinpoint its direction precisely in the following way: examine the QRS complexes recorded in all six leads of the hexaxial reference figure and identify the lead with the most equiphasic, lowest amplitude QRS. The axis of this lead on the hexaxial reference figure must be perpendicular to the heart's electrical axis. In other words, the heart's axis must be located at a point within the identified quadrant that is 90 degrees away from the axis of the lead with the most equiphasic QRS.

IDENTIFICATION OF COMMON CARDIAC ARRHYTHMIAS

Systematic Electrocardiogram Analysis

Health professionals approach ECG interpretation in many different ways. No one method is correct; the important factor is to use a consistent, systematic approach.[5] Box 19-2 outlines one approach.

Step One

The ECG strip is analyzed for the presence of all waves and complexes. In the process, it is noted whether the parts of the complexes look the same from beat to beat.

Step Two

The ventricular activity is analyzed. The rate of ventricular contractions is calculated (see Clinical Focus 19-1), and the rhythm

---

BOX 19-2

Steps in Electrocardiogram Analysis

Step 1: Identify specific waves
Step 2: Analyze QRS complexes
    Rate
    Rhythm
    Shape
Step 3: Analyze P waves
    Rate
    Rhythm
    Shape
Step 4: Assess AV relationship
    Ratio of P waves to QRS complexes
    Location of P wave with respect to QRS complex
    PR interval

CLINICAL FOCUS 19-2

Chronic Bronchitis with Chronic Hypoxemia: Effect on the Cardiac Axis

A 60-year-old man with a long history of cigarette smoking and chronic obstructive pulmonary disease visits your clinical facility for an evaluation. This patient is chronically hypoxemic and hypercapnic, with room air PaO_2 of 50 mm Hg and $PaCO_2$ of 60 mm Hg. A standard ECG reveals a strongly negative QRS complex in lead I and a more positive than negative QRS complex in aV_F. Explain this finding.

Discussion

Referring to Figure 19-15, these QRS recordings reveal a right axis deviation. In other words, the mean direction of current flow in the ventricles aims toward the +90-degree to +180-degree quadrant. A strongly negative QRS in lead I indicates that the heart's current is flowing almost 180 degrees away from the lead I positive electrode. This finding is consistent with the patient's history. Chronic hypoxemia is associated with hypoxic pulmonary vasoconstriction. This patient also may have a component of emphysema that destroys alveolar capillary bed tissue. Such destruction decreases the cross-sectional area of the pulmonary vascular bed. Hypoxemic vasoconstriction and destruction of the vascular bed increase pulmonary vascular resistance, overworking the right ventricle. Consequently, the right ventricle hypertrophies over time. Its increased muscle mass generates more electrical activity than normal during ventricular depolarization, drawing the cardiac vector toward itself; this is manifested on the ECG as a right axis deviation. This ECG finding and the patient's medical history point to the severity and advanced nature of this patient's pulmonary disease. This patient may benefit from long-term oxygen therapy at home to decrease hypoxic pulmonary vasoconstriction, which would decrease right ventricular work.

---

is assessed. Rhythm regularity is determined by comparing the R-R intervals with each other, using an ECG caliper or a blank sheet of paper and pencil. If the variation between the shortest and longest R-R interval is less than 0.16 second, the ECG rhythm is regular; a greater variation is called irregular.[1] Irregular rhythms may be slightly or grossly irregular.

The QRS shapes are then inspected to determine whether they are identical and of the expected polarity, considering the monitoring lead. Two QRS complexes of different polarity indicate the presence of an ectopic focus (see Chapter 18). Wide QRS complexes indicate slowed conduction velocity, which may be due to an ectopic focus in the ventricles or an abnormal conduction path.

Step Three

Atrial activity is analyzed. The atrial rate is calculated by counting P waves, using the same method as for QRS complexes.

The P wave and QRS rates should be identical if normal sinus node pacing is present. More P waves than QRS complexes means not all atrial impulses are conducted to the ventricles. Atrial rhythm is checked in the same way as the QRS rhythm. The P wave shape is checked to determine whether it is of the expected polarity. Changes in polarity indicate shifts in pacemaker sites.

Step Four

The AV electrical relationship is assessed. Is the AV conduction ratio a normal 1:1 (e.g., one P wave followed by one QRS complex)? If the ratio is 2:1 or greater, not all atrial impulses are conducted, and an AV conduction impairment may exist. Alternatively, the atrial rate may be so high that the AV node blocks some atrial impulses because of its normal refractory nature. Does the P wave precede or follow the QRS complex? A P wave following the QRS may mean the impulse originates in the AV node. A prolonged PR interval (>0.2 second) means the impulse conduction velocity from the sinoatrial (SA) node to the ventricles is slowed.

Normal Sinus Rhythm

Normal sinus rhythm (NSR) (Figure 19-16) occurs when the sinus node initiates each depolarizing impulse at a rate of 60 to 100 per minute, and each impulse is conducted normally through the atria and ventricles. The result is coordinated atrial

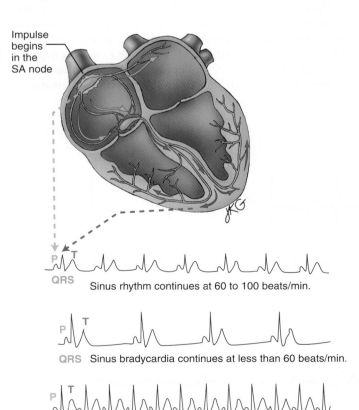

Figure 19-16 Sinus rhythm, sinus bradycardia, and sinus tachycardia. (From Aehlert B: *ECGs made easy*, ed 4, St Louis, 2011, Mosby.)

and ventricular contractions. In Figure 19-16, P waves, QRS complexes, and T waves are clearly defined and normal. The P wave-to-QRS complex ratio is 1:1. Also, the spacing between QRS complexes is relatively constant, indicating a regular rhythm. The PR interval, measured from the beginning of the P wave to the beginning of the first QRS deflection, is about four small squares, or 0.16 second. This interval is in the normal range, indicating a normal impulse-conduction time between the SA node and the ventricles. In a 6-second time frame (30 large squares), there are seven QRS complexes; the heart rate is 70 beats per minute.

Abnormal Sinus Rhythms

The term arrhythmia means "without rhythm." However, the term is used in this book to include breaks in the regularity of normal rhythms.

Tachycardia

Sinus tachycardia is defined in adults as a heart rate greater than 100 beats per minute.[4] The SA node is the pacemaker, and its impulses travel in a normal manner to the ventricles (see Figure 19-16); therefore, P, QRS, and T waves appear normal, as in NSR. The PR intervals shorten in severe tachycardia, as does the space between the T wave and the next P wave. The rhythm is usually regular.

Sinus tachycardia is the normal response of a healthy heart to an increased demand for blood flow in exercise. It also may be caused by fever (increase of 10 beats per minute per degree Fahrenheit increase)[4]; anxiety; pain; and stimulants such as coffee, tea, alcohol, and nicotine. Anything that increases sympathetic stimulation causes tachycardia. Beta-adrenergic drugs such as epinephrine cause tachycardia because they mimic sympathetic stimulation. Sympathetic stimulation, tachycardia, and increased cardiac output are normal compensatory responses to abnormal conditions such as anemia, hypoxia, and hypovolemia.

A rapid heart rate increases the heart's workload and oxygen requirements. In individuals with partially blocked coronary arteries, tachycardia may increase the heart's oxygen requirements above the level that can be supplied by blood flow. This may cause myocardial ischemia and can precipitate myocardial infarction.[1] Treatment of sinus tachycardia, if necessary, is always directed at the underlying cause. Strong vagal stimulation such as carotid sinus massage may slow the heart rate momentarily. Beta-blocking drugs such as propranolol block sympathetic cardiac beta receptors and are sometimes used to slow the heart rate.

Bradycardia

Sinus bradycardia is defined in adults as a heart rate less than 60 beats per minute.[4] The SA node is the pacemaker. SA node impulses follow normal conduction pathways to the ventricles. Consequently, ECG waves and complexes appear normal, as in NSR (see Figure 19-16). Normal PR intervals and QRS widths indicate a normal impulse-conduction time; the SA node simply fires at rates that are slower than normal. The rhythm is usually regular.

Resting heart rates less than 60 beats per minute are normal during sleep and in physically conditioned individuals. A trained heart has increased contractility and ejects larger volumes of blood with each stroke; therefore, a normal cardiac output can be maintained at a lower heart rate. In abnormal conditions, excessive vagal stimulation or sympathetic nervous system inhibition may cause sinus bradycardia.

Carotid sinus syndrome is a condition in which the pressure receptors in the fork of the common carotid artery are oversensitive. These receptors contain many vagal nerve endings. Even slight pressure on the neck near the carotid artery may severely slow or momentarily stop the heartbeat and induce syncope (fainting).[4] Vomiting, straining against a closed glottis (Valsalva maneuver), or suctioning the pharynx and trachea with a catheter causes increased vagal stimulation (vagovagal reflex), slowing the sinus node discharge rate.

A bradycardia of 50 to 59 beats per minute is usually asymptomatic. Trained athletes often have even lower resting heart rates (e.g., in the mid to upper 40s). Such conditioned individuals can tolerate low heart rates because their stroke volumes are large enough that they still maintain normal cardiac outputs. In nonathletes, rates of 30 to 45 beats per minute often generate symptoms such as hypotension, weakness, dizziness, and sweating, which are signs of inadequate blood flow. Syncope may occur if blood flow to the brain is too low.

In patients with acute myocardial infarction, mild bradycardia may be beneficial because it decreases the heart's workload and oxygen requirements. However, severe bradycardia in myocardial infarction may allow enough time for an irritable ectopic focus to take over the pacemaker function. This situation can produce serious, life-threatening arrhythmias.[1]

Symptomatic bradycardias require prompt treatment to prevent the dangerous consequences of low blood flow and serious cardiac arrhythmias. Parasympathetic-blocking drugs (also known as cholinergic blockers) such as atropine reduce the inhibition of the sinus node, increasing the heart rate. Severe bradycardia may require artificially implanted pacemakers.

Sinus Arrhythmia

Sinus arrhythmia (Figure 19-17) is defined as irregularly generated sinus node impulses, all of which are normally conducted throughout the heart. Sinus node impulses alternate between faster and slower rates, commonly increasing during inspiration and decreasing during expiration. The pacemaker and conduction times are normal, and all ECG components appear normal. The only abnormality is the irregular spacing between QRS complexes (see Figure 19-19). Sinus arrhythmias are usually of no clinical significance and do not require treatment.[1]

Premature Atrial Contraction

Premature atrial contractions (PACs) (Figure 19-18) occur when an ectopic focus fires. An ectopic focus fires before the SA node would normally fire, causing an early atrial contraction (identified as P′ on the ECG [see Figure 19-18]). Ventricular QRS complexes are normal because all impulses are conducted normally into the ventricles. However, QRS complexes are irregularly spaced because of the PAC. PACs may originate from a single ectopic focus or from multiple ectopic foci in the atria.

The size, shape, and polarity of the P′ wave may vary depending on the location of the ectopic focus. If the ectopic site is near the SA node, the P′ wave appears normally positive (upright). If the ectopic site is near the AV node, the P′ wave is negative (inverted) because the atria depolarize in a direction that is opposite from normal. Sometimes PACs occur so prematurely

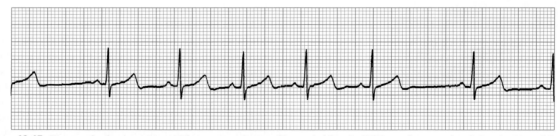

Figure 19-17 Sinus arrhythmia at 54 to 88 beats per minute. (From Aehlert B: *ECGs made easy,* ed 4, St Louis, 2011, Mosby.)

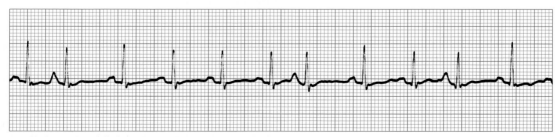

Figure 19-18 Sinus tachycardia with three PACs. From the left, beats 2, 7, and 10 are PACs. (From Aehlert B: *ECGs made easy,* ed 4, St Louis, 2011, Mosby.)

that the P′ wave is located on top of the T wave, distorting its shape.

If the ectopic focus discharges too early, the AV node may still be refractory from the preceding beat. Subsequently, the AV node fails to conduct the ectopic impulse to the ventricles. In such a situation, a QRS complex does not follow the P′ wave, and the PAC is called a **nonconducted (blocked) PAC**.[3]

Because the PAC usually depolarizes the SA node prematurely, the timing of the SA node's discharge is reset in step with the PAC. In other words, the point at which the SA node was forced to depolarize early becomes a new starting point for the next SA node cycle. This change causes the next normal P wave (following the PAC) to appear later than it would have if the SA node's rhythm had not been disturbed.

Emotional stress, alcohol, caffeine, tobacco, electrolyte imbalances, and sympathetic stimulation may cause PACs in normal hearts. Various drugs may also produce irritable foci in the atria, causing PACs. In ischemic heart disease, insufficient coronary blood flow may increase the irritability of atrial muscle and produce PACs. Occasional isolated PACs are not clinically significant. Frequent PACs in patients with heart disease are a warning sign of increasing atrial muscle irritability and potentially serious atrial arrhythmias.[1] Drugs that suppress atrial excitability, such as sodium channel inhibitors (e.g., quinidine) or calcium channel blockers (e.g., verapamil), may be used to manage PACs.

Supraventricular Arrhythmias

Atrial Flutter

Atrial flutter (Figure 19-19) is a type of **supraventricular tachycardia** caused by a single ectopic pacemaker located

above the AV node firing at a rate of 200 to 350 beats per minute.[4] Because the ectopic focus is located above the ventricles, the arrhythmia is called supraventricular. Commonly, the ventricular contraction rate is about half the atrial rate (about 150 beats per minute) because the normal refractory nature of the AV node prevents many of the atrial impulses from entering the ventricles. Otherwise, the ventricles would not have adequate filling time, and cardiac output would decrease significantly.

Typically, the ventricular rhythm is regular (see Figure 19-19) if the refractory nature of the AV node remains constant. Ventricular QRS complexes often appear at regular intervals because of the constant AV conduction ratio (see Figure 19-19). The P waves in atrial flutter are replaced by atrial flutter waves, often described as saw-toothed in appearance. Flutter waves may precede, be buried in, or follow the QRS complexes. They are superimposed on T waves and ST segments.

Atrial flutter is most commonly seen in older people with advanced rheumatic heart disease, especially if the disease affects mitral and tricuspid valves.[1] The automaticity of atrial muscle tends to increase in these conditions. Symptoms of atrial flutter include sensations of palpitations in the chest (caused by the rapid ventricular rate), nervousness, and anxiety. If the ventricular rate is extremely high, cardiac output may decrease as a result of inadequate ventricular filling time. This may cause confusion, dizziness, and possibly fainting. In people who have impaired coronary blood flow, atrial flutter may worsen myocardial ischemia or cause an infarction by increasing ventricular oxygen consumption.

Atrial flutter is sometimes treated with cardioversion. In cardioversion, an electrical shock synchronized with the heart rate is delivered to the chest surface, causing a depolarizing current to pass through the heart. If cardioversion is successful, atrial flutter is converted to NSR.

Atrial Fibrillation

Atrial fibrillation (Figure 19-20) is caused by uncoordinated, chaotic electrical discharge from numerous ectopic foci in the atria (Figure 19-21). These atrial impulses occur about 300 to 600 times per minute, typically averaging about 400 per minute.[1] The random discharge of many ectopic foci creates irregular, fine fibrillatory waves; P waves are totally absent (see Figure 19-20). As in atrial flutter, the refractory nature of the AV node prevents many of these atrial impulses from reaching the ventricles; thus, the ventricular rate is much slower. Because AV nodal stimulation is random and erratic, impulse conduction to the ventricles is unpredictable, and the ventricular rhythm is grossly irregular, as illustrated in Figure 19-20. Although QRS complexes are normal, their spacing is highly variable. The hallmark of atrial fibrillation is a totally irregular ventricular rhythm accompanied by fine, irregular undulations of the ECG baseline.

Atrial fibrillation may occur as a progression of atrial flutter. An enlarged, distended atrium predisposes it to develop ectopic foci because atrial enlargement lengthens conduction times. The more stretched the muscle, the more time is required for impulses to spread over the atria. This lengthened

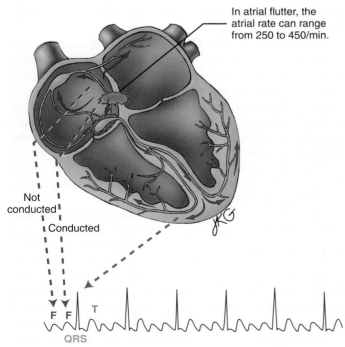

Figure 19-19 Atrial flutter. *F,* Flutter wave. (From Aehlert B: *ECGs made easy,* ed 4, St Louis, 2011, Mosby.)

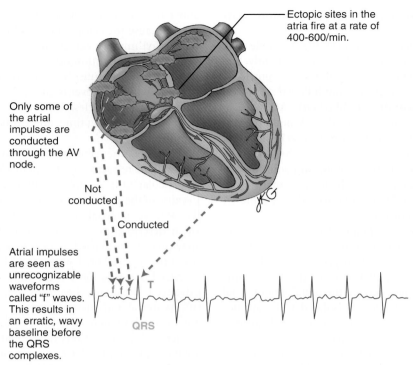

Ectopic sites in the atria fire at a rate of 400-600/min.

Only some of the atrial impulses are conducted through the AV node.

Not conducted

Conducted

Atrial impulses are seen as unrecognizable waveforms called "f" waves. This results in an erratic, wavy baseline before the QRS complexes.

Figure 19-20 Atrial fibrillation. *f,* Fibrillatory wave. (From Aehlert B: *ECGs made easy,* ed 4, St Louis, 2011, Mosby.)

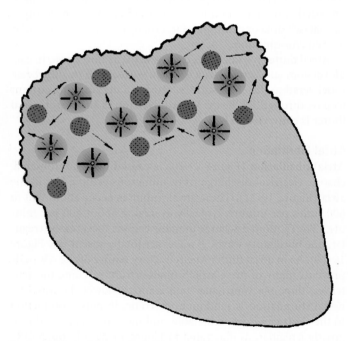

Figure 19-21 Atrial ectopic foci in atrial fibrillation. (From Seidel JC, editor: *Basic electrocardiography: a modular approach,* St Louis, 1986, Mosby.)

conduction time may allow some muscle fibers to repolarize while other atrial fibers are still depolarizing. The depolarizing areas restimulate the repolarized areas, propagating a vicious cycle of unorganized fibrillation. Any condition that increases atrial pressures, such as congestive heart failure, mitral valve stenosis, and chronically high pulmonary vascular resistance, may enlarge the atria.

The uncoordinated, chaotic fibrillation of the atria means they have no functional pumping action; instead, they quiver with no distinct contraction or relaxation phases. The "atrial kick" that normally adds to ventricular filling at the end of ventricular diastole is lost. Consequently, the ventricles fill incompletely, causing a reduction of the stroke volume and cardiac output by 20% to 30%.[4]

Incomplete ventricular filling is exaggerated when two ventricular contractions occur quite close together in time. Inadequate filling time coupled with the loss of the atrial kick may reduce the stroke volume so much that no pulse can be felt in a peripheral artery. In such a situation, the ventricular beat can be heard with a stethoscope placed on the chest, but a peripheral pulse cannot be felt. This phenomenon is known as a **pulse deficit** and is a characteristic feature of atrial fibrillation. Therefore, in patients with atrial fibrillation, the heart rate should be monitored with a stethoscope or an ECG machine, and the peripheral pulse should be palpated.

The reduction in cardiac output in atrial fibrillation may produce symptoms of confusion, dizziness, hypotension, and fainting. A major concern in atrial fibrillation is the stasis, or pooling, of blood in the atria caused by the lack of coordinated pumping action. This sluggish blood movement predisposes to blood clot (thrombus) formation. The thrombus may break loose from the atrium and travel downstream, in which case it is called a **thromboembolism**. If it originates from the right atrium, it may plug a vessel in the lungs (pulmonary embolism), or if it originates from the left atrium, it may plug a vessel in the brain, causing a stroke. For this

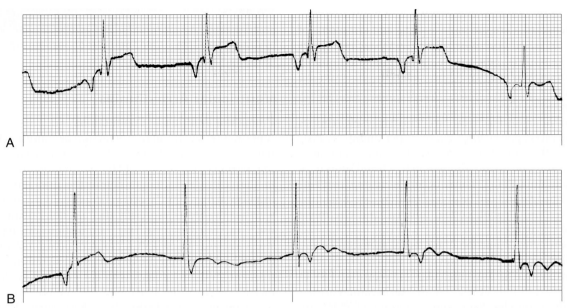

Figure 19-22 Junctional escape rhythm. Continuous strips. **A,** Note the inverted (retrograde) P waves before the QRS complexes. **B,** Note the change in the location of the P waves. In the first beat, the retrograde P wave is seen before the QRS. In the second beat, no P wave is seen. In the remaining beats, the P wave is seen after the QRS complexes. (From Aehlert B: *ECGs made easy*, ed 4, St Louis, 2011, Mosby.)

reason, patients with atrial fibrillation are often given antico-agulant drugs.[6]

Treatment of atrial fibrillation is generally aimed at reducing the rapid ventricular response and restoring normal sinus rhythm. Calcium channel–blocking drugs (diltiazem or verapamil) may be given to control heart rate, and the antiarrhythmic drug amiodarone (which inhibits myocardial Na^+ and K^+ channels) may be given to reduce atrial irritability and restore normal sinus rhythm.[6] Electrical cardioversion also may be used to convert atrial fibrillation to NSR if the patient displays serious symptoms.

CONCEPT QUESTION 19-4

Why do chronic congestive heart failure and high atrial pressures predispose a person to the development of atrial fibrillation?

Junctional Arrhythmias

The cardiac muscle immediately surrounding the AV node is called the AV junction; the preferred term for rhythms arising from the AV node and junctional area is junctional rhythms. If the sinus node fails to generate impulses, the AV junction may assume the role of the pacemaker. This kind of junctional self-pacing is called a **junctional escape rhythm**. Because the firing rate of the AV junction is 40 to 60 impulses per minute, a junctional escape rhythm is generally slower than normal sinus rhythm (Figure 19-22).

In a junctional rhythm, the electrical impulse travels to the ventricles through normal pathways; the QRS complex is normal in shape and duration. However, the impulse must travel in a backward, or retrograde, direction to depolarize the atria. Retrograde atrial conduction causes P wave changes characteristic of junctional rhythms: the P wave may be (1) inverted (as shown in Figure 19-22), (2) hidden, or (3) retrograde.

Inverted P waves are of negative polarity, caused by the backward direction of the atrial depolarizing current (see Figure 19-22). If inverted P waves occur immediately before the QRS complex, they originated high in the AV junctional area. Because the distance the impulse travels to depolarize the ventricles is shorter than normal, the PR interval is quite short (usually <0.12 second).[1]

Hidden P waves originate in the midjunctional area, which means the travel distance for the impulse that causes atrial and ventricular depolarization is about the same. Thus, atria and ventricles depolarize at approximately the same time, and the QRS complex completely hides the P wave. No P wave appears on the ECG, and no PR interval exists.

Electrical impulses arising from the lower AV junction produce retrograde P waves, or P waves following the QRS complex. The impulse travel distance from its origin to the ventricles is shorter than the distance to the atria. Thus, atria depolarize slightly later than the ventricles, producing the retrograde P wave.

An irritable ectopic focus in the junctional fibers causes a **premature junctional contraction**. A premature junctional contraction may be difficult to distinguish from a PAC and is caused by similar mechanisms.

Junctional tachycardias occur when junctional fibers pace the heart at rates greater than 100 beats per minute. Junctional tachycardia may be paroxysmal (occurring in intermittent spasms) or nonparoxysmal. In nonparoxysmal junctional tachycardia, the heart rate may reach 150 beats per minute.[1] The rhythm is usually regular, and the QRS configuration is normal (Figure 19-23). Signs and symptoms of nonparoxysmal junctional tachycardia are the same as signs and symptoms of atrial tachycardias. Nonparoxysmal junctional tachycardia is caused by enhanced AV junction excitability, most commonly resulting from digitalis toxicity.[1] Other causes include excessive administration of beta-adrenergic drugs and ischemic damage to the AV junctional fibers.

Paroxysmal junctional tachycardia (PJT) may result in bursts of rapid heart rates approaching 240 beats per minute. A PAC usually initiates the onset. Paroxysms may last for a few minutes or for hours. Parasympathetic stimulation by carotid sinus neck massage usually stops PJT. PJT may occur for no apparent reason in healthy people and can be precipitated by catecholamine drugs, overexertion, alcohol, coffee, tobacco, and electrolyte and acid-base imbalances.[1]

Because paroxysmal junctional and atrial tachycardias are difficult to differentiate when P waves are not clearly present, the term **paroxysmal supraventricular tachycardia (PSVT)** is commonly used to indicate paroxysmal tachycardias arising from above the ventricles. Signs and symptoms of PSVT are similar to signs and symptoms of nonparoxysmal junctional tachycardia except symptoms are exaggerated in extremely high ventricular rates.

In patients with no underlying ischemic heart disease, treatment of PSVT involves the following, in sequence: (1) vagal parasympathetic stimulation (e.g., carotid sinus massage), (2) intravenous adenosine administration, and (3) intravenous calcium channel blockers (e.g., verapamil). Parasympathetic stimulation also can be accomplished by breath holding (Valsalva maneuver), coughing, and gag-reflex stimulation. More recently, adenosine has been found to be effective in terminating PSVT. Adenosine inhibits the AV conduction velocity and prolongs the AV nodal refractory period. Verapamil has similar effects but tends to produce more hypotension.[6]

Ventricular Arrhythmias

Premature Ventricular Contractions

A **premature ventricular contraction or complex (PVC)** is initiated by an ectopic focus in the ventricles below the branching portion of the bundle of His. An abnormally irritable focus in the ventricle discharges before the next normal SA node impulse arrives. PVCs occur occasionally in healthy people with healthy hearts, especially after alcohol, caffeine, or tobacco use.[1] Increased sympathetic stimulation during emotional stress also may cause PVCs. Isolated, occasional PVCs in otherwise healthy people are of no clinical significance. However, frequent PVCs in patients with coronary artery disease signal increased ventricular irritability and the potential appearance of life-threatening arrhythmias, such as ventricular tachycardia (VT) and ventricular fibrillation (VF).

Because an ectopic focus in the ventricles generates a PVC, the QRS complex is not preceded by a P wave (Figure 19-24). Besides appearing before the next expected normal QRS, a PVC also has a wide (>0.12 second), bizarre appearance. The wide QRS shows that depolarization occurred over abnormal conduction pathways, slowing the impulse velocity. The bizarre shape shows that depolarization occurred in an abnormal direction and sequence. However, the bizarre quality of the PVC varies, depending on the location of the ectopic focus. An ectopic focus located high in the ventricles near the bifurcation of the bundle of His may produce a PVC that appears normal. An ectopic impulse arising from a low point in the ventricles depolarizes the ventricles in an abnormal direction, creating a markedly

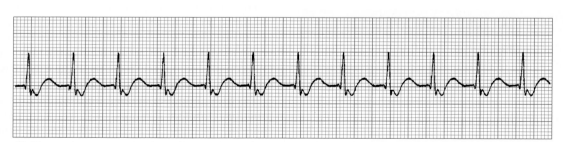

Figure 19-23 Junctional tachycardia at 120 beats per minute. (From Aehlert B: *ECGs made easy*, ed 4, St Louis, 2011, Mosby.)

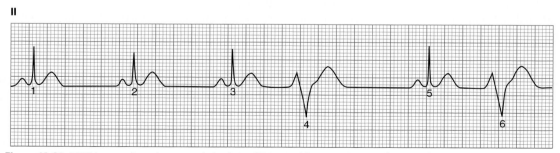

Figure 19-24 PVC in an otherwise normal rhythm. (From Aehlert B: *ECGs made easy*, ed 4, St Louis, 2011, Mosby.)

bizarre complex, as shown in Figure 19-24. Figure 19-25 shows two differently shaped PVCs, the first of positive polarity and the second of negative polarity; this indicates the presence of ectopic foci located in different areas of the ventricles. These are called **multifocal PVCs**, as opposed to **unifocal PVCs**. Multifocal PVCs indicate increased ventricular irritability and have more serious clinical implications than unifocal PVCs.

CONCEPT QUESTION 19-6

Why do multifocal PVCs indicate a more serious ventricular irritability than unifocal PVCs?

PVCs have the following characteristics:
- They occur prematurely.
- Their shape differs from normal QRS complexes.
- They generate T waves of opposite polarity from normal.
- The QRS complex is wide.
- P waves are unrelated to the PVC.
- A full compensatory pause occurs after the PVC.

The compensatory pause occurs because the abnormal ventricular impulse does not enter the atrium to depolarize the SA node (i.e., the SA nodal rhythm is undisturbed). When the SA node fires in its normal sequence, its P wave is obliterated by the PVC, and its impulse arrives at the ventricles while they are still refractory. The ventricles are not stimulated again until the next normal SA nodal impulse arrives. The interval between the two visible P waves on either side of a PVC (see Figure 19-24) is twice the interval between two normally sequenced P waves.

Hypoxia, acidosis, hypokalemia, and myocardial infarction increase myocardial irritability and may cause PVCs. The more irritable the ventricles, the greater the incidence of PVCs. A PVC alternating every other beat with a normal QRS complex is called **bigeminy**. When three or more PVCs occur in a row, VT is present. Frequent PVCs (more than six per minute) in the presence of acute myocardial infarction are treated by oxygen therapy and coronary vasodilators to relieve tissue hypoxia. In addition, antiarrhythmic drugs such as lidocaine are given to decrease ventricular irritability, although this does not cure the underlying disease process.[6]

Ventricular Tachycardia

Ventricular tachycardia (VT) (Figure 19-26) is a successive series of PVCs occurring at a rate of 100 to 250 per minute. VT may occur in short bursts or be sustained (>30 seconds).[6] VT is most common in patients with myocardial infarction or coronary artery disease. P waves are generally not visible, and all QRS complexes are wide and bizarre in appearance (see Figure 19-26).

VT is a sign of extremely serious ventricular irritability and instability and is usually considered life-threatening. Rapid ventricular rates reduce ventricular filling time and reduce cardiac output significantly, causing severe hypotension and

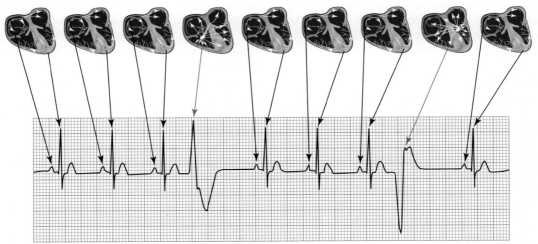

Figure 19-25 Multifocal PVCs. Ectopic foci arise from different points in the ventricles. (From Shade B, Wesley K: *Fast and easy ECGs: a self-paced learning program,* New York, 2007, McGraw-Hill.)

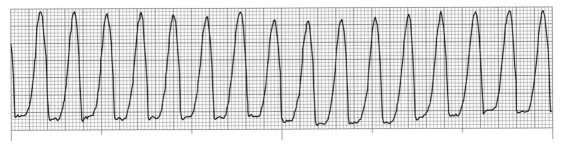

Figure 19-26 Monomorphic ventricular tachycardia. (From Aehlert B: *ECGs made easy,* ed 4, St Louis, 2011, Mosby.)

loss of consciousness. A major danger is the potential for VT to progress into VF. Erratic ectopic impulses may stimulate the ventricles during their vulnerable period of repolarization, creating electrical ventricular chaos. Treatment of VT consists of intravenous lidocaine or amiodarone infusion to reduce ventricular irritability.[6] If these antiarrhythmic drugs are unsuccessful, electrical countershock (cardioversion) is generally used.

Torsades de pointes is a special type of VT in which the polarity of the wide QRS complexes rhythmically changes between positive and negative, at heart rates of 200 to 250 beats per minute.[6] This French term means "twisting of the points" and aptly describes the QRS twisting around the ECG isoelectric baseline. In contrast to the uniform shape and amplitude of QRS complexes in other forms of VT, in torsades de pointes, the QRS complexes wax and wane as they twist around the ECG baseline.

Torsades de pointes occur in conditions that delay ventricular repolarization, as manifested by a prolonged QT interval. It may be caused by electrolyte imbalances such as hypocalcemia and hypomagnesemia and by prolonged use of drugs that delay repolarization, such as lidocaine, quinidine, and procainamide.[6] Therefore, torsades de pointes requires different treatment than other VTs—antiarrhythmic drugs worsen the problem. Treatment options include overdriving the ventricular rhythm by electrical pacing or by isoproterenol (a sympathomimetic drug) infusion and intravenous magnesium sulfate infusion.[6] Direct electrical countershock is used if other methods are ineffective. Torsades de pointes may revert spontaneously to NSR but may also degenerate to VF. The underlying cause (e.g., electrolyte imbalances, drug overdose) must be removed to treat this arrhythmia successfully.

Ventricular Fibrillation

Ventricular fibrillation (VF) is the most lethal of all cardiac arrhythmias and is equivalent to full cardiac arrest. As in atrial fibrillation, many ectopic foci throughout the ventricles fire in a completely unorganized, unsynchronized manner. The ventricles are reduced to a nonfunctional, quivering muscle mass with no pumping ability. Cardiac output decreases to zero, and death occurs in minutes. The ECG (Figure 19-27) reveals no recognizable waves or complexes. Fibrillation may be fine (low amplitude) or coarse (high amplitude). Coarse VF means the heart is fibrillating vigorously.

People who develop VF lose consciousness rapidly and die unless emergency treatment is initiated immediately. No drug can convert VF to a normal rhythm. The only effective treatment for VF is strong, electrical countershock (**defibrillation**), which must be administered with no delay if it is to be successful. Automatic external defibrillators (AED) and implantable cardioverter-defibrillators (ICD) have facilitated early defibrillation. In defibrillation, a strong depolarizing current (electrical shock) passing through the heart abruptly terminates all electrical activity in all myocardial fibers, allowing the most viable pacemaker (hoped to be the sinus node) to reestablish the rhythm. Coarse VF is generally more successfully defibrillated than fine VF. Epinephrine should be given intravenously to induce vigorous fibrillation if initial defibrillation attempts are unsuccessful.[6]

If VF persists or returns after several defibrillation attempts, antiarrhythmic drugs (usually lidocaine or amiodarone) are given to depress ventricular irritability.[6] Because VF is equivalent to cardiac arrest, cardiopulmonary resuscitation (CPR) (i.e., external cardiac compression and artificial ventilation) must be implemented between defibrillation attempts.

Circus Reentry in Ventricular Fibrillation

The cardiac impulse normally travels throughout the ventricles quite rapidly and then dies out because all muscle is refractory at that time and cannot propagate the impulse further. However, several abnormal factors, including the following, may alter the way ventricles depolarize, predisposing them to develop a fibrillating pattern: (1) lengthened conduction pathways, (2) decreased conduction velocity, and (3) shortened refractory time.[4] A lengthened conduction pathway may allow the portion of muscle depolarized first to repolarize before the rest of the ventricular muscle is finished depolarizing. Because heart muscle tends to wrap around the ventricles in a circular fashion, the last muscle to depolarize may be adjacent to recovered, repolarized muscle. The depolarizing stimulus reenters the newly repolarized muscle and is propagated around the circle repeatedly. This phenomenon is called **circus movement (circus reentry)**.

A decreased conduction velocity may lead to circus reentry in a similar way. The shortened refractory time of ventricular muscle also allows the propagation of circus movement. Dilated hearts in patients with congestive heart failure lengthen conduction pathways. Ischemia, or infarction, of the Purkinje system slows the conduction velocity. Certain drugs and cell injury may shorten refractory times. Various abnormal conditions predispose the ventricles to abnormal depolarization patterns and fibrillation.

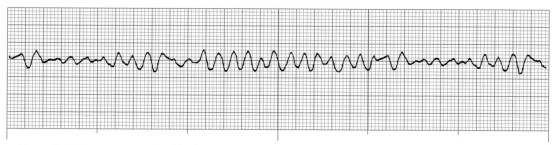

Figure 19-27 Coarse ventricular fibrillation. (From Aehlert B: *ECGs made easy,* ed 4, St Louis, 2011, Mosby.)

Atrioventricular Conduction Blocks

Injury to the AV node causes interference with normal conduction between the atria and ventricles. The AV node and bundle of His represent the only electrical connection between atrial and ventricular muscle. Hypoxia, edema, or physical damage to the AV node–bundle complex may cause delayed conduction. Some drugs also may depress AV conduction.

AV blocks are generally categorized as first-degree, second-degree, or third-degree blocks. In **first-degree AV block**, all sinus nodal impulses are conducted to the ventricles, but the conduction time is slowed through the AV node–bundle complex. This slowed conduction is marked by an increase of the PR interval greater than 0.2 second (Figure 19-28). All QRS complexes have normal configurations.

In **second-degree AV block**, some but not all SA nodal impulses are conducted to the ventricles. In type I second-degree block (Figure 19-29), the PR intervals gradually lengthen until a QRS complex fails to appear after the P wave (nonconducted P wave). Following the nonconducted P wave, the PR interval is shorter, only to lengthen progressively again until another P wave fails to conduct to the ventricles. This type of second-degree block is also known as **Mobitz type I (Wenckebach) block**.[6] Type II second-degree block, also called **Mobitz**

type II block, is characterized by constant PR intervals but with various conduction ratios. For example, there may be only four QRS complexes for every five P waves (5:4 conduction ratio), or there may be one QRS for every two P waves (2:1 conduction ratio). In both types of second-degree blocks, QRS complexes are normal.

In **third-degree AV block (complete heart block)**, no SA nodal impulses are transmitted to the ventricles (Figure 19-30). No relationship exists between P waves and QRS complexes; the atria and ventricles are electrically isolated from one another, and each establishes its own rhythm. In this situation, the ventricles must establish their own pacemaker because all SA nodal impulses are blocked. Ventricular self-pacing in this situation is called a **ventricular escape rhythm**, which is generally less than 40 beats per minute.[6] Depending on the location of the ectopic pacemaker, the QRS complexes may appear normal or widened and bizarre. Generally, the ectopic pacemaker emerges just below the block in the AV bundle; the closer this pacemaker is to the bundle, the more stable it is in producing a reliable rhythm.[6]

Third-degree block may cause a significant decrease in cardiac output and blood pressure, with subsequent dizziness and fainting. In Stokes-Adams syndrome, the ventricular escape pacemaker fails to take over immediately after the

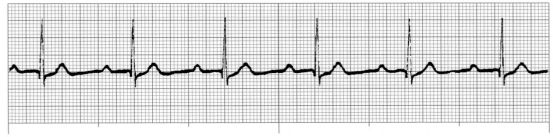

Figure 19-28 Sinus rhythm at 60 beats per minute with first-degree AV block. (From Aehlert B: *ECGs made easy,* ed 4, St Louis, 2011, Mosby.)

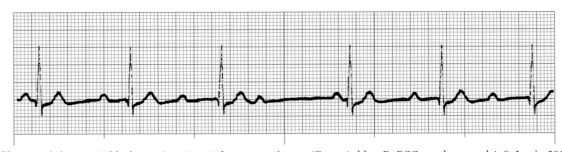

Figure 19-29 Second-degree AV block type I at 43 to 60 beats per minute. (From Aehlert B: *ECGs made easy,* ed 4, St Louis, 2011, Mosby.)

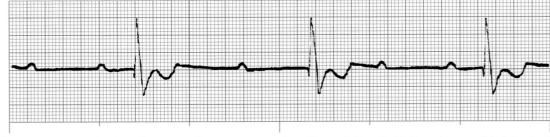

Figure 19-30 Third-degree AV block with a ventricular escape pacemaker. (From Aehlert B: *ECGs made easy,* ed 4, St Louis, 2011, Mosby.)

onset of third-degree block. Consequently, loss of blood flow to the brain causes fainting. This condition can lead to complete ventricular asystole and death if an escape pacemaker does not eventually take over. In such instances, surgical insertion of an artificial cardiac pacemaker is necessary. Intravenous infusion of atropine (a parasympathetic blocking drug) and beta-adrenergic catecholamines also may be indicated to help reverse the conduction block while the patient waits for pacemaker insertion.[6] Treatment for first-degree and second-degree blocks generally consists of withholding drugs known to slow cardiac conduction.

CONCEPT QUESTION 19-7

Why is the heart rate in third-degree AV block so much slower than the normal heart rate?

▌ POINTS TO REMEMBER

- ECG waves and complexes are voltage changes that can be monitored by at least 12 different electrode systems called leads, providing 12 different perspectives on the heart's electrical activity.
- Abnormally high amplitude waves and complexes are associated with increased muscle mass (hypertrophy).
- The heart's mean cardiac vector (MCV), or mean direction of current flow, is aimed at the greatest average muscle mass.
- The heart's MCV can be determined by analyzing the QRS polarity recorded in two leads with axes perpendicular to each other.
- Factors that cause arrhythmias include dilated, stretched heart muscle; tissue hypoxia; tissue death (infarction); electrolyte imbalances; abnormal sympathetic or parasympathetic tone; various stimulants (caffeine, tobacco, alcohol); and drugs.

- The general approach for treating arrhythmias is to treat the underlying cause and provide symptomatic treatment if necessary.
- Atrial fibrillation is associated with irregularly spaced QRS complexes and pulse deficits.
- Premature ventricular contractions of different polarity recorded by the same lead indicate a dangerously irritable ventricular muscle.
- Complete heart block requires the ventricles to establish their own pacemaker, which produces a severe bradycardia.
- Ventricular fibrillation is the most life-threatening of all arrhythmias and can be treated only by electrical countershock (defibrillation).

References

1. Huszar RJ: *Basic dysrhythmias: interpretation and management*, ed 3, St Louis, 2002, Mosby.
2. Conover MB: *Understanding electrocardiography*, ed 8, St Louis, 2003, Mosby.
3. Dubin D: *Rapid interpretation of EKG's*, ed 6, Tampa, 2000, Cover Publishing.
4. Hall JE: *Guyton and Hall textbook of medical physiology*, ed 12, Philadelphia, 2011, Saunders.
5. Brown KR, Jacobsen S: *Mastering dysrhythmias: a problem-solving guide*, Philadelphia, 1988, FA Davis.
6. Olgin JE, Zipes DP: Specific arrhythmias: diagnosis and treatment. In Bonow RO, et al, editors: *Braunwald's heart disease: a textbook of cardiovascular medicine*, ed 9, Philadelphia, 2011, Saunders.

CHAPTER 20

Control of Cardiac Output and Hemodynamic Measurements

CHAPTER OUTLINE

OBJECTIVES

After reading this chapter you will be able to:

- Describe how various physiological factors affect preload, afterload, and contractility
- Distinguish between factors that affect venous return and cardiac output
- Describe the way in which cardiac output and venous return are interdependent
- Use combined cardiac and venous return curves to illustrate the compensatory interaction between the heart and vasculature during abnormal hemodynamic conditions
- Explain why decreased left ventricular contractility leads to pulmonary edema
- Explain why various clinical hemodynamic measurements are indicators of preload, afterload, and contractility
- Develop diagnostic classifications based on analysis of hemodynamic data
- Develop a general therapeutic approach based on analysis of hemodynamic data

KEY TERMS

cardiac function curve
cardiac index (CI)
hemodynamic
hyperdynamic
inotropic factors
left ventricular end-diastolic pressure (LVEDP)
mean arterial pressure (MAP)
mean circulatory filling pressure

mean pulmonary artery pressure (MPAP)
percutaneous catheterization
pulmonary artery end-diastolic pressure (PAEDP)
pulmonary vascular resistance index (PVRI)
right ventricular end-diastolic pressure (RVEDP)
stroke volume index
systemic vascular resistance index (SVRI)
venous return curve

FACTORS CONTROLLING CARDIAC OUTPUT

Cardiac output is the quantity of blood the left ventricle pumps into the aorta each minute. Venous return is the quantity of blood the veins return to the right atrium each minute. Cardiac output and venous return both refer to the same blood flow under steady-state conditions. The heart cannot pump any more blood than it receives from the veins. It follows that blood flowing from the veins into the heart determines the cardiac output. To understand how cardiac output is regulated, one must understand the relationship between the two subdivisions of the cardiovascular system: the heart and the vascular system.

Cardiac output is determined by (1) peripheral circulatory factors that affect venous return, such as vascular resistance and blood volume, and (2) the heart's ability to pump the amount of blood it receives through the veins. The factors affecting venous return are normally the most important in controlling cardiac output in healthy people. The built-in Frank-Starling mechanism in the normal heart automatically adjusts to any amount of blood returning from the veins. Any increase in venous return is immediately pumped into the aorta. Only in pathological conditions does the heart fail to pump all of the blood it receives—in which case pumping ability becomes the factor that determines cardiac output.[1]

Cardiac Factors

Cardiac output is the product of stroke volume and heart rate. A stroke volume of 75 mL and a heart rate of 72 beats per minute produce a cardiac output of 5400 mL or 5.4 L per minute. Stroke volume is determined by three factors: (1) preload, (2) afterload, and (3) contractility.

Preload: Frank-Starling Mechanism

An increased venous return increases the end-diastolic or filling volume of the ventricles. The greater the end-diastolic volume, the more the ventricular muscle fibers are stretched. This load, or stretch, placed on myocardial fibers just before contraction is the heart's preload. According to the Frank-Starling law, an increase in preload causes myocardial fibers to contract with greater force and eject a greater stroke volume (see Chapter 17). Within physiological limits, the ventricles pump all the blood they receive without allowing it to dam in the atria and veins. Figure 20-1 is a Frank-Starling curve, also known as a **cardiac function curve**.

Another mechanism related to muscle fiber stretch also influences cardiac output. When increased venous return stretches the right atrial wall, it stretches the sinoatrial node, increasing its impulse generation frequency by 10% to 20%.[1] Myocardial fiber stretch increases cardiac output by increasing both contraction force and heart rate, although the Frank-Starling mechanism is the most important in this regard.

In clinical practice, measurement of right atrial and left atrial pressures is used to estimate the preload. These pressures represent the right and left ventricular "loading" or "filling"

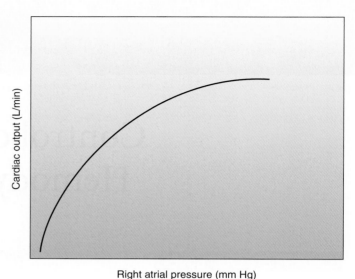

Figure 20-1 Frank-Starling cardiac function curve.

pressures and are equivalent to **right ventricular end-diastolic pressure (RVEDP)** and **left ventricular end-diastolic pressure (LVEDP)**. These preload pressures are indicators of muscle fiber length. However, high preload pressures may not significantly increase muscle fiber length if ventricular compliance is abnormally low or ventricular expansion is restricted by high external pressure, as might occur with pericardial fluid buildup or high intrapleural pressures during mechanical ventilation. Such factors must be considered when atrial pressures are used to assess ventricular preload.

CONCEPT QUESTION 20-1

Explain the effects of heart failure on preload.

Afterload

Afterload can be thought of as ventricular outflow resistance; it is the resistance opposing ejection of the ventricular stroke volume into the pulmonary artery or the aorta. Clinical indicators of left and right ventricular afterload are **mean arterial pressure (MAP)** and **mean pulmonary artery pressure (MPAP)**. Any factor that affects blood pressure affects afterload; for example, vasoconstriction increases afterload, and vasodilation decreases it.

The pumping effectiveness of the healthy heart is not influenced by afterload as much as it is by preload. Blood pressure (afterload) must increase to a very high level before stroke volume diminishes. For example, an abrupt increase in arterial resistance decreases the ventricle's ejected stroke volume for the first few beats, causing higher volumes of blood to be left in the ventricles at the end of systole. As a result, blood flowing into the ventricles during diastole stretches myocardial fibers more than before. The increased stretch enhances the healthy ventricle's contraction force, restoring the original stroke volume. In this way, the Frank-Starling mechanism helps the ventricle accommodate an increased afterload, maintaining a constant stroke volume. As one might predict, an increase in afterload increases myocardial work and oxygen consumption for a given cardiac output.

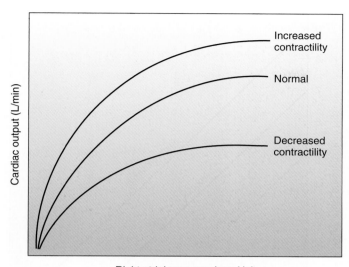

Figure 20-2 Effect of contractility on the cardiac function curve.

Contractility and Ejection Fraction

The force of myocardial muscle fiber contraction for a given preload and afterload is known as the heart's contractility. In other words, the heart's response to changes in preload while the afterload is constant is a measure of contractility. A heart with increased contractility produces a greater stroke volume for a given preload (filling pressure) than a heart with normal contractility. This means that the ventricle ejects a larger fraction of its end-diastolic volume as contractility increases—that is, the ejection fraction increases. Ejection fraction is thus a measure of ventricular contractility. The heart's normal ejection fraction is approximately 60% of the end-diastolic volume under resting conditions; in strenuous exercise, it may increase to 90%.[1]

The concept of contractility is shown in the Frank-Starling curves in Figure 20-2. These curves are also known as cardiac function curves. The greater the heart's contractility, the greater is its workload and oxygen demand. Factors influencing the heart's contractility are called **inotropic factors**. Positive inotropic factors increase the heart's contractility; negative inotropic factors decrease contractility.

Vascular Factors

Vascular factors affecting venous blood return are the most important factors in regulating cardiac output in the normal heart.[1] Venous blood flow returning to the right atrium is equal to the sum of all venous blood flows from all parts of the peripheral circulation.

This concept can be understood by considering the effects of exercise and the resultant increase in tissue metabolism. An increased rate of metabolism is evidenced by increased tissue oxygen consumption, which dilates arterioles and increases local blood flow. As a result, venous flow from exercising muscles increases, adding to the overall venous return to the right atrium. Consequently, the heart's muscle fibers stretch as preload increases, causing stroke volume and cardiac output to increase in proportion to the additional venous return. Thus, the heart does not dictate the amount of blood to be pumped into the circulation each minute; instead, incoming venous flow dictates the amount of blood the heart must pump. The healthy heart reacts by adjusting its stroke volume to match exactly the amount of blood it receives.

Long-term peripheral vascular resistance is a very important factor in determining venous return and cardiac output levels. The effect of chronically increased peripheral vascular resistance is to reduce the cardiac output level, whereas a chronic decrease in vascular resistance increases the cardiac output.[1] In the long-term, cardiac output and peripheral vascular resistance change in opposite directions.

Blood volume is also an important vascular factor in determining cardiac output. For example, severe hemorrhage decreases the circulating volume to such a low level that there is not enough pressure to push blood back to the heart; the heart is underfilled, and cardiac output decreases. In the end, the major vascular factors that determine venous return and cardiac output are (1) right atrial pressure, which represents a force hindering venous blood return to the heart; (2) mean filling pressure of the systemic circulation, which is the force pushing blood back to the heart; and (3) vascular resistance to blood flow between the peripheral vessels and the right atrium.[1]

Venous Return Curves

As discussed earlier, the cardiovascular system consists of cardiac and vascular subdivisions. The Frank-Starling curve (see Figure 20-1) is relevant to the cardiac subdivision; it illustrates the relationship between cardiac output and right atrial pressure. The **venous return curve** (Figure 20-3) is relevant to the vascular subdivision; it illustrates the relationship between right atrial pressure and venous return. A positive feedback relationship exists between the cardiac and vascular subdivisions: In the cardiac subdivision, an increase in right atrial pressure causes an increase in cardiac output (Frank-Starling mechanism); in the vascular subdivision, an increase in cardiac output secondary to increased contractility causes a decrease in right atrial pressure, which enhances venous return.[2] At any given point in time, the right atrial pressure is common to both cardiac and vascular subdivisions, simultaneously playing a different role in each.

The venous return curve shows that if cardiac output were to suddenly fall to zero (as it would in cardiac arrest) and if all neural circulatory reflexes were abolished, right atrial pressure would increase to a maximum of about 7 mm Hg, reflecting the overall static equilibrium between venous and arterial

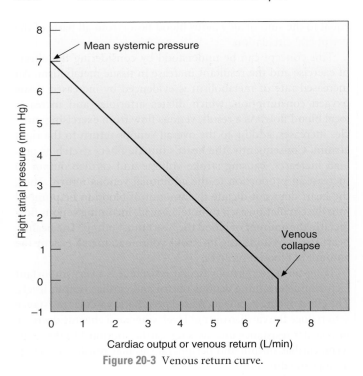

Figure 20-3 Venous return curve.

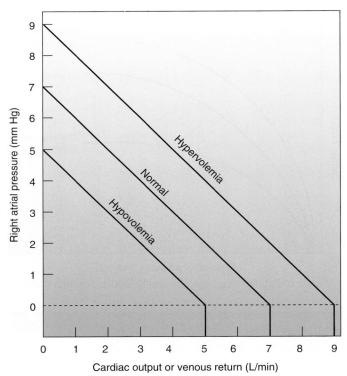

Figure 20-4 Effect of blood volume on the venous return curve.

pressures.[1] This hypothetical vascular equilibrium pressure established under static, no-flow conditions is called the **mean circulatory filling pressure**. The vascular equilibrium pressure in this hypothetical situation is lower than the simple average of pressures in venous and arterial vessels because the veins are highly distensible and serve as a large reservoir in which blood pools.

The mean circulatory filling pressure is determined by two major factors: the blood volume and intravascular space, or the size of the vascular "container." The intravascular space is determined mainly by vessel diameter, which is a factor of (1) the elastic recoil force of the vessels and (2) vessel smooth muscle tone, or the degree of vasoconstriction present.[3] When blood is circulating normally, the average pressure at the venous end of the systemic capillaries is about equal to the theoretical mean circulatory filling pressure.[3] The difference between this pressure and right atrial pressure is the pressure gradient that drives venous return.[1] If the heart fails to pump all the blood it receives from the veins, blood dams up in the right atrium and increases its pressure, which decreases the pressure gradient that drives venous return. As a result, venous inflow of blood falls to match the failing heart's reduced pumping capacity. On the other hand, if cardiac contractility increases and the heart pumps out more blood than it receives, right atrial pressure falls, increasing the pressure gradient that drives venous return.

If the heart pumps blood so vigorously that right atrial pressure falls below zero (see Figure 20-3), venous return and cardiac output stop rising. The reason for this phenomenon is that as the heart contracts more powerfully, it generates an increasingly greater subatmospheric pressure in the right atrium and the inferior vena cava, collapsing this great vein just before it enters the thoracic cavity; that is, the higher abdominal cavity pressure surrounding the vein caves in its walls just before it

enters the chest. As a result, venous return and cardiac output cannot increase further.

Effect of Blood Volume and Arteriolar Resistance on Venous Return Curve. Figure 20-4 illustrates the effect of increased and decreased blood volume on the venous return curve. The mean circulatory filling pressure, hypothetically equal to intravascular pressure during circulatory standstill, depends only on vessel wall recoil (compliance) and blood volume. For a given vessel compliance, increased blood volume (hypervolemia) increases the mean circulatory filling pressure; decreased blood volume (hypovolemia) decreases mean circulatory filling pressure. Figure 20-4 illustrates this concept, showing mean circulatory filling pressures of 9 mm Hg for hypervolemia, 7 mm Hg for normovolemia, and 5 mm Hg for hypovolemia. In other words, the more the vascular space is filled, the "tighter" the vessels become; this increases the mean circulatory filling pressure and shifts the venous return curve up and to the right. Conversely, the less the vascular space is filled, the "looser" the system becomes, lowering the mean circulatory filling pressure and shifting the venous return curve down and to the left.

Figure 20-5 illustrates the effect of arteriolar resistance on the venous return curve. Because the arterioles contain only about 3% of the total blood volume, their constriction or dilation does not significantly affect mean circulatory filling pressure.[4] Therefore, the venous return curves representing different arteriolar resistances in Figure 20-5 have different slopes but converge on the same mean circulatory filling pressure "hinge" point (7 mm Hg). (These curves assume that blood volume and vascular compliance remain constant.) Figure 20-5 shows that a decrease in arteriolar resistance allows more blood to flow through systemic capillaries, into the veins, and into the right

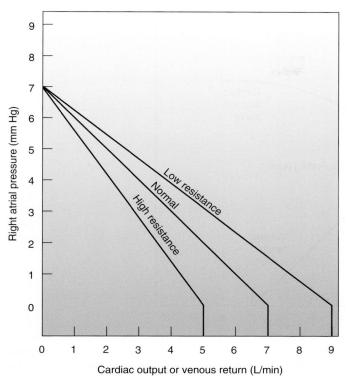

Figure 20-5   Effect of vascular resistance on the venous return curve.

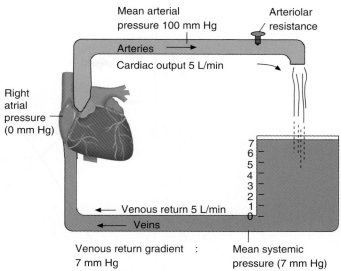

Figure 20-6 Coupling of the heart and systemic vasculature. Notice that factors affecting venous return and cardiac output are simultaneously resolved at one right atrial pressure. (Modified from Green JF: *Fundamental cardiovascular and pulmonary physiology*, ed 2, Philadelphia, 1987, Lea & Febiger.)

atrium. This rotates the curve about its mean circulatory filling pressure hinge point (7 mm Hg) in an upward direction; the decrease in the curve's slope denotes less resistance (higher cardiac output for a given right atrial pressure). Conversely, high arteriolar resistance decreases the amount of blood that can flow through systemic capillaries each minute and reduces blood return to the right atrium; this rotates the venous return curve around the same hinge point in a downward direction; the increased slope of the curve denotes greater resistance (lower cardiac output for a given right atrial pressure).

Coupling of the Heart and Vasculature: Guyton Diagram

Figure 20-6 shows the coupling of the heart and systemic blood vessels. The blood pressure at the venous end of the systemic capillaries is represented by the 7-mm high blood column at the right of the figure. The pressure at the bottom of the blood column is the mean circulatory filling pressure (7 mm Hg). Right atrial pressure is 0 mm Hg, so a pressure gradient of 7 mm Hg exists between the venous end of the capillaries and the right atrium. This gradient supplies the force or "push" to move blood through the veins to the right atrium.[1]

At any given instant, the cardiovascular system operates at a certain point on the cardiac output curve and at a certain point on the venous return curve; these two points must be identical because the heart operates at only one right atrial pressure. That is, all factors that regulate venous return and cardiac output are simultaneously resolved at this single right atrial pressure. A variation in either cardiac output or venous return causes the other one to change. For example, increased sympathetic

nervous activity produces an increase in cardiac contractility and increases the cardiac output; this lowers right atrial pressure, increasing the venous return pressure gradient. Consequently, venous blood flow to the heart increases. Reduced vascular resistance, as occurs with exercise, increases venous return and increases the right atrial pressure; this increases the heart's preload and, in accordance with the Frank-Starling mechanism, increases the cardiac output. In normal, steady-state conditions, venous blood flow into the right atrium dictates the amount of blood that the heart must pump. The healthy heart has more than adequate reserve to respond to any amount of blood entering it. As stated earlier, only in an abnormal condition (e.g., loss of contractility, or heart failure) is the heart's ability to pump the primary determinant of cardiac output.

Both venous return and cardiac output curves can be superimposed on the same graph, forming a Guyton diagram (Figure 20-7)[2]; this requires the axes of the venous return curve to be reversed (compare with Figure 20-3). The point at which the cardiac function and venous return curves intersect identifies the right atrial pressure common to both the cardiac and the vascular subdivisions of the cardiovascular system. This intersection is the cardiovascular system's equilibrium or operating point, the point at which cardiac output and venous return are equal. The Guyton diagram in Figure 20-3 represents the normal circulation in which a right atrial pressure of about 2 mm Hg is associated with a cardiac output and venous return of about 5 L per minute.

Effect of Contractility Changes

Figure 20-8 illustrates the effect of increased and decreased myocardial contractility on the cardiovascular system. Point *A* is the normal operating point. In a hypothetical situation

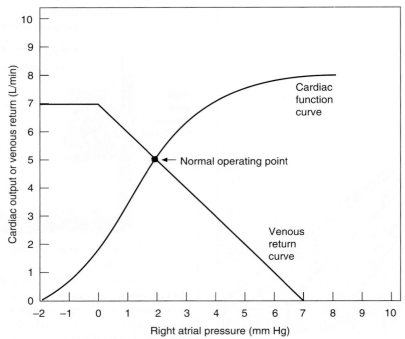

Figure 20-7 Combined cardiac and venous return curves (Guyton diagram). Factors regulating venous return and cardiac output are simultaneously resolved at one right atrial pressure, the normal operating point. This point represents a right atrial pressure of about 2 mm Hg and a cardiac output of about 5 L per minute.

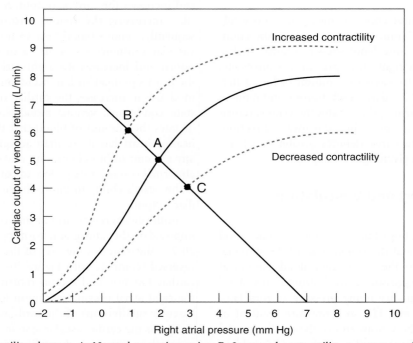

Figure 20-8 Effects of contractility changes. **A,** Normal operating point. **B,** Increased contractility pumps more blood from the right atrium, increasing cardiac output while decreasing right atrial pressure. **C,** Decreased contractility decreases cardiac output, allowing blood to dam in the right atrium, increasing right atrial pressure.

in which only contractility increases (constant blood volume and vascular resistance), the cardiac function curve moves up and to the left, intersecting the venous return curve at point B. This point represents a new equilibrium in which the heart pumps more blood from the right atrium, decreasing right atrial pressure and increasing the gradient for venous return.

Consequently, venous return increases to match the increased cardiac output. In the end, cardiac output and venous return are greater at a lower right atrial (preload) pressure, which is the hallmark of increased contractility.

Conversely, if myocardial contractility suddenly decreases (assuming a constant blood volume and vascular resistance),

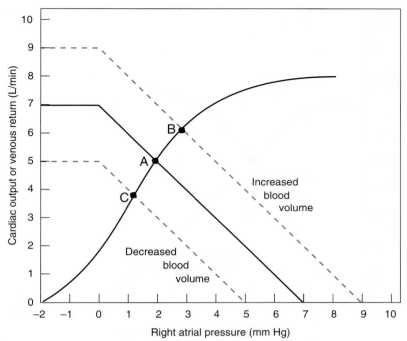

Figure 20-9 Effects of blood volume changes. **A,** Normal operating point. **B,** Increased volume increases filling (right atrial) pressure and cardiac output. **C,** Decreased volume does the opposite.

cardiac output decreases. The cardiac function curve moves down and to the right, intersecting the venous return curve at point *C* in Figure 20-8. This point represents a new equilibrium in which the heart pumps less blood than normal from the right atrium, and right atrial pressure increases. The resulting decrease in the venous return pressure gradient is consistent with the decreased cardiac output. In this situation, cardiac output and venous return are lower at a higher right atrial pressure, which is a hallmark of decreased contractility (e.g., congestive heart failure). (The term "congestive" refers to the congestion or pooling of blood in the veins.)

Effects of Blood Volume Changes

An increased blood volume (as occurs with intravenous fluid infusion) increases vascular pressures throughout the system; mean circulatory filling pressure increases, causing the venous return curve to shift up and to the right, intersecting the cardiac function curve at point *B* (Figure 20-9). Cardiac output increases, moving from point *A* to point *B* in Figure 20-9. In this way, cardiac output increases to accommodate the increased venous return; however, this increase does not represent greater contractility because the position of the cardiac function curve stays constant in this example. As venous blood flow into the heart increases, the heart responds according to the Frank-Starling law by contracting with greater force, but its ejection fraction does not change.

A sudden blood volume loss such as occurs with hemorrhage has the opposite effect. Venous pressures fall and myocardial fibers are less stretched; in accordance with the Frank-Starling law, cardiac output decreases. The venous return curve shifts down and to the left to a new equilibrium point (point *C* in Figure 20-9).

Effect of Peripheral Arteriolar Resistance Changes

An increased arteriolar resistance produces complex changes in the Guyton diagram because both cardiac and venous return curves shift simultaneously. To understand the general concept, it is helpful to consider the hypothetical effect of an increased arteriolar resistance alone, with the right atrial pressure and cardiac force of contraction remaining constant (Figure 20-10). Under such circumstances, an increased resistance would cause the venous return curve to rotate down and to the left, pivoting around its constant right atrial pressure hinge point (mean circulatory filling pressure) on the graph's horizontal axis. At the same time, the cardiac function curve would shift down and to the right because at a constant right atrial pressure and force of contraction, the heart would pump less blood against a greater resistance or afterload. The right atrial pressure would stay constant in this hypothetical example because of proportional decreases in both cardiac output and venous return. The new equilibrium point *B* would be formed below the original point *A*.

However, Figure 20-10 artificially separates the effects of vascular resistance from the effects of subsequent compensatory factors. It does not take into account the normal physiological response of the healthy heart to an increase in afterload. As explained previously, an increased afterload raises the heart's end-systolic volume, increasing the preload; in response, the Frank-Starling mechanism increases the healthy heart's contracting force and stroke volume. The resulting increase in arterial pressure overcomes the increased arteriolar resistance and maintains the cardiac output at a normal level. However, if the heart has poor contractility and is already overstretched, an increased vascular resistance may induce acute cardiac failure.

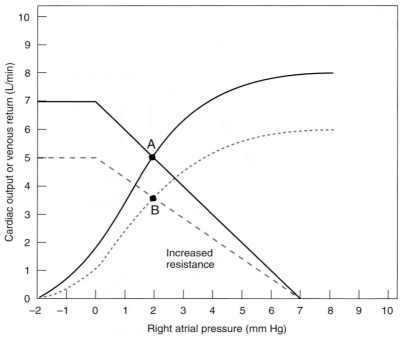

Figure 20-10 Effect of increased arteriolar resistance. **A,** Normal operating point. **B,** At a constant preload (right atrial pressure), the heart pumps less against higher resistance.

Effect of Therapeutic Interventions

To anticipate how cardiovascular drugs and intravenous fluids affect the cardiac output and venous return curves, one must consider the effect of the intervention on each curve separately. To assess the effect of an intervention on the cardiac output curve, one need only answer the question: Does the intervention increase, decrease, or not affect the heart's contractility? For example, drugs that increase sympathetic tone (e.g., epinephrine) or inhibit parasympathetic tone (e.g., atropine) or that increase intracellular calcium ion concentration (e.g., digitalis) increase the heart's contractility and move the cardiac output curve up and to the left. Drugs that inhibit sympathetic tone (e.g., beta blockers) or block the cell membrane calcium ion channels (e.g., calcium channel blockers) decrease myocardial contractility and move the cardiac output curve down and to the left.

To assess the effect of an intervention on the venous return curve, one need only answer the question: Does the intervention change the relationship between intravascular space and the blood volume? Such an intervention entails a change either in blood volume (intravenous fluids or diuretic drugs) or in the vascular space (vasoconstrictor or vasodilator drugs). Intravenous fluid infusion would move the venous return curve up and to the right, which would increase the mean circulatory filling pressure and increase the cardiac output (it would intercept the cardiac output curve at a higher level). Diuretics would move the venous return curve down and to the left, which would decrease the mean circulatory filling pressure and cardiac output (it would intercept the cardiac output curve at a lower level). Vasodilator drugs would decrease the slope of the venous return curve, increasing the cardiac output for a given right atrial pressure (the venous return curve would intercept

the cardiac output curve at a higher point). Vasoconstrictor drugs would have the opposite effect.

Normal Compensatory Response to Sudden Loss of Contractility

Acute myocardial infarction suddenly reduces the heart's contractility and pumping ability (usually the left ventricle), and cardiac output acutely decreases. Momentarily, blood flows into the left ventricle at a higher rate than it is pumped out, causing blood to dam up in the left atrium, the pulmonary vasculature, and ultimately the right ventricle and atrium. Increased right atrial pressure is reflected throughout the systemic venous circulation. A new low-flow state develops in which cardiac output and venous return are again equal, with higher venous pressures and lower arterial pressures than normal. This situation, called acute uncompensated heart failure, is shown in Figure 20-11 (see point B).

The body's immediate response is a massive sympathetic nervous discharge. Sympathetic stimulation is helpful in two ways: (1) it immediately increases the damaged heart's contractility or inotropic state, and (2) it causes systemic arterial and venous vasoconstriction. Improved contractility shifts the cardiac function curve slightly up and to the left. At the same time, vasoconstriction "tightens" the blood vessels, shifting the venous return curve up and to the right. Over the long-term, blood volume increases because the kidney conserves water in response to the chronically low blood pressure. The combination of (1) improved contractility, (2) vasoconstriction, and (3) renal fluid retention creates a new compensated equilibrium point (see point C in Figure 20-11). This is known as compensated heart failure. Cardiac output is restored to normal values, but this requires higher left ventricular filling pressures than

CLINICAL FOCUS 20-1

Physical Examination Findings in Left Ventricular Failure

The physical examination of a patient with acute left ventricular failure may reveal some or all of the following signs and symptoms:

- The patient complains of dyspnea.
- Fine crackles (breath sounds) are heard on auscultation.
- Symptoms worsen when the patient lies flat (this is known as orthopnea).
- Systemic blood pressure is low.
- Skin is cool and clammy.
- Neck veins (jugular veins) are pulsating and distended in the sitting position.
- Palpation reveals an enlarged liver (hepatomegaly).
- Ankles and lower legs are swollen (pedal edema).

Dyspnea and fine crackles are caused by the same mechanism: left heart pumping failure and blood backup into the pulmonary veins and capillaries. The resulting hydrostatic pulmonary edema produces fine, moist crackles on inspiration and impairs oxygenation; in addition, engorged alveolar capillaries decrease lung compliance and increase work of breathing. A supine position increases venous return because of gravitational forces, which overloads the failing ventricle even more. Ventricular pumping failure reduces blood flow and pressure; coupled with reflex vasoconstriction, this underperfuses the tissues, and the skin becomes cool and clammy to the touch. Severe left heart failure produces right heart failure, causing blood backup into the right atrium and systemic venous system. High venous pressures are responsible for jugular venous distention; engorged, enlarged liver; and leg and ankle edema. This kind of heart failure could be caused by an acute myocardial infarction or valvular disease such as mitral or aortic valve stenosis.

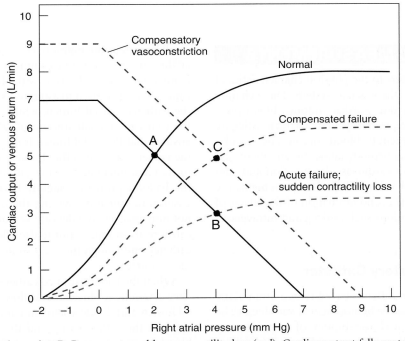

Figure 20-11 A, Normal operating point. **B,** Response to sudden contractility loss (*red*). Cardiac output falls acutely, increasing right atrial pressure. **C,** Sympathetic activity increases contractility (*blue*) and causes vasoconstriction (*green*), restoring cardiac output to near normal but at a higher right atrial pressure.

normal. As a result, the pressures in the pulmonary vasculature, right heart, and systemic veins are higher than normal. In compensated heart failure, a higher right atrial pressure is required to achieve a cardiac output of 5 L per minute (see point *C* in Figure 20-11) than in the normal heart (see point *A*).

Figure 20-12, *A,* shows a sudden reduction in cardiac output to 2.5 L per minute with subsequent increases in right atrial and venous pressures (compare with Figure 20-6). Figure 20-12, *A,* corresponds with point *B* on the graph in Figure 20-11. Figure 20-12, *B,* illustrates an improved pumping ability caused by the inotropic influence of sympathetic stimulation and increased blood volume. This compensated state corresponds with point *C* in Figure 20-11.

CONCEPT QUESTION 20-4

In what way would physical findings in pure right heart failure differ from findings in combined right and left heart failure?

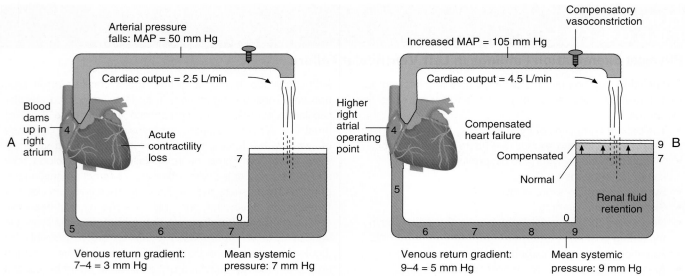

Figure 20-12 A, Acute loss of contractility decreases cardiac output, allowing blood to back up in the right atrium. This decreases the pressure gradient for venous return. **B,** Compensatory sympathetic activity improves contractility and causes vasoconstriction, both of which improve blood pressure and cardiac output. Renal fluid retention increases the venous return pressure gradient. Cardiac output is now near normal but requires higher right atrial pressure. (See Figure 20-11.) (Modified from Green JF: *Fundamental cardiovascular and pulmonary physiology,* ed 2, Philadelphia, 1987, Lea & Febiger.)

HEMODYNAMIC MEASUREMENTS

The term **hemodynamic** refers to the physical characteristics of actively circulating blood in the vascular system. These characteristics include blood flow rate (cardiac output), blood pressures, and vascular resistance. Hemodynamic characteristics are determined by cardiac contractility, blood volume, and vascular smooth muscle tone. Clinical hemodynamic measurements are valuable in the assessment of cardiovascular function and adequacy of intravascular fluid volume. These measurements are also valuable in the monitoring and evaluation of the effects of various therapeutic interventions such as drug and intravenous fluid therapy.

Use of Pulmonary Artery Catheter

A pulmonary artery catheter, often referred to as a Swan-Ganz catheter, can be used to measure hemodynamic variables. (The mechanical characteristics and capabilities of a pulmonary artery catheter are discussed in Chapter 6.) Figure 20-13 illustrates a typical quadruple-lumen, balloon-tipped pulmonary artery catheter. It may be surgically inserted into the heart and pulmonary vessels via the internal jugular vein (Figure 20-14). This vein provides a direct path to the right atrium. Other potential insertion sites leading to the right atrium include the subclavian vein, the femoral vein in the groin, and the basilic or median cubital veins in the right arm.[5] The process of surgically puncturing the skin to gain vascular access to insert the catheter is called **percutaneous catheterization**.

When the catheter is properly placed, the proximal port communicates with the right atrium through the proximal lumen (see Figure 20-13). The distal port communicates with a small branch of the pulmonary artery through the distal lumen at the catheter's tip. On gaining vascular access, the catheter is introduced into the vein with the balloon deflated; at that time, a syringe is used to aspirate a small amount of blood from the catheter's distal lumen, which is flushed gently back into the vein with a small amount of saline solution.[5] This process ensures that the distal lumen is open and unobstructed. When the catheter tip enters the thoracic vein, the balloon is inflated to its recommended volume (about 1.5 mL); at this volume, the balloon protrudes slightly beyond the hard catheter tip, cushioning but not covering the distal opening. The balloon not only protects the delicate vascular endothelium and endocardium from injury, but it also allows blood flow to float the catheter tip through the heart to its proper position in the pulmonary artery.[5]

When the balloon-tipped catheter wedges in a small pulmonary arteriole, it blocks blood flow between the catheter's distal lumen and the downstream left atrium. Because blood flow between the catheter's tip and the left atrium is stopped, the blood pressure measured through the distal lumen is about the same as the left atrial pressure. As explained in Chapter 6, this is called the pulmonary capillary wedge pressure (PCWP). The PCWP is a clinical indicator of left ventricular filling pressure or preload. Similarly, right atrial pressure, or central venous pressure, measured from the proximal port is a clinical indicator of right ventricular preload.

The proximal and distal catheter lumens are connected to pressure transducers, which are mechanical devices that convert pressure fluctuations to electrical signals. The electrical signals are displayed as pressure waveforms on a monitoring screen; pressure is displayed on the vertical axis, and time is displayed on the horizontal axis.

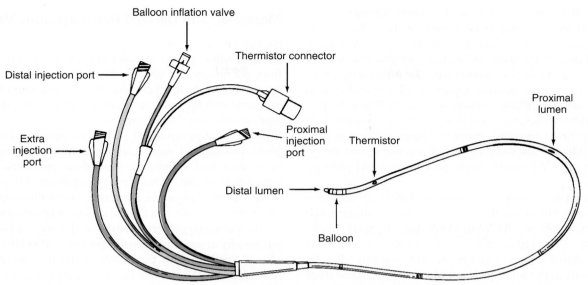

Figure 20-13 Quadruple channel pulmonary artery catheter (Swan-Ganz catheter). (From Martin L: *Pulmonary physiology in clinical practice: the essentials for patient care and evaluation,* St Louis, 1987, Mosby.)

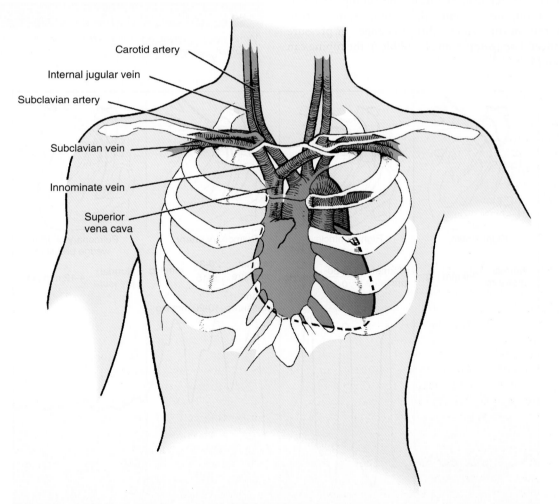

Figure 20-14 Anatomical location of major veins for inserting a pulmonary artery catheter. Common insertion sites are the subclavian and internal jugular veins. (From Daily EK, Schroeder JS: *Techniques in bedside hemodynamic monitoring,* ed 5, St Louis, 1994, Mosby.)

Figure 20-15 shows examples of different pressure waveforms recorded from the distal lumen of the catheter as it passes through the heart and pulmonary artery. Waveform shapes aid in catheter insertion because they give information about the location of the catheter tip. The pulmonary artery waveform in the third panel of Figure 20-15 is recorded from the distal lumen when the balloon is deflated. When the balloon is inflated, blocking blood flow, the PCWP waveform in the right panel is recorded. Proper catheter position is confirmed by inflating and deflating the balloon and noting abrupt changes from PCWP waveforms to pulmonary artery pressure waveforms.

The pulmonary artery waveform in Figure 20-15 has a clear, sharp upstroke on the left, falling to a distinct notch in the downstroke on the right. This dicrotic notch marks the closure of the pulmonary semilunar valves as the heart enters the diastolic phase (see Chapter 17). A similar dicrotic notch appears in the aortic pressure waveform measured from a catheter placed in a systemic artery. In the systemic arterial catheter, often called an arterial line, the dicrotic notch marks closure of the aortic semilunar valves. The absence of a dicrotic notch recorded from either a pulmonary or a systemic artery catheter usually means the tubing system is overdamped. Damping prevents the tubing system from immediately transmitting small, abrupt changes in pressure to the transducer. For example, an air bubble in the tubing can cause overdamping.

Measured and Derived Hemodynamic Variables

Measured Variables

Cardiac output, pressures, and heart rate are directly measured from pulmonary and systemic arterial catheters. Directly measured variables are listed in Table 20-1. Cardiac output is directly measured with the pulmonary artery catheter using the thermo-dilution technique (see Chapter 6).

Right atrial pressure and PCWP are influenced by vascular blood volume and ventricular contractility. As stated earlier, increased blood volume increases these pressures. Increased contractility means the heart pumps more blood from the atria, decreasing these pressures. Decreased contractility has the opposite effect; blood dams in the atria, increasing their pressures.

The pulmonary artery pressure at the very end of diastole, **pulmonary artery end-diastolic pressure (PAEDP)**, normally almost equalizes with the PCWP if the pulmonary vascular resistance (PVR) is normal (see Figure 20-15). For this reason, PAEDP is sometimes used in place of PCWP in the estimation of left ventricular filling pressure. However, when PVR is high, PAEDP is much higher than PCWP and does not accurately reflect left ventricular filling pressure.

CONCEPT QUESTION 20-5

Why does increased PVR affect the difference between PAEDP and PCWP?

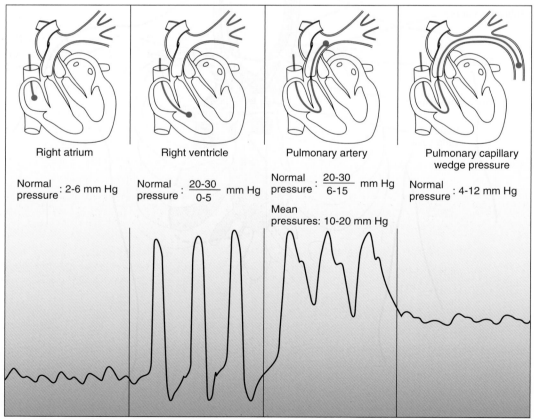

Right atrium	Right ventricle	Pulmonary artery	Pulmonary capillary wedge pressure
Normal pressure: 2-6 mm Hg	Normal pressure: $\frac{20\text{-}30}{0\text{-}5}$ mm Hg	Normal pressure: $\frac{20\text{-}30}{6\text{-}15}$ mm Hg Mean pressures: 10-20 mm Hg	Normal pressure: 4-12 mm Hg

Figure 20-15 Normal pressure waveforms derived from the pulmonary artery catheter as it is floated into position. (From Wilkins RL, Sheldon RL, Krider SJ: *Clinical assessment in respiratory care*, ed 3, St Louis, 1995, Mosby.)

Mean pulmonary and systemic artery pressures are indicators of right and left ventricular afterloads. The ventricles must overcome MPAP and MAP to eject their stroke volumes. These pressures are influenced by vascular blood volume and vessel diameter. Decreased left ventricular contractility also affects the MPAP, as blood backs up through the pulmonary vasculature.

CONCEPT QUESTION 20-6

Why does decreased left ventricular contractility affect MPAP?

Derived Variables

Other physiologically important information can be calculated from directly measured hemodynamic variables. Table 20-2 lists these calculated hemodynamic variables.

The **cardiac index (CI)** is the cardiac output divided by the body surface area (BSA) in square meters. BSA is related to height and weight and is correlated with body mass (see the DuBois body surface area chart in Appendix IV). People of different sizes can be compared by indexing the cardiac output to BSA. For example, a basketball player who is 7 feet tall has a higher cardiac output than an average person who is 5 feet, 10 inches tall. Both individuals have similar CIs, which are obtained by dividing cardiac output by BSA. A CI less than 2.5 L/min/m^2 indicates a generalized state of low blood flow and poor peripheral circulation, implying poor myocardial contractility or greatly reduced blood volume.[6]

The stroke volume is the cardiac output divided by the heart rate. Abnormally low contractility reduces stroke volume. Very high heart rates also may reduce the stroke volume because the ventricles have inadequate filling time during diastole. The **stroke volume index** relates stroke volume to body size. Similar to a low CI, a low stroke volume index implies poor myocardial contractility.

Systemic vascular resistance (SVR) and the **systemic vascular resistance index (SVRI)** are indicators of left ventricular afterload. The left ventricle must overcome SVR to eject its stroke volume. Increased SVR is caused by arteriolar vessel constriction; decreased SVR is caused by vasodilation. Likewise, PVR and the **pulmonary vascular resistance index (PVRI)** are indicators of right ventricular afterload and are caused by changes in pulmonary vessel diameters. The SVRI and PVRI calculations use CI rather than cardiac output in the denominator.

The driving pressures that produce blood flow through systemic and pulmonary circulations are first calculated to determine SVR and PVR. These pressure gradients are divided by the blood flow—that is, the cardiac output. This method works because resistance is measured in terms of pressure per unit of flow (mm Hg/L/min).

The systemic circulation driving pressure is equal to the difference between MAP (the beginning point of the systemic circulation) and mean right atrial pressure (the end point of the systemic circulation). This difference divided by cardiac

TABLE 20-1

Directly Measured Hemodynamic Variables

Measurement	Normal Range
Pulmonary Artery Catheter	
Right atrial pressure or central venous pressure (RAP, CVP)	<6 mm Hg
Pulmonary artery pressure (PAP)	20-30/6-15 mm Hg
Mean pulmonary artery pressure (MPAP)	10-20 mm Hg
Pulmonary capillary wedge pressure (PCWP)	4-12 mm Hg
Cardiac output (CO)	4-8 L/min
Heart rate (HR)	60-100 beats/min
Systemic Arterial Catheter	
Arterial pressure (BP)	120/80 mm Hg
Mean arterial pressure (MAP)	80-100 mm Hg

TABLE 20-2

Calculated Hemodynamic Variables

Variable	Normal Range	Formula
Cardiac index (CI)	2.5-4.0 L/min/m^2	CO/BSA
Stroke volume (SV)	60-130 mL/beat	CO/HR
Stroke volume index (SVI) or stroke index (SI)	30-50 mL/m^2	SV/BSA
Systemic vascular resistance (SVR)	900-1400 dynes • sec • cm^{-5}	([MAP – RAP]/CO) × 80
Systemic vascular resistance index (SVRI)	1700-2600 dynes • sec • cm^{-5}	([MAP – RAP]/CI) × 80
Pulmonary vascular resistance (PVR)	100-250 dynes • sec • cm^{-5}	([MPAP – PCWP]/CO) × 80
Pulmonary vascular resistance index (PVRI)	200-450 dynes • sec • cm^{-5}	([MPAP – PCWP]/CI) × 80
Left ventricular stroke work index (LVSWI)	40-75 g-m/m^2/beat	SI × (MAP – PCWP) × 0.0136
Right ventricular stroke work index (RVSWI)	4-8 g-m/m^2/beat	SI × (MPAP – CVP) × 0.0136

CO, Cardiac output; *BSA,* body surface area in square meters derived from the Dubois body surface area chart; *HR,* heart rate; *SV,* stroke volume; *MAP,* mean arterial pressure; *RAP,* right atrial pressure; *MPAP,* mean pulmonary artery pressure; *PCWP,* pulmonary capillary wedge pressure; *CVP,* central venous pressure.

output yields SVR in mm Hg/L/min. Multiplying the SVR by 80 changes mm Hg/L/min to centimeter-gram-second (CGS) units of measure, commonly designated in the clinical setting as dynes · sec · cm^{-5} (see Table 20-2 and Chapter 6).

The driving pressure for the pulmonary circulation is also the difference between the circulation's beginning pressure (MPAP) and ending pressure (PCWP). Dividing this difference by the cardiac output and multiplying by 80 gives PVR in CGS resistance units.

CONCEPT QUESTION 20-7

What factors may increase the numerical difference between MPAP and PCWP?

Left and right ventricular stroke work indices indicate left and right ventricular contractility and oxygen consumption. Stroke work index is a measure of how hard the ventricle must contract to move blood through the vascular system. In terms of classic physics, work is done when a force moves a mass a given distance (work = force × distance). In the heart, force is the average pressure the ventricle generates, and distance is the volume of blood ejected (stroke volume). The differences between the ventricles' end-diastolic pressures and their corresponding MAPs are the average pressures the ventricles must generate to eject their stroke volumes during contraction. Clinical indicators of end-diastolic pressures for the right and left ventricles are the right atrial pressure and PCWP. The pressure that the left ventricle generates during contraction is the numerical difference between MAP and PCWP, and for the right ventricle, it is the difference between MPAP and the right atrial pressure. Multiplying both pressure differences by the stroke indices produces the stroke work index for the left and right ventricles. The multiplication of the stroke work index by 0.0136 converts the units to gram-meters/m^2/beat, which is the standard unit used in medicine to express cardiac work (see Table 20-2).

If the left ventricle loses its contractility, it cannot perform much work because it cannot pump much blood; the left ventricular stroke work index decreases. At the same time, myocardial oxygen consumption decreases because the heart performs less work. Table 20-3 summarizes the clinical hemodynamic indicators of the heart's preload, afterload, and contractility.

Significance of Pulmonary Capillary Wedge Pressure Measurement

The two main clinical reasons for measuring PCWP are to (1) measure pulmonary capillary hydrostatic pressure and (2) estimate the filling pressure of the left ventricle. PCWP is an estimate of left atrial pressure and is thus an estimate of left ventricular filling pressure. Although the PCWP is the pressure in the small arteries just before the pulmonary capillary beds, it reflects left atrial pressure. When the catheter balloon is inflated, there is no flow between the catheter tip and the left atrium; therefore, PCWP and left atrial pressure are essentially identical. Under these circumstances, PCWP is a good estimator of left atrial pressure.

CONCEPT QUESTION 20-8

Assuming normal blood volume and valvular function, what does an elevated PCWP imply?

Capillary Hydrostatic Pressure

PCWP is the pressure in the pulmonary capillaries that tends to force fluid into the interstitial space. Normally, this force of 6 to 12 mm Hg is opposed by capillary osmotic forces, and with the help of lymphatic removal of interstitial fluid, pulmonary edema is prevented.

When the PCWP increases to greater than 18 mm Hg, early clinical signs of pulmonary edema generally appear on the chest

TABLE 20-3

Clinical Indicators of Preload, Afterload, and Contractility

Cardiac Factor	Clinical Indicator	Influencing Factors
Preload		
Left ventricle	PCWP	Blood volume, contractility, intrapleural pressure (positive pressure ventilation)
Right ventricle	RAP (CVP)	
Afterload*		
Left ventricle	MAP, SVR, SVRI	Vessel diameter, blood volume and viscosity, contractility*
Right ventricle	MPAP, PVR, PVRI	
Contractility		
Left ventricle	LVSWI, SV, SVI, CI	Functional muscle mass, electrolyte balance (K$^+$, Ca^{++}), sympathetic neural activity, acid-base balance
Right ventricle	RVSWI	

PCWP, Pulmonary capillary wedge pressure; *RAP (CVP),* right atrial (central venous) pressure; *MAP,* mean arterial pressure; *SVR,* systemic vascular resistance; *SVRI,* systemic vascular resistance index; *MPAP,* mean pulmonary artery pressure; *PVR,* pulmonary vascular resistance; *PVRI,* pulmonary vascular resistance index; *LVSWI,* left ventricular stroke work index; *SV,* stroke volume; *SVI,* stroke volume index; *CI,* cardiac index; *RVSWI,* right ventricular stroke work index.
*Decreased left ventricular contractility influences right ventricular afterload.

x-ray image. At a PCWP greater than 25 mm Hg, the chest x-ray film shows obvious evidence of pulmonary edema.[6] The PCWP provides valuable information about the effects of intravenous fluid infusions in hemodynamically unstable patients.

Left Ventricular Preload

Ideally, the PCWP equals the left atrial pressure, which equals the left ventricular end-diastolic pressure (LVEDP). LVEDP is normally proportional to the left ventricular end-diastolic volume (LVEDV). The true concept of preload refers to fiber length, not ventricular pressure. A reasonable assumption is that LVEDV is directly related to muscle fiber length. However, increased ventricular diastolic pressure may not translate

into increased volume or increased fiber length in abnormal circumstances. For example, any factor that restricts ventricular expansion during diastole alters the relationship between pressure and volume. Such factors include (1) an already overstretched, distended ventricle; (2) pericardial tamponade; (3) myocardial infarction scaring (stiff ventricle); and (4) the increased pressure surrounding the heart during positive pressure mechanical ventilation, especially in the presence of high levels of positive end expiratory pressure (PEEP). In these cases, LVEDP is elevated, which increases left atrial pressure and PCWP; however, these high pressures reflect a restriction to the ability of the left ventricle to expand, not increased volume or fiber length.

CLINICAL FOCUS 20-2

Interpretation of Pulmonary Capillary Wedge Pressure in the Presence of Mechanical Ventilation and Positive End Expiratory Pressure

The relationship between PCWP and left ventricular filling pressure is especially important in mechanically ventilated patients with PEEP. True left ventricular filling pressure is the pressure distending the ventricular wall—that is, the pressure inside the ventricle minus the pressure outside the ventricle. The pressure outside the ventricle is the surrounding intrathoracic pressure. Figure 20-16, *A*, represents normal, spontaneous breathing conditions when LVEDP is 6 mm Hg. The pulmonary artery catheter senses this pressure as PCWP of 6 mm Hg. The intrathoracic pressure is –5 mm Hg, producing a transmural (across the wall) filling pressure of 11 mm Hg. In Figure 20-16, *B*, mechanical ventilation and PEEP have increased mean intrathoracic pressure from –5 mm Hg to +10 mm Hg for a total increase of 15 mm Hg. About half of this pressure increase (7.5 mm Hg) is transmitted into the ventricle,

increasing LVEDP from 6 mm Hg to 13.5 mm Hg. The pulmonary artery catheter measures PCWP of 13.5 mm Hg, an apparent increase in filling pressure. However, the transmural filling pressure is only 3.5 mm Hg, an actual decrease in filling pressure compared with spontaneous breathing. (The transmural filling pressure is obtained by subtracting the new intrathoracic pressure [10 mm Hg] from LVEDP [13.5 mm Hg].) In this case, increased PCWP inaccurately signaled an increase in left ventricular filling pressure. PCWP must be interpreted with caution when mechanical ventilation with PEEP is used. A clinical rule of thumb is to subtract about one half (with normal lung compliance) to one fourth (with low lung compliance) of PEEP from PCWP to estimate true filling pressure. Generally, this adjustment needs to be made only when PEEP is greater than 15 cm H$_2$O.

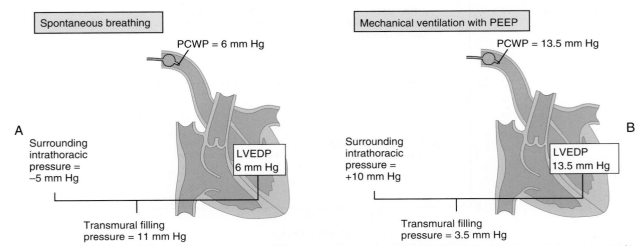

Figure 20-16 **A,** PCWP is proportional to true left ventricular filling pressure; that is, as transmural filling increases, PCWP increases in direct proportion. **B,** PCWP is not proportional to true left ventricular filling pressure. Although LVEDP and PCWP increased from **A** to **B,** the transmural ventricular filling pressure actually decreased.

CLINICAL APPLICATION OF HEMODYNAMIC MEASUREMENTS

Use of Ventricular Function Curves

Infusion of known quantities of fluid into the veins and the recording of changes in filling pressure and cardiac output provide the necessary information to construct a ventricular function curve in the clinical setting. This process is known as a fluid challenge—the heart is challenged with fluid, and the change in the heart's output is measured. This procedure helps to identify the filling pressure that produces the greatest cardiac output. A typical left ventricular function curve in the clinical setting plots PCWP on the horizontal axis and CI on the vertical axis. As fluid is infused, PCWP increases, resulting in an increased CI (Starling principle). The PCWP that corresponds to the greatest ventricular output is the optimum filling pressure. Fluids can be administered to maintain the maximum cardiac output.

In the 1970s, Forrester et al.[6] identified four distinct quadrants on the ventricular function graph that correlated with specific clinical signs in patients with myocardial infarctions. (This analysis also can be applied to hemodynamic conditions not associated with myocardial infarction.) Figure 20-17 identifies the four hemodynamic subsets. Forrester found that people with PCWP greater than 18 mm Hg had clinical signs of pulmonary edema and that people with CI less than 2.2 L/min/m^2 had clinical signs of peripheral hypoperfusion.

This analysis provides insight into a person's hemodynamic condition. A PCWP of 5 mm Hg and CI of 1.5 L/min/m^2 are consistent with a loss of blood volume, as is found with hemorrhage (see subset *III* in Figure 20-17). A PCWP of 25 mm Hg and CI of 1.5 L/min/m^2 are consistent with left ventricular pumping failure (see subset *IV* in Figure 20-17). Hypervolemia,

also called fluid overload, is characterized by high PCWP but increased peripheral perfusion (see subset *II* in Figure 20-17). Subset I is associated with normal pulmonary and peripheral perfusion status. An exception occurs in patients with septic shock, who often experience massive vasodilation. These patients may have abnormally high cardiac output even though preload (PCWP) is normal or low. These patients also fall into subset I; their hemodynamic status is characterized as **hyperdynamic**; cardiac output is abnormally high secondary to greatly reduced SVR. Although pulmonary capillary pressure is often normal, patients with septic shock may nevertheless have pulmonary edema because sepsis is associated with alveolar capillary membrane injury and high permeability. Figure 20-18 shows examples of conditions described by the four hemodynamic subsets.

Principles of Clinical Management

A major goal in clinical management of critically ill patients is maintaining adequate tissue oxygenation, which must be kept in mind when hemodynamic information is interpreted. Figure 20-19 illustrates hemodynamic and pulmonary factors that determine oxygen delivery to the tissues. Arterial oxygen content is determined by the lung's ability to transfer oxygen into the blood and by the blood's hemoglobin concentration. Cardiac output is determined by the heart rate and stroke volume. Stroke volume is determined by preload, afterload, and contractility.

Hemodynamic monitoring provides information about all oxygen delivery determinants, allowing the identification of any abnormal components. A rational treatment strategy aimed specifically at correcting the basic abnormality can then be developed. Continuous hemodynamic monitoring allows

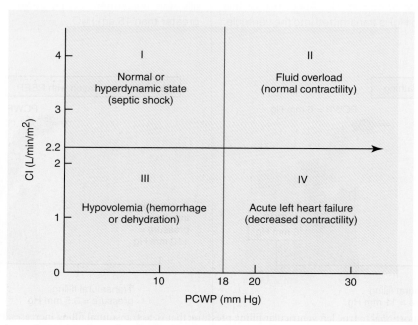

Figure 20-17 Forrester's four hemodynamic subsets (*I-IV*). The intersection of the lines representing PCWP and CI is determined by the hemodynamic environment.

constant assessment of the effectiveness of corrective therapy and allows modifications according to patient response. Respiratory therapists, nurses, and physicians must understand the way changes in both hemodynamic and pulmonary factors affect tissue oxygenation. An understanding of the way various therapies, including drugs, intravenous fluids, and mechanical ventilation, may affect hemodynamic variables is essential.

Once hemodynamic monitoring data are analyzed and the abnormal variables are identified, the general nature of the abnormality becomes apparent. A logical course of corrective action then follows.

Abnormal Preload

If PCWP is elevated, clinicians should investigate factors in the patient that cause high preload, such as hypervolemia and ventricular failure. High intrapleural pressure induced by mechanical ventilation also could be a cause of elevated PCWP, although this does not increase the preload. If hypervolemia is the cause, measures that reduce blood volume are

needed, such as administration of diuretic drugs. Ventricular failure may be addressed by at least two different approaches: (1) administration of vasodilator drugs to reduce ventricular afterload and (2) administration of drugs that increase contractility (inotropic drugs). Both drugs improve pumping effectiveness and reduce preload. If high mechanical ventilation pressures are the problem, measures to reduce mean intrapleural pressures are taken. Similarly, when PCWP is low, especially if accompanied by a low cardiac output, intravenous fluids should be infused. Figure 20-20 illustrates these general principles of management.

Abnormal Afterload

If SVR and SVRI are elevated, the patient is examined to discover the presence of factors that increase afterload, e.g., vasoconstriction increases SVR, which increases ventricular afterload. The likely cause of vasoconstriction must be identified next. Sympathetic vasoconstriction is a compensatory response to a decrease in cardiac output and blood pressure.

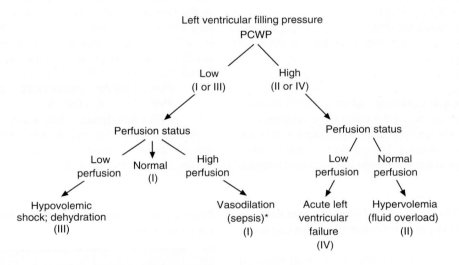

Figure 20-18 Diagnostic examples of the four hemodynamic subsets (*I-IV*; see Figure 20-17). This flowchart assumes normal pulmonary vascular resistance.

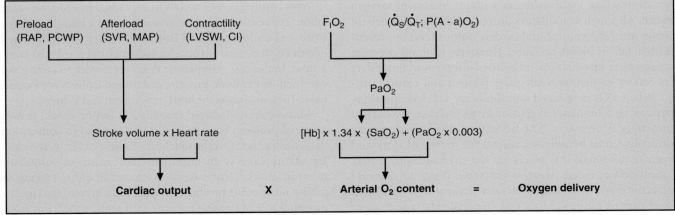

Figure 20-19 Determinants of oxygen delivery to the tissues.

CLINICAL FOCUS 20-3

Differentiating Myocardial Infarction from Pulmonary Embolus

An elderly woman is brought back from surgery after repair of a fractured femur. Her course was uneventful until 8 hours later when she developed severe shortness of breath and central chest pain. She is now very anxious and breathes with large tidal volumes and a rapid respiratory rate. She is admitted to the intensive care unit where pulmonary artery and systemic arterial catheters are inserted. Monitoring data from the pulmonary artery catheter are as follows:

Right atrial pressure = 20 mm Hg
Pulmonary artery pressure = 52/30 mm Hg
MPAP = 45 mm Hg
PCWP = 6 mm Hg
Cardiac output = 5 L/min
Other vital signs are as follows:
Heart rate = 128 beats/min
Respiratory rate = 33 breaths/min
Blood pressure = 115/88 mm Hg
Are these findings consistent with a myocardial infarction and acute left heart failure?

Discussion

Myocardial infarction and pulmonary embolus often produce similar signs and symptoms: central chest pain, dyspnea, and respiratory distress. Myocardial infarction reduces ventricular contractility and stroke volume. The condition is expected to cause blood to dam up in the left atrium, which should produce increased PCWP. The high PCWP should be transmitted to the pulmonary artery, increasing pulmonary artery pressure.

A large pulmonary embolus pumped into the pulmonary artery would lodge in an arterial branch, blocking blood flow. This condition would also increase pulmonary artery pressure because it creates resistance to right ventricular output. However, pressure downstream from the embolus would not be elevated; it may actually be decreased if overall blood flow is decreased. Pulmonary embolus should increase pulmonary artery pressure but not PCWP. (PCWP is actually left atrial pressure, downstream from the embolus.)

From the hemodynamic data, you know this patient has a pulmonary problem, not a left-sided cardiac problem. A myocardial infarction cannot be causing this patient's symptoms and hemodynamic abnormalities. A highly significant feature of the hemodynamic data is the difference between pulmonary artery diastolic pressure and PCWP (30 mm Hg − 6 mm Hg = 24 mm Hg). These two pressures are normally almost identical. This high pressure difference shows that PVR is high. Calculation of PVR confirms this:

$$PVR = ([MPAP - PCWP] \times 80) \div Cardiac\ output$$
$$PVR = ([45 - 6] \times 80) \div 5$$
$$PVR = 624\ dynes \bullet sec \bullet cm^{-5}$$

A normal PVR is 100 to 250 dynes • sec • cm^{-5}. Anticoagulant and possibly clot-dissolving drugs are indicated for this patient. Oxygen therapy and pain medication are also needed.

Both left ventricular failure and severe blood loss may decrease cardiac output and blood pressure; either condition can result in increased SVR.

In left ventricular failure, the increased afterload imposed by vasoconstriction increases myocardial work and oxygen demand, possibly worsening ventricular failure. Such circumstances call for vasodilator drugs to better balance the heart's oxygen supply and demand.[5,6] If the resistance to ejection is reduced, the percentage of ventricular volume ejected for a given contraction force increases without increasing oxygen demand. Although vasodilators decrease SVR, the subsequent increase in stroke volume and cardiac output tend to prevent a further fall in blood pressure. However, if blood pressure decreases after vasodilation, infusion of intravenous fluids may be necessary to maintain adequate preload and cardiac output.[5] When SVR is reduced and fluids are infused, inotropic drugs can be administered cautiously to increase myocardial contractility if necessary. The benefits of drugs that increase contractility must be weighed against the increased work and oxygen requirement this places on the myocardium; it may be appropriate to use negative inotropic drugs to decrease contractility and myocardial oxygen demand.[5] If increased SVR is caused by blood loss and hypovolemia, administration of intravenous fluids and possibly blood is indicated.

Restoration of the blood volume eliminates compensatory vasoconstriction.

CONCEPT QUESTION 20-9

What factors tend to diminish the further decline in blood pressure when vasodilator drugs are given to patients with left ventricular failure with compensatory systemic vasoconstriction?

Abnormally low SVR and SVRI are caused by excessive vasodilation. The resulting decrease in blood pressure leads to underperfused and underoxygenated tissues. Coronary perfusion may be decreased, and cause myocardial ischemia and a reduced cardiac output. In this case, vasopressor drugs are needed to induce vasoconstriction. Perfusion pressure and oxygen delivery are increased to vital organs such as the heart, brain, liver, and kidneys.

Massive sepsis-induced vasodilation (septic shock) presents a special problem because it may not respond to conventional vasoconstrictors. Overproduction of nitric oxide by the vascular endothelium is an important mechanism of vasodilation in septic shock.[7] Nitric oxide synthase inhibitors (agents that inhibit nitric oxide production) have been investigated for their potential role in treating patients with septic shock, but studies have yielded controversial results.

CLINICAL FOCUS 20-4

Different Treatments for Systemic Hypotension

Two patients in the intensive care unit have pulmonary artery catheters in place, and both have very low systemic blood pressures. PCWPs are as follows:

    Patient A: PCWP = 3 mm Hg

    Patient B: PCWP = 30 mm Hg

    Would your general approach to therapy be the same or different for these two patients?

Discussion

Based on PCWPs, your therapeutic approaches should be different. Hypotension in patient A is probably associated with low circulating blood volume (hypovolemia) because left ventricular filling pressure is only 3 mm Hg. Hypotension in patient B is probably caused by left ventricular pumping failure because left ventricular filling pressure is extremely elevated. In other words, low filling pressure in patient A produces a low cardiac output and systemic hypotension. Treatment involves intravenous fluid administration. Low cardiac output and hypotension in patient B are caused by decreased ventricular contractility. Subsequently, blood dams in the left atrium and pulmonary vasculature; pulmonary edema is probably present. Treatment is aimed at improving cardiac function; this generally entails vasodilators to decrease resistance to ventricular ejection and drugs that increase contractility. As cardiac output improves, blood is pumped from the left atrium, relieving high pulmonary vascular pressures.

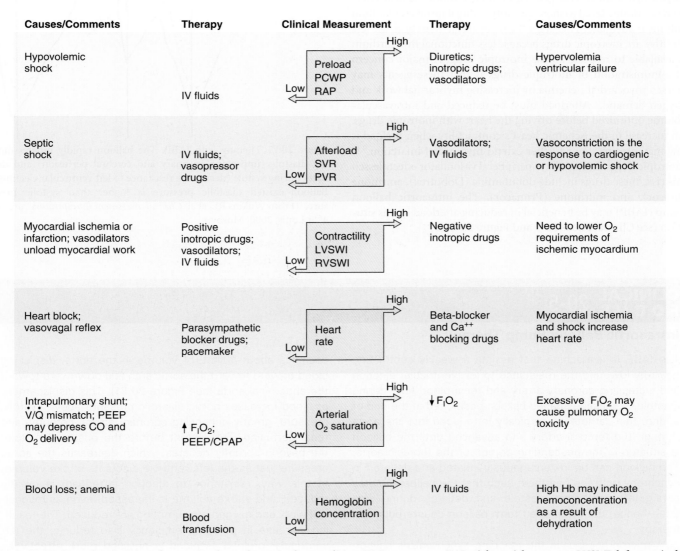

Figure 20-20 General principles of managing hemodynamic abnormalities. *IV,* Intravenous; *RAP,* right atrial pressure; *LVSWI,* left ventricular stroke work index; *RVSWI,* right ventricular stroke work index; *V̇/Q̇* , ventilation-perfusion; *CO,* cardiac output; *FIO$_2$,* fractional concentration of oxygen in inspired gas; *CPAP,* continuous positive airway pressure.

Abnormal Contractility

A low left ventricular stroke work index and low cardiac output indicate abnormally low myocardial contractility. Myocardial ischemia and myocardial infarction decrease cardiac contractility. Myocardial ischemia is caused by inadequate coronary blood flow because of either low perfusion pressure or coronary artery occlusion.

Myocardial infarction means functional heart muscle mass is reduced, which decreases contractility. The initial approach to this problem is generally intravenous fluid infusion if fluid overload and pulmonary edema are not present.[8] In some failing hearts, PCWP may need to be maintained above normal levels to sustain an adequate cardiac output.[5] On the other hand, if cardiogenic pulmonary edema is present, diuretics may be required to reduce fluid volume; diuretics are especially indicated in chronic heart failure in which compensatory renal fluid retention results in hypervolemia. After fluid volume has been optimized, afterload-reducing agents, or vasodilator drugs, are used to reduce myocardial work and oxygen requirements. Inotropic drugs may then be administered to increase contractility if intravascular fluid volume is adequate. The larger the myocardial infarction, the less effective are inotropic drugs because less functional myocardium is available to respond to the inotropic drug. A major concern in administration of inotropic drugs is that these agents may worsen myocardial ischemia by increasing myocardial work and oxygen demand.[9] Afterload must be reduced and intravascular volume optimized before driving the heart with inotropic drugs. An increase in the ischemic heart's contractility when preload is low may precipitate or further extend myocardial infarction.[9,10] Inotropic drugs that also have peripheral vasodilator effects lessen this risk; these drugs include dobutamine (Dobutrex), amrinone (Inocor), and milrinone (Primacor). The intraaortic balloon pump (IABP) may be beneficial in reducing afterload in this situation (see Clinical Focus 20-5 and Figure 20-21).

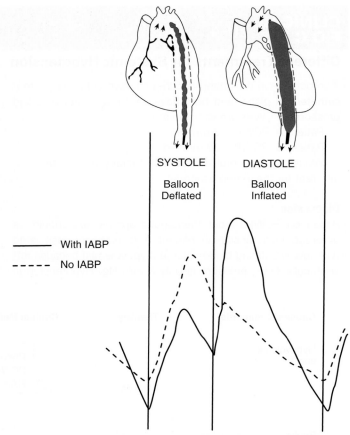

Figure 20-21 Therapy with IABP. The balloon rapidly inflates during diastole (improving coronary and cerebral perfusion) and deflates during systole (decreasing resistance to left ventricular ejection). Balloon-assisted diastolic pressure is higher than systolic pressure. (From Wilkins RL, et al: *Clinical assessment in respiratory care*, ed 4, St Louis, 2000, Mosby.)

CLINICAL FOCUS 20-5

Intraaortic Balloon Pump Therapy

The IABP is a machine that assists a weakly contracting heart by lowering the resistance to left ventricular ejection and increasing coronary artery and renal blood flow during diastole. A sausage-shaped balloon positioned at the end of a long, thin catheter is surgically introduced into the aorta through the femoral artery and advanced until the balloon is situated in the descending portion of the thoracic aorta. The balloon can be instantaneously inflated and deflated in synchrony with the heartbeat such that the balloon inflates during left ventricular diastole and deflates during systole—hence, the often used term balloon counterpulsation therapy.

A microprocessor in the machine synchronizes balloon pulsations with the electrocardiogram pattern. As the balloon instantaneously inflates during diastole, it suddenly occupies about 40 mL of volume in the aorta, displacing blood upward toward the aortic arch and downward toward the abdominal aorta (see Figure 20-21). This displacement of blood increases aortic diastolic pressure above systolic pressure, greatly enhancing coronary artery, cerebral, and renal perfusion. The instant before the onset of systole, the balloon abruptly deflates, which decreases the aortic pressure just as the left ventricle ejects its stroke volume. In this way, resistance to ejection (afterload) is greatly reduced, and stroke volume is increased, even as myocardial work and oxygen consumption are reduced. The resulting increase in pumping efficiency also reduces the left ventricular preload as blood is pumped more effectively; this decreases pulmonary capillary pressure and helps resolve pulmonary edema.

TABLE 20-4

Expected Hemodynamic Changes in Specific Clinical Conditions

Condition	Evidence of Pulmonary Edema	PCWP	PAP	PVR	CO	SVR	MAP
Hypovolemic shock	No	Decreased	Variable	Normal	Decreased	Increased	Decreased
Septic shock	Often	Normal/ decreased	Variable	Variable	Increased	Decreased	Decreased
Cardiogenic shock (left ventricular failure)	Yes	Increased	Increased	Normal	Decreased	Increased	Decreased
Pulmonary embolus	No	Normal	Increased	Increased	Variable	Normal	Normal
Acute respiratory distress syndrome	Yes	Normal/ decreased	Variable	Variable	Variable	Variable	Variable
Dehydration	No	Decreased	Decreased	Variable	Decreased	Increased	Decreased
Mechanical ventilation with PEEP*	Dependent on accompanying condition	Increased	Normal/ increased	Normal/ increased	Normal/ increased	Normal/ increased	Normal/ decreased

PCWP, Pulmonary capillary wedge pressure; *PAP*, pulmonary artery pressure; *PVR*, pulmonary vascular resistance; *CO*, cardiac output; *SVR*, systemic vascular resistance; *MAP*, mean arterial pressure; *PEEP*, positive end-expiratory pressure.
*Effect of mechanical ventilation depends on left ventricular function and mean intrathoracic pressure.

Patients with myocardial ischemia may benefit from negative rather than inotropic drugs because these agents reduce myocardial work and oxygen requirements. For the same reason, these patients also may benefit from drugs that reduce the heart rate. Such drugs include beta-receptor and calcium channel–blocking agents. These drugs produce some degree of vasodilation, lessening the decrease in stroke volume that would otherwise be associated with reduced contractility.

CONCEPT QUESTION 20-10

Why does giving a vasodilator drug possibly prevent the decrease in cardiac output that can occur when only contractility-reducing drugs are administered?

Drugs that dissolve blood clots (fibrinolytic therapy) improve the survival of patients with acute coronary artery occlusion, especially if the drug is given within 2 hours of the occlusion.[11] If given early enough, these drugs restore blood flow to the ischemic area of the heart before infarction can occur. Fibrinolytic intravenous drugs include tissue plasminogen activator (tPA) and streptokinase.

Other causes of decreased myocardial contractility include electrolyte (particularly potassium and calcium ions) and acid-base imbalances. Treatment involves infusing appropriate electrolytes and correcting acid-base disturbances. Oxygen administration is also essential to maximize myocardial oxygenation. Figure 20-20 provides the general principles of management based on hemodynamic information. Table 20-4 lists expected hemodynamic values in specific clinical conditions. Table 20-5 lists examples of drugs that alter hemodynamic values.

TABLE 20-5

Hemodynamic Effects of Cardiovascular Drugs

Therapeutic Objective	Class	Drug Examples	Considerations
Increase contractility	Inotropic agents	Digoxin, dopamine, dobutamine, epinephrine, isoproterenol, amrinone, milrinone	All increase myocardial work and oxygen requirements Epinephrine and isoproterenol greatly increase heart rate
Decrease contractility, decrease myocardial oxygen requirements	Negative inotropic agents	Verapamil, diltiazem, nicardipine, propranolol, atenolol, carvedilol	Propranolol and atenolol block beta receptors Carvedilol blocks beta and alpha$_1$ receptors Other drugs block calcium channels Verapamil is a coronary vasodilator All drugs tend to decrease heart rate
Decrease preload, decrease pulmonary edema	Diuretic agents	Furosemide, torsemide	Very potent, rapid-acting diuretics are associated with K$^+$ loss
Increase preload, restore blood volume and oxygen-carrying capacity and cardiac output	Intravenous fluids and blood transfusions		Starling principle is applied
Decrease afterload, decrease myocardial workload and oxygen requirements, increase cardiac output	Vasodilator agents	Nitroprusside, nitroglycerin, hydralazine, phentolamine, prazosin, captopril, lisinopril	Nitroprusside is a very potent systemic vasodilator; nitroglycerin is a coronary vasodilator; lisinopril and potent captopril are ACE inhibitors
Increase afterload, increase perfusion pressure	Vasopressor agents	Phenylephrine, epinephrine, norepinephrine, dopamine, metaraminol	Epinephrine, norepinephrine, and dopamine also increase myocardial contractility

ACE, Angiotensin-converting enzyme.

CLINICAL FOCUS 20-6

Therapeutic Options for Abnormal Hemodynamic Conditions

Case 1

A 60-year-old man comes into the emergency department complaining of severe chest pain. He has a medical history of a myocardial infarction that occurred 3 years ago. He is pale, sweating, and anxious. He seems to be in no respiratory distress. His vital signs are as follows:

Blood pressure: 130/80 mm Hg

Heart rate: 100 beats/min

Respiratory rate: 16 breaths/min

The electrocardiogram findings show signs of an acute myocardial infarction, and he is admitted to the intensive care unit. Several hours later, his blood pressure decreases to 100/75 mm Hg, and his heart rate increases to 125 beats per minute. His skin is cool and clammy, and his respiratory rate is 22 breaths per minute. You now hear fine, crackling breath sounds over both lung fields with your stethoscope. A pulmonary artery catheter is inserted, and the following data are gathered:

Right atrial pressure: 12 mm Hg

Pulmonary artery pressure: 42/25 mm Hg

MPAP: 31 mm Hg

PCWP: 23 mm Hg

CLINICAL FOCUS 20-6

Therapeutic Options for Abnormal Hemodynamic Conditions—cont'd

Cardiac output: 3.5 L/min
Systemic blood pressure: 100/75 mm Hg
Room air arterial blood gas values are as follows:
pH = 7.48
PCO_2 = 33 mm Hg
HCO_3^- = 24 mEq/L
PaO_2 = 65 mm Hg
SaO_2 = 0.92
Hemoglobin = 14 g/dL
BSA = 1.75 m^2
What is your interpretation?

Discussion

This patient is experiencing acute left ventricular pump failure. He does not have a severe oxygen transfer problem in the lung as evidenced by the PaO_2 and F_IO_2 values. The cool, clammy skin is a clinical sign of hypoperfusion. The decrease in blood pressure and increased heart rate mean the heart's pumping efficiency is worsening; an increased rate is needed to sustain the cardiac output because stroke volume is decreasing. Rapid heart rates are dangerous in cases of myocardial ischemia because the decreased diastolic time leads to decreased coronary perfusion. Fine, crackling breath sounds are associated with pulmonary edema; this is consistent with left ventricular failure and damming of blood in the pulmonary capillaries. The following hemodynamic data confirm these suspicions:

High PCWP: Left ventricular contractility loss, pump failure, pulmonary edema of cardiac origin
CI: 3.5 ÷ 1.75 m^2 = 2.0 L/min/m^2 (subset *IV* in Figure 20-17, consistent with acute left heart failure)
PVR: (31 − 23) ÷ 3.5 = 2.29
2.29 × 80 = 183.2 dynes • sec • cm^{-5} (normal)

Left heart failure, not abnormal PVR, is causing the high pulmonary artery pressure; left heart failure also accounts for the increased right atrial pressure.

Stroke index: Stroke volume/BSA =
(3500 mL/min ÷ 125) ÷ 1.75 m^2 = 16 mL/m^2
Left ventricular stroke work index:
(83.3 − 23) × 16 × 0.0136 = 13.1 g-m/m^2/beat

Low left ventricular stroke work index confirms decreased left ventricular contractility (see Table 20-2).

SVR: (83.3 − 12) ÷ 3.5 × 80 = 1630 dynes • sec • cm^{-5}

High SVR is consistent with systemic vasoconstriction, a compensatory response to decreased cardiac output; this increases myocardial oxygen consumption.

Oxygen delivery is as follows:

$$\textbf{Cardiac output} \times ([\textbf{Hemoglobin} \times \textbf{1.34} \times \textbf{SaO}_2] +$$
$$[\textbf{PaO}_2 \times \textbf{0.003}]) \times \textbf{10} = \textbf{3.5} \times$$
$$(\textbf{17.26} + \textbf{0.195}) \times \textbf{10} = \textbf{611 mL / min}$$

Normal oxygen delivery is about 1000 mL per minute (see Chapter 7); the low oxygen delivery in this case is mainly a function of the low cardiac output. Your main goal is to increase oxygen delivery; although you need to administer oxygen, the main method for increasing oxygen delivery focuses on the cardiovascular system. Your general goals with regard to the cardiovascular system include the following:

1. Decrease myocardial work and oxygen requirements, while improving cardiac output—you must decrease SVR (afterload) and therefore will administer vasodilators.
2. Increase myocardial contractility—after reducing afterload, you may administer inotropic drugs to increase cardiac output further without overworking the heart.
3. Decrease PCWP to allow resolution of pulmonary edema and improve oxygenation—therapy administered in the first two steps addresses this goal. Improved pumping effectiveness decreases left atrial and pulmonary vascular pressures.

Case 2

A 55-year-old woman is admitted to the hospital for a severe urinary tract infection. She has a normal blood pressure and a temperature of 101° F. She is placed on intravenous antibiotics and fluids. Several days later, she develops a respiratory rate of 30 breaths per minute and a temperature of 103° F. Her blood pressure is now 83/50 mm Hg. She appears to be in respiratory distress and has fine, crackling breath sounds. Chest x-ray shows evidence of pulmonary edema in both lungs. In the intensive care unit, a Swan-Ganz catheter is inserted, and the following data are obtained:

Cardiac output = 7.5 L/min
SVR = 500 dynes • sec • cm^{-5}
CI = 4.5 L/min/m^2
MAP = 61 mm Hg
PCWP = 6 mm Hg
Pulmonary artery pressure = 25/10 mm Hg
MPAP = 15 mm Hg

What type of problem is this patient experiencing, and why does she have pulmonary edema?

Discussion

The pulmonary edema is not caused by high pulmonary capillary pressures because PCWP is normal. Although CI is above normal, the patient has systemic hypotension; this is caused by low SVR (see Table 20-2 for normal values). Considering the history of her illness, you should suspect septic shock; the urinary tract infection has probably developed into a generalized septicemia, which explains the low SVR, high CI, and pulmonary edema. Bacterial endotoxins dilate the systemic vasculature, decreasing afterload and increasing cardiac output. These endotoxins also injure the alveolar capillary membrane, increasing its permeability. Even at normal capillary pressures, pulmonary edema is present; this edema may be called noncardiogenic edema or high permeability pulmonary edema. Treatment includes intravenous fluids to maintain blood pressure, antibiotics, and vasopressors.

Nesiritide: Defeating Maladaptive Compensatory Responses to Heart Failure

As noted in Chapter 17, the renin-angiotensin-aldosterone system (RAAS) is activated in heart failure in response to decreased cardiac output and blood pressure. In addition, the sympathetic nervous system (SNS) is activated, elevating plasma levels of norepinephrine. These two neuroendocrine systems are initially compensatory and help restore cardiovascular stability; angiotensin II and norepinephrine cause peripheral vasoconstriction, and aldosterone promotes renal sodium retention, which causes water retention. Although these systems help restore blood pressure, they soon become maladaptive and cause further cardiovascular dysfunction.[12] Increased circulating norepinephrine and angiotensin II are toxic to vascular endothelial and myocardial cells; they induce proliferation and hypertrophy of these cells leading to vascular and ventricular remodeling. Aldosterone also induces similar remodeling changes, all of which have adverse effects on cardiac function. The goal of modern therapy in heart failure is the inhibition of the RAAS and SNS, which explains why angiotensin-converting enzyme inhibitors (e.g., lisinopril), beta blockers (e.g., atenolol), and aldosterone inhibitors (e.g., spironolactone) have beneficial effects.[12]

The natural physiological antagonists of the RAAS are atrial natriuretic peptide and B-type natriuretic peptide (BNP); these peptides are secreted by atrial and ventricular muscle cells in response to the increased pressure and stretch that occurs in heart failure. These peptides inhibit aldosterone and renin release, promoting sodium diuresis (and subsequent water loss) and vasodilation. BNP promotes a balanced dilation of both arteries and veins, reducing preload and afterload. However, in heart failure, the body favors mechanisms that maintain blood pressure; the RAAS and SNS predominate, leading to remodeling and progressive worsening of left ventricular function. In the last decade, a recombinant human BNP, nesiritide, has been approved for use in managing heart failure. Nesiritide reduces blood levels of aldosterone, renin, and epinephrine and produces a balanced arterial venous dilation; it was thought to combat the deleterious effects of ventricular remodeling and reduce myocardial work, while improving cardiac output. However, a more recent large study (7141 patients) of the effects of nesiritide in acute decompensated heart failure revealed that nesiritide was not superior to placebo treatment.[12]

POINTS TO REMEMBER

- Factors that affect venous return are the most important in controlling cardiac output in a normal healthy heart.
- Only when the heart fails as a pump does cardiac contractility become the major factor determining cardiac output.
- The heart's stroke volume is determined by preload, afterload, and contractility.

- Preload relates to the cardiac fiber precontraction length, afterload relates to ventricular outflow resistance, and contractility relates to the force and velocity with which muscle fibers shorten.
- Clinical indicators of preload are PCWP (left ventricle) and right atrial pressure (right ventricle).
- Indicators of right and left ventricular afterload are PVR and SVR.
- Indicators of right and left ventricular contractility are right ventricular stroke work index and left ventricular stroke work index.
- Preload, afterload, and contractility affect the cardiac function curve; blood volume, vessel diameter, and vessel compliance affect the venous return curve.
- PCWP greater than 18 mm Hg is usually associated with some degree of pulmonary edema.
- A CI less than 2.2 L/min/m^2 is associated with clinical symptoms of hypoperfusion.
- A sudden loss of ventricular contractility leads to compensatory systemic vasoconstriction, which is often treated with vasodilator drugs to reduce cardiac work and oxygen demands.
- The renin-angiotensin-aldosterone system and sympathetic nervous system are generally maladaptive compensatory mechanisms in chronic heart failure and are generally targeted for inhibition in treatment strategies.

References

1. Hall JE: *Guyton and Hall textbook of medical physiology*, ed 12, Philadelphia, 2011, Saunders.
2. Brengelmann GL: A critical analysis of the view that right atrial pressure determines venous return, *J Appl Physiol* 94(3):849, 2003.
3. Little RC: *Physiology of the heart and circulation*, ed 3, Chicago, 1985, Year Book Medical Publishers.
4. Berne RM, et al: *Physiology*, ed 5, St Louis, 2005, Mosby.
5. Darovic GO: *Handbook of hemodynamic monitoring*, ed 2, St Louis, 2004, Saunders.
6. Forrester JS, et al: Medical therapy of acute myocardial infarction by application of hemodynamic subsets (first of two parts), *N Engl J Med* 295(24):1356, 1976.
7. Baker J, et al: Administration of the nitric oxide synthase inhibitor NG-methyl-L-arginine hydrochloride (546C88) by intravenous infusion for up to 72 hours can promote the resolution of shock in patients with severe sepsis: results of a randomized, double-blind, placebo-controlled multicenter study (study no. 144-002), *Crit Care Med* 32(1):1, 2004.
8. Holmes CL, Walley KR: The evaluation and management of shock, *Clin Chest Med* 24(4):775, 2003.
9. Mattu A, Martinez JP, Kelly BS: Modern management of cardiogenic pulmonary edema, *Emerg Med Clin North Am* 23(4):1105, 2005.
10. Chatterjee K, De Marco T: Role of nonglycosidic inotropic agents: indications, ethics, and limitations, *Med Clin North Am* 87(2):391, 2003.
11. Antman EM, Morrow DA: ST-segment elevation myocardial infarction: management. In Bonow RO, et al, editors: *Braunwald's heart disease: a textbook of cardiovascular medicine*, ed 9, Philadelphia, 2011, Saunders.
12. O'Conner CM, et al: Effect of nesiritide in patients with acute decompensated heart failure, *N Engl J Med* 365(1):32, 2011.

SECTION III

THE RENAL SYSTEM

CHAPTER 21

Filtration, Urine Formation, and Fluid Regulation

OBJECTIVES

After reading this chapter you will be able to:

- Describe the anatomy of the nephron
- Differentiate between the terms filtrate and urine and reabsorption and secretion
- Explain how glomerular filtration rate and urine output are related
- Explain how autoregulation of the glomerular filtration rate and renal blood flow are related

- Explain how the nephron processes the tubular filtrate to excrete a concentrated or dilute urine
- Describe why it is important that the kidney's countercurrent multiplier mechanism maintains a high osmotic pressure deep in the medulla
- Explain how aldosterone, natriuretic peptides, and antidiuretic hormone influence extracellular fluid volume
- Describe the mechanisms whereby various classes of diuretic drugs work

KEY TERMS

afferent arteriole
aldosterone
angiotensin
antidiuretic hormone (ADH)
atrial natriuretic hormone (ANH)
Bowman's capsule
collecting duct
cortex
efferent arteriole
filtration fraction
glomerulus
isotonic

juxtaglomerular apparatus
juxtaglomerular cells
loop of Henle
macula densa
medulla
nephron
peritubular capillaries
proximal convoluted tubule
renal corpuscle
renin
tubular transport maximum
vasa recta

FUNCTIONAL ANATOMY OF THE KIDNEYS

Kidneys are generally thought of as excretory organs that produce and eliminate urine. Perhaps a more accurate view of the kidneys is that they process and condition the blood plasma, returning it to the general circulation after removing unwanted substances. The kidneys function to maintain homeostasis of the entire body fluid environment. Because they control body fluid volume and composition, the kidneys are in a position to compensate for other organ system deficiencies. For example, if blood pressure decreases as a result of hemorrhage or cardiac failure, the kidneys conserve water, increasing the blood volume and pressure. If the lungs fail to regulate carbon dioxide excretion properly, the kidneys adjust acid and base excretion accordingly to restore acid-base balance. This chapter presents the basic principles of urine formation and the mechanisms for conserving and eliminating individual body fluid constituents.

Gross Anatomy

The kidneys are paired, bean-shaped organs that are located on the posterior abdominal wall behind the peritoneal membrane; hence, the kidneys are called retroperitoneal organs (Figure 21-1, *A*). A fat pad surrounding the renal capsule protects the kidneys from mechanical shock (Figure 21-1, *B*). Blood vessels and nerves enter the medial concave border of the kidney at the hilum (Figure 21-2). The kidney contains an outer **cortex** and inner **medulla** (see Figure 21-2). A ureter from each kidney carries urine to the bladder.

Nephron Anatomy

The **nephron** is the basic functional unit of the kidney. This structure is responsible for filtering the blood plasma, eliminating only the unwanted substances, and returning the remainder to the circulation. These unwanted substances include urea (a by-product of amino acid metabolism), creatinine (from muscle cells), uric acids (from nucleic acids), bilirubin (from hemoglobin breakdown), and metabolites of assorted hormones; in addition, the kidneys eliminate various toxins and foreign substances, whether produced by the body or ingested.[1]

Each kidney contains between 0.4 million and 1.2 million nephrons.[2] Because the kidney cannot regenerate new nephrons, normal aging and disease reduce their number such that a normal 80-year-old individual has about 40% fewer functioning nephrons than he or she did at age 40.[1] The nephron is composed of the following structures, listed in the order in which fluid flows through them: (1) Bowman's capsule, (2) proximal convoluted tubule, (3) loop of Henle, (4) distal convoluted tubule, and (5) collecting duct (Figure 21-3).

Bowman's Capsule

The beginning of the proximal tubule is called **Bowman's capsule** (a hollow sphere composed of epithelium, deeply indented to form a double-walled pouch). A small **afferent arteriole** enters this spherical pouch and branches diffusely to form a

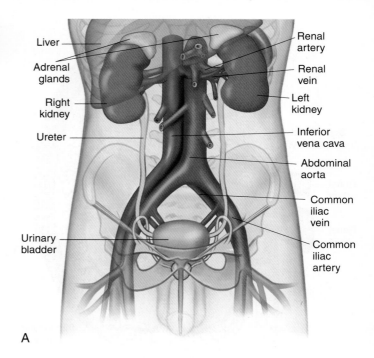

A

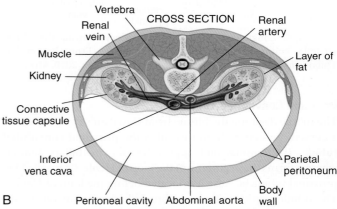

B

Figure 21-1 **A,** Location of the kidneys in the abdominal cavity. **B,** Kidneys located behind the parietal peritoneum of the abdomen. (From Patton KT, Thibodeau GA: *Anatomy & physiology,* ed 7, St. Louis, 2010, Mosby.)

dense tuft of capillaries called the **glomerulus**. The glomerulus is in intimate contact with the inner capsular wall. Glomerular capillaries contain thousands of minute pores, or fenestrations, rendering them highly permeable to all plasma constituents except large protein molecules. Blood leaves the glomerulus by way of the **efferent arteriole**, formed by the convergence of the glomerular capillaries. The glomerulus and its surrounding double-walled capsule are collectively called the **renal corpuscle** (see Figure 21-3). This entire structure is located in the renal cortex. The epithelial layer forming the inner pouch of Bowman's capsule (the visceral layer) and the fenestrated glomerular capillary endothelium form the glomerular filtration membrane. The first step of urine formation occurs when glomerular hydrostatic pressure (about 60 mm Hg)[1] forces plasma through the glomerular filtration membrane. The resulting filtrate enters Bowman's capsule.

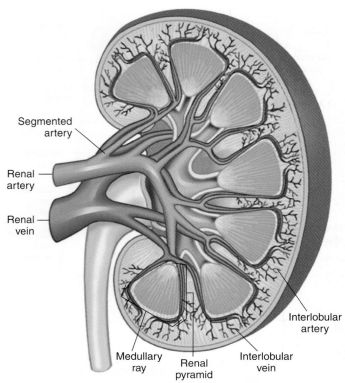

Figure 21-2 Longitudinal section of the kidney showing the cortex, medulla, and vascular and tubular structures. (From Patton KT, Thibodeau GA: *Anatomy & physiology*, ed 7, St. Louis, 2010, Mosby.)

Proximal Convoluted Tubule

The tubule draining the filtrate from Bowman's capsule follows a curved, twisted path and is called the **proximal convoluted tubule**. Its terminal end approaches the medullary border, where it forms the beginning of the loop of Henle. (It is called the proximal tubule because it is located before the loop of Henle.) The tubule's epithelium has a brushlike border of numerous fine microvilli facing its luminal side (see Figure 21-3). These microvilli greatly increase the luminal wall surface area.

Loop of Henle

The **loop of Henle** consists of a straight descending limb, a sharp hairpin turn, and an ascending limb (see Figure 21-3). About 70% to 80% of the glomeruli are located in the outer cortex (cortical nephrons) and have short loops of Henle that never reach the medulla.[1] The remaining nephrons located deeper in the cortex near the medullary border are called juxtamedullary nephrons. These nephrons have long loops dipping deep into the medulla.

Distal Convoluted Tubule

As the name implies, the distal convoluted tubule is beyond, or distal, to the loop of Henle. It resides in the renal cortex with Bowman's capsule and the proximal tubule.

Collecting Duct

The distal tubules of several nephrons connect with a long, straight tubule called the **collecting duct**. These ducts extend

deep into the medulla, where they converge with other ducts at the renal papilla. At this location, a funnel-like structure called the minor calyx receives the filtrate.

Renal Vasculature

Because the kidneys must eventually filter all the blood plasma, they receive an extremely high blood flow relative to their mass (about 20% of the cardiac output).[1] Renal arteries enter the hilum and eventually subdivide to form afferent arterioles entering Bowman's capsule (see Figure 21-3).

The kidneys have two capillary beds: the glomerulus and **peritubular capillaries**. The peritubular capillaries are branches of the efferent arteriole, which was formed by the convergence of the glomerular capillaries. The peritubular capillaries closely surround proximal and distal convoluted tubules. The **vasa recta** are a branch of the peritubular circulation that surrounds the loop of Henle (see Figure 21-3).

Because of the moderately high resistance of the efferent arteriole, the glomerular capillaries are a high-pressure bed, and the peritubular capillaries are a low-pressure bed. As a result, glomerular capillaries act as filtration vessels, and peritubular capillaries act as absorption vessels. The vasa recta receive only 1% to 2% of the renal blood flow.[1] Medullary blood flow is quite sluggish, in contrast to rapid cortical blood flow.

Juxtaglomerular Apparatus

Near their glomerular entry and exit points, afferent and efferent arterioles contain cuffs of smooth muscle that control vessel diameter. At these points, the distal convoluted tubule abuts both arterioles.[1] The densely packed distal tubular cells in this area are called the **macula densa**; the smooth muscle cuffs of the afferent and efferent arterioles are called **juxtaglomerular cells**. The macula densa and juxtaglomerular cells are collectively known as the **juxtaglomerular apparatus** (see Figure 21-3). When systemic blood pressure decreases, cells of the juxtaglomerular apparatus secrete **renin**, an enzyme that activates **angiotensin**, which ultimately leads to widespread systemic arteriole constriction.

Basic Theory of Nephron Function

The nephron clears the blood plasma of metabolic products such as urea, creatinine, and uric acid. The nephron also clears the plasma of substances that accumulate in the body in excess quantities, such as sodium, potassium, chloride, and hydrogen ions.

The nephron accomplishes its function in the following way: First, it filters about 20% of the renal blood plasma through the glomerular membrane into the proximal tubules[1]; next, it reabsorbs most of the filtrate's water and electrolytes and all of the glucose back into the peritubular capillaries. The remaining filtrate (water and waste products) stays in the tubules and is eliminated in the urine. In addition, the nephron actively secretes certain substances directly into the tubular filtrate; urine contains both filtered and secreted substances.

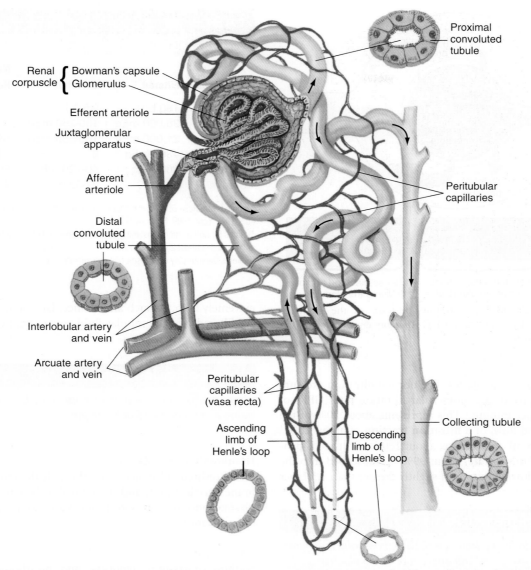

Figure 21-3 Components of the nephron. (From Thibodeau GA, Patton KT: *Anatomy & physiology,* ed 3, St Louis, 1996, Mosby.)

FORMATION OF GLOMERULAR FILTRATE

Filtration Pressure

Filtration is the movement of water and solutes from the plasma in the glomerulus, across the glomerular membrane, and into Bowman's capsule. Filtration occurs because of a pressure gradient between glomerular capillary blood and the capsular filtrate. The main factor establishing this pressure gradient is the hydrostatic pressure of the glomerular blood (Figure 21-4). This pressure is about 60 mm Hg, much higher than capillary pressures anywhere else in the body.[1] The major cause of this high pressure is the high resistance of the efferent arteriole.

Figure 21-4 illustrates the various factors that affect glomerular filtration pressure. Blood osmotic pressure and capsular hydrostatic pressure oppose filtration. The net filtration

pressure equals the sum of forces pushing fluid out of the glomerular capillaries minus the sum of forces pushing fluid back into the glomerular capillaries, as the following equation shows:[1]

60 mm Hg	**–**	**(18 mm Hg + 32 mm Hg)**	**=**	**10 mm Hg**
Glomerular hydrostatic pressure		Capsular hydrostatic pressure	Glomerular osmotic pressure	Net filtration pressure

The reason for the relatively high osmotic pressure in glomerular blood (32 mm Hg) is that the process of filtration concentrates the blood; that is, water is filtered out of the blood, leaving plasma proteins behind.

Glomerular filtration occurs much more rapidly than filtration in other tissue capillaries because (1) the glomerular membrane is about 100 to 500 times more permeable than other capillaries[1] and (2) glomerular hydrostatic pressure is much

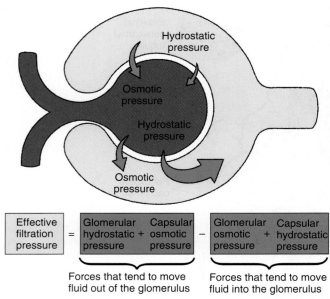

Figure 21-4 Forces affecting filtration pressure in the glomerulus. (From Thibodeau GA, Patton KT: *Anatomy & physiology*, ed 3, St Louis, 1996, Mosby.)

TABLE 21-1

Net Daily Reabsorptive Work Performed by the Kidneys*

Substance	Filtered	Excreted	Net Reabsorption (%)
Water	180 L	0.5-3 L	98-99
Na^+	26,000 mEq	100-250 mEq	>99
Cl^-	21,000 mEq	100-250 mEq	>99
HCO_3^-	4800 mEq	0	≈100
K^+	800 mEq	40-120 mEq	85-95[†]
Urea	54 g	27-32 g	40-50

Modified from Rose BD: *Clinical physiology of acid-base and electrolyte disorders*, ed 3, New York, 1989, McGraw-Hill.
*Values for normal men consuming a typical Western diet. The filtered load of water and solutes is about 25% less in women.
[†]Reflects the interplay of reabsorption and secretion of K^+.

higher than in other capillaries. The normal filtration pressure of 10 mm Hg produces a glomerular filtration rate (GFR) of about 125 mL per minute.[1] This represents about 20% of the glomerular blood flow, or a **filtration fraction** of about 20%.[1] At a GFR of 125 mL per minute, about 180 L of filtrate is produced daily. Of this filtrate, about 99% is reabsorbed into the blood for a total urine output of slightly greater than 1.5 L per day.

CONCEPT QUESTION 21-1

Explain why there is a difference between osmotic pressures in afferent arteriole blood and efferent arteriole blood and why this is important.

Filtrate Constituents

Glomerular filtrate is quite similar in composition to interstitial fluids of body tissues. It contains no red blood cells and only about 0.03% protein (about $\frac{1}{240}$ of the protein in plasma).[1] Glomerular filtrate is the same as plasma except it contains almost no proteins.

Threshold Substances
Threshold substances in the filtrate are totally reabsorbed unless they are present in amounts greater than normal.[1] All actively reabsorbed substances have a maximum rate at which they can be reabsorbed; this is called the **tubular transport maximum**. If the tubular transport maximum is exceeded, these substances are excreted in the urine. Substances with a threshold tubular transport maximum include glucose, amino acids, phosphates, and sulfates. For example, urine normally contains no glucose, unless the plasma glucose concentration is

extremely high. In such an instance, large amounts of glucose are filtered into the tubular fluid, exceeding the tubular reabsorption capacity.

CONCEPT QUESTION 21-2

Explain why a person with diabetes may have glucose in the urine and be prone to dehydration.

Nonthreshold Substances
Nonthreshold substances pass through the glomerular membrane into the filtrate and are not reabsorbed, regardless of their plasma concentration. Creatinine is an example of a nonthreshold substance.[1]

Electrolytes
Sodium, potassium, chloride, and bicarbonate are almost totally reabsorbed from the tubules. Table 21-1 shows the reabsorption percentage for these electrolytes.

Determinants of Glomerular Filtration Rate

As shown in the previous discussion, anything affecting (1) glomerular pressure, (2) plasma osmotic pressure, or (3) Bowman's capsular pressure affects the GFR. The renal blood flow and vessel diameter of afferent and efferent arterioles affect the three factors just listed and the GFR.

Renal Blood Flow
Increased renal blood flow increases the glomerular pressure and enhances filtration. It also enhances the GFR for another reason. Under normal conditions, glomerular blood protein concentration greatly increases as water passes through the filtration membrane into Bowman's capsule. The subsequent increase in plasma osmotic pressure slows the filtration rate. Conversely, when blood flow is rapid, it spends less time in the glomerulus, and less water leaves the plasma. Consequently, the

increase in plasma osmotic pressure and its inhibitory effect on the filtration rate are less severe.[1]

Afferent Arteriole Constriction

Afferent arteriole constriction decreases glomerular blood flow and glomerular filtration pressure. As a result, GFR decreases. Arteriole dilation has the opposite effect.

Efferent Arteriole Constriction

Efferent constriction increases glomerular outflow resistance and increases glomerular capillary pressure and the filtration rate. However, severe efferent arteriole constriction decreases blood flow through the glomerulus, allowing more water to be filtered into Bowman's capsule. The subsequent increase in plasma osmotic pressure counteracts the filtration pressure, and the overall effect may be to slow the GFR.[1]

Autoregulation of Glomerular Filtration Rate

GFR remains fairly constant between arterial pressures of 75 mm Hg and 160 mm Hg.[1] A constant GFR is important to eliminate waste products and reabsorb solutes appropriately. With an excessively slow GFR, filtrate passes so slowly through the tubules that most of it is reabsorbed; hence the kidneys fail to eliminate waste products adequately. An extremely rapid GFR does not give the tubules enough time to reabsorb needed substances, and the kidneys lose too much water and solute in the urine.

Two specialized feedback mechanisms automatically maintain a constant GFR between arterial blood pressures of 75 mm Hg and 160 mm Hg: (1) the afferent arteriolar vasodilator feedback mechanism and (2) the efferent arteriolar vasoconstrictor feedback mechanism.[1] The juxtaglomerular apparatus controls both mechanisms.

Afferent Vasodilator Feedback Mechanism

A low GFR allows the tubules to reabsorb too much sodium and chloride ions from the filtrate. The specialized macula densa cells in the distal tubule sense the low sodium chloride concentration in the filtrate, which elicits a signal that causes afferent arteriole dilation.[1] As a result, glomerular blood flow and GFR increase.

Efferent Vasoconstrictor Feedback Mechanism

In response to a decrease in the filtrate's sodium chloride concentration, juxtaglomerular cells of both afferent and efferent arterioles release the enzyme renin; juxtaglomerular cells are major storage sites for renin.[1] Renin is an enzyme that acts on circulating angiotensinogen and converts it to angiotensin I.[1] A proteolytic enzyme called angiotensin-converting enzyme (ACE) converts angiotensin I to angiotensin II, a potent vasoconstrictor that preferentially constricts the kidney's efferent arterioles.[1] Consequently, glomerular capillary pressure increases, increasing the GFR. Together, the afferent vasodilator and efferent vasoconstrictor mechanisms keep GFR constant in the face of wide blood pressure swings.

CONCEPT QUESTION 21-3

Tumors of the juxtaglomerular apparatus may cause excessive renin production. Explain the unwanted consequences and why drugs classified as angiotensin-converting enzyme (ACE) inhibitors may be beneficial in this condition.

Autoregulation of Renal Blood Flow

The same mechanisms just described also regulate renal blood flow. The most important autoregulatory mechanism in this regard is the afferent vasodilator mechanism. As described in the previous section, decreased blood flow tends to reduce GFR, which elicits afferent arteriolar dilation. Blood flow is restored toward normal. However, this mechanism is primarily designed to regulate GFR; autoregulation of renal blood flow is merely incidental.[1]

A severe decrease in blood pressure causes efferent arteriole constriction. Although this constriction helps maintain GFR, it reduces renal blood flow. In this way, renal blood flow is more poorly regulated than GFR.

Myogenic Reflex Mechanism

Most arterioles in the body contract their smooth muscle to resist stretching in the face of increased blood pressure and vascular wall tension. This phenomenon, called the myogenic reflex mechanism, brings renal blood flow and GFR back to normal when blood pressure is too high.[1] When vessel walls are stretched, calcium ions are allowed to move into vascular smooth muscle cells, facilitating contraction; the opposite effect occurs when blood pressure is low.[2] The importance of the myogenic reflex mechanism in the autoregulation of renal blood flow and GFR is unclear.[1,2]

CONCEPT QUESTION 21-4

How might efferent arteriole constriction in response to blood loss eventually increase the kidney's fluid reabsorption capacity and restore the blood volume?

PROCESSING THE GLOMERULAR FILTRATE

Reabsorption and Secretion in the Tubules

In Figure 21-5, the glomerular filtrate entering juxtamedullary nephron tubules flows (1) into Bowman's capsule, (2) through the proximal tubule, (3) through the loop of Henle, (4) through the distal tubule and past the juxtaglomerular apparatus, and (5) through the collecting duct. (Note the large osmotic pressure gradient in the interstitial fluid from the corticomedullary boundary to the papilla deep in the medulla.) In the juxtamedullary nephrons, Henle's loop and the vasa recta extend deep into the medulla's high osmotic pressure environment. As explained later, this design provides a mechanism for concentrating the filtrate, eliminating a maximum amount of unwanted solute with a minimum loss of water.

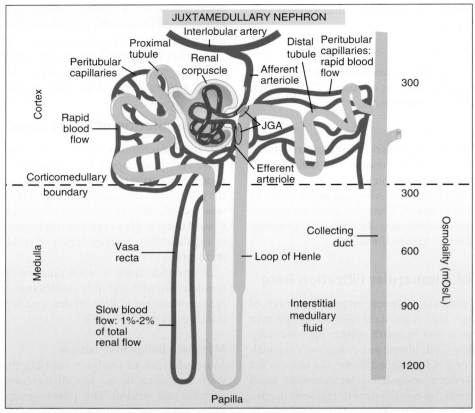

Figure 21-5 Juxtamedullary nephron. *JGA,* Juxtaglomerular apparatus.

Proximal Tubules

About 20% of the plasma of the glomerular capillary blood is filtered into Bowman's capsule and then enters the proximal tubules (Figure 21-6). The low pressure and high blood flow rate of the peritubular capillaries, combined with the blood's high osmotic pressure, provide an excellent reabsorption mechanism. (The process of filtration greatly increases the osmotic pressure of efferent arteriole blood, which is increased further with efferent vasoconstriction.)

About 65% of the filtrate volume is reabsorbed into the peritubular capillaries.[1] The extensive brush border surface area on the luminal side of proximal tubule cells facilitates this reabsorption process. All amino acids and glucose are reabsorbed in conjunction with the active reabsorption of sodium.

Descending Loop of Henle

The remaining 35% of the filtrate volume enters the descending limb of Henle's loop (Figure 21-7), where it is **isotonic** with the peritubular interstitial fluid. The descending limb is freely permeable to water and moderately permeable to most ions.[1] Thus, as the filtrate moves to the bottom of Henle's loop, its osmotic pressure equalizes with that of the surrounding medullary interstitial fluid.

CONCEPT QUESTION 21-5

Characterize the volume and concentration of solutes in the tubular filtrate at the bottom of the loop of Henle.

Ascending Loop of Henle

After it flows around the papillary tip of Henle's loop, the filtrate moves up the ascending limb, flowing in a direction opposite to that of the filtrate in the descending limb (a process called countercurrent flow) (Figure 21-8). This portion of Henle's loop is highly impermeable to water, especially in its thick portion.

Cells of the ascending limb actively pump sodium ions out of the filtrate into the interstitial fluid. Because this portion of Henle's loop is impermeable to water, water cannot follow sodium ions, and the filtrate becomes mildly hypotonic with respect to the interstitial fluid outside of the tubule (see Figure 21-8).

The way in which the kidney maintains a high osmotic pressure in the interstitial fluid deep in the medulla is explained as follows:

1. The sodium ions pumped out of the ascending loop of Henle immediately diffuse into the descending limb of Henle's loop and the vasa recta. The oppositely directed flow in these structures carries the sodium down to the papilla (see Figure 21-8).
2. Blood flow in the vasa recta is quite sluggish. As a result, it cannot effectively remove solutes from the deep medullary region.
3. New quantities of sodium continually flow from the proximal tubule into the loop of Henle. This influx of sodium, combined with the continual reabsorption of sodium from the ascending limb, is known as the countercurrent multiplier.[1] The resulting high osmotic pressure in the medulla is necessary for excreting a concentrated urine, as explained in the next section.

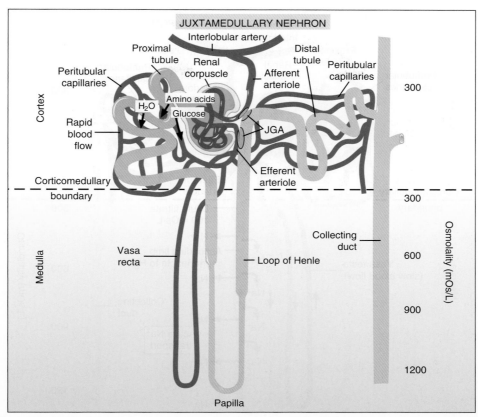

Figure 21-6 Reabsorption of fluid and solutes in the proximal tubules. About 65% of the filtrate volume is reabsorbed at this point. *JGA*, Juxtaglomerular apparatus.

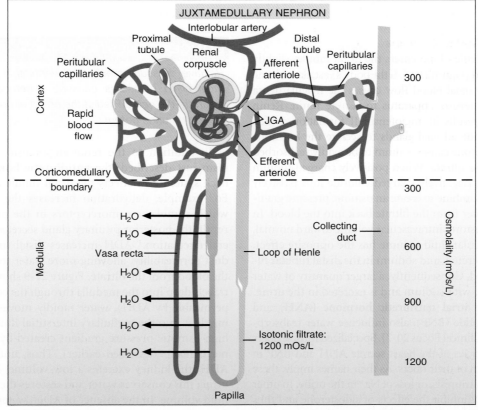

Figure 21-7 The filtrate becomes more concentrated as it flows down the descending limb of the loop of Henle.

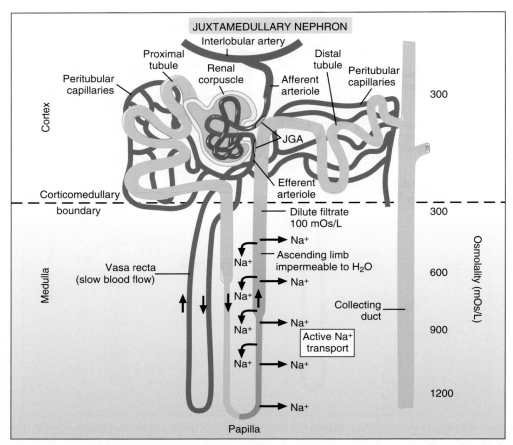

Figure 21-8 Active Na⁺ transport out of the ascending limb of the loop of Henle. Countercurrent flow in the descending limbs of Henle's loop and the vasa recta carry Na⁺ back down to the papilla, maintaining high osmotic pressure in this region.

Distal Tubules and Collecting Ducts

The filtrate leaving Henle's loop enters the distal tubules slightly dilute, as just described (Figure 21-9). If the body's vascular volume is too low, decreased renal blood flow causes the macula densa cells of the juxtaglomerular apparatus to secrete renin. Renin secretion ultimately results in angiotensin II formation, which causes the cortex of the adrenal glands to secrete the hormone **aldosterone**.[1] Aldosterone causes sodium to be avidly reabsorbed from the distal tubular filtrate. When positively charged sodium ions leave the filtrate, negatively charged chloride ions passively follow. These events combine to create an osmotic pressure gradient that reabsorbs water from the filtrate back into the blood. In this way, the kidney restores intravascular volume toward normal.

Excessive extracellular fluid volume has the opposite effect. Aldosterone is not secreted, and sodium in the distal tubular filtrate is not reabsorbed. Consequently, a larger quantity of water remains in the tubule with sodium and is excreted in the urine.

Other hormones, **atrial natriuretic hormone (ANH)** and B-type natriuretic peptide (BNP), also influence water reabsorption (see Chapter 20, Clinical Focus 20-7). Specialized muscle fibers in the atria and ventricles of the heart secrete ANH and BNP in response to overstretch of their fibers. As their names imply, these hormones promote natriuresis, or loss of Na⁺ in the urine. In other words, ANH and BNP inhibit the effects of aldosterone and thus tend to prevent water reabsorption and increase urine volume.[1,3]

CONCEPT QUESTION 21-6

Positive pressure mechanical ventilation tends to decrease atrial filling pressures because it decreases venous blood return to the heart. Predict the effect of positive pressure ventilation on urine output.

In addition to the renin-angiotensin-aldosterone mechanism just described, the **antidiuretic hormone (ADH)** feedback system also affects the distal tubule and collecting duct. For example, dehydration increases the blood's osmolality, which stimulates osmoreceptors in the pituitary gland. As a result, the posterior pituitary gland secretes ADH into the general circulation.[1] ADH increases distal tubule and collecting duct permeability, allowing more water to be reabsorbed into the blood from the filtrate. Figure 21-9 shows that as the filtrate travels deep into the medulla through the collecting duct (made permeable by ADH), water rapidly moves out of the collecting duct into the medullary interstitial fluid in response to the high osmotic pressure gradient created by the countercurrent mechanism (described earlier). Thus, under the influence of ADH, the kidney excretes a low-volume, highly concentrated urine; this conserves water and restores the body's extracellular fluid volume. In the absence of ADH, water remains trapped in the collecting duct, and the kidney excretes a large volume of

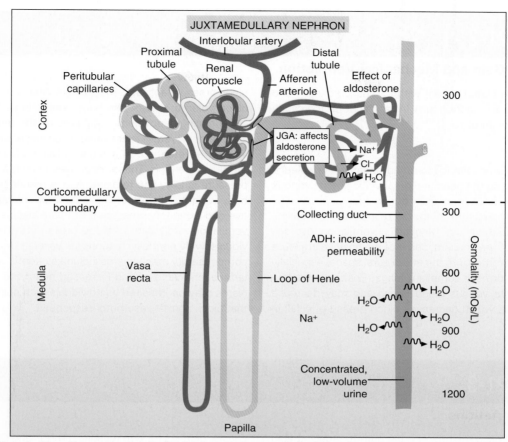

Figure 21-9 The relatively dilute filtrate entering the distal tubules is further adjusted for solute concentration under the influence of aldosterone and ADH. Aldosterone increases Na^+ (and water) reabsorption; ADH increases water reabsorption.

CLINICAL FOCUS 21-1

Effect of Heart Failure on Fluid Volume

The blood volume of patients with chronic congestive heart failure is often increased by as much as 20% and more rarely as much as 40%.[1] A weakly contracting heart may not generate high enough arterial pressure for adequate renal perfusion and urine output. As explained in this chapter, the body responds to low renal perfusion pressure by secreting aldosterone and ADH. Consequently, the kidney reabsorbs large quantities of water, increasing the blood volume. The kidneys keep retaining the fluid volume until the heart either fails from fluid overload or responds by increasing the cardiac output sufficiently to achieve a normal urine output (Frank-Starling law). This mechanism of increasing the blood volume is one of the most important circulatory compensations for heart failure. It allows even a poorly contracting heart to sustain adequate perfusion pressures. However, this same mechanism may produce pulmonary edema and poor blood oxygenation. To treat the edema of congestive heart failure, physicians often prescribe diuretic drugs.

dilute urine. It should now be apparent why the mechanisms that maintain the high corticomedullary osmotic gradient are essential for excreting concentrated urine.

CONCEPT QUESTION 21-7

Diabetes insipidus is characterized by a lack of ADH secretion. Predict the consequences of this condition.

URINE OUTPUT AND SYSTEMIC BLOOD PRESSURE

Systemic blood pressure affects the volume of urine output. Therefore, urine output is a clinical indicator of perfusion adequacy. Decreased blood pressure, regardless of the reason, temporarily decreases GFR, eliciting the efferent vasoconstrictor mechanism, as described previously. As a result, glomerular pressure increases, and more fluid is filtered into Bowman's capsule; this increases the osmotic pressure of blood flowing out of the efferent arteriole into the peritubular capillaries. Consequently, the peritubular capillaries reabsorb greater quantities of water from the tubules. In addition, aldosterone and ADH secretion greatly increase water reabsorption, as described in the preceding section. The result is excretion of a small amount of concentrated urine.

CLINICAL FOCUS 21-2

Body Weight Gain and Mechanical Ventilation

A mechanically ventilated patient with a spinal cord injury and quadriplegia gains 8 lb in 24 hours. What might be the cause of such a rapid weight gain?

Discussion

The normally subatmospheric (so-called negative) intrapleural pressure surrounding the heart and great veins assists venous blood return to the heart, especially during spontaneous inspiration; that is, as pressure in the pleural cavity decreases, blood is pulled into the chest. Mechanical ventilation reverses this favorable pressure gradient; some of the positive pressure in the lung is transmitted into the intrapleural space, especially in patients with normally compliant lungs. Positive intrapleural pressure resists venous blood return and may decrease the cardiac output, which decreases blood pressure. A fall in

blood pressure activates mechanisms that attempt to increase blood volume; that is, the body responds as though it were experiencing hypovolemia. As a result, the renin-angiotensin-aldosterone system is activated, causing sodium reabsorption and water retention. In addition, ADH is secreted, adding to the fluid retention. These responses persist as long as blood pressure is low. The retained fluid is manifested as a gain in body weight. This effect is exaggerated if high levels of positive end expiratory pressure (PEEP) are also used. Mechanical ventilation rarely causes blood pressure to decrease in individuals with normally responsive vascular systems. Normal compensatory mechanisms include systemic vasoconstriction (arterial and venous) and increased heart rate. These mechanisms may be impaired in individuals with spinal cord injuries that block normal vasomotor responses.

CLINICAL FOCUS 21-3

Diuretic Drug Actions

Diuretic drugs increase the rate of urine output, reducing fluid volume in the body. Diuretic drugs are used clinically in treating conditions such as cardiogenic pulmonary edema and systemic hypertension; therefore, patients in coronary and respiratory intensive care units often receive diuretic drugs. Diuretic drugs produce their effect mainly by increasing the concentrations of osmotically active substances in the filtrate of renal tubules. As a result, water remains in the tubules and is excreted in the urine. Several different types of drugs accomplish this action.

Osmotic Diuretics

Osmotic diuretics are substances that freely pass through the glomerular membrane into the tubular filtrate but are not easily reabsorbed by the peritubular capillaries. Mannitol is an example of an osmotic diuretic; its site of action is mainly in the proximal tubules. Mannitol elevates the osmotic pressure of the filtrate, keeping water inside the tubules to be excreted as urine. In addition to their diuretic activity, these drugs are effective in treating cerebral edema in patients with head injuries; high blood osmotic pressure tends to cause fluid to move out of the cerebral tissues into the blood, decreasing brain swelling and intracranial pressure.

Loop Diuretics

Loop diuretics include furosemide (Lasix), torsemide (Demadex), and ethacrynic acid (Edecrin). They block active sodium and chloride transport out of the ascending limb of Henle's loop (the main mechanism for Na^+ and Cl^- reabsorption). This

causes diuresis for two reasons: (1) Na^+ and Cl^- remain in the tubules and act as osmotic diuretics, and (2) because sodium transport out of the ascending limb of Henle's loop is blocked, osmotic pressure of medullary interstitial fluid diminishes. Consequently, the interstitium of the medulla reabsorbs less water from the collecting duct, and more fluid passes into the urine. These drugs are effective, quick-acting agents useful in treating edema of congestive heart failure. Urine output may increase by 25 times for several minutes.[1] Dehydration and excessive potassium loss are complications. (Potassium loss occurs because most potassium is reabsorbed by cotransport with sodium.)

Thiazides

Thiazide-type drugs, such as chlorothiazide, also inhibit Na^+ reabsorption from the tubular filtrate. They act primarily on the distal tubule but are much less potent than loop diuretics.

Carbonic Anhydrase Inhibitors

Drugs in this class, such as acetazolamide (Diamox), inhibit the reaction between CO_2 and H_2O, primarily in the proximal tubular cell, decreasing the amount of H^+ that the tubule cell secretes into the filtrate. This means (1) less Na^+ than normal is reabsorbed from the filtrate (i.e., some Na^+ is reabsorbed by exchanging it for H^+) and (2) less HCO_3^- can be reabsorbed from the filtrate owing to the scarcity of H^+ with which to react. The osmotic effect of increased Na^+ and HCO_3^- in the filtrate causes more water to be lost in the urine. The loss of HCO_3^- in the urine (bicarbonate diuresis) can reduce the blood pH.

CLINICAL FOCUS 21-3

Diuretic Drug Actions—cont'd

Potassium-Sparing Agents: Aldosterone Inhibitors

Spironolactone (Aldactone) is an example of a potassium sparing diuretic; this drug competes with aldosterone for receptor sites in the distal and collecting tubules, decreasing Na^+ reabsorption; Na^+ remains in the tubules and acts as an osmotic diuretic agent. Because aldosterone promotes K^+ secretion into the tubules, these drugs prevent K^+ loss because of their aldosterone-inhibiting activity.

Sodium Channel Blockers

Sodium channel blockers act on the luminal membrane of the collecting duct; an example is amiloride. This drug directly blocks the reabsorption of Na^+ from the collecting duct filtrate by blocking the sodium channels in the luminal membrane of the collecting duct. Na^+ ions remain in the filtrate and act as an osmotic diuretic. Because less Na^+ is reabsorbed from the filtrate into the tubule cell, the Na^+-K^+ pump in the nonluminal membrane of the tubule cell is less active; this pump normally transports Na^+ out of the cell and into the blood while transporting K^+ from the blood into the cell. The ultimate result of blocking Na^+ entry on the luminal side of the tubule cell is that less K^+ is pumped into the cell from the nonluminal side; as a result, K^+ remains in the blood. In this way, sodium channel blockers are also potassium-sparing diuretics.[1]

Conversely, increased blood pressure slightly raises GFR (despite autoregulatory mechanisms) and presents the tubules with more solutes than can be reabsorbed. These solutes are excreted in the urine, "pulling" water with them because of an osmotic gradient. As a result, urine output increases. Doubling the systemic arterial blood pressure increases urine output seven to eight times greater than normal.[1]

POINTS TO REMEMBER

- The kidneys continually filter about 20% of the circulating blood plasma into the tubules and then return 99% of it to the general circulation after removing waste products and excess substances.
- Filtrate refers to the water and solutes filtered out of the blood at the glomerulus, whereas urine refers to about 1% of the filtrate that is excreted from the body.
- Reabsorption occurs when substances are reclaimed from the filtrate and returned to the blood; secretion refers to the active transport of substances from renal tubule cells into the filtrate.
- The nephron tubules reabsorb most of the filtrate into the blood by active transport or passive diffusion mechanisms.
- The kidneys contain autoregulatory feedback mechanisms that maintain a constant GFR in the face of large systemic blood pressure changes.
- Renal blood flow is not as precisely regulated as GFR; autoregulation of GFR generally occurs even at the expense of renal blood flow regulation.
- Urine output is directly related to blood pressure and cardiac output and is an indicator of their adequacy.
- The regulation of the body's fluid volume is extremely important for sustaining adequate blood flow, preventing edema.

References

1. Hall JE: *Guyton and Hall textbook of medical physiology*, ed 12, Philadelphia, 2011, Saunders.
2. Nielsen S, et al: Anatomy of the kidney. In Taal MW, et al, editors: *Brenner and Rector's the kidney*, ed 9, Philadelphia, 2011, Saunders.
3. Slotki IN, Skorecki KL: Disorders of sodium balance. In Taal MW, et al editors: *Brenner and Rector's the kidney*, ed 9, Philadelphia, 2011, Saunders.

Electrolyte and Acid-Base Regulation

OBJECTIVES

After reading this chapter you will be able to:

*   Explain why sodium reabsorption tends to take priority over reabsorption of other ions, and why this may lead to acid-base and electrolyte imbalances under certain conditions
*   Describe how the kidney reabsorbs sodium through primary and secondary active transport
*   Explain why plasma chloride ion imbalances lead to acid-base and potassium ion imbalances
*   Explain why acid-base imbalances cause potassium ion imbalances
*   Explain why potassium imbalances cause acid-base imbalances

*   Describe how chloride and potassium ion reabsorption is tied to sodium ion reabsorption
*   Describe how the kidney either reabsorbs or excretes bicarbonate to compensate for respiratory acid-base disturbances
*   Explain why urinary buffers must be present for the kidney to secrete hydrogen ions in conditions of acidemia
*   Explain why diuretics that block sodium reabsorption tend to cause potassium and chloride depletion
*   Explain why dehydration leads to alkalemia
*   Explain why individuals who are chronically hypercapnic tend to be hypochloremic
*   Explain how renal failure affects acid-base, fluid, and electrolyte balance

ammonia buffer system
blood urea nitrogen (BUN)
chronic renal failure
cotransport
countertransport
glomerulonephritis
nephrotic syndrome

phosphate buffer system
postrenal failure
primary active transport
secondary active transport
sodium-potassium-adenosine triphosphatase (Na+,K+-ATPase)
    pump
uremia

RENAL ELECTROLYTE REGULATION

Sodium, potassium, and chloride regulation are intimately related to acid-base regulation. The regulation of these electrolytes is also important for maintaining normal fluid volume, nerve-impulse transmission, and muscle contraction. For the kidney to reabsorb water and other substances from the tubular lumen into the peritubular capillary blood, the substance first must be transported across the tubular epithelium into the renal interstitial fluid and then through the peritubular capillary membrane into the blood. Substances cross the tubular epithelial cells either by active transport through the cell membranes themselves (transcellular pathway) or by passive diffusion through the junctional spaces between the cells (paracellular pathway).[1] Active transport requires adenosine triphosphate (ATP) for an energy source and can move a substance "uphill" across a cell membrane, against its concentration gradient. Such transport is called **primary active transport** if it is coupled directly to the ATP energy source; it is called **secondary active transport** if it is indirectly linked to the energy source, for example, if the process of primary active transport of one ion creates an electrical gradient that affects the movement of an oppositely charged ion.

Sodium and Chloride Regulation

Sodium is the major osmotically active substance in the extracellular fluid, which means wherever sodium goes, water follows. Na^+ along with Cl^-, the most abundant anion, determine the extracellular fluid volume.[2] About 26,000 mEq of Na^+ passes through the glomerular membrane into the tubular filtrate daily. However, daily Na^+ intake averages only about 150 mEq.[1] Therefore the kidney's main job is to reabsorb Na^+, not to excrete it. Because of the major role of Na^+ in maintaining fluid balance, the body places a priority on Na^+ reabsorption, even at the expense of imbalances in other electrolytes. As noted in Chapter 21, greater than 99% of the Na^+ in the filtrate is reabsorbed. Na^+ is reabsorbed from the tubular filtrate by two mechanisms: (1) primary active transport and (2) secondary active secretion of H^+ and K^+ ions.

Primary Active Transport of Sodium

Primary active transport accounts for most Na^+ reabsorption from the tubular filtrate and occurs in all tubules except the descending loop of Henle.[1] On the nonluminal side of the tubular epithelial cell (Figure 22-1), the **sodium-potassium-adenosine**

triphosphatase (Na+-K+-ATPase) pump actively transports Na^+ ions out of the cell, into the interstitial fluid, and ultimately into the peritubular capillary blood. The membrane protein forming this pump hydrolyzes ATP molecules to generate the energy necessary to actively transport Na^+ ions out of the cell. K^+ ions are simultaneously transported into the cell from the interstitial fluid, but more Na^+ ions are pumped out of the cell than K^+ ions are pumped in. This process keeps Na^+ concentration in the tubule cell very low and creates a negatively charged intracellular environment.

Because $[Na^+]$ is comparatively much higher in the tubular filtrate, and Na^+ is a positively charged ion, both chemical diffusion and electrostatic forces favor its movement from the tubular lumen into the cell, down its concentration and electrostatic gradients.[1] Specialized sodium-carrier proteins in the luminal membrane of the tubule cell facilitate this process by binding with Na^+ ions and releasing them inside of the tubule cell. Cl^- ions passively follow Na^+ ions, which maintains the filtrate's electrical neutrality. That is, the transport of the positively charged Na^+ ion out of the filtrate into the tubular cell leaves the tubular lumen negatively charged with respect to the extracellular fluid and the blood; this electrostatic gradient causes Cl^- (the most abundant anion in the filtrate) to diffuse passively through paracellular pathways (between the tubule cells) into the interstitial space and ultimately into the capillary blood.[1] Cl^- diffusion also occurs because of a concentration gradient; that is, Na^+ transport out of the filtrate creates an osmotic gradient for water reabsorption from the tubular lumen, which concentrates Cl^- ions in the filtrate. Cl^- thus passively diffuses out of the filtrate in response to both electrostatic and chemical diffusion forces.[1]

The brush border on the luminal side of the epithelial cell provides an extensive surface area for Na^+ transport. Sodium-carrier proteins in these membranes are also important in secondary active reabsorption, or cotransport.

Secondary Active Secretion of Hydrogen and Potassium

Reabsorption of Na^+ by way of the active secretion of H^+ and K^+ ions is a more complex process. For H^+ secretion (Figure 22-2), the process proceeds in the following manner: First, carbon dioxide (CO_2) from the peritubular capillary blood diffuses into the tubular cells, where it reacts with water (in the presence of carbonic anhydrase) and forms H^+ ions. The H^+ ion in the tubule cell and Na^+ ion in the filtrate simultaneously combine with opposite ends of a protein-carrier molecule in the luminal border of the cell membrane. Na^+ diffusion into the cell, down

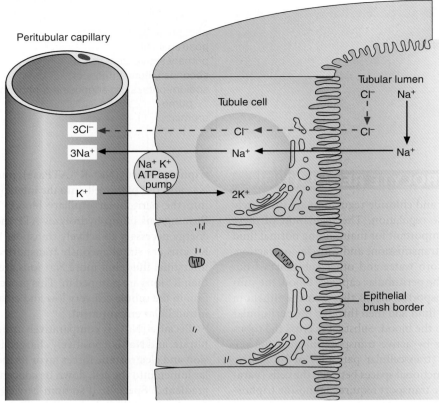

Figure 22-1 Na$^+$ reabsorption through primary active transport. Na$^+$ diffuses from the filtrate and into the tubule cell in response to its concentration gradient and the electrostatic attraction of the cell's negatively charged interior. The Na$^+$-K$^+$-ATPase pump helps generate this intracellular negativity by pumping out more Na$^+$ than it pumps in K$^+$. Cl$^-$ passively accompanies Na$^+$ (cotransport).

its concentration and electrostatic gradients (described previously), provides the energy for H$^+$ transport into the filtrate (see Figure 22-2). This process is called **countertransport** because the transported ions move in opposite directions. Figure 22-2 shows that the HCO$_3^-$ ion generated by the reaction between CO$_2$ and water accompanies Na$^+$ transport out of the cell and into the peritubular capillaries. In this way, Na$^+$ reabsorption from the filtrate occurs without Cl$^-$ reabsorption. A similar countertransport mechanism is involved in the secondary active secretion of K$^+$ into the tubules in exchange for Na$^+$ (Figure 22-3). This mechanism of potassium secretion is more likely to occur in the presence of alkalemia when H$^+$ is scarce; this is the reason alkalemia tends to cause K$^+$ depletion (hypokalemia).

Normally, a relatively small amount of the total Na$^+$ reabsorption occurs by way of active H$^+$ and K$^+$ secretion mechanisms. In H$^+$ and K$^+$ secretion, HCO$_3^-$ ion rather than Cl$^-$ ion is reabsorbed into the blood with Na$^+$. Cl$^-$ ion shortage (as may occur with diuretic therapy) increases the demand for H$^+$ and K$^+$ secretion as a mechanism for reabsorbing sodium.

Secondary Active Transport of Chloride

In most of the tubular segments, Cl$^-$ ions are reabsorbed with Na$^+$ ions by passive diffusion as described earlier. In the thick segment of the loop of Henle, Cl$^-$ ions are transported in a secondary active transport process also known as **cotransport**. In this mechanism, the same carrier protein referred to previously

that combines with Na$^+$ in the luminal tubular membrane simultaneously combines with Cl$^-$. As Na$^+$ diffuses down its electrochemical gradient into the tubule cell, it pulls Cl$^-$ with it. This secondary active transport of Cl$^-$ requires no ATP energy source; it simply uses the force of the Na$^+$ ions' "downhill" diffusion into the cell to energize the process. In addition to Cl$^-$, a significant amount of K$^+$ is reabsorbed with Na$^+$ through the same mechanism; for each Na$^+$ ion, two Cl$^-$ ions and one K$^+$ ion are cotransported by a membrane carrier protein known as the 1 sodium, 2 chloride, 1 potassium cotransporter.[1]

Potassium Regulation

Precise control of extracellular [K$^+$] is extremely important because cardiac muscle cells are very sensitive to slight concentration changes; an elevation of only 3 to 4 mEq/L in the plasma [K$^+$] can cause lethal arrhythmias.[1] The maintenance of K$^+$ balance depends mainly on renal excretion, which must adapt quickly to large variations in K$^+$ intake to prevent lethal hyperkalemia. Because more than 98% of total body K$^+$ is in the cells, the intracellular compartment is a K$^+$ reservoir in hyperkalemia and a source of K$^+$ in hypokalemia; redistribution of K$^+$ between intracellular and extracellular fluid compartments is an important part of controlling extracellular K$^+$ levels.[1] After a normal meal, a person's K$^+$ level would increase to lethal levels if most of the K$^+$ did not rapidly move to the intracellular

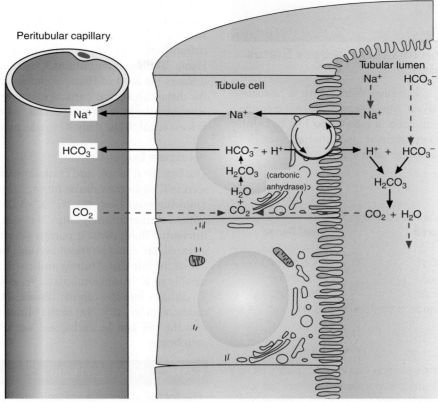

Figure 22-2 Na^+ reabsorption through secondary active secretion of H^+. Through the countertransport process, Na^+ is reabsorbed with HCO_3^- rather than Cl^-. This increases the blood's HCO_3^- concentration. This process plays a more predominant role in Na^+ reabsorption when the Cl^- ion concentration is low.

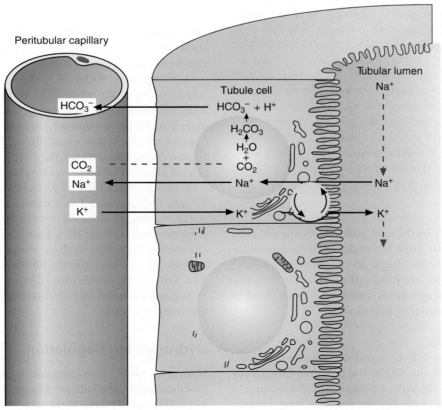

Figure 22-3 Na^+ reabsorption through secondary active secretion of K^+. This mechanism of Na^+ reabsorption is most likely to occur in the presence of alkalemia when the H^+ ion is unavailable for exchange with Na^+. Alkalemia tends to cause hypokalemia.

CLINICAL FOCUS 22-1

Effect of Hypochloremia on Acid-Base Status and Potassium Balance

A woman with chronic congestive heart failure is hospitalized in the intensive care unit. She is receiving diuretic drugs, has a nasogastric suction tube in place, and has been on a low-salt diet before hospitalization. Her arterial blood gas results reveal the following acid-base status:

pH = 7.51
$PaCO_2$ = 43 mm Hg
HCO_3^- = 33 mEq/L

Her plasma electrolyte results are as follows:

	Measured	Normal Range
Na^+	140 mEq/L	137-147 mEq/L
K^+	3.0 mEq/L	3.5-4.8 mEq/L
Cl^-	89 mEq/L	98-105 mEq/L
CO_2	34 mEq/L	25-33 mEq/L

What are the mechanisms contributing to this patient's metabolic alkalosis?

Discussion

Diuretic drugs, nasogastric suction (removal of gastric HCl), and low-salt diets contribute to hypochloremia. (Note the low Cl^- concentration.) Hypochloremia places a greater demand than normal on the secondary active H^+ and K^+ secretion mechanisms for Na^+ reabsorption. Consequently, greater than normal amounts of H^+ and K^+ are secreted into the tubular fluid in exchange for Na^+. This process rids the body of H^+ and K^+, while adding HCO_3^- every time Na^+ is reabsorbed; this explains the patient's metabolic alkalosis and hypokalemia. It also helps explain the reciprocal relationship between Cl^- and HCO_3^- concentrations. Low $[Cl^-]$ leads to increased HCO_3^- reabsorption with Na^+ ions. Hypochloremia may cause metabolic alkalosis and hypokalemia. As long as the Cl^- ion remains scarce in the tubular filtrate, HCO_3^- continues to be reabsorbed with Na^+, and the alkalosis continues. Infusion of a KCl solution is needed to correct this alkalosis by supplying the necessary Cl^- for Na^+ reabsorption. This allows HCO_3^- diuresis to occur and simultaneously corrects the hypokalemia.

impairs K^+ (and Cl^-) reabsorption; overuse of loop diuretics can cause hypokalemia and hypochloremia. Approximately another 25% of the filtrate's K^+ is reabsorbed by the same cotransport mechanism in the ascending limb of the loop of Henle. The small amount of K^+ remaining in the filtrate after it leaves the loop of Henle is almost completely reabsorbed by the distal tubule and cortical segments of the collecting ducts. However, the kidneys must excrete a quantity of K^+ in the urine at least equal to the daily K^+ intake to avoid hyperkalemia.

Potassium Excretion

The late distal tubule and cortical portion of the collecting duct secrete K^+ into the tubular filtrate. This secretion occurs in the following way: First, the Na^+,K^+-ATPase pump in the nonluminal cell membrane pumps Na^+ out of the cell and into the interstitial fluid, while it pumps K^+ into the cell, increasing its intracellular concentration. Second, because the luminal border of the late distal tubule and cortical collecting duct is permeable to K^+ (unlike tubular cells elsewhere in the nephron), K^+ diffuses into the tubular filtrate. Thus, for the K^+ secretion mechanism to work, Na^+ in the filtrate must continually diffuse into the cell and be exchanged for K^+ at the nonluminal cell membrane.

CONCEPT QUESTION 22-1

Predict the effect of a low-sodium diet on the kidney's secretion of K^+ and on the blood $[K^+]$.

Control of Potassium Excretion

Because it greatly influences cardiac impulse conduction (see Chapter 18 and nervous system function, extracellular fluid $[K^+]$ regulation is especially important. K^+ ion excretion is controlled by (1) extracellular fluid $[K^+]$ and (2) aldosterone secretion by the adrenal gland cortex.[2]

A rising extracellular $[K^+]$ directly stimulates tubular K^+ secretion, especially when $[K^+]$ is already above the normal range. It does so by stimulating the Na^+,K^+-ATPase pump, increasing K^+ uptake through the nonluminal tubule cell membrane. Conversely, low extracellular $[K^+]$ depresses the rate of K^+ secretion. Extracellular fluid $[K^+]$ also directly affects the rate of aldosterone secretion by the adrenal cortex.[1] Aldosterone also activates the Na^+,K^+-ATPase pump, pumping more K^+ into the tubular cell as it pumps more Na^+ out of the cell. A functioning aldosterone system is extremely important in regulating extracellular $[K^+]$. Diseases that abnormally increase aldosterone secretion, such as primary aldosteronism, greatly increase K^+ secretion into the filtrate, causing severe hypokalemia. Conversely, diseases that destroy the adrenal glands, such as Addison's disease, stop aldosterone production and produce severe hyperkalemia.

compartment. K^+ uptake by the cells, and thus its lowered concentration in extracellular fluid, is stimulated by insulin, aldosterone, and beta-adrenergic drugs, all of which activate the Na^+,K^+-ATPase pump present in all cell membranes.[1] For this reason, albuterol (a beta$_2$ agonist) is sometimes administered to individuals with life-threatening hyperkalemia.

Potassium Reabsorption

About 65% of K^+ in the filtrate is reabsorbed into the blood by cotransport with Na^+ and Cl^- in the proximal tubules (by way of the 1 sodium, 2 chloride, 1 potassium cotransporter).[1] Anything that blocks Na^+ reabsorption, such as a loop diuretic,

Hydrogen Ion Regulation

Numerous HCO_3^- ions continually pass across the glomerular membrane into the tubular filtrate, removing base from the blood. The tubular cells at the same time secrete large numbers of H^+ ions into the filtrate, removing acid from the blood. If the amount of H^+ ions secreted matches the amount of HCO_3^- ions filtered, there is no net loss of acid or base. A difference in these filtration and secretion rates means there is a net loss of acid or base.

Tubular Hydrogen Ion Secretion

All parts of the nephron's tubular system actively secrete H^+ except the thin segments of the loop of Henle. About 95% of H^+ secretion occurs via secondary active transport; the remaining 5% occurs via primary active transport.[1]

Secondary active secretion of H^+ occurs mainly in the proximal tubules, loop of Henle, and early distal tubules. This process is the same as that described for the Na^+ reabsorption mechanism (see Figure 22-2). First, CO_2 in the peritubular blood plasma freely diffuses into the tubular cell, where it reacts instantly with water under the influence of carbonic anhydrase. As a result, carbonic acid forms and dissociates into HCO_3^- and H^+ ions. The H^+ ions are secreted into the tubular filtrate by the Na^+-H^+ countertransport mechanism described previously (see Figure 22-2). The luminal brush border of the tubule cell is impermeable to HCO_3^-; therefore HCO_3^- cannot follow H^+, and intracellular $[HCO_3^-]$ increases. In this way, a concentration gradient for HCO_3^- diffusion is formed, and it diffuses out of the cell along with newly reabsorbed Na^+ into the interstitial fluid and peritubular capillary blood. Generally, for every H^+ ion secreted, one HCO_3^- ion enters the blood.

Primary active secretion accounts for a small amount of H^+ secretion, occurring in the late distal tubule and the entire length of the collecting duct. In this process, a specific transport protein in the tubule cell luminal membrane, hydrogen-transporting ATPase, pumps the H^+ formed by the reaction between CO_2 and water into the filtrate. The only difference between this process and secondary active secretion is that H^+ ions are transported across the luminal membrane by an active hydrogen pump instead of by countertransport with Na^+ ions. Although this mechanism accounts for only about 5% of the total H^+ secreted, it is much more powerful than the secondary active secretion mechanism. Primary active transport can concentrate H^+ ions in the filtrate 900-fold compared with a maximum of about 3-fold to 4-fold for the secondary process.[1] This extreme H^+ ion concentrating ability can reduce urine pH to a maximum of about 4.5. All tubular H^+ secretion stops below this pH level.[1]

Hydrogen Ion Secretion and Bicarbonate Ion Reabsorption

The H^+ ion secreted into the filtrate immediately reacts with the HCO_3^- ion (see Figure 22-2). (Remember that numerous HCO_3^- ions are filtered out of the blood at the glomerulus.) When the HCO_3^- ion buffers the secreted H^+ ion, H_2CO_3 and ultimately CO_2 and water are formed. All cell membranes are freely permeable to CO_2; CO_2 immediately diffuses into the tubular cell where it instantly reacts with water under the influence of carbonic anhydrase. Again, the CO_2 hydrolysis reaction produces a HCO_3^- ion; the intracellular concentration of HCO_3^- thus increases, and it diffuses into the interstitial fluid. In this way, the filtrate's HCO_3^- ions are "reabsorbed" into the blood,

although the reabsorbed HCO_3^- ion is not the same ion that was in the filtrate.

Normally, H^+ secretion slightly exceeds the rate of HCO_3^- filtration at the glomerulus. This means that the titration of HCO_3^- against H^+ in the tubular filtrate is incomplete, leaving a slight excess of H^+. Thus, the excreted urine is usually slightly acidic.[1]

Renal Compensation for Respiratory Acidosis

In respiratory acidosis, the ratio of dissolved CO_2 to HCO_3^- ions increases (see Chapter 10). As a result, the rate of H^+ secretion increases relative to the rate of HCO_3^- filtration into the tubules (Figure 22-4). When arterial blood PCO_2 is elevated, relatively more CO_2 diffuses into the tubule cell from the blood, generating more H^+ ions, which are secreted into the filtrate. All available HCO_3^- ions react with these H^+ ions and are reabsorbed, as described previously. The remaining H^+ ions are excreted in the urine, carrying with them a different urinary buffer anion from the filtrate (discussed in a later section). In this way, for every H^+ secreted, one HCO_3^- ion is gained by the blood, which is the desired response to acidosis (i.e., elimination of acid and retention of base). In this way the normal kidney compensates for respiratory acidosis.

Renal Compensation for Respiratory Alkalosis

In respiratory alkalosis, the rate of HCO_3^- filtration into the tubules exceeds the rate of tubular H^+ secretion. Because of their high numbers, not all HCO_3^- ions in the filtrate have a H^+ ion with which to react (Figure 22-5). Because of the impermeability of the luminal tubular membrane to HCO_3^-, these ions are trapped in the filtrate and pass into the urine, carrying with them positive ions such as Na^+ or K^+. This is the desired response to alkalosis (i.e., elimination of base and reduced secretion of acid) and is the mechanism whereby the kidney compensates for respiratory alkalosis.

Role of Urinary Buffers

Not many H^+ ions can be excreted in the urine in the free form. Free H^+ ions rapidly reduce the filtrate pH to 4.5, a level below which H^+ secretion mechanisms cannot function.[1] Therefore, filtrate buffers are necessary for normal H^+ ion excretion. The primary urinary buffer is HCO_3^- as already described. The two other major buffer systems that transport excess H^+ ions in the urine are the **phosphate buffer system** and **ammonia buffer system**.

Phosphate Buffers

Phosphate buffers in the tubular filtrate include HPO_4^{-2} and $H_2PO_4^-$. Because these buffer anions are poorly reabsorbed from the filtrate, they become concentrated and powerful as water is reabsorbed. The phosphate buffer system's pK_a is 6.8, a pH level close to that of the tubular filtrate.[1] This means the phosphate buffer system operates in its most effective range in the tubular filtrate (see Chapter 10). The function of the phosphate buffer system is illustrated in Figure 22-6.

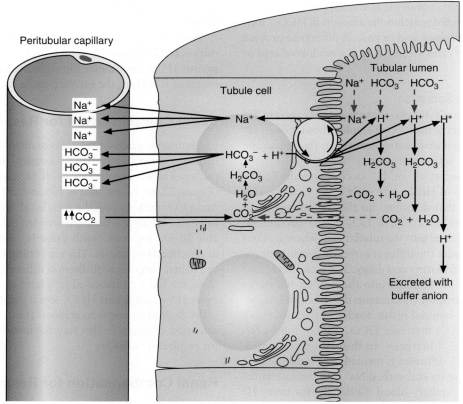

Figure 22-4 Renal response to respiratory acidosis. All HCO_3^- in the filtrate is returned to the blood, where it counteracts plasma carbonic acid.

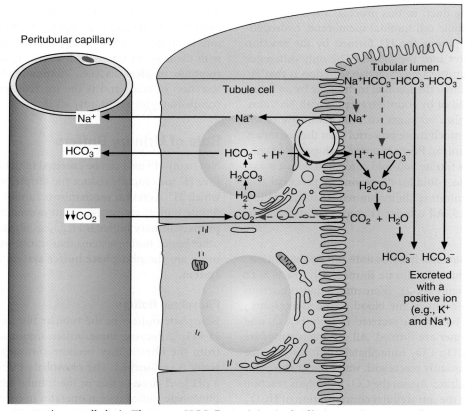

Figure 22-5 Renal response to respiratory alkalosis. The excess HCO_3^- remaining in the filtrate requires greater than normal amounts of K^+ secretion to maintain tubular electroneutrality. Respiratory alkalosis creates hypokalemia.

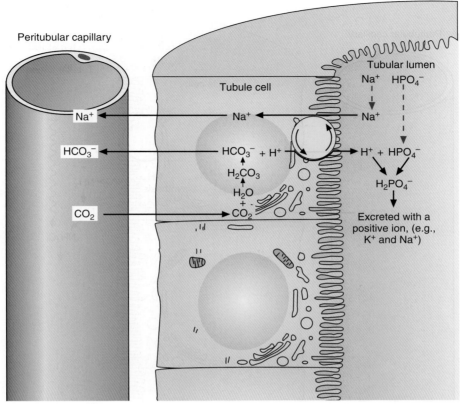

Figure 22-6 Phosphate buffer system. Besides reacting with HCO_3^- ions, excess H^+ combines with urinary phosphate buffers.

Ammonia Buffer System

The ammonia buffer system consists of the ammonia molecule (NH_3) and ammonium ion (NH_4^+). Most of the tubular epithelium synthesizes NH_3, which diffuses into the filtrate (Figure 22-7). The NH_3 molecule buffers the H^+ ion in the filtrate, forming NH_4^+. Every time this process occurs, the filtrate NH_3 concentration decreases, causing more NH_3 to diffuse out of the tubule cell, which stimulates more NH_3 synthesis. In this way, the amount of free H^+ in the filtrate controls the rate of NH_3 synthesis.

The NH_4^+ ion must be excreted with a negative ion in the filtrate to maintain electroneutrality. The most abundant filtrate anion, Cl^-, tends to be excreted with NH_4^+ as the NH_4Cl molecule (ammonium chloride). Ammonium chloride is an extremely weak acid and does not lower the filtrate pH much. Without the ammonia secretion mechanism, the excess H^+ ions in the filtrate would react with Cl^- ions, forming the strong acid, HCl. Filtrate pH would then quickly decrease below 4.5 and stop the tubule cells from secreting more H^+ ions.

People with chronic acidosis (e.g., patients with chronic obstructive pulmonary disease [COPD] and chronic CO_2 retention) produce large amounts of NH_3 in their kidneys to buffer excess H^+ ions. Because the resulting NH_4^+ ions require an equally large amount of Cl^- excretion, these patients tend to become hypochloremic. As discussed previously, hypochloremia interferes with Na^+ reabsorption because the main mechanism for reabsorbing Na^+ involves simultaneous Cl^- reabsorption. Therefore, to reabsorb Na^+ (always a first priority), people with

chronic acidosis rely more on the secondary H^+ and K^+ secretion mechanisms. This reliance tends to deplete the body's H^+ and K^+ stores, producing hypokalemia and a relative alkalemia; that is, even though blood pH may be in the normal range in this situation, it is on the alkalotic side of normal.

Potassium and Acid-Base Balance

Hypokalemia Caused by Alkalosis

The kidney's main task in Na^+ ion regulation is to reabsorb it from the filtrate. (Greater than 99% of it is reabsorbed.) The kidneys reabsorb sodium even if this causes other electrolyte imbalances. For example, in a state of alkalosis, the tubule cells rely more heavily on the potassium-secreting mechanism to reabsorb Na^+ (see Figure 22-3). In other words, the relative shortage of H^+ ions forces the kidney to secrete more K^+ ions; this is a major reason alkalosis tends to cause hypokalemia. Also, in alkalosis, the glomerulus filters more HCO_3^- ions into the filtrate than can be matched by tubular H^+ ion secretion (see Figure 22-5). Because H^+ is scarce and Na^+ reabsorption is a high priority, the tubules secrete more K^+ than normal to accompany the excess HCO_3^- in the urine.

Alkalosis Caused by Hypokalemia

Similarly, a state of hypokalemia also can cause alkalosis. For example, diuretic therapy or lack of dietary K^+ intake may cause hypokalemia. The tubules must then secrete inappropriately large amounts of H^+ ions to reabsorb Na^+ via the

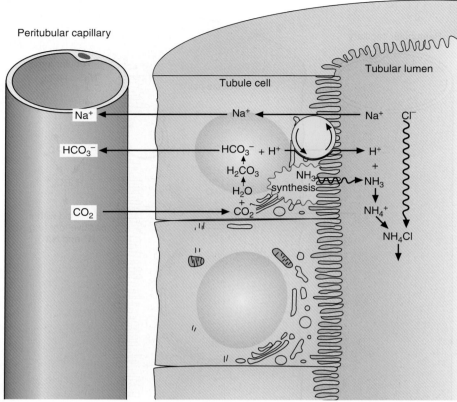

Figure 22-7 Ammonia buffer system. The tubule cell synthesizes ammonia, which diffuses into the tubular lumen according to its concentration gradient. H^+ reacts with the NH_3 molecule, forming NH_4^+, which requires excretion of a Cl^- ion. Chronic acidosis, in which the ammonia system is highly active, leads to hypochloremia.

countertransport mechanism (see Figure 22-2), which normally accounts for a relatively small percentage of Na^+ reabsorption. Consequently, alkalosis occurs. Hypokalemic alkalosis is compounded by a coexisting state of dehydration.[3] Dehydration produces a profound stimulus for Na^+ reabsorption, which (coupled with hypokalemia) intensifies the kidney's need to secrete H^+. Overuse of diuretic drugs can lead to such a condition.

Acidosis Caused by Hyperkalemia

Conversely, hyperkalemia has the opposite effect. The high plasma $[K^+]$ in hyperkalemia stimulates increased K^+ secretion into the filtrate, as described earlier. This increased filtrate K^+ competes with H^+ for the filtrate's buffer anions. As a result, the tubules secrete inappropriately low amounts of H^+, leading to an increased plasma $[H^+]$ and acidemia.

Intracellular Mechanisms Affecting Plasma Hydrogen Ion Concentration and Potassium Ion Concentration

The relationship of $[K^+]$ and plasma pH has a further explanation at the cellular level in the body.[4] These interrelationships are illustrated in red blood cells in Figure 22-8 (the same relationships are also present in all of the body's cells). Plasma hypokalemia creates a concentration gradient that favors intracellular K^+ diffusion out of the cell (Figure 22-8, A). The resulting intracellular negativity causes a net movement of plasma H^+ into the cell. The reduction in plasma $[H^+]$ produces alkalemia.

Conversely, in alkalemia (Figure 22-8, B), intracellular H^+ ions diffuse out of the cell in response to a H^+ ion concentration gradient, and plasma K^+ diffuses into the cell. The movement of K^+ into the cell causes hypokalemia.

Similarly, in acidemia (Figure 22-8, C), the plentiful plasma H^+ diffuses into the cell, and K^+ diffuses out of the cell, producing hyperkalemia. Conversely, hyperkalemia causes K^+ to move into the cell and H^+ to move out of the cell, causing acidemia (Figure 22-8, D).

Because of these intracellular-extracellular K^+ shifts, the plasma $[K^+]$ on a clinical laboratory report must be interpreted carefully. In the examples in Figure 22-8, total body stores of K^+ do not change; K^+ merely shifts between fluid compartments. However, consider the acidotic condition in Figure 22-8, C, in which plasma $[K^+]$ increases. In response to the increasing $[K^+]$, the kidneys excrete more K^+, causing more K^+ to diffuse out of the cells into the plasma. Thus, plasma $[K^+]$ may be normal or high, but total body K^+ stores may actually be depleted. Similarly, low $[K^+]$ in alkalemia (see Figure 22-8, B) does not always mean the body's K^+ stores are depleted.

CONCEPT QUESTION 22-2

Of two hypokalemic patients, which one probably has the most severe depletion of K^+ stores: patient A, who is alkalemic, or patient B, who is acidemic?

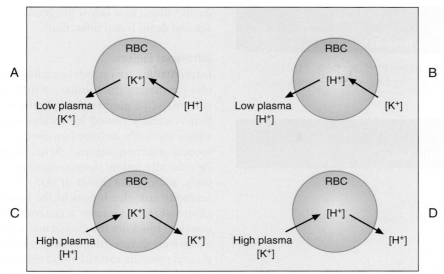

Figure 22-8 Plasma pH and K^+ ion interactions. **A,** Hypokalemia causes alkalemia. **B,** Alkalemia causes hypokalemia. **C,** Acidemia causes hyperkalemia. **D,** Hyperkalemia causes acidemia. *RBC,* Red blood cell.

SPEED OF RENAL ACID-BASE CORRECTION

The blood buffers can readjust pH in seconds, whereas the lungs can readjust pH in minutes. In contrast, the renal mechanisms require hours to days to readjust pH. Although the kidneys are slow to act, they are much more powerful and complete in their ability to restore a normal pH. In contrast to the blood buffers and respiratory system, the kidneys can continue to act until pH is readjusted almost exactly to normal rather than a certain percentage of the way.[1] The kidneys are important, not for their speed but for their ability to compensate for acid-base disturbances more completely.

HARMFUL EFFECTS OF FLUID, ELECTROLYTE, AND ACID-BASE IMBALANCES

Volume Depletion

Inadequate fluid intake or diuretic therapy may cause general dehydration. A state of dehydration generally causes the tubules to reabsorb sodium aggressively, augmenting the H^+ and K^+ secretion mechanisms. Diuretic drugs, especially loop diuretics that block sodium reabsorption such as furosemide (Lasix), may additionally cause Cl^- and K^+ loss, placing an even greater demand on the tubules to secrete H^+. (Remember that reabsorption of Cl^- and K^+ depends heavily on cotransport with sodium.) These mechanisms combine to cause metabolic alkalosis and hypokalemia, adversely affecting cardiac depolarization and nerve impulse conduction. Alkalemia caused by volume loss is often called contraction alkalosis.

Chloride and Potassium Imbalances

Causes of hypochloremia and hypokalemia are listed in Boxes 22-1 and 22-2. With regard to hypochloremia, patients with

BOX 22-1

Causes of Hypochloremia

- Low-salt diets
- Diuretic therapy
- Nasogastric suction
- Chronic CO_2 retention (COPD)

COPD, Chronic obstructive pulmonary disease.

BOX 22-2

Causes of Hypokalemia

- Lack of dietary intake
- Diarrhea
- Diuretic therapy
- Alkalosis (e.g., ventilator induced)

congestive heart failure are often on low-salt diets and taking diuretic drugs to prevent fluid retention and edema; this the body's Cl^- stores. Critically ill patients on ventilators usually have nasogastric suction tubes placed that empty the stomach to prevent regurgitation and aspiration of vomitus; this causes loss of gastric HCL. In another example, a patient with COPD and chronic hypercapnia may have a paradoxically alkalotic pH, which would appear to be "overcompensation." However, this condition is not overcompensation for respiratory acidosis; instead, it reflects chronic Cl^- depletion as a result of increased NH_3 buffering activity (loss of NH_4Cl in the urine). Alkalosis occurs because the lack of Cl^- ions causes the kidney to rely more heavily on H^+ ion secretion to reabsorb Na^+.

Severe diarrhea (see Box 22-2) may cause hypokalemia and acidosis because the lower bowel is rich in K^+ and HCO_3^- ions. Respiratory alkalosis is sometimes a complication of inappropriate ventilator therapy; regardless of its cause, alkalosis causes hypokalemia because the kidneys respond to low [H+] by secreting more K+ (see Figure 22-5).

Harmful Effects of Potassium Imbalances, Acidosis, and Alkalosis

Box 22-3 lists harmful effects of K+ imbalances, and Box 22-4 lists adverse effects of acidosis and alkalosis. The main clinical effect of acidosis is central nervous system depression, whereas the major effect of alkalosis is overexcitability of the central and peripheral nervous systems.

EFFECTS OF RENAL FAILURE

Renal failure falls into two general physiological categories: (1) acute renal failure and (2) chronic renal failure.[1] Renal failure usually interferes with electrolyte and water balance, causing sodium and fluid retention. In severe instances, the kidney fails to excrete adequate amounts of fixed acids and nitrogenous waste products. In complete renal failure without treatment, patients soon die.

Acute Renal Failure

Acute renal failure falls into three categories:[1] (1) decreased blood supply, as might occur in heart failure or hemorrhage; (2) intrarenal failure, or abnormalities within the kidney itself; and (3) postrenal failure, which refers to obstruction to urine outflow from the kidney.

Reduced Renal Blood Flow

If renal blood flow remains greater than 20% to 25% of normal, kidney cell ischemia is generally not severe enough to cause cell death.[1] Blood flow below this level can cause hypoxic cell damage and death (renal infarction).

Intrarenal Failure

Intrarenal failure includes conditions that injure the glomerular capillaries, the tubular epithelium, and the renal interstitium. Acute **glomerulonephritis** is an example of a disease that is usually caused by an abnormal immune reaction in which the body develops antibodies to group A beta streptococci microorganisms.[1] Renal manifestations of the disease usually follow streptococcal infections elsewhere in the body, such as the throat or skin. The streptococcal antigen-antibody complex lodges in the basement membrane of the glomerulus; this causes a general inflammatory glomerular reaction, blocking the glomerular capillaries or making them excessively permeable. High glomerular permeability allows plasma proteins and red blood cells to leak into the filtrate. As a result, plasma oncotic pressure decreases, which accounts for pleural effusions in the chest that often accompany acute glomerulonephritis.[5] (That is, plasma oncotic pressure may become so low that it can no longer keep fluids from leaking out of the vascular space into the pleural cavity.) In severe instances, total renal shutdown occurs. The acute inflammation usually disappears in a few weeks to a few months.[1]

Another form of intrarenal failure is tubular necrosis. Certain poisons and severe renal ischemia can cause tubular necrosis (death of tubular epithelial cells).[1] Renal poisons include carbon tetrachloride and mercury compounds. In addition, tetracycline antibiotics and some anticancer drugs are toxic to the nephron.[1] Dead epithelial cells slough away from their attachments and plug the tubules, preventing the normal flow of filtrate. Severe renal ischemia, usually caused by acute cardiovascular failure, also can kill tubular epithelial cells and plug the tubular lumen.

Postrenal Failure

Postrenal failure occurs when obstructions to renal outflow occur. If this involves only one kidney, the other kidney can usually maintain normal fluid and electrolyte balance. If obstruction affects both kidneys and persists for several days, it can lead to irreversible kidney damage.[1] Causes of obstruction include kidney stones and blood clots of the ureters, which also may block the bladder opening or the urethra.[1]

Blood Transfusion Reactions

Severe immune reactions to blood transfusion can cause acute renal failure. Transfusion reactions are characterized by the destruction of many red blood cells, releasing hemoglobin into the plasma. The hemoglobin molecule is small enough to pass through the glomerular membrane but may not be adequately reabsorbed by the proximal tubules. Excess hemoglobin in the filtrate precipitates and blocks the tubules.[1]

All of the foregoing forms of acute renal failure prevent the normal flow of filtrate through the tubules. Consequently, the kidneys retain sodium and fluid because they cannot excrete these substances. As a result, body tissues become edematous, and blood pressure increases.[1]

Chronic Renal Failure

Chronic renal failure is characterized by a decrease in the number of functional nephrons. In chronic glomerulonephritis, the glomerular filtration membrane progressively thickens and becomes fibrotic, rendering the affected glomeruli functionless.[1] This condition reduces the kidney's filtering capacity.

In pyelonephritis, the renal pelvis becomes inflamed, eventually extending back into the renal tubules. Bacteria commonly cause pyelonephritis, especially fecal bacteria that contaminate the urinary tract.[1] If unchecked, the resulting infection progressively destroys many nephrons.

Arteriosclerotic disease reduces blood flow through the renal arteries and may lead to the ischemic death of many nephrons. The kidney tissue becomes fibrotic and greatly reduced in size. This process occurs to some extent in the aging kidney, decreasing renal blood flow to about 45% of normal by the age of 80.[1]

Physiological Effects of Chronic Renal Failure

Generally, the kidneys can maintain adequate function with only one third of the normal number of nephrons. Further reduction in functioning nephrons increases the body's retention of waste products, especially urea and creatinine. The tubular filtrate load of solutes in the remaining functional nephrons increases greatly, exceeding the kidney's reabsorption capacity. Consequently, the solutes remaining in the filtrate act as osmotic diuretics, increasing each nephron's filtrate flow and urine output. Despite significant renal impairment, total urine output often paradoxically increases.[1] In other words, the increase in each nephron's urine output outweighs the effect of decreased nephron numbers. The high flow rate of filtrate through the remaining functional tubules impairs the kidney's urine-concentrating ability. Flow is too rapid through the collecting ducts for adequate water reabsorption to occur. Consequently, the kidneys excrete dilute urine, manifested by a decrease in the urine's specific gravity.[1]

If a person with complete renal shutdown continues to ingest food and water, extracellular concentrations of nitrogenous waste products, sodium, potassium, and fixed acids rapidly increase. The most important effects of retaining these substances are the following:[1] (1) general edema secondary to salt and water retention; (2) metabolic acidosis caused by the kidney's failure to excrete fixed acids; (3) high blood concentrations of nitrogenous compounds such as urea, creatinine, and uric acid, which are end products of protein breakdown; and (4) increased blood concentration of phenols, sulfates, phosphates, and potassium. This condition is called **uremia** because of the high urea concentrations in all body fluids. After about one week of renal failure, patients develop a confused mental state that may progress to a condition known as uremic coma. Acidosis, which depresses the central nervous system, is apparently responsible for the coma.[1]

CONCEPT QUESTION 22-3

Predict the respiratory consequences of renal failure that is accompanied by uremia.

Nephrotic Syndrome

Nephrotic syndrome is characterized by increased glomerular membrane permeability and subsequent loss of plasma proteins into the urine. This syndrome may occur in the absence of other renal abnormalities but is usually associated with some degree of renal failure.[1] Any condition that increases glomerular permeability can cause nephrotic syndrome. Low plasma protein concentration lowers plasma osmotic pressure, causing generalized interstitial edema and fluid collection in body cavities such as the abdomen (ascites), pleural space (pleural effusion), and pericardial space (pericardial effusion).

Goodpasture's Syndrome

Goodpasture's syndrome is an autoimmune disease affecting glomerular and pulmonary alveolar basement membranes.[5] The body forms circulating antibodies against these structures, causing hemorrhage and fibrosis. Patients with this disease develop hemoptysis (coughing up of blood) and hematuria (blood in the urine). Goodpasture's syndrome targets primarily the kidney; the lung's alveoli become involved because of a cross-reaction.[5]

Goodpasture's syndrome affects mainly young adult males over the age of 16 years. This rare syndrome causes renal and respiratory failure. The prognosis is quite poor; average survival after the appearance of the first symptom is about six months.[5]

RENAL FUNCTION TESTS

Renal Clearance Tests

Renal clearance tests are used to assess the ability of the kidneys to clear the plasma of a specific substance. Intravenous pyelography (IVP) involves the injection of an iodine-containing substance intravenously and watching the subsequent rise in urinary iodine concentration over the next several minutes.[1] Since iodine is opaque to x-rays, urinary iodine outlines the renal pelvis on x-ray pictures. Lack of renal pelvis shadows on the x-ray film (pyelogram) indicates that the patient has poor renal clearance.

Blood Urea Nitrogen and Creatinine

Common blood tests of renal function are **blood urea nitrogen (BUN)** and creatinine tests. Normal BUN concentration ranges from 8 to 20 mg/dL; blood creatinine concentration ranges from 0.6 to 1.2 mg/dL.[6] Urea is synthesized in the liver from ammonia, a by-product of protein (amino acid) catabolism. Urea is constantly formed and must be excreted by the kidneys. BUN increases in kidney failure as a result of decreased tubular filtration capacity. In extreme instances, BUN may increase to 300 mg/dL.[1]

Creatinine, another end product of protein catabolism, is constantly formed in muscle tissues. The quantity of creatinine produced is proportional to the body's muscle mass. Blood creatinine concentration may be elevated in kidney and muscle diseases. When BUN and creatinine are elevated in renal failure, metabolic acidosis is usually also present.

CLINICAL FOCUS 22-2

Artificial Kidney: Hemodialysis

The artificial kidney, or dialysis machine, has been used clinically for many years to sustain the lives of patients with complete renal failure. The basic principle of hemodialysis involves the diffusion of substances through a semipermeable membrane from areas of high concentration to areas of low concentration. In the hemodialysis process, the patient's blood passes through tiny channels formed by thin semipermeable membranes. On the other side of the membrane is a dialyzing solution containing specific concentrations of various solutes. The composition of the dialyzing fluid is such that unwanted substances diffuse out of the blood and into the solution.

Dialyzing fluid contains neither urea nor creatinine. Because the patient's plasma has high concentrations of these substances, they rapidly diffuse out of the blood and into the dialysis fluid. The solute composition of dialysis solution is chosen to correct the abnormalities caused by renal failure. $[Na^+]$ and $[K^+]$ are less in dialyzing fluid than in plasma, causing a net loss of these ions. Conversely, $[HCO_3^-]$ is higher in dialysis fluid. As a result, HCO_3^- diffuses into the plasma, counteracting the metabolic acidosis of renal failure.

During the dialysis procedure, blood is withdrawn through a large-bore intravascular catheter at a rate of about 300 mL per minute and pumped through the dialysis machine. A small portion of the patient's cardiac output flows continuously through the dialysis machine until the plasma is adequately cleared of unwanted substances. The entire process usually lasts about 3 to 4 hours and may be needed up to three times per week.

CONCEPT QUESTION 22-4

Explain the mechanism by which renal failure may precipitate ventilatory failure in a patient who has advanced COPD.

POINTS TO REMEMBER

- Electrolyte and acid-base balance are important for proper nerve and cardiac impulse conduction.
- The kidney compensates for respiratory acid-base disturbances mainly by titrating filtered HCO_3^- against secreted H^+.

- Respiratory acidosis increases tubular H^+ secretion, which reacts with and reabsorbs all filtrate HCO_3^-.
- Respiratory alkalosis decreases H^+ secretion, allowing excess filtrate HCO_3^- to be eliminated in the urine.
- The priority the body places on sodium reabsorption sometimes causes imbalances in other ions, especially K^+ and H^+ ions.
- Factors that interfere with sodium reabsorption usually cause K^+ and acid-base imbalances.
- The presence of buffers in the filtrate is important in excreting excess H^+ ions.
- Acid-base balance and potassium balance are interrelated such that alkalosis and hypokalemia mutually augment each other; the same is true for acidosis and hyperkalemia.
- Diuretic drugs often cause electrolyte imbalances and acid-base imbalances.
- Renal failure generally impairs the kidneys' ability to excrete adequate amounts of sodium, fixed acids, and end products of protein breakdown (e.g., urea and creatinine).
- Renal failure is characterized by fluid retention, metabolic acidosis, and high blood concentrations of urea and creatinine.
- Respiratory consequences of renal failure include hyperventilation in an attempt to compensate for metabolic acidosis; renal failure may precipitate ventilatory failure in patients with preexisting respiratory disease.

References

1. Hall JE: *Guyton and Hall textbook of medical physiology*, ed 12, Philadelphia, 2011, Saunders.
2. Mount DB: Transport of sodium, chloride, and potassium. In Taal MW, et al, editors: *Brenner and Rector's the kidney*, ed 9, Philadelphia, 2011, Saunders.
3. Masoro EJ, Siegel PD: *Acid-base regulation: physiology and pathophysiology*, Philadelphia, 1971, Saunders.
4. Filley G: *Acid-base and blood gas regulation*, Philadelphia, 1971, Lea & Febiger.
5. Fraser RG, et al: *Fraser and Pare's diagnosis of diseases of the chest*, ed 4, Philadelphia, 1999, Saunders.
6. Hristova EN, Henry JB: Metabolic intermediates, inorganic ions and biochemical markers of bone metabolism. In McPherson RA, Pincus MR, editors: *Henry's clinical diagnosis and management by laboratory methods*, ed 21, Philadelphia, 2006, Saunders.

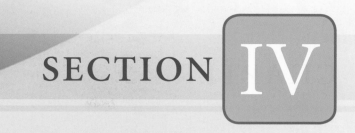

INTEGRATED RESPONSES
IN EXERCISE AND AGING

CHAPTER 23

Cardiopulmonary Response to Exercise in Health and Disease

OBJECTIVES

After reading this chapter you will be able to:
- Describe why continual regeneration of adenosine triphosphate (ATP) is necessary to sustain exercise
- Explain how aerobic and anaerobic metabolic processes differ in their ability to generate ATP
- Explain how oxygen consumption and carbon dioxide production differ in aerobic metabolism of carbohydrates and fats
- Explain why the changes in respiratory, cardiovascular, and metabolic processes are different below than above the anaerobic threshold

- Explain how caloric expenditure is related to oxygen consumption
- Use exercise test data to differentiate cardiac and pulmonary limitations to exercise
- Explain why sedentary and athletically trained individuals differ in their ability to perform exercise
- Use exercise test data to differentiate obstructive and restrictive pulmonary limitations to physical activity
- Use exercise test data to prescribe appropriate physical activity in cardiopulmonary rehabilitation programs

KEY TERMS

adenosine triphosphate (ATP)
aerobic
anaerobic
anaerobic glycolysis
anaerobic threshold
breathing reserve (BR)
creatine phosphate (CP)
glycogen
heart rate reserve (HRR)
indirect calorimetry
maximum exercise ventilation ($\dot{V}_E$max)
maximum heart rate (HR_{max})

maximum oxygen consumption ($\dot{V}O_2$max)
metabolic cart
metabolic equivalent (MET)
O_2 pulse
pyruvic acid
respiratory quotient (RQ)
steady state
$\dot{V}CO_2 / \dot{V}O_2$
$\dot{V}_E / \dot{V}CO_2$
$\dot{V}_E / \dot{V}O_2$
ventilatory equivalents for carbon dioxide and oxygen
V-slope method

PHYSIOLOGY OF EXERCISE

Strenuous exercise greatly increases the body's requirements for oxygen delivery and carbon dioxide elimination. Close coupling between increased metabolic activity and cardiopulmonary function is necessary to supply adequate oxygen to exercising muscles and maintain a normal blood acid-base balance. This coupling is schematically represented in Figure 23-1.

Normal exchange of O_2 and CO_2 between muscle cells and the air requires the following:[1] (1) efficient alveolar ventilation, (2) pulmonary blood flow matched to ventilation, (3) adequate blood hemoglobin content, (4) adequate cardiac pump function, (5) systemic blood flow matched to tissue requirements, and (6) ventilatory control mechanisms sensitive to arterial blood gas changes. These factors normally interact in a finely coordinated fashion, responding precisely to the metabolic needs of exercising muscle.

Normally, respiratory and cardiac reserve capacities are so large that only great physiological impairment reduces daily functioning ability. Exercise testing is clinically important because it stresses all physiological systems, revealing their capacity to respond. Respiratory and cardiac impairments produce characteristically different patterns of response to exercise, allowing cardiovascular and pulmonary limitations to be differentiated. The purpose of this chapter is to provide a physiological basis for evaluating exercise performance, not to provide a definitive guide for interpreting exercise test results.

Metabolism during Exercise

The source of energy for skeletal muscle contraction is **adenosine triphosphate (ATP)**. The structure of the ATP molecule is symbolized as follows:[2]

$$\text{Adenosine} - PO_3^- \sim PO_3^- \sim PO_3^-$$

The bonds between the PO_3^- radicals, designated by the symbol $\sim$, are high-energy phosphate bonds. The process of metabolism breaks these bonds, releasing the energy needed to form and break cross-bridges between the muscle's actin and myosin myofibrils, as described in Chapter 17; in this way, muscle fibers shorten and generate force. During exercise conditions, each high-energy bond stores about 7300 calories (7.3 kcal) per mole of ATP molecules.[2] The hydrolysis of the first PO_3^- bond produces 7300 calories, generating adenosine diphosphate (ADP) in the process. Hydrolysis of the remaining PO_3^- bond yields yet another 7300 calories and creates adenosine monophosphate (AMP) for a total energy release of about 14.6 kcal/mol.[2]

ATP stores in skeletal muscle are extremely small and can sustain strenuous muscular activity for only about 3 seconds.[2] Therefore ATP molecules must be reconstituted continuously during exercise through **aerobic** (with oxygen) and **anaerobic** (without oxygen) metabolic processes.

The energy required for sustained exercise is derived from internal and external mechanisms.[3] Internal mechanisms include anaerobic production of ATP, O_2 release from hemoglobin, and dissolved O_2 uptake from plasma and tissue fluids. External mechanisms involve the delivery of atmospheric O_2 molecules to the tissues. Atmospheric O_2 is relatively unimportant for power surges of a few seconds and the first few minutes of exercise. Internal mechanisms are crucial for initiating exercise because of the delay involved in transporting atmospheric O_2 to the tissues. As exercise continues, energy production becomes primarily dependent on the adequate delivery of atmospheric O_2 to the tissues. As exercise intensity reaches maximum limits, internal anaerobic sources of energy become increasingly important.

Aerobic Metabolism

Aerobic metabolism of carbohydrates (glucose), fats (fatty acids), and proteins (amino acids) provides the major energy

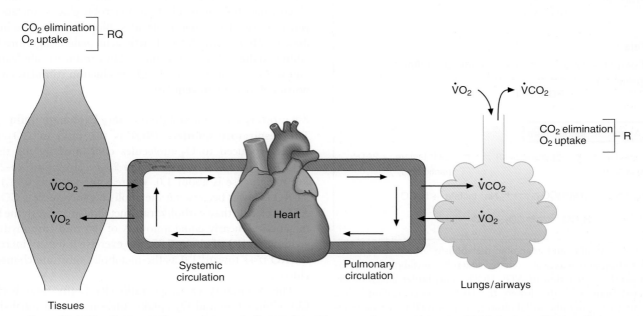

Figure 23-1 Ventilatory-cardiovascular-metabolic coupling. The gas-exchange pathway is a highly integrated series of steps.

source for ATP synthesis.[2] During exercise, stored **glycogen** in the muscles breaks down into glucose. Glucose breaks down into **pyruvic acid**, which reacts with O_2 in the cell's mitochondria, forming ATP, CO_2, and water; thus the aerobic or oxidative process of ATP synthesis consumes O_2 and generates CO_2.

Aerobic metabolism of fatty acids also produces ATP molecules. For a given rate of ATP production, fat metabolism requires more O_2 than carbohydrate metabolism (Figure 23-2). This means carbohydrate metabolism uses O_2 more efficiently and requires less cardiovascular work per mole of ATP synthesis. However, fat metabolism generates less CO_2 per mole of ATP produced than carbohydrate metabolism (see Figure 23-2); in other words, fat metabolism requires less ventilatory work than carbohydrate metabolism in generating a given amount of energy.[2]

Anaerobic Metabolism and Lactic Acid Production

Anaerobic metabolic processes occur in the absence of O_2. An example of anaerobic metabolism is the breakdown of **creatine phosphate (CP)**, which, similar to the ATP molecule, possesses a high-energy phosphate bond:

$$Creatine \sim PO_3^-$$

The breakdown of this bond supplies the immediate energy for ATP resynthesis from ADP, as shown:

$$Creatine \sim PO_3^- + ADP \rightarrow creatine + ATP$$

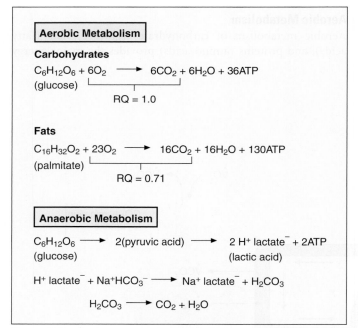

Figure 23-2 Aerobic and anaerobic metabolism. About midway between resting and maximal exercise, anaerobic metabolism supplements aerobic generation of ATP. HCO_3^- ions buffer anaerobically generated lactic acid; this lowers the HCO_3^- concentration, while generating CO_2. Aerobic metabolism generates ATP much more efficiently than anaerobic metabolism.

However, this process produces only enough ATP to fuel muscle contraction for 8 to 10 seconds during heavy exercise.[2]

If the cardiovascular system does not supply enough O_2 for aerobic metabolism, glucose from muscle glycogen is metabolized in a process called **anaerobic glycolysis**. In this process, pyruvic acid is metabolized anaerobically into lactic acid and ATP (see Figure 23-2). The lactic acid subsequently diffuses into the interstitial fluid and blood, creating lactic acidosis, a form of metabolic acidosis. Increased blood lactic acid concentration indicates the presence of anaerobic metabolism, implying inadequate O_2 delivery to the tissues.

Anaerobic Threshold

As exercise intensity increases, energy requirements gradually increase until aerobic metabolism alone can no longer meet the demand for ATP resynthesis. Consequently, the body must rely on anaerobic metabolism to generate additional ATP. The onset of anaerobic metabolism, the **anaerobic threshold**, normally occurs at about 50% to 65% of the body's **maximum oxygen consumption ($\dot{V}O_2max$)**.[3] Because fat cannot be metabolized anaerobically, less fat is used as exercise intensity increases.[2] The major energy sources at maximal exercise are aerobic and anaerobic glucose metabolism. For this reason, the body's glucose stores limit exercise endurance. Sustained exercise such as marathon running may totally deplete glucose stores, explaining the reason some marathon runners suddenly fatigue or "hit the wall" after about 20 miles.

Figure 23-2 shows that aerobic metabolism produces ATP far more efficiently than anaerobic metabolism. In aerobic metabolism, one molecule of glucose produces 36 molecules of ATP compared with only two molecules of ATP in anaerobic glucose metabolism. In addition, anaerobic glucose metabolism generates two lactic acid molecules. Blood bicarbonate immediately buffers newly formed lactic acid, generating more CO_2, adding to the CO_2 already produced by aerobic metabolism (see Figure 23-2). This increased CO_2 production stimulates a proportional increase in ventilation.[3]

Respiratory Quotient and Respiratory Exchange Ratio

The **respiratory quotient (RQ)** is the ratio of CO_2 molecules produced to O_2 molecules consumed by the tissues ($\dot{V}CO_2 / \dot{V}O_2$), as shown in Figure 23-1.[2] (In Figure 23-2, the RQ for glucose is about 1.0, whereas for fat, it is 0.71.) The fat RQ is lower because fat metabolism generates less CO_2 per ATP molecule than carbohydrate metabolism. At rest, the body metabolizes nearly equal amounts of fats and carbohydrates, yielding an RQ of about 0.85.[2] As exercise intensity increases, the RQ rises toward 1.0 as the metabolic substrate changes to glucose.

The respiratory exchange ratio (R) is the ratio between CO_2 elimination and O_2 uptake, measured from inhaled and exhaled gases at the mouth (see Figure 23-1).[2] In steady-state conditions, R equals RQ. The **steady state** is characterized by a CO_2 elimination rate that matches the CO_2 production rate; likewise, the lung's O_2 uptake rate equals the tissue's O_2 consumption rate in steady-state conditions. During short bursts of maximal exercise such as the 100-yard dash, RQ and R are different because tissue O_2 consumption and CO_2 production momentarily exceed the lung's O_2 uptake and CO_2 elimination. Like RQ, R increases as exercise intensity increases; the onset of anaerobic metabolism further increases R as bicarbonate reacts with lactic acid and generates more CO_2.

CONCEPT QUESTION 23-3

As exercise intensity increases, CO_2 production and alveolar ventilation increase steadily. Why does the rate of alveolar ventilation rise increase abruptly after anaerobic metabolism begins?

Exercise Testing Methods

Exercise tests in the laboratory involve treadmills or bicycle ergometers that provide the subject with graded exercise over a period of time. In a graded exercise test, the workload is progressively increased in a series of stages by increasing the treadmill speed (and its angle from the floor) or by increasing the bicycle's pedal resistance. For example, the subject may exercise at a certain treadmill speed and angle for 3 minutes, after which the speed and angle are increased for the next 3 minutes, and so on. The subject exercises through a well-defined series of stages, each more difficult than the last, until maximum capacity is reached. During this time, a machine called a **metabolic cart** measures the inhaled and exhaled O_2 and CO_2 concentrations, tidal volume (V_T), respiratory rate, and minute ventilation.

To obtain these measurements, the subject breathes through a specially designed mouthpiece attached to the metabolic cart by large-bore tubes. Nose clips prevent breathing through the nose. The lips must be sealed tightly around the mouthpiece to prevent mixing of respiratory gases with atmospheric air. An electrocardiogram (ECG) machine measures the heart rate (HR) and ECG pattern during the exercise test. Depending on the data desired, various other physiological parameters may be measured. Table 23-1 lists physiological measurements grouped according to the invasiveness of the test and the monitoring equipment needed.

CLINICAL FOCUS 23-1

Arterial Carbon Dioxide Pressure during Exercise

In an exercise testing laboratory, a well-trained, long-distance runner undergoes an exercise test. At rest, she has a $PaCO_2$ of 40 mm Hg, R of 0.8, and minute ventilation of 6.5 L per minute. After 5 minutes of running on the treadmill, the following measurements are obtained:

$\dot{V}CO_2$ = 960 mL/min

$\dot{V}O_2$ = 1200 mL/min

Minute ventilation = 33 L/min

From these data, do you expect her $PaCO_2$ to be low, normal, or high?

Discussion

Because this athlete's $\dot{V}_E$ increased more than five times over the resting measurement, you may be inclined to predict a low $PaCO_2$. However, her R remained unchanged at 0.8, as the following calculation shows:

$$\dot{V}CO_2/\dot{V}O_2 = 960/1200 = 0.8$$

The increase in $\dot{V}_E$ perfectly matched her increased metabolic CO_2 production and $\dot{V}O_2$. Although her $\dot{V}_E$ increased greatly, it was an appropriate increase, proportional to metabolic demands. In other words, this athlete was not hyperventilating, even at a $\dot{V}_E$ of 33 L per minute. Therefore, her $PaCO_2$ is expected to remain unchanged. $PaCO_2$ remains remarkably constant in normal individuals during mild to moderate exercise.

TABLE 23-1

Measurements during Graded Exercise Testing

Level of Rest	Measurements
Group 1	No mouthpiece
	Patient response and symptoms
	Heart rate
	Blood pressure
	ECG
	SaO_2 by oximetry
Group 2	Mouthpiece, oxygen, and carbon dioxide analyzer
	Respiratory rate
	Tidal volume
	Minute ventilation
	End-tidal gas measurements
	$\dot{V}O_2$ and O_2 pulse
	$\dot{V}CO_2$
	Respiratory exchange ratio
Group 3	Arterial line
	Blood gas values: PaO_2, $PaCO_2$, and pH
	HCO_3^- and lactate
	V_D/V_T
Group 4	Right-sided heart catheter
	Pulmonary artery pressures
	Cardiac output
	Mixed venous PO_2 and SO_2

Modified from Martin L: *Pulmonary physiology in clinical practice: the essentials for patient care and evaluation*, St Louis, 1987, Mosby.
ECG, Electrocardiogram; *SaO₂*, arterial oxygen saturation; *V̇O₂*, oxygen consumption per minute; *O₂ pulse*, oxygen consumption per heartbeat; *V̇CO₂*, carbon dioxide production per minute; *PaO₂*, arterial oxygen pressure; *PaCO₂*, arterial carbon dioxide pressure; *pH*, measure of blood H⁺ concentration; *HCO₃⁻*, blood bicarbonate; *V_D/V_T*, dead space-to-tidal volume ratio; *PO₂*, oxygen pressure; *SO₂*, oxygen saturation.

Physiological Changes during Exercise

Oxygen Consumption, Cardiac Output, and Blood Pressure

Figure 23-3 represents the exercise performance of a normal person. $\dot{V}O_2$ increases linearly with the work rate from rest to maximal exercise. The slope of $\dot{V}O_2$ increase is about the same for all normal people; it is unaffected by training, age, or gender.[1] Because $\dot{V}O_2$ depends primarily on the amount of work done by exercising muscle, $\dot{V}O_2$ can be predicted from the work rate.[2,3]

As exercise intensifies, contracting muscles consume ever greater amounts of ATP, which means aerobic ATP regeneration requires an increasingly greater O_2 supply from the blood flow. Cardiac output rises to meet this demand by increasing stroke volume (SV) and heart rate. SV increases to its maximum value within the first half of the tolerable work rate range (at about 45% of the maximum $\dot{V}O_2$).[3] From that point on, SV remains fairly constant; the only way the heart can increase its output further is to increase its rate of contraction. The early increase in SV is the result of an increased ejection fraction rather than greater diastolic filling; sympathetic nervous stimulation and circulating epinephrine increase systolic ejection.[3] Heart rate increases linearly with O_2 requirements until the **maximum heart rate (HR$_{max}$)** is achieved (Figure 23-4).

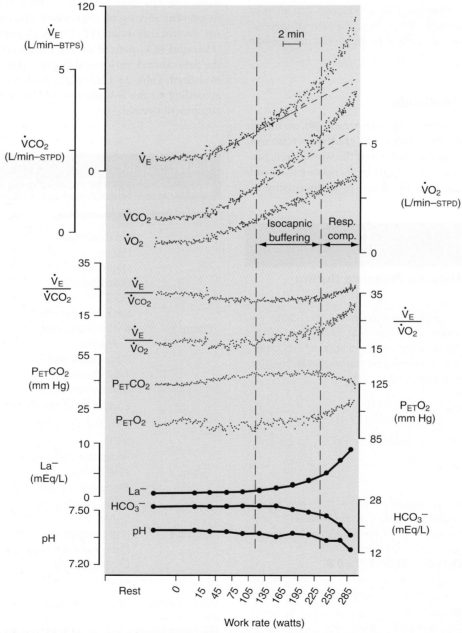

Figure 23-3 Breath-by-breath physiological changes during exercise from rest to maximal exertion in minute ventilation ($\dot{V}_E$), carbon output ($\dot{V}CO_2$), oxygen uptake ($\dot{V}O_2$), ventilatory equivalent for carbon dioxide ($\dot{V}_E/\dot{V}CO_2$), ventilatory equivalent for oxygen ($\dot{V}_E/\dot{V}O_2$), end-tidal PCO_2 ($P_{ET}CO_2$), end-tidal PO_2 ($P_{ET}O_2$), arterial blood lactate, bicarbonate, and pH. *BTPS,* Body temperature and pressure, saturated; *STPD,* standard temperature and pressure, dry. (From Mason RJ, et al, editors: *Textbook of respiratory medicine,* ed 4, St Louis, 2005, Saunders.)

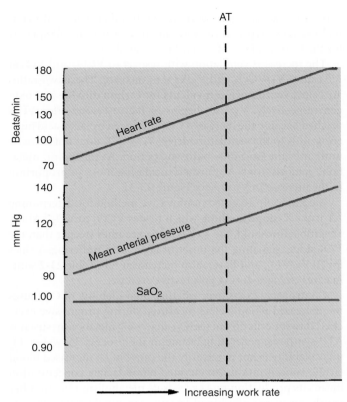

Figure 23-4 Changes in heart rate, systemic blood pressure, and SaO_2 during exercise from rest to maximal exertion. *AT*, Aerobic threshold. (From Martin L: *Pulmonary physiology in clinical practice: the essentials for patient care and evaluation,* St Louis, 1987, Mosby.)

As cardiac output increases with exercise, systolic blood pressure rises significantly (often ≥200 mm Hg). Diastolic pressure changes little, if at all, in normal, healthy people because the peripheral vasculature dilates significantly in response to increased O_2 demand, which greatly reduces vascular resistance.[2,3] Thus, the pulse pressure (systolic - diastolic) increases significantly, forcing open all of the capillaries in working skeletal muscle. In heavy exercise, up to 80% of the cardiac output is diverted to skeletal muscle, making possible greatly increased O_2 delivery and $\dot{V}O_2$ rates.

HR_{max} is age related and does not change with fitness. The predicted HR_{max} for adults is as follows:[4]

$HR_{max} = 220 - Age\ (years)$

HR_{max}, and thus, cardiac output are reduced in older persons because their hearts are less responsive to beta-adrenergic stimulation.[4] An unconditioned person and a conditioned athlete of the same age have the same HR_{max}, but the conditioned athlete has a much greater SV and therefore a much higher cardiac output at HR_{max}. For a given amount of submaximal exercise, a conditioned person's HR is much lower than the HR of a sedentary person. This explains why a sedentary person reaches the HR_{max} sooner and at much lower exercise intensity than an athlete. Because the unconditioned person's cardiac output is lower at the HR_{max}, maximum O_2 delivery and $\dot{V}O_2$ are also lower.

Carbon Dioxide Production, Respiratory Exchange Ratio, and Minute Ventilation

The increased metabolic activity of exercising muscles raises not only the $\dot{V}O_2$ but also the $\dot{V}CO_2$. Before the anaerobic threshold is reached, $\dot{V}CO_2$ increases linearly and parallel with $\dot{V}O_2$. Thus, R remains constant. The ventilation rate and depth rise to accommodate the increase in $\dot{V}CO_2$, producing a linear increase in $\dot{V}_E$ parallel with $\dot{V}CO_2$ and $\dot{V}O_2$ (see Figure 23-3, before anaerobic threshold).

Although it is generally accepted that increased $\dot{V}CO_2$ during exercise is the stimulus for the higher $\dot{V}_E$, some evidence suggests that a neurally mediated, muscle-derived signal plays a role. Apparently, peripheral muscle receptors send signals to the central nervous system, increasing blood pressure, HR, and ventilation. These signals are enhanced by muscle ischemia but are not present in ischemia alone without exercise.[5] Thus, muscle movement appears to be partly responsible for the increased $\dot{V}_E$ of exercise.

The ventilatory response to exercise was discussed in Chapter 11. The immediate hyperpnea of exercise has long been a controversial subject and remains incompletely understood.[3] The abrupt increase in $\dot{V}_E$ at the onset of exercise (phase I) occurs long before any chemical or humoral change can occur in the body. Rather than being geared to a chemoreceptor reflex mechanism, the abrupt increase in ventilation appears to be a response to anticipated future metabolic demand. Evidence points to a sophisticated internal respiratory controller that integrates multiple afferent and efferent signals to predict the level of metabolic activity that will occur and then adjusts ventilation before the fact.[6] A study of children with congenital central hypoventilation syndrome revealed that passive leg motion induced by a motor-driven ergocycle increased $\dot{V}_E$, although these children had no $\dot{V}_E$ response to inhaled CO_2.[7] Increased $\dot{V}_E$ occurred immediately with the first breath after the onset of pedaling motion in children with congenital central hypoventilation syndrome and normal controls. This study supports the idea that muscle or joint receptors play a role in exercise hyperpnea.

Normal people increase $\dot{V}_E$ by increasing both V_T and respiratory rate. Early in exercise, a higher V_T produces most of the increase in $\dot{V}_E$. After about 60% to 70% of the vital capacity is reached, V_T plateaus, and increased respiratory rate is responsible for additional $\dot{V}_E$ increases.[8]

Figure 23-5 shows that dead space-to-tidal volume ratio (V_D/V_T) decreases as exercise progresses. The initial steep reduction in V_D/V_T reflects early increases in V_T with respect to the fixed anatomical dead space. V_D/V_T decreases from normal values of 0.3 to 0.4 at rest to 0.15 to 0.2 in exercise, in part due to a larger V_T but also because of significant blood flow diversion to previously underperfused upper lung zones.[3,8] As the respiratory rate begins to account for more of the increase in $\dot{V}_E$, the decline in V_D/V_T is less steep.

Events Occurring after Anaerobic Threshold

As shown in Figure 23-3, the anaerobic threshold is the point at which the $\dot{V}CO_2$ slope becomes steeper than the $\dot{V}O_2$ slope, indicating an increase in CO_2 generation rate. This increase in

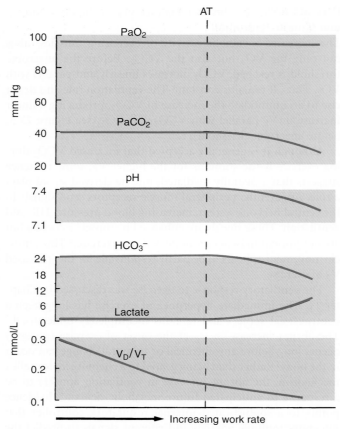

Figure 23-5 Changes in arterial blood gases, blood lactate, and V_D/V_T ratio during exercise from rest to maximal exertion. (From Martin L: *Pulmonary physiology in clinical practice: the essentials for patient care and evaluation,* St Louis, 1987, Mosby.)

CO_2 generation is due to the bicarbonate buffering of anaerobically produced lactic acid.[3,4] The increased generation of CO_2 stimulates ventilation, and the $\dot{V}_E$ slope rises in parallel with the $\dot{V}CO_2$ slope, maintaining a constant $PaCO_2$. In the end, the amount of CO_2 exhaled per minute increases with respect to the amount of O_2 taken up by the lungs, and R increases. The new $\dot{V}_E$ slope has two phases. For some time, immediately after an aerobic threshold (AT) appears, the $\dot{V}_E$ slope rises to match the increased $\dot{V}CO_2$ slope. This short phase is referred to as isocapnic buffering, in which ventilation increases in concert with CO_2, momentarily compensating for the evolving lactic acidosis (see Figure 23-3).

As bicarbonate stores diminish and arterial pH falls, ventilation is stimulated more intensely, causing a second-phase increase in $\dot{V}_E$, out of proportion with the $\dot{V}CO_2$ increase. (See the steeper $\dot{V}_E$ slope after the second *dotted vertical line* in Figure 23-3.) The sharper rise in $\dot{V}_E$ relative to $\dot{V}CO_2$ represents hyperventilation; thus, $PaCO_2$ falls, as is reflected by the decrease in $P_{ET}CO_2$. (Recall that $P_{ET}CO_2$ is normally about equal to $PaCO_2$.) At the same time, $P_{ET}O_2$ also increases because the increase in $\dot{V}_E$ supplies O_2 to the lungs more rapidly than it can be taken up.

As exercise intensity progresses to maximum levels, arterial pH falls further as blood lactate increases and bicarbonate

concentration falls (see Figure 23-5). In other words, at maximal exercise, hyperventilation fails to compensate adequately for the lactic acidosis of anaerobic metabolism.

The increased ventilation with respect to $\dot{V}CO_2$ and $\dot{V}O_2$ at AT causes $\dot{V}_E/\dot{V}CO_2$ and $\dot{V}_E/\dot{V}O_2$ to increase. These two ratios are called **ventilatory equivalents for carbon dioxide and oxygen** respectively. $\dot{V}_E/\dot{V}O_2$ begins to increase soon after AT is reached because the increased CO_2 produced by lactic acid buffering adds to the ventilatory drive. $\dot{V}_E/\dot{V}CO_2$ does not increase until after the isocapnic buffering period. At this point, metabolic acidosis drives $\dot{V}_E$ further, increasing it out of proportion to the increase in $\dot{V}CO_2$ (see Figure 23-3).

A commonly accepted noninvasive method for determining AT is the **V-slope method**, which relates $\dot{V}CO_2$ to $\dot{V}O_2$.[4] At the anaerobic threshold, the $\dot{V}CO_2$ slope becomes steeper than the $\dot{V}O_2$ slope, signaling the onset of lactic acid buffering. Values for R, $\dot{V}_E/\dot{V}O_2$, and $P_{ET}O_2$ also increase at AT. Table 23-2 summarizes changes during progressive exercise.

Controversy exists over whether unavailability of O_2 causes the increased blood lactate measured during progressive exercise.[3] If tissue cells do not use O_2, anaerobic metabolism sustains ATP synthesis, generating lactate in the process. However, O_2 unavailability is not necessarily the cause of an increased blood lactate concentration. An elevated blood lactate concentration means its production rate exceeds its metabolism rate. In other words, an increase in blood lactate may simply reflect that its metabolism rate cannot keep up with its production, not that O_2 is unavailable. Therefore, blood lactate concentration may not accurately reflect the degree of O_2 limitation.[3] Nevertheless, the onset of lactic acidosis is delayed in exercising subjects breathing high O_2 concentrations. In addition, high workloads elicit lower than normal blood lactate concentrations when patients are breathing supplemental O_2. Conversely, the lactate threshold is reached sooner and maximum lactate concentration is higher when a patient is breathing a low fractional concentration of oxygen in inspired gas (F_IO_2). These findings provide strong evidence that anaerobic threshold is an O_2-dependent mechanism.[9]

Arterial Blood Gases

Figure 23-5 shows that arterial blood gases remain remarkably constant up to the anaerobic threshold. As discussed earlier, $[HCO_3^-]$ and pH decrease after reaching AT as HCO_3^- buffers lactic acid; about 22 mEq of CO_2 are evolved for each 1 mEq of lactic acid buffered.[3] Hyperventilation does little to raise PaO_2 and has even less effect on SaO_2 (see Figure 23-4); that is, room air F_IO_2 limits the increase in PaO_2, and SaO_2 is already near its maximum level under normal resting conditions (refer to the oxygen-hemoglobin equilibrium curve in Chapter 8). Thus, arterial oxygen content does not increase significantly from rest to maximal exercise. For these reasons, increased O_2 delivery to the tissues depends entirely on the increase in cardiac output in normal individuals.

Oxygen Diffusion Capacity

O_2 diffusion capacity almost triples with exercise.[2] At rest, blood flow through many pulmonary capillaries is extremely

TABLE 23-2

Physiological Changes during Exercise as Work Rate Increases

Measured Value	Reason for Change
Before Anaerobic Threshold	
Expired Gas	
$\dot{V}O_2$ rate increases linearly	Need for aerobic ATP regeneration increases linearly
$\dot{V}CO_2$ rate increases at the same rate as $\dot{V}O_2$	CO_2 is a by-product of aerobic ATP regeneration
$\dot{V}_E$ rate increases at the same rate as $\dot{V}CO_2$	$\dot{V}_E$ matches CO_2 production to maintain acid-base homeostasis
R ($\dot{V}CO_2/\dot{V}O_2$) is constant	$\dot{V}O_2$ and $\dot{V}CO_2$ rates increase equally
$P_{ET}O_2$ is constant	O_2 uptake from the lungs equals inspired O_2
$P_{ET}CO_2$ is constant	CO_2 exhaled equals CO_2 produced
$\dot{V}_E/\dot{V}O_2$ is constant	$\dot{V}_E$ and $\dot{V}O_2$ rates increase equally
$\dot{V}_E/\dot{V}CO_2$ is constant	$\dot{V}_E$ and $\dot{V}CO_2$ rates increase equally
Blood	
Lactic acid concentration is constant	Metabolism is mainly aerobic
Heart Rate and Cardiac Output	
Rates of increase are linear	O_2 delivery keeps pace with $\dot{V}O_2$
At Anaerobic Threshold	
Expired Gas	
$\dot{V}O_2$ rate increases linearly	Aerobic ATP regeneration needs continue to increase linearly
$\dot{V}CO_2$ increases at a greater rate than $\dot{V}O_2$	Lactic acid buffering by HCO_3^- accelerates $\dot{V}CO_2$
$\dot{V}_E$ increases at a greater rate than $\dot{V}O_2$	$\dot{V}_E$ responds proportionately to $\dot{V}CO_2$ increase
R increases	Increased $\dot{V}_E$ causes CO_2 elimination rate to exceed O_2 uptake rate
$P_{ET}O_2$ and $\dot{V}_E/\dot{V}O_2$ increase	$\dot{V}_E$ increases more than $\dot{V}O_2$
$P_{ET}CO_2$ and $\dot{V}_E/\dot{V}CO_2$ are constant	$\dot{V}_E$ matches CO_2 production (isocapnic buffering)
Blood	
Lactic acid concentration increases	Anaerobic metabolism begins to supplement aerobic ATP regeneration
Heart Rate and Cardiac Output	
Rates of increase are linear	O_2 delivery keeps pace with $\dot{V}O_2$ requirements
Anaerobic Threshold to Maximal Exercise	
Expired Gas	
$\dot{V}O_2$ increases linearly to plateau ($\dot{V}O_2$max)	O_2 needs continue to increase linearly
	$\dot{V}O_2$max is limited by maximum heart rate
$\dot{V}CO_2$ increases at a greater rate than $\dot{V}O_2$	Lactic acid buffering and CO_2 generation rate continue to increase
$\dot{V}_E$ increases at a greater rate than $\dot{V}CO_2$	Development of metabolic (lactic) acidosis stimulates $\dot{V}_E$ further (respiratory compensation)
R continues to increase	CO_2 elimination rate continues to increase more than O_2 uptake rate
$P_{ET}O_2$ and $\dot{V}_E/\dot{V}O_2$ increase more sharply	Added stimulation from metabolic acidosis increases $\dot{V}_E$ disproportionately to $\dot{V}O_2$
$P_{ET}CO_2$ decreases and $\dot{V}_E/\dot{V}CO_2$ increases	Added stimulation from metabolic acidosis increases $\dot{V}_E$ disproportionately relative to $\dot{V}CO_2$ (compensatory hyperventilation)

TABLE 23-2	
Physiological Changes during Exercise as Work Rate Increases—cont'd	
Measured Value	**Reason for Change**
Blood	
Lactic acid concentration increases	Continued increase in anaerobic metabolism supplements aerobic ATP regeneration
$[HCO_3^-]$ decreases	HCO_3^- is used up in lactic acid buffering
Heart Rate and Cardiac Output	
Linear rates increase to plateau (HR_{max})	O_2 delivery keeps pace with O_2 requirements until age-determined HR_{max} is achieved

$\dot{V}O_2$, Oxygen consumption per minute; $\dot{V}CO_2$, carbon dioxide production per minute; *ATP,* adenosine triphosphate; $\dot{V}_E$, minute ventilation; *R,* respiratory exchange ratio in the lungs; $P_{ET}O_2$, end-tidal gas oxygen pressure; $P_{ET}CO_2$, end-tidal gas carbon dioxide pressure; HCO_3^-, blood bicarbonate; $\dot{V}O_2max$, maximum attainable oxygen consumption; HR_{max}, maximum attainable heart rate.

slow or even stopped. During exercise, increased cardiac output perfuses all capillaries to their maximum capacities, greatly increasing the surface area for diffusion. In addition, increased pulmonary vascular pressure produces a more uniform vertical distribution of pulmonary blood flow, greatly improving apical perfusion and increasing the diffusion surface area.[8]

Oxygen Cost of Work

After a steady state is reached during exercise, $\dot{V}O_2$ can be predicted from the work rate (watts) whether the exercising individual is trained or untrained, old or young, male or female.[9] The linear relationship between $\dot{V}O_2$ and work rate (Figure 23-6) has a slope of about 10 mL $\dot{V}O_2$/watt. This relationship reflects the fact that the same number of O_2 molecules is always used to generate the specific number of ATP molecules needed to produce a particular muscular contraction force. For this reason, the terms $\dot{V}O_2$ and work rate can be used interchangeably. In other words, work efficiency is relatively constant in people in steady-state exercise. Work efficiency is expressed as follows:[9]

$$\text{Efficiency} = \frac{\text{External work done / min}}{\text{Body's energy cost / min}}$$

In this calculation, the external work and energy cost of performing the work are converted to their caloric equivalents. $\dot{V}O_2$ can be converted to its caloric equivalent if the following information is known: (1) the number of calories produced when the body metabolizes 1 g of carbohydrate, fat, or protein and (2) the amount of O_2 used in the process. (Such conversions are the basis for **indirect calorimetry**, a process for determining the resting energy expenditure and caloric nutritional needs in critically ill patients.) Likewise, the work rate (watts) can be converted to caloric equivalents from its relationship with $\dot{V}O_2$. The normal work efficiency for lower extremity bicycle work is about 0.30, or 30%.[9]

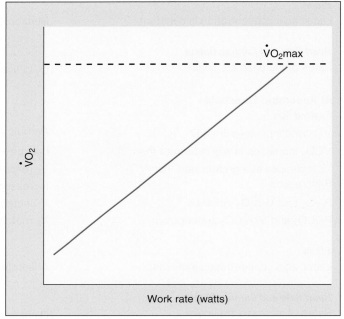

Figure 23-6 $\dot{V}O_2$ increases linearly with the work rate until $\dot{V}O_2$max is reached. $\dot{V}O_2$ can be predicted from the work rate.

In clinical practice, work is generally not measured in watts; instead, it is measured in milliliters per minute of $\dot{V}O_2$ per kilogram of body weight. The average resting $\dot{V}O_2$/kg for a 70-kg, 40-year-old man is about 3.5 mL O_2/min/kg, a value known as a **metabolic equivalent (MET)**.[4] The number of METs associated with a given level of work is calculated by first measuring the total O_2 consumed per minute and dividing by body weight (kg); the result is then divided by 3.5. For example, 35 mL O_2/min/kg is equal to 10 METs. However, estimating $\dot{V}O_2$ from the work rate is inaccurate if the exercising subject fails to reach a steady state—a state in which tissue $\dot{V}O_2$ and O_2 uptake in the lungs are equal. In addition, $\dot{V}O_2$ may not increase linearly with the work rate in patients with cardiovascular disease.

Oxygen Debt

The body cannot store much O_2. During heavy exercise of short duration, the body consumes most of the stored O_2 in the lungs, blood, and muscle fibers within about one minute, and the lungs cannot take up O_2 fast enough to meet the body's requirements; this creates an O_2 debt. The debt is repaid in the immediate recovery period as the subject hyperventilates, and the lungs take up much greater amounts of O_2 than the muscles normally require at rest. O_2 taken up during the recovery phase is used to reconstitute the high-energy ATP system and to metabolize lactic acid.[2]

Normal Exercise-Limiting Factors

Cardiac Factors

At maximal exercise, HR may triple compared with rest, and SV may double, producing a cardiac output up to six times above normal.[3,4] O_2 delivery and $\dot{V}O_2$ increase to the same degree. Nevertheless, cardiac capacity is the factor that normally limits exercise; ventilatory capacity does not limit the ability of normal, healthy people to perform work.[1,2]

Cardiac capacity is determined chiefly by the maximum attainable HR. Early in exercise, SV reaches a maximum value, whereas HR continues to increase. O_2 delivery and $\dot{V}O_2$ reach maximum limits because HR does so. Because healthy individuals can generally attain their predicted HR_{max}, the **heart rate reserve (HRR)** is normally zero during maximal exercise.[1] HRR is calculated as shown:

$$\textbf{HRR} = \textbf{Predicted HR}_{max} - \textbf{Observed HR}_{max}$$

If SV is abnormally low, HR_{max} is reached prematurely, limiting the maximum amount of O_2 that can be delivered and consumed.

A measure of the heart's efficiency in terms of O_2 delivered or consumed is the **O_2 pulse**, measured in milliliters of O_2 consumed per heart beat, as the following shows:

$$\textbf{O}_2 \textbf{ pulse} = \dot{\textbf{V}}\textbf{O}_2/\textbf{HR}$$

The O_2 pulse increases only when work rate increases, theoretically because blood flow distribution to working tissues improves, allowing for greater O_2 extraction per unit of blood. An increase in O_2 pulse is thus a marker for improved blood flow distribution.[3] Fick's equation (see Chapter 8) can be rearranged as follows to show that the O_2 pulse is equal to SV multiplied by the arterial-venous O_2 content difference:

$$\textbf{CO} \times \textbf{C(a} - \bar{\textbf{v}})\textbf{O}_2 = \dot{\textbf{V}}\textbf{O}_2$$

Substituting SV × HR for CO:

$$\textbf{SV} \times \textbf{HR} \times \textbf{C(a} - \bar{\textbf{v}})\textbf{O}_2 = \dot{\textbf{V}}\textbf{O}_2$$

Rearranging for the O_2 pulse gives the following:

$$\dot{\textbf{V}}\textbf{O}_2/\textbf{HR} = \textbf{SV} \times \textbf{C(a} - \bar{\textbf{v}})\textbf{O}_2$$

The O_2 pulse (left side of the preceding equation) increases early in exercise as SV increases. As SV peaks, increased tissue O_2 extraction (i.e., increased $C[a-\bar{v}]O_2$) accounts for further O_2 pulse increases. The O_2 pulse plateaus as HR_{max} is approached. A low SV produces a low O_2 pulse because the heart rate is high in relation to $\dot{V}O_2$.

CONCEPT QUESTION 23-5

Explain why the O_2 pulse of a sedentary, unconditioned person is lower than the O_2 pulse of a trained athlete.

Pulmonary Factors

During maximal exercise, $\dot{V}_E$ may be as high as 150 L per minute, about 25 times resting $\dot{V}_E$. The respiratory rate approximately triples, whereas the V_T increases about sixfold, up to about 60% or 70% of the vital capacity.[8] Despite these large increases, normal, healthy people still do not attain their measured maximum voluntary ventilation (MVV) during maximal exercise.[8] The **breathing reserve (BR)** is usually defined as the difference between MVV and **maximum exercise ventilation ($\dot{V}_E$max)**,[8] as the following equation shows:

$$\textbf{BR} = \textbf{MVV} - \dot{\textbf{V}}_\textbf{E}\textbf{max}$$

BR represents a theoretical potential for increasing ventilation further once the point of maximum exercise is reached. MVV (measured over 12 to 15 seconds) is normally 20% to 50% larger than the ventilation an individual attains during maximal exercise.[8,10-12] MVV is commonly estimated by multiplying the forced expiratory volume in 1 second (FEV_1) by 40 (MVV = $FEV_1 \times 40$).[13] Does this mean normal people have the potential to increase their ventilation by an additional 20% to 50% once they reach the point of maximum exercise? They probably cannot. The maximum ventilation that can be voluntarily sustained for 15 minutes or longer corresponds to 55% to 80% of the MVV in normal people.[10,12] Electromyographic studies show signs of diaphragmatic fatigue in normal people who are ventilating at greater than 70% of the MVV, a level commonly attained during maximal exercise. If $\dot{V}_E$max is compared with the maximal sustainable ventilation over the same time frame, BR is quite small, even in normal subjects. Nevertheless, BR calculated in the traditional way (MVV − $\dot{V}_E$max) is an important quantitative indicator of ventilatory reserve; it is higher in normal people and lower in people with pulmonary disease. Although respiratory muscle fatigue may occur during maximal exercise in normal subjects, it is not clear that this fatigue actually limits exercise.[10]

Some studies show that maximum ventilatory capacity may be an exercise-limiting factor in elite, world-class athletes.[13,14] Trained athletes in these studies were able to exercise at intensities beyond levels that elicited $\dot{V}O_2$max. This supramaximal exercise was predicted to require 115% of the measured $\dot{V}O_2$max. These athletes were able to sustain supramaximal exercise to the extent that they could increase their minute ventilation. In other words, although they reached their maximum cardiac capacity, these athletes were able to use their remaining ventilatory capacity to exercise further. In this sense, ventilatory capacity was the factor that determined maximal exercise intensity.

Physically Conditioned versus Physically Unconditioned

The maximum heart rates of physically fit and unfit people of the same age are the same. Physically conditioned and unconditioned people performing the same amount of work consume the same amounts of O_2 because $\dot{V}O_2$ is linearly related to the work rate regardless of conditioning, age, or gender. What then is the defining difference between physically conditioned and unconditioned people?

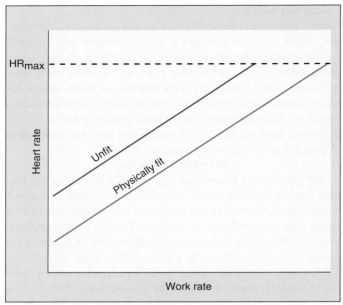

Figure 23-7 A given work rate elicits a faster heart rate in an unfit person than in a fit person. An unfit person achieves a maximum heart rate sooner and at a relatively low work rate.

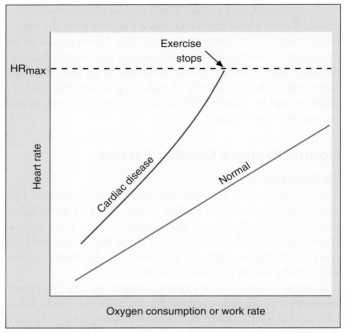

Figure 23-8 Cardiac disease limits the increase in stroke volume during exercise. Consequently, the heart rate must increase out of proportion to the increases in $\dot{V}O_2$ and the work rate in order to increase the cardiac output. (Note the nonlinear increase in the heart rate.) The maximum heart rate is reached early at a low work rate and $\dot{V}O_2$.

These differences have been mentioned in previous sections. A physically conditioned person has a much greater SV than an unconditioned person. For this reason, a physically fit person generates a much higher cardiac output during maximal exercise, although HR_{max} is the same for both people if they are the same age. This means the conditioned person delivers adequate O_2 to the muscles at a lower HR than the unconditioned person.

At a given work rate, the unconditioned individual has a higher HR than the conditioned person (Figure 23-7). Although the same amount of O_2 is required to perform the work, the lower SV of the unconditioned person requires a faster HR. During maximal exercise, determined by HR_{max}, the unconditioned person has a relatively low work output, cardiac output, oxygen-delivery rate, and $\dot{V}O_2$max. For these reasons, $\dot{V}O_2$max is an indicator of fitness. The average $\dot{V}O_2$max of an untrained 20-year-old person is about 40 to 50 mL/min/kg and that of a 60-year-old person is about 28 to 35 mL/min/kg. The $\dot{V}O_2$max of highly trained athletes is 1.5 to 1.7 times greater than that of nonathletes.[13,15]

Physical training programs raise $\dot{V}O_2$max by increasing the heart's muscle mass, SV, and cardiac output. Such cardiac hypertrophy and increased pumping effectiveness occur only with aerobic, endurance types of training, not with short, high-energy sprint types of training.[2] Training increases the amount of O_2 the muscles can extract from the blood, partly because muscle capillary density is increased and distribution of blood flow to working muscles is improved and partly because of an enhanced capacity of trained muscles to use O_2.[3] At the cellular level, trained muscles have larger and more numerous mitochondria and increased levels of aerobic enzymes; these factors combined with an increased capillary density enhance carbohydrate metabolism and ATP production.[3]

CONCEPT QUESTION 23-6

After a 12-week exercise conditioning program, your resting HR decreases from 72 beats per minute to 58 beats per minute. What is the physiological explanation?

PHYSIOLOGICAL BASIS FOR CLINICAL EXERCISE TESTING

Differentiating Cardiac and Pulmonary Causes of Exercise Intolerance

Cardiopulmonary exercise testing is widely used to distinguish between circulatory and ventilatory exercise limitations.[16] Cardiac and pulmonary defects produce their own unique kinds of abnormal test results, allowing the contribution of each system to exercise intolerance to be evaluated.

Cardiac Disease

The heart limits exercise when it fails to pump enough blood to meet the body's O_2 needs and the ventilatory reserve is not yet exhausted. Low cardiac output means either HR or SV fail to increase adequately. Most commonly, cardiac diseases limit increases in SV, causing the body to rely on a higher HR to keep pace with increasing O_2 requirements. As a result, HR rises at an ever-increasing pace in a nonlinear fashion with respect to $\dot{V}O_2$; HR is abnormally high for a given cardiac output (Figure 23-8). This produces a low O_2 pulse ($\dot{V}O_2$/HR). Because HR increases more rapidly than $\dot{V}O_2$ increases, the O_2 pulse reaches a maximum value early and plateaus (Figure 23-9). Although

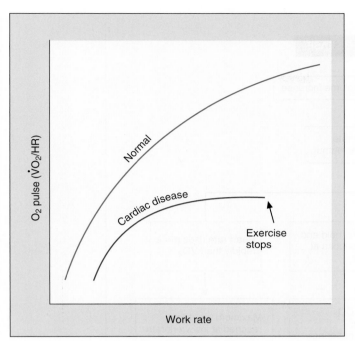

Figure 23-9 Abnormally low stroke volume in cardiac disease causes the maximum heart rate and maximum $\dot{V}O_2$ to be reached early during exercise. This produces a low O_2 pulse that plateaus early.

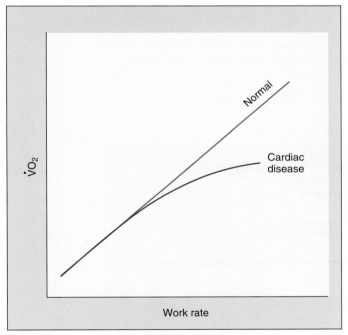

Figure 23-10 In cardiac disease, the inadequate increase in cardiac output during exercise means O_2 delivery increases inadequately, which limits the increase in $\dot{V}O_2$.

cardiac output increases during exercise, it cannot keep pace with increasing tissue O_2 needs. This inadequate increase in cardiac output means O_2 delivery increases at an inadequate rate, which limits the increase in $\dot{V}O_2$. Consequently, the relationship between $\dot{V}O_2$ and work rate is not linear, as it is in healthy people (Figure 23-10).[1]

Low cardiac output and O_2 delivery cause people to reach anaerobic threshold and generate lactic acid at low work rates. The subsequent buffering of this acid by bicarbonate increases CO_2 generation. Consequently, $\dot{V}_E$ requirements increase, and the patient develops dyspnea early in exercise. Low cardiac output also reduces pulmonary blood flow with respect to ventilation, increasing alveolar dead space and V_D/V_T. This further increases the $\dot{V}_E$ required to maintain CO_2 homeostasis. Figure 23-11 summarizes the typical consequences of exercise in a patient with cardiac disease.

Pulmonary Disease

The lungs limit exercise when they cannot provide the increased $\dot{V}_E$ required to do more work, while the cardiovascular system is still functioning below maximum capacity. In the following sections, the discussion of pulmonary problems is limited to obstructive and restrictive lung diseases.

Severe airflow obstruction greatly reduces MVV because high airway resistance slows maximum expiratory flow during rapid respiratory rates. This increased resistance prevents the lungs from emptying to normal resting levels during exercise. As a result, the lungs develop increased end expiratory volumes; this decreases inspiratory capacity (IC), further limiting ventilatory capacity.[17] MVV may be so low that it is matched or exceeded by $\dot{V}_E$max.[8] Individuals with severe obstruction reach their ventilation limits before they reach their maximum HR or predicted $\dot{V}O_2$max. In other words, they are more limited in their ability to eliminate CO_2 than in their ability to make O_2 available to the tissues. The mechanical pulmonary apparatus simply cannot move air fast enough to satisfy ventilatory demands of exercise.

Abnormal ventilatory mechanics in obstructive disease produces significant ventilation-perfusion ($\dot{V}/\dot{Q}$) mismatches. Certain lung regions are hypoventilated, whereas others are hyperventilated. In COPD, the degree to which alveolar ventilation is reduced is less than the degree to which dead space ventilation is increased, which results in a greater than normal V_D/V_T. A greater V_D/V_T decreases ventilatory efficiency, requiring a higher total $\dot{V}_E$ to maintain a normal $\dot{V}_A$ and CO_2 elimination rate. Consequently, $\dot{V}_E/\dot{V}CO_2$ and $\dot{V}_E/\dot{V}O_2$ are increased. Patients with COPD usually have a higher resting $\dot{V}_E$ than healthy people for the same metabolic rate.[18] The higher resting $\dot{V}_E$ combined with a lower MVV leaves less ventilatory reserve available to accommodate the demands of exercise. The BR (MVV − $\dot{V}_E$max) remaining at maximal exercise is often zero in patients with advanced COPD (Figure 23-12).

Because MVV depends on patient effort and motivation, it is often indirectly estimated from FEV_1. Various studies show that MVV in normal subjects and patients with COPD is accurately estimated by the following formula:[19-21]

$$\mathbf{MVV = FEV_1 \times 40}$$

If ventilatory capacity alone limits exercise, low breathing reserve and high HR reserve are expected at the point of maximal exercise. Also, a low $\dot{V}O_2$max is expected because HR_{max} is not achieved, limiting O_2 delivery. V_D/V_T remains elevated and relatively constant with increasing exercise rather than decreasing, as in normal people.[18] (This is manifested as a relatively

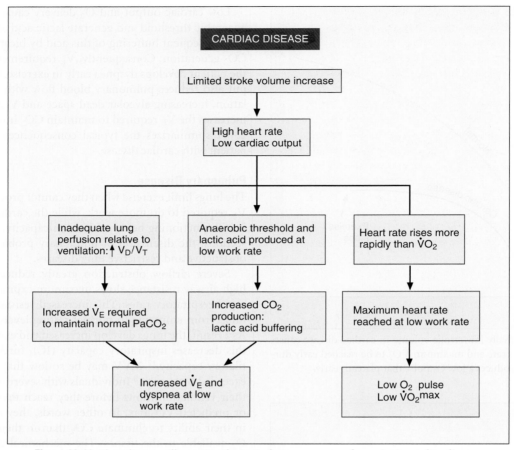

Figure 23-11 Flow diagram illustrating the typical consequences of exercise in cardiac disease.

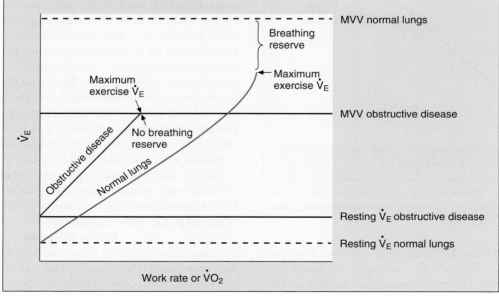

Figure 23-12 Ventilatory limitation to exercise. In lung disease, resting minute ventilation is high, and MVV is low, decreasing the ventilatory capacity. Ventilation at maximal exertion is near or equal to MVV, leaving little or no breathing reserve. Severe dyspnea stops exercise at a low work rate and submaximum heart rate. This limits $\dot{V}O_2$max.

constant difference between $PaCO_2$ and $P_{ET}CO_2$.) A patient with pulmonary limitations stops exercising because of severe dyspnea as BR approaches zero (see Figure 23-12).

During pulmonary-limited exercise, the anaerobic threshold generally occurs in the normal range, about midway between resting $\dot{V}O_2$ and predicted $\dot{V}O_2max$. However, ventilatory capacity may limit obstructed patients so severely that dyspnea prevents them from exercising to levels necessary for anaerobic metabolism.[1] Nevertheless, studies show that most patients with COPD reach the anaerobic threshold and develop metabolic acidosis during maximal exercise.[18] Abnormal lung mechanics prevent $\dot{V}_E$ from responding adequately to the subsequent decrease in pH and increase in CO_2. Consequently, acidosis worsens rapidly after anaerobic metabolism begins.

Depending on the disease severity, PaO_2 may increase, remain constant, or decrease with exercise.[18] Exercise improves $\dot{V}/\dot{Q}$ in some instances (because of improved lung perfusion), increasing the PaO_2. A decreasing PaO_2 during exercise distinguishes emphysema from chronic bronchitis. Emphysema is characterized by a destruction of the capillary vascular bed. High blood flow during exercise exceeds the alveolar capillary membrane O_2 diffusion capacity, causing PaO_2 to decrease. PaO_2 remains constant or increases with exercise in pure chronic bronchitis because the membrane surface area is not affected in this disease.

Restrictive disease such as pulmonary fibrosis is characterized by a nonuniform distribution of inflammatory scar tissue throughout the alveoli, creating alternating areas of low and normal compliance. Scar tissue may replace the capillary bed in severely involved units or merely thicken the alveolar capillary membrane. The result is a high V_D/V_T, a reduced surface area for gas exchange, impaired diffusion, and overall low lung compliance. Low lung compliance decreases all lung volumes and capacities, especially IC. The small IC limits the patient's ability to increase the V_T during exercise. Consequently, the breathing rate increases earlier in exercise and to a much greater extent than normal. As a result, the V_T/IC ratio increases and approaches 1.0. During maximal exercise in restrictive disease, the breathing rate usually exceeds 50 breaths per minute.[1] As with obstructive disease, $\dot{V}_E$ max often nearly equals MVV, reducing BR.

As exercise progresses in patients with restrictive diseases, the limited diffusion capacity leads to a decrease in PaO_2. This occurs because an increased cardiac output decreases the time that capillary blood is in contact with alveolar gas; there is not enough time for alveolar O_2 to diffuse into the capillary blood. As with obstructive disease, dyspnea usually causes the patient to stop exercising before HR_{max} is reached, lowering the $\dot{V}O_2max$. Box 23-1 summarizes exercise test abnormalities in patients who have obstructive and restrictive lung diseases.

Exercise Tests and Prescription in Cardiopulmonary Rehabilitation

Exercise is an essential component of cardiopulmonary rehabilitation programs. The major benefit of exercise in this setting is that exercise leads to decreased myocardial work (HR) for a given level of activity. Exercise test results identify appropriate

---

BOX 23-1

Typical Exercise Test Abnormalities in Pulmonary Disease

Obstructive and Restrictive Disease
Low breathing reserve
Low maximum $\dot{V}O_2$
High V_D/V_T
High heart rate reserve
Inadequate $\dot{V}_E$ response to lactic acidosis
High $(PaCO_2 - P_{ET}CO_2)$
High $P(A-a)O_2$
High $\dot{V}_E/\dot{V}CO_2$ and $\dot{V}_E/\dot{V}O_2$

Restrictive Disease
High V_T/IC ratio
Breathing rate >50 breaths/min during maximal exercise
Systematic decreases in PaO_2 and increases in $P(A-a)O_2$ as work rate increases

$\dot{V}O_2$, Oxygen consumption per minute; V_D/V_T, dead space-to-tidal volume ratio; $\dot{V}_E$, minute ventilation; P_ACO_2, alveolar carbon dioxide pressure; $P_{ET}CO_2$, end-tidal gas carbon dioxide pressure; $P(A-a)O_2$, alveolar-arterial oxygen pressure difference; $\dot{V}CO_2$, carbon dioxide production per minute; V_T, tidal volume; IC, inspiratory capacity; PaO_2, arterial oxygen pressure.

---

training heart rates. Patients can then monitor their own HR and choose appropriate exercise intensities.

Depending on the factor that limits exercise, patients may benefit from endurance training, controlled breathing and relaxation exercises, and exercises while breathing supplemental O_2.[22] For endurance training such as walking or bicycling, exercise intensity should be high enough to produce a HR greater than 60% but less than 80% of the predicted HR_{max}. About 30 minutes of exercise at this intensity every other day is needed to achieve the classic training effect (i.e., decreased HR for a given submaximal workload). The Karvonen equation is commonly used to compute a target HR range for endurance training in cardiac patients; this method adds from 45% to 85% of the difference between HR_{max} and resting HR to the resting heart rate as follows:[23]

Target HR range = 0.45 to 0.85 $(HR_{max} - HR_{rest}) + HR_{rest}$

Exercise testing is valuable for assessing the effectiveness of cardiopulmonary rehabilitation programs; initial test results establish a physiological baseline that can be compared with test results obtained after a rehabilitation program is completed. Such comparative quantitative data objectively demonstrates patient outcome and progress, which helps justify the medical necessity of rehabilitation programs to third-party payers such as Medicare and private insurance companies.

For example, if the resting HR is 60 beats per minute and HR_{max} obtained during an exercise stress test is 130 beats per minute, the difference is 70 beats per minute ($130 - 60 = 70$). This difference is then multiplied by 0.45 and 0.85 and added to the resting HR to define the target HR range:

$0.45 (70) = 32 + 60 = 92$
$0.85 (70) = 60 + 60 = 120$

Target HR range for endurance training is 92 to 120 beats per minute.

CLINICAL FOCUS 23-2

Origin of Exercise Limitation

Case 1

A 58-year-old woman with a history of cigarette smoking undergoes an exercise test to evaluate dyspnea on exertion. She weighs 70 kg. Pulmonary function tests reveal moderate airway obstruction and MVV of 42 L per minute. ECGs show no ischemic abnormalities. Treadmill exercise test data are obtained and show the following:

	At Rest	0% Grade—1.7 mph	5% Grade—1.7 mph	10% Grade—1.7 mph	12% Grade—2.5 mph
$\dot{V}O_2$ (mL/min)	340	825	985	1130	1372
$\dot{V}CO_2$ (mL/min)	295	660	808	949	1180
$\dot{V}_E$(L/min)	10	27	33	38	40
P(A-a)O_2 (mm Hg)	16	13	12	19	21
HR (beats/min)	75	96	100	113	120

Further measurements were not made because the patient became severely dyspneic and could not continue exercising. Did this patient achieve the anaerobic threshold or the maximum heart rate, or both? Did cardiac or pulmonary factors limit exercise?

Discussion

The AT marks the onset of lactic acid production. The subsequent decrease in pH is normally expected to stimulate ventilation, causing $\dot{V}_E$ to increase more rapidly than $\dot{V}CO_2$. Also, $\dot{V}CO_2$ is expected to increase more rapidly than $\dot{V}O_2$ at AT. Examination of the data indicates this did not happen; $\dot{V}CO_2$ and $\dot{V}_E$ increased fourfold, and RQ did not rise above 1.0. (In the last stage, RQ = 1180 ÷ 1372, which equals 0.86.) Therefore, the anaerobic threshold apparently was not reached.

This patient's maximum predicted heart rate is as follows: 220 – 58 = 162 beats/min. A significant HRR exists at maximal exercise capacity. Normally, HRR is about zero during maximal exercise. Conversely, little BR exists during maximal exercise; $\dot{V}_E$ max is about 95% of MVV (40 ÷ 42 = 0.95), leaving a BR of 5%. Normally, a BR between 20% and 50% of MVV exists during maximal exercise. This patient's exercise is limited by pulmonary, not cardiac, factors. The following factors support this conclusion: (1) failure to reach the anaerobic threshold, (2) large HRR, and (3) extremely small BR. The appropriate increase in the heart rate and O_2 pulse ($\dot{V}O_2$/HR) during exercise rules out cardiac limitation. This woman's complaint of dyspnea on exertion must be related to pulmonary disease.

Case 2

A 60-year-old man with a history of smoking undergoes an exercise test to evaluate dyspnea and substernal chest pain on exertion. A resting 12-lead ECG reveals no abnormalities. Pulmonary function tests show a mildly obstructive pattern. MVV is 130 L per minute. The patient exercises on a bicycle ergometer for about 3 minutes, with no added workload. The workload is then gradually increased in 1-minute increments. The patient stops exercising after 7 minutes because of chest pains. ST segment depression occurs on the ECG in the last 2 minutes of exercise. The following results are obtained during maximal exercise:

	Predicted	Measured
$\dot{V}O_2$max (mL/min)	2250	1485
HR$_{max}$ (beats/min)	160	149
$\dot{V}O_2$ at AT (mL/min)	>900	550
$\dot{V}_E$max (L/min)	—	91

Following are resting versus maximal exercise data:

	Resting	Maximal Exercise
PaO$_2$ (mm Hg)	85	113
P(A-a)O_2 (mm Hg)	16	9

Is cardiac disease or pulmonary disease responsible for this patient's exertional dyspnea and exercise limitation?

Discussion

Data relevant to cardiac (see Figure 23-11) and pulmonary function (see Box 23-1) are as follows:

Cardiac

HR$_{max}$ = 92% of predicted: 149/160 = 0.92
$\dot{V}O_2$max = 66% of predicted: 1485/2250 = 0.66
Predicted O_2 pulse = 2250/160 = 13.9 mL O_2/beat
Actual O_2 pulse = 1485/149 = 9.97 mL O_2/beat
Anaerobic threshold at $\dot{V}O_2$ = 550 mL/min (37% of $\dot{V}O_2$max)
Heart rate reserve = 8%

Pulmonary

$\dot{V}_E$max = 70% of MVV: 91/130 = 0.7 (BR = 30%)
PaO$_2$ increased with exercise
P(A-a)O_2 decreased with exercise

CLINICAL FOCUS 23-2

Origin of Exercise Limitation—cont'd

Evidence for a low SV includes the following: (1) predicted HR_{max} almost reached early in exercise at a low $\dot{V}O_2max$ and (2) O_2 pulse lower than predicted. Achieving the anaerobic threshold at only 37% of the measured $\dot{V}O_2max$ means O_2 delivery to the muscles is too low to meet the workload's requirement. ST segment depression indicates myocardial ischemia, which further decreases contractility and SV.

Conversely, $\dot{V}_E$ max is only 70% of MVV. Considerable potential exists for increasing $\dot{V}_E$ further during maximal exercise. The increasing PaO_2 and decreasing $P(A-a)O_2$ mean that $\dot{V}/\dot{Q}$ improves with exercise (a normal phenomenon).

The combined evidence suggests an oxygen-delivery problem not related to lung function. In other words, inappropriately low cardiac output causes anaerobic metabolism and lactic acid production at low work rates. Lactic acid increases the $\dot{V}_E$ requirement, accounting for the exertional dyspnea. Normal BR and normal response of PaO_2 and $P(A-a)O_2$ to exercise confirm the absence of pulmonary limitation.

It is more accurate to use the actual HR_{max} obtained from an exercise test rather than the predicted HR_{max}.[23] An alternative, even more accurate method (recommended for both cardiac patients and healthy adults) is based on oxygen consumption reserve ($\dot{V}O_2R$), which is the difference between $\dot{V}O_2max$ measured during a stress test and the resting O_2 consumption:[23]

$$\dot{V}O_2R = \dot{V}O_2max - \dot{V}O_2rest$$

The target training $\dot{V}O_2$ range is determined by adding 45% to 85% of the $\dot{V}O_2R$ to the $\dot{V}O_2rest$. $\dot{V}O_2$ is a measure of workload, as discussed earlier, and can be expressed in terms of METs. METs associated with workloads have been estimated for various exercise modalities, which facilitates the exercise prescription process.

Because people with severe ventilatory limitations may be unable to exercise at intensities required to reach the anaerobic threshold, one might question whether exercise can improve cardiovascular fitness. However, studies of endurance training in patients with varying degrees of ventilatory impairment show improved endurance in all patients, regardless of pulmonary disease severity.[24] All patients can experience cardiovascular benefits from cardiopulmonary rehabilitation programs, regardless of lung function. Conversely, habitual aerobic exercise in older, fit adults does not slow the normal functional decline in the aging lung. A study of highly fit adults 67 to 73 years of age revealed normal deterioration rates in $\dot{V}O_2max$ and pulmonary mechanics.[25]

POINTS TO REMEMBER

- The source of energy for skeletal muscle activity is ATP, which must be continually regenerated.
- Ventilation and blood flow supply adequate O_2 for aerobic synthesis of ATP until the demands of heavy exercise exceed the oxygen-delivery capacity of the cardiovascular system, after which anaerobic metabolism supplements aerobic ATP generation.
- Maximum ventilation capacity never limits exercise capacity in healthy individuals; exercise is normally limited by maximum cardiac output capacity, which is limited by the maximum achievable HR.

- Breathing reserve is defined as the difference between the measured MVV and the ventilation achieved in maximal exercise.
- The ventilation achieved in maximal exercise is normally about 70% of the MVV; breathing reserve is normally about 30%.
- HRR is defined as the difference between predicted HR_{max} and HR achieved in maximal exercise.
- HR achieved in maximal exercise is normally about 100% of the predicted HR_{max}; thus, HRR is normally about 0%.
- Conditioned and unconditioned healthy individuals of the same age have the same HR_{max}, but a conditioned individual has a much greater cardiac SV and thus a much greater maximal cardiac output and exercise capacity.
- Pulmonary limitation to exercise is characterized by achievement of MVV while HR is still below its predicted maximum.
- Cardiac limitation to exercise is characterized by a nonlinear relationship between HR increase and $\dot{V}O_2$ increase such that the predicted HR_{max} is attained prematurely.
- Anaerobic threshold is marked by a sharper increase in CO_2 production and ventilation due to bicarbonate buffering of lactic acid.

References

1. Wasserman K, et al: *Principles of exercise testing and interpretation: including pathophysiology and clinical applications*, Philadelphia, 2004, Lippincott Williams & Wilkins.
2. Hall JE: *Guyton and Hall textbook of medical physiology*, ed 12, Philadelphia, 2011, Saunders.
3. Sietsema KE: Clinical exercise testing. In Mason RJ, et al, editors: *Murray and Nadel's textbook of respiratory medicine*, ed 5, Philadelphia, 2010, Saunders.
4. Chaitman BR: Exercise stress testing. In Bonow RO, et al, editors: *Braunwald's heart disease: a textbook of cardiovascular medicine*, ed 9, Philadelphia, 2011, Saunders.
5. Clark AL, Piepoli M, Coats AJ: Skeletal muscle and the control of ventilation on exercise: evidence for metabolic receptors, *Eur J Clin Invest* 25(5):299, 1995.
6. Poon CS, Tin C, Yu Y: Homeostasis of exercise hyperpnea and optimal sensorimotor integration: the internal model paradigm, *Respir Physiol Neurobiol* 159(1):1, 2007.

7. Gozal D, et al: Ventilatory responses to passive leg motion in children with congenital central hypoventilation syndrome, *Am J Respir Crit Care Med* 153(2):761, 1996.

8. Truwit J: Pulmonary disorders and exercise, *Clin Sports Med* 22(1):161, 2003.

9. Whipp BJ: The bioenergetic and gas exchange basis of exercise testing, *Clin Chest Med* 15(2):173, 1994.

10. Fitting JW: Respiratory muscle fatigue limiting physical exercise? *Eur Respir J* 4(1):103, 1991.

11. Pierce AK, et al: Exercise ventilatory patterns in normal subjects and patients with airway obstruction, *J Appl Physiol* 25(3):249, 1968.

12. Freedman S: Sustained maximum voluntary ventilation, *Respir Physiol* 8(2):230, 1970.

13. Booher MA, Smith BW: Physiological effects of exercise on the cardiopulmonary system, *Clin Sports Med* 22(1):1, 2003.

14. Norton KI, et al: Exercise stimulus increases ventilation from maximal to supramaximal intensity, *Eur J Appl Physiol Occup Physiol* 70:115, 1995.

15. Cerretelli P, Prampero PE: Gas exchange in exercise. In Farhi LE, Tenney SM, editors: *Handbook of physiology: the respiratory system*, vol IV, Washington, DC, 1987, American Physiological Society.

16. Palange P, et al: Cardiopulmonary exercise testing in the evaluation of patients with ventilatory vs circulatory causes of reduced exercise tolerance, *Chest* 105(4):1122, 1994.

17. Babb TG, et al: Effect of mild-to-moderate airflow limitation on exercise capacity, *J Appl Physiol* 70(1):223, 1991.

18. Gallagher CG: Exercise limitation and clinical exercise testing in chronic obstructive pulmonary disease, *Clin Chest Med* 15:305, 1994.

19. Miller WF, Johnson RL, Wu N: Relationships between maximal breathing capacity and timed expiratory capacities, *J Appl Physiol* 14:510, 1959.

20. Miller WF, Scacci R: Pulmonary function assessment for determination of pulmonary impairment and disability evaluation, *Clin Chest Med* 2(3):327, 1981.

21. Dillard TA, Hnatink OW, McCumber TR: Maximum voluntary ventilation: spirometric determinants in chronic obstructive pulmonary disease patients and normal subjects, *Am Rev Respir Dis* 147(4):870, 1993.

22. Folgering H, von Herwaarden C: Exercise limitations in patients with pulmonary diseases, *Int J Sports Med* 15(3):107, 1994.

23. Womack L: Cardiac rehabilitation secondary prevention programs, *Clin Sports Med* 22(1):135, 2003.

24. Frankel JE, et al: Exercise in the elderly: research and clinical practice, *Clin Geriatr Med* 22(2):239, 2006.

25. McClaran SR, et al: Longitudinal effects of aging on lung function at rest and exercise in healthy active fit elderly adults, *J Appl Physiol* 78(5):1995, 1957.

CHAPTER 24

Effects of Aging on the Cardiopulmonary System

OBJECTIVES

After reading this chapter you will be able to:

- Explain why health care of elderly people has taken on increasingly greater importance in the twenty-first century
- Explain why older people are more prone to falls and how this phenomenon is related to pulmonary health
- Explain why elderly people are more predisposed to infections than younger people
- Describe the nature of major age-related physiological changes of the respiratory and cardiovascular systems

- Describe the nature of the body's compensatory responses to age-related cardiopulmonary changes
- Explain why the PaO_2 of a healthy elderly person is lower than the PaO_2 of a younger person when both individuals are breathing room air
- Explain why an elderly person has a lower maximum cardiac output and oxygen consumption during exercise than a younger person
- Explain the major benefits of an exercise program for elderly individuals

KEY TERMS

baby boomers
kyphoscoliosis

senile emphysema

IMPLICATIONS OF AN AGING POPULATION

People are increasingly surviving to older ages than they did in previous generations, owing to modern advances in medicine that affect old age mortality and because of improved diet and exercise habits. In addition, with the aging of **baby boomers** (individuals born in the post World War II era, generally between 1946 and 1964), increasingly greater numbers of people in the United States are entering the 65 years and older age bracket. According to the U.S. Census Bureau, the elderly population (≥65 years old) increased more than 10-fold between 1900 and 2000 (from 3.1 million to 35 million), whereas the general population only tripled in the same time span.[1] Elderly people account for about 12% of the U.S. population. In 1900, the median age (half of the population younger and half older) was 23 years; in 2000, the median age was 35 years. The elderly population as a whole is aging; the fastest growing age group

in the United States as well as the world is the oldest-old—80 years old and older.[1,2] It is predicted that by 2050, the number of people in the world 60 years old or older will exceed, for the first time in history, the number of people younger than age 15.[2]

The aging population has significantly influenced the focus of health care.[3] Health of older people typically worsens with increasing age because of increased vulnerability to accidents and disease. The demand for long-term health care facilities and home-based health care is ever increasing.

The clinician must be able to distinguish between the effects of normal aging and the effects of disease to treat elderly patients effectively; effects of aging and disease are often combined. It is difficult to sort and assess the subtle effects of other factors such as smoking history, environmental pollution, and physical activity. Separating the effects of normal aging from the effects of disease is complicated because age increases susceptibility to disease. Increased propensity for developing disease, especially more severe disease, is the most important physiological change of aging.[3] The lung function of a healthy 70-year-old is about half that of a 30-year-old; renal function declines by about the same amount. Although decreased reserve capacity does not affect activities of daily living, it greatly affects the ability of older people to recover from severe illnesses.[3]

Neuromuscular systems that maintain upright posture become less effective with age; this leads to postural instability and a predisposition to falls, which are more likely to produce fractures because of bone mass loss and greater bone fragility.[3] Danger of falling is exacerbated by sensory impairments such as poor eyesight, hearing loss, and balance disorders. In addition, loss of muscular mass and strength, arthritis, orthopedic problems, blood pressure instability, and medications contribute to the tendency to fall. Bone fractures lead to immobility, and when combined with an impaired gag reflex and a less effective mucociliary clearance mechanism, the susceptibility to respiratory infection and pneumonia increases.[3]

CONCEPT QUESTION 24-1

Why would decreased mobility subsequent to a fall and bone fracture increase an elderly person's risk for developing pneumonia?

Effects of Aging on the Respiratory System

Structural Changes

Aging changes the compliance of the lungs and chest wall. The chest wall progressively stiffens as the thoracic cage joints and attachments calcify and become less mobile.[3,4] With advancing age, vertebral column deformities produce some degree of **kyphoscoliosis** (abnormal front-to-back and side-to-side curvature of the spine).[5] Simultaneously, intercostal and diaphragmatic muscles atrophy, losing strength and endurance. These changes combine to decrease upper and lower rib cage and abdominal expansion.[5,6]

In contrast to the chest wall, the lung becomes more compliant with age as it loses elastic tissue and recoil force. As a result, the chest wall expands slightly, which mildly increases lung volumes at end-tidal exhalation (functional residual capacity [FRC]) and at maximal effort exhalation (residual volume [RV]). These changes lead to slight hyperinflation and a mildly increased anterior-posterior chest diameter (barrel chest).[3,4]

CONCEPT QUESTION 24-2

Why does increased lung compliance as a result of aging lead to a barrel chest shape?

Loss of elastic recoil forces also allows small noncartilaginous airways to remain at larger diameters after normal expiration, increasing the anatomical dead space volume and the dead space-to-tidal volume ratio (V_D/V_T); in addition, alveolar ducts and alveoli become wider, shallower, and less complex in shape, resulting in a marked decrease in gas-exchange surface area.[4] These changes are suggestive of emphysema—hence the misleading term **senile emphysema.** Anatomical changes are much more extensive and debilitating in clinically significant pulmonary emphysema than they are in the healthy aged lung.

Functional Changes

Table 24-1 summarizes functional respiratory changes with aging. Loss of elastic tissue with subsequent loss of alveolar complexity decreases gas-exchange surface area and diffusion capacity. Small noncartilaginous airways become more prone to compression and collapse during forced expiration as they lose the tethering effect of surrounding elastic fibers. This tendency toward collapse decreases maximum expiratory flow rates, especially in effort-independent portions of the forced vital capacity (FVC). Expiratory flow limitation is the most consistent effect of aging during moderate and heavy exercise.[4] As the lung ages, total lung capacity remains relatively constant, while residual volume increases; this causes vital capacity to decrease by about 30 mL per year after age 30 years.[7]

The volume expired in the first second of the FVC (forced expiratory volume in 1 second [FEV_1]) decreases progressively and linearly with age, paralleling the decline in FVC so that FEV_1/FVC changes only to a small degree in a healthy elderly person.[4,8] FEV_1 decreases about 30 mL per year after age 25 years.[5] Apparently, habitual physical exercise and high aerobic capacity do not slow this normal deterioration in lung function[9]; however, cigarette smoking accelerates it. Smoking cessation brings the rate of FEV_1 decline back to a more normal rate.[10]

In a clinical study comparing three healthy older age groups, maximal rib cage expansion, abdominal expansion, FVC, and FEV_1 were measured in subjects (1) 75 to 79 years old, (2) 80 to 84 years old, and (3) 85 years old and older.[5] Significant decreases in all measurements were noted between groups 1 and 2 and groups 1 and 3, but there were no differences between the two oldest groups, groups 2 and 3. The investigators attributed this finding to a "survival effect." In other words, very old age eliminates weaker elements of the population, and further deterioration over time does not occur rapidly. The same study found a significant correlation between expansion parameters (e.g., upper rib cage, lower rib cage, and abdominal expansion) and FVC and FEV_1. The authors concluded that a decrease in thoracic and abdominal expansion ability may be a simple but reliable index of ventilatory impairment and respiratory weakness in elderly persons.[5]

A different study showed that airway hyperresponsiveness to methacholine (a parasympathetic drug that elicits bronchospasm) may be linked to accelerated pulmonary function decline in middle-aged and older men.[11] In this study, responsiveness to inhaled methacholine was a significant predictor of the FEV_1 decline rate. Drugs that reduce nonspecific airway hyperresponsiveness, such as inhaled corticosteroids, may slow the progression of deteriorating lung function in older patients who have hyperreactive airways.[11]

The tendency for small airways to collapse during expiration leads to an increase in the closing volume (i.e., the lung volume at which small airways in gravity-dependent lung regions close [see Chapter 3]).[4] At about 65 years of age, the closing capacity (closing volume plus RV) equals FRC in seated subjects. This

TABLE 24-1

Changes in Respiratory Function with Aging

Function	Mechanism	Clinical Manifestation
Mechanics of ventilation	Loss of lung elastic recoil; decreased chest wall compliance	↓ VC; ↑ RV; no change in TLC; ↓ expiratory flow rates
	Decreased respiratory muscle mass and strength	↓ Maximal inspiratory and expiratory force
Perfusion, ventilation, and gas exchange	Decreased uniformity of ventilation with small airway closure during tidal breathing, especially in the supine position; ↓ cardiac output; ↓ $C\bar{v}O_2$	↑ $P(A\text{-}a)O_2$; ↓ PaO_2; no change in $PaCO_2$ or pH
	Increased physiological dead space	None (slightly ↑ $\dot{V}_E$)
	Decreased alveolar surface area	↓ D_LCO
Exercise capacity	Decreased aerobic work capacity of skeletal muscle; deconditioning	↓ Maximum $\dot{V}O_2$
	Decreased efficiency of ventilation	↑ $\dot{V}_E/\dot{V}O_2$
Regulation of ventilation	Decreased responsiveness of central and peripheral chemoreceptors	↓ $\dot{V}_E$ and $P_{0.1}$ responses to hypoxia and hypercapnia
Sleep and breathing	Decreased ventilatory drive	↑ Frequency of apneas, hypopneas, and desaturation episodes during sleep
	Decreased upper airway muscle tone	Snoring; ↑ incidence of obstructive sleep apnea
	Decreased arousal and cough reflexes	↑ Susceptibility to aspiration and pneumonia
Lung defense mechanisms	Decreased upper airway function; decreased mucociliary clearance	↑ Susceptibility to aspiration and pneumonia
	Decreased humoral and cellular immunity	↑ Susceptibility to infection; ↓ clinical response to infection

Modified from Pierson DJ, Kacmarek RM: *Foundations of respiratory care,* New York, 1992, Churchill Livingstone.
VC, Vital capacity; *RV,* residual volume; *TLC,* total lung capacity; *P(A-a)O_2,* alveolar-arterial PO_2 difference; *PaO_2,* arterial oxygen pressure; *PaCO_2,* arterial carbon dioxide pressure; *pH,* measure of blood H⁺ concentration; *C̄vO_2,* mixed venous oxygen content; *V̇_E,* expired minute ventilation; *D_LCO,* diffusing capacity for carbon monoxide; *V̇O_2,* oxygen consumption; *P_{0.1},* mouth occlusion pressure.

means that during tidal ventilation, some small airways close at end-expiration, and the alveoli they supply are not ventilated continuously. Thus, at rest, older people ventilate their upper lung regions more than their lower lung regions; this is the opposite of the lung's blood flow distribution. The resulting low $\dot{V}/\dot{Q}$ ratio in the lung bases leads to arterial hypoxemia and an increased $P(A\text{-}a)O_2$ (see Table 24-1). This $\dot{V}/\dot{Q}$ mismatch is the major mechanism whereby PaO_2 declines with age.[7,8] During exercise, however, increased tidal volumes improve $\dot{V}/\dot{Q}$ ratios of lung bases, which elevates PaO_2 and decreases $P(A\text{-}a)O_2$.[8]

CONCEPT QUESTION 24-3

By what mechanism would exercise improve the $\dot{V}/\dot{Q}$ ratio of the lung bases in an elderly individual?

The overall deterioration of ventilation mechanics with age can decrease maximum voluntary ventilation and maximum achievable ventilation during heavy exercise by as much as 40% (see Table 24-1).[3] Inefficient gas exchange, as manifested by an increased V_D/V_T ratio, increases the ventilation required for each 1 L of oxygen consumption ($\dot{V}_E/\dot{V}O_2$).[4] However, age decreases the maximum oxygen consumption during peak exercise mainly because the skeletal muscle mass is reduced,

not because ventilatory or cardiac abnormalities exist.[12] Despite decreased respiratory function in elderly persons, exercise is still limited by the heart's maximum pumping capacity; only in habitually active elderly subjects who achieve high oxygen consumption does the respiratory system likely place some degree of limitation on exercise capacity.[4]

The ventilatory response to hypercapnia and hypoxia decreases by as much as 50% in subjects 64 years old and older.[8] This decreased responsiveness may impair the ability of older people to accommodate the effects of acute or chronic pulmonary disease.

Aging is associated with a significantly increased risk of community-acquired pneumonia and influenza.[3] Overall immune competence decreases with age (see Table 24-1). Although a healthy elderly individual can mount immune responses, they are not as robust and enduring as in a younger person.[3] The increased incidence of cancer in older people is further evidence of a weakened immune system.[13] However, decreased immune function is probably responsible for the decreased incidence of autoimmune diseases in elderly individuals.[3]

CONCEPT QUESTION 24-4

Predict the effectiveness of vaccines in older people.

CLINICAL FOCUS 24-1

An 85-year-old man is recovering from cardiopulmonary bypass surgery. He was successfully removed from the ventilator 5 days ago with no difficulty and is out of the intensive care unit and on the general floor of the hospital. He has been on oxygen at a rate of 2 L per minute via nasal cannula, and he is now undergoing a room air breathing trial. Pulse oximeter indicates 90% saturation breathing room air. You tell the attending physician that this corresponds with PaO_2 of about 60 mm Hg. The physician believes that this indicates marginal oxygenation ability, but you believe oxygenation is acceptable, given the age of the patient. Are you correct?

Discussion

For reasons discussed in this chapter, PaO_2 normally declines with age. However, proposed prediction equations for computing PaO_2 as a function of age vary widely; for example, for an 85-year-old man, predicted values range from 63 to 84 mm Hg.[22] Some studies showed that the decrease in PaO_2 with age is not linear; there is a steady decline up to age 70 to 74, but PaO_2 then increases slightly between ages 75 and 90.[22] At any rate, a room air PaO_2 of 60 mm Hg for an 85-year-old man is not grossly abnormal.

Airway clearance mechanisms are less effective in older patients (see Table 24-1). Impaired respiratory mechanics and weakened respiratory muscles decrease cough effectiveness. Even in healthy older people, mucociliary clearance rates are slowed. In addition, inflammatory responses and humoral and cell-mediated immunity decrease with age.[3] All of these factors place elderly persons at greater risk for developing pneumonia with any respiratory illnesses.

Effects of Aging on the Cardiovascular System

Box 24-1 outlines age-related changes in cardiovascular structure and function. Distinguishing between the normal effects of aging and cardiac disease (quite common in older people) is difficult.

Structural Changes

Age changes heart muscle, valvular, and vascular structures (see Box 24-1). Heart mass, primarily the left ventricle, increases gradually between 25 and 80 years of age, even in people free of cardiovascular disease or hypertension.[14] This gradual hypertrophy is probably caused by the increased afterload imposed by increasing arterial wall stiffness. In addition, increased collagen deposition in the heart muscle stiffens the ventricles, making them less distensible during diastolic filling.[3,14,15]

With age, the heart valve leaflets thicken and calcify (see Box 24-1). Mitral and aortic valves are most commonly affected; mitral valve calcification is particularly common in older

BOX 24-1

Age-Related Changes in Cardiovascular Structure and Function

Structure
Myocardial
Increased mass
Increased LV wall thickness
Increased collagen connective tissue

Valvular
Increased aortic and mitral valve thickness
Increased circumference of all valves
Calcification of valve leaflets

Arterial
Increased wall thickness
Increased collagen content

Function
Heart Rate
Slightly decreased resting heart rate
Decreased maximum heart rate in exercise
Degeneration of sinus node
Decreased sinus node intrinsic rate

LV Systolic
Essentially unchanged maximal cardiac output
Increased stroke volume index
Prolonged duration of ventricular contraction

LV Diastolic
Decreased ventricular compliance
Slowed rate of ventricular relaxation
Decreased early diastolic filling rate
Increased dependence on atrial contraction for diastolic filling
Higher diastolic filling pressure

Cardiac Fiber
Unchanged peak contractile force
Greater dependence on Starling mechanism for contractile force during exercise
Reduced removal of intracellular Ca^{++} after contraction
Decreased responsiveness to beta-adrenergic stimulation

Vascular
Decreased compliance
Increased pulse pressure
Increased vascular resistance

Modified from Duncan AK, et al: Cardiovascular disease in elderly patients, *Mayo Clin Proc* 71:184, 1996.
LV, Left ventricle.

women.[14] Calcification may cause mild mitral valve regurgitation (backflow) during systole, increasing atrial size and the incidence of atrial fibrillation and conduction defects.[14] Atrial fibrillation is the most prevalent arrhythmia of elderly patients, occurring in approximately one third of older patients undergoing surgery.[3]

CONCEPT QUESTION 24-5

Why does increased atrial size in an elderly person predispose to the development of atrial fibrillation?

Age thickens the inner layer of arterial walls and increases their collagen content. In the process, the arteries stiffen, and systolic pressure increases.[3] This change increases the pulse pressure.[16]

Functional Changes

Box 24-1 outlines age-related changes in myocardial function. The most important physiological change is the delay in ventricular filling, which can decline by 50% at age 80.[3] Ventricular filling becomes much more dependent on atrial contraction, primarily because the left ventricular wall becomes thickened and stiffened. Systolic function is normally preserved.

The resting heart rate is only slightly reduced, in contrast to a more markedly reduced maximum achievable heart rate during exercise. These reductions are caused by loss of sinus node pacemaker cells (approaching 90% by age 80)[3] and by decreased myocardial responsiveness to beta-adrenergic stimulation.[12,17]

The combination of reduced ventricular filling and a slower heart rate contributes to postural hypotension, which is common in 20% of elderly individuals.[3] This phenomenon also contributes to instability and falls by making an individual susceptible to fainting. Generally, the cardiovascular system of an elderly person has a decreased capacity to adjust to position changes to maintain a constant blood pressure. Elderly people are especially prone to postural hypotension after large meals and during any volume-depleting stress, such as diarrhea or diuretic therapy.[3] Volume depletion or dehydration is a very common disorder in frail elderly individuals because of decreased fluid intake.

CONCEPT QUESTION 24-6

Why would a frail elderly individual have a tendency to decrease fluid intake and develop dehydration?

Although vascular resistance increases with age, two mechanisms maintain an appropriate cardiac output at rest and during exercise: (1) compensatory left ventricular hypertrophy and (2) more vigorous atrial contraction, which increases ventricular filling pressure.[12,18] Enhanced atrial activity increases the end-diastolic volume, ensuring an adequate stroke volume.[19] The stroke volume index increases during exercise because cardiac output is sustained at a lower maximum heart rate, although at higher filling pressures.

Two factors probably contribute to the age-related slowing of ventricular filling during the early diastolic phase (see Box 24-1): (1) decreased ventricular compliance and (2) impaired ventricular relaxation after systole.[15] The latter involves interference with the actin-myosin inactivation process. Age impairs the ability of the sarcoplasmic reticulum to take up Ca^{++} ions from the muscle fiber after contraction. The result is intracellular Ca^{++} overload, leading to impaired diastolic relaxation.[15] Studies have shown that calcium channel–blocking drugs improve left ventricular diastolic filling in older subjects without hindering systolic function.[14,15]

CONCEPT QUESTION 24-7

Explain the mechanism whereby calcium channel–blocking drugs might improve ventricular diastolic filling.

Although healthy older people have lower maximum heart rates, they increase their cardiac outputs appropriately during exercise by increasing the preload and thus, stroke volume. To accomplish this, older people rely more heavily on atrial contraction. The major age-related impairments are (1) increased vascular resistance, (2) reduced response to beta-adrenergic stimulation, and (3) hampered ventricular relaxation. The body's major adaptations are (1) left ventricular hypertrophy and (2) increased atrial contribution to diastolic filling. The maximum oxygen consumption is reduced in fit, older people mainly because of decreased skeletal muscle mass.[12,16] Well-designed exercise programs of low to moderate intensity are extremely important in maintaining muscle mass and physical function in older people. Regardless of functional limitations, exercise programs can improve flexibility, strength, muscle mass, and mobility in older people; exercise also promotes psychological well-being and is about as effective as antidepressants in treating depression in elderly persons.[20,21] A simple walking program is a safe, effective activity for many older people.

POINTS TO REMEMBER

- Elderly people represent a greater proportion of the general population than ever before.
- Age decreases immune competence and the effectiveness of lung clearance mechanisms and increases susceptibility to pneumonia.
- A major concern in elderly people is postural instability and falls that result in bone fractures, immobility, and subsequent pulmonary complications.
- Advancing age reduces ventilatory capacity in healthy people primarily by altering lung and chest wall structures.
- Despite reduced ventilatory capacity in elderly people, ventilation does not limit exercise in healthy older people.
- A major cardiac change in aging is delayed ventricular filling secondary to decreased ventricular compliance, resulting in greater dependence on active atrial contraction to fill the ventricles.
- Age-related impairments to cardiac function include increased vascular resistance, reduced myocardial responsiveness to beta-adrenergic stimulation, and delayed ventricular relaxation.

- The body compensates for age-related cardiac impairments by increasing left ventricular muscle mass and increasing atrial contraction strength.
- Cardiac output and maximum oxygen consumption are lower in elderly persons than in younger persons primarily because the oxygen-consuming muscle mass is reduced.

References

1. Hobbs F, Stoops N: *Demographic trends in the 20th century, U.S. Census Bureau, Census 2000 Special Reports, Series CENSR-4,* Washington, DC, 2002, US Government Printing Office.
2. United Nations Department of Economic and Social Affairs, Population Division: *World population ageing: 1950-2050 (ST/ ESA/ SER.A/207),* New York, 2002, United Nations Publications.
3. Minaker KL: Common clinical sequelae of aging. In Goldman L, Schafer AI, editors: *Goldman's Cecil medicine,* ed 24, Philadelphia, 2012, Saunders.
4. Lovering AT, Haverkamp HC, Eldridge MW: Responses and limitations of the respiratory system to exercise, *Clin Chest Med* 26(3):439, 2005.
5. Pfitzenmeyer P, et al: Lung function in advanced age: study of ambulatory subjects aged over 75 years, *Gerontology* 39(5):267, 1993.
6. Tolep K, et al: Comparison of diaphragm strength between healthy adult elderly and young men, *Am J Respir Crit Care Med* 152(2):677, 1995.
7. Erb BD: Elders in the wilderness. In Auerbach PS, editor: *Wilderness medicine,* ed 5, Philadelphia, 2007, Mosby.
8. Levitzky MG: *Pulmonary physiology,* ed 7, New York, 2007, McGraw-Hill Medical.
9. McClaran SR, et al: Longitudinal effects of aging on lung function at rest and exercise in healthy active fit elderly adults, *J Appl Physiol* 78(5): 195, 1995.
10. Burchfiel CM, et al: Effects of smoking and smoking cessation on longitudinal decline in pulmonary function, *Am J Respir Crit Care Med* 151(6):1778, 1995.
11. O'Connor GT, Sparrow D, Weiss ST: A prospective longitudinal study of methacholine airway responsiveness as a predictor of pulmonary-function decline: the Normative Aging Study, *Am J Respir Crit Care Med* 152(1):87, 1995.
12. Swine C: Aging of heart function in man, *Presse Med* 21(26):1216, 1992.
13. Gyetko MR, Toews GB: Immunology of the aging lung, *Clin Chest Med* 14(3):379, 1993.
14. Duncan AK, et al: Cardiovascular disease in elderly patients, *Mayo Clin Proc* 71(2):184, 1996.
15. Arrighi JA, et al: Improvement of the age-related impairment in left ventricular diastolic filling with verapamil in the normal human heart, *Circulation* 90(1):213, 1994.
16. Hall JE: *Guyton and Hall textbook of medical physiology,* ed 12, Philadelphia, 2011, Saunders.
17. Chaitman BR: Exercise stress testing. In Bonow RO, et al, editors: *Braunwald's heart disease: a textbook of cardiovascular medicine,* ed 9, Philadelphia, 2011, Saunders.
18. Mahler DA, Cunningham LN, Curfman GD: Aging and exercise performance, *Clin Geriatr Med* 2(2):433, 1986.
19. Limacher MC: Aging and cardiac function: influence of exercise, *South Med J* 87(5):S13, 1994.
20. Singh MA: Exercise and aging, *Clin Geriatr Med* 20(2):201, 2004.
21. Frankel JE, et al: Exercise in the elderly: research and clinical practice, *Clin Geriatr Med* 22(2):239, 2006.
22. Janssens JP: Aging of the respiratory system: impact on pulmonary function tests and adaptation to exertion, *Clin Chest Med* 26(3):469, 2005.

Symbols and Abbreviations Used in Cardiopulmonary Physiology

GENERAL SYMBOLS

P	Pressure (gas or blood)
$\overline{X}$	Dash above any symbol indicates mean value
$\dot{X}$	Dot above a symbol usually indicates volume per unit of time (flow rate)
f	Frequency per unit of time (e.g., breaths per minute)
max	Maximum
[x]	Brackets around any symbol indicate concentration

PRIMARY GAS SYMBOLS

P	Pressure
V	Volume
$\dot{V}$	Gas flow rate (e.g., L per minute, L per second)
F	Fractional concentration of a gas (expressed as a decimal (e.g., 21% = 0.21)

SECONDARY GAS SYMBOLS (SUBSCRIPTS TO PRIMARY SYMBOLS)

I	Inspired (e.g., F_IO_2)
E	Expired (e.g., F_ECO_2)
$\overline{E}$	Mixed or mean expired
A	Alveolar
T	Tidal
D	Dead space
B	Barometric
L	Lung

PRIMARY BLOOD SYMBOLS

Q	Blood volume
$\dot{Q}$	Blood flow rate (e.g., L per minute)
C	Content (concentration) in blood
S	Saturation in blood (expressed as a decimal fraction or percentage)

SECONDARY BLOOD SYMBOLS (SUBSCRIPTS TO PRIMARY SYMBOLS)

a	Arterial
v	Venous
$\overline{v}$	Mixed or mean venous blood
c′	Pulmonary end-capillary blood

LUNG VOLUMES AND CAPACITIES

VC	Vital capacity
IC	Inspiratory capacity
TLC	Total lung capacity
FRC	Functional residual capacity
VT	Tidal volume
IRV	Inspiratory reserve volume
ERV	Expiratory reserve volume
RV	Residual volume
RV/TLC%	Percentage of TLC represented by RV

PULMONARY FUNCTION SPIROMETRY

FVC	Forced vital capacity (exhaled)
FEV_T	Volume of gas exhaled in a specific time interval during the FVC maneuver (e.g., FEV_1 = volume exhaled in the first second of the FVC)
FEV_1/FVC, or $FEV_1\%$	Fraction or percentage of the FVC exhaled in the first second
$FEF_{200-1200}$	Forced expiratory flow or average flow between the first 200 mL and 1200 mL of the FVC (L per second)
$FEF_{25\%-75\%}$	Forced expiratory flow or average flow during the middle 50% of the FVC (L per second)
PEFR, or PF	Peak expiratory flow rate, sometimes shortened to "peak flow" (L per second)
$\dot{V}max$	Maximum expiratory flow (lung volume at which $\dot{V}max$ is measured is usually specified (e.g., $\dot{V}max$ 50% is the maximum instantaneous flow as a subject exhales through the 50% point of the FVC; measured in L per second)
MVV	Maximum voluntary ventilation (L per minute)

VOLUME AND VENTILATION MEASUREMENTS

V_D	Dead space volume
V_A	Alveolar volume
$\dot{V}_D$	Dead space ventilation per minute (L per minute or mL per minute)
$\dot{V}_A$	Alveolar ventilation per minute (L per minute or mL per minute)
$\dot{V}_E$	Total expired ventilation per minute or minute ventilation (L per minute or mL per minute)
V_{Danat}	Anatomical dead space (conducting airways) volume
V_{DA}	Alveolar dead space volume
$\dot{V}CO_2$	Carbon dioxide production per minute (mL per minute)
$\dot{V}O_2$	Oxygen consumption per minute (mL per minute)
R	Respiratory exchange ratio in the lungs (carbon dioxide excretion divided by oxygen uptake or $\dot{V}CO_2/\dot{V}O_2$)
RQ	Respiratory quotient; refers to gas-exchange ratio at the tissue level (carbon dioxide production divided by oxygen consumption, or $\dot{V}CO_2/\dot{V}O_2$)

PRESSURE TERMS IN VENTILATORY MECHANICS (USUALLY MEASURED IN CM H_2O)

P_{aw}	Airway pressure
P_{ao}	Pressure at the airway opening (e.g., pressure at the mouth or endotracheal tube); equal to atmospheric pressure during spontaneous unassisted breathing
P_{pl}	Intrapleural pressure
P_A	Alveolar pressure
P_{bs}	Pressure at the body surface (equal to P_{ao} or atmospheric pressure during spontaneous unassisted breathing)
P_L	Transpulmonary pressure; distending pressure of the lungs ($P_L = P_A - P_{pl}$)
P_w	Transthoracic pressure; pressure across the chest wall ($P_w = P_{pl} - P_{bs}$)
P_{rs}	Transrespiratory pressure; pressure across the respiratory system, that is, lungs plus chest wall ($P_{rs} = P_A - P_{bs}$); also equal to pressure across the airways or transairway pressure—between the airway opening and alveoli—during spontaneous unassisted breathing ($P_{rs} = P_A - P_{ao}$); unofficial symbol: P_{TA} for "transairway pressure"

FLOW-PRESSURE RELATIONSHIPS

R	Resistance (pressure/flow)
R_{aw}	Airway resistance (cm H_2O/L/sec)

VOLUME-PRESSURE RELATIONSHIPS

C	Compliance (volume/pressure)
E	Elastance (pressure/volume)
C_L	Lung compliance (L/cm H_2O)
C_{st}	Static compliance; measurement performed in the absence of airflow
C_{dyn}	Dynamic compliance; measurement performed during airflow
C/FRC	Specific compliance; compliance divided by the lung volume at which it is measured, usually FRC

DIFFUSION

D_LCO	Diffusion capacity of the lung for carbon monoxide (mL/min/mm Hg)
D_LCO/V_L	Diffusion capacity per unit of lung volume

BLOOD GASES AND CONTENTS (PRESSURES MEASURED IN MM HG)

P_AO_2	Alveolar gas oxygen pressure
PaO_2	Arterial blood oxygen pressure
$P\bar{v}O_2$	Mixed venous blood oxygen pressure
$P_{ET}O_2$	End-tidal exhaled gas oxygen pressure
P_ACO_2	Alveolar gas carbon dioxide pressure
$P_{ET}CO_2$	End-tidal exhaled gas carbon dioxide pressure
$P_{\bar{E}}CO_2$	Mixed expired gas carbon dioxide pressure (dead space plus alveolar gas)
$Pc'O_2$	Pulmonary end-capillary oxygen pressure
SaO_2	Arterial oxygen saturation (expressed as decimal fraction or percentage)
$S\bar{v}O_2$	Mixed venous oxygen saturation (expressed as decimal fraction or percentage)
pH	Measure of blood H^+ concentration ($pH = -\log[H^+]$)
$[HCO_3{}^-]$	Blood bicarbonate ion concentration (mEq/L)
CaO_2	Arterial oxygen content (mL/dL)
$C\bar{v}O_2$	Mixed venous oxygen content (mL/dL)
$Cc'O_2$	Pulmonary end-capillary oxygen content (mL/dL)
$P(A-a)O_2$	Alveolar-arterial oxygen pressure difference
$C(a-\bar{v})O_2$	Arterial-mixed venous oxygen content difference (mL/dL)

VENTILATION-PERFUSION RELATIONSHIPS

$\dot{V}_A/\dot{Q}_C$	Alveolar ventilation per minute divided by pulmonary capillary blood flow per minute (expressed as a decimal fraction)
$\dot{Q}_S/\dot{Q}_T$	Shunt fraction; fraction of the cardiac output that is not exposed to alveolar ventilation
V_D/V_T	Dead space fraction; fraction of the tidal volume or minute ventilation that is not exposed to alveolar capillary blood flow

SYMBOLS RELEVANT TO EXERCISE PHYSIOLOGY AND TESTING

$\dot{V}O_2max$	Maximum attainable oxygen consumption at maximal exercise (mL per minute)
HR_{max}	Maximum attainable heart rate
$\dot{V}_Emax$	Maximum ventilation attained during maximal exercise (L per minute)
HRR	Heart rate reserve (predicted HR_{max} minus actual measured HR)
BR	Breathing reserve ($MVV - \dot{V}_Emax$)
O_2 pulse	Oxygen consumption per heartbeat ($\dot{V}O_2$/HR)
MET	Average resting oxygen consumption per kilogram body weight (mL O_2/min/kg); one MET = 3.5 mL/min/kg
AT	Aerobic threshold
$\dot{V}_E/\dot{V}O_2$	Ventilatory equivalent for oxygen ([L/min $\dot{V}_E$]/[L/min $\dot{V}O_2$])
$\dot{V}_E/\dot{V}CO_2$	Ventilatory equivalent for carbon dioxide ([L/min $\dot{V}_E$]/[L/min $\dot{V}CO_2$])

HEMODYNAMIC MEASUREMENTS (PRESSURES MEASURED IN MM HG)

Measured

RAP	Right atrial pressure
CVP	Central venous pressure (equal to RAP)
PAP	Pulmonary artery pressure
PAEDP	Pulmonary artery end-diastolic pressure
MPAP	Mean pulmonary artery pressure
PCWP	Pulmonary capillary wedge pressure
LVEDP	Left ventricular end-diastolic pressure
LVEDV	Left ventricular end-diastolic volume
BP	Blood pressure (systemic unless otherwise specified)
MAP	Mean arterial pressure (systemic unless otherwise specified)
CO	Cardiac output
HR	Heart rate

Calculated (I, Index, Expresses the Value per Square Meter of BSA, Body Surface Area)

SV and SVI	Stroke volume and stroke volume index (SVI = SV/BSA)
CI	Cardiac index (CI = CO/BSA)
SW and SWI	Stroke work and stroke work index (SWI = SW/BSA)
LVSW and LVSWI	Left ventricular stroke work and left ventricular stroke work index (LVSWI = LVSW/BSA)
RVSW and RVSWI	Right ventricular stroke work and right ventricular stroke work index (RVSWI = RVSW/BSA)
PVR and PVRI	Pulmonary vascular resistance and pulmonary vascular resistance index (PVRI = PVR/BSA)
SVR and SVRI	Systemic vascular resistance and systemic vascular resistance index (SVRI = SVR/BSA)

Units of Measurement

WEIGHT

Kilograms	Grams	Milligrams	Micrograms	Nanograms
0.001	1	1000	1,000,000	1,000,000,000
Kilograms	**Grams**	**Pounds**		
1	1000	2.2		

VOLUME

Liters	Deciliters	Milliliters
1	10	1000
0.1	1	100
0.0001	0.01	1 (equal to 1 cubic centimeter [cc])

LENGTH

Meters	Centimeters	Millimeters	Micrometers	Nanometers
1	100	1000	1,000,000	1,000,000,000
0.1	1	10	10,000	10,000,000
0.001	0.1	1	1000	1,000,000
Centimeters	**Millimeters**	**Inches**	**Feet**	
1	10	0.3937	0.03281	
0.1	1	0.03937	0.00328	
2.54	25.4	1	0.0833	
30.48	304.8	12	1	

PRESSURE

mm Hg	cm H_2O	psi
1	1.36	0.01934
0.735	1	0.01422
51.7	70.34	1

1 atmosphere of pressure at sea level = 760 mm Hg = 1034 cm H_2O = 14.7 psi.

Equation Derivations

VENTILATION EQUATION

The alveolar ventilation equation illustrates mathematically that P_ACO_2 and alveolar ventilation are inversely related (e.g., if $\dot{V}_A$ is halved, P_ACO_2 doubles, or if $\dot{V}_A$ doubles, P_ACO_2 is halved). The derivation of this equation is as follows:

Carbon dioxide production ($\dot{V}CO_2$) is equal to dead space and alveolar ventilation multiplied by their respective fractional carbon dioxide concentrations (F_DCO_2 and F_ACO_2), as the following shows:

1. $$\dot{V}CO_2 = (F_DCO_2 \times \dot{V}_D) + (F_ACO_2 \times \dot{V}_A)$$

The dead space is not in contact with blood flow and therefore receives no carbon dioxide from the blood. Therefore, F_DCO_2 is equal to that of atmospheric air (0.0003) and can be ignored. All carbon dioxide in the lung comes from alveolar gas, as the following shows:

2. $$\dot{V}CO_2 = F_ACO_2 \times \dot{V}_A$$

The fractional carbon dioxide concentration in the alveoli (F_ACO_2) can be converted to P_ACO_2, as the following shows (see Chapter 7):

3. $$P_ACO_2 = F_ACO_2 \times (P_B - 47)$$

Solving for F_ACO_2 is as follows:

4. $$F_ACO_2 = P_ACO_2/(P_B - 47)$$

Substituting this new term for F_ACO_2 in equation 2 is as follows:

5. $$\dot{V}CO_2 = (P_ACO_2/P_B - 47) \times \dot{V}_A$$

Rearranging is as follows:

6. $$\dot{V}CO_2 \times (P_B - 47) = P_ACO_2 \times \dot{V}_A$$

$\dot{V}CO_2$ is constant if the metabolic rate remains constant. Likewise, ($P_B - 47$) is a constant. Thus, the left side of equation 6 is constant: $\dot{V}CO_2 \times (P_B - 47) = K$, in which K is a constant. Substituting K for the left side of equation 6 is as follows:

7. $$P_ACO_2 \times \dot{V}_A = K$$

Equation 7 illustrates the inverse relationship between P_ACO_2 and $\dot{V}_A$; doubling or halving $\dot{V}_A$ has the opposite effects on P_ACO_2.

PCO$_2$ EQUATION

Equation 6 can be solved for P_ACO_2 as follows:

8. $$P_ACO_2 = \frac{\dot{V}CO_2 \times (P_B - 47)}{\dot{V}_A}$$

A complicating factor in equation 8 is that conventionally $\dot{V}CO_2$ is measured in milliliters per minute at 0° C, 760 mm Hg, and 0% relative humidity (standard temperature and pressure, dry, or STPD conditions), whereas $\dot{V}_A$ is measured in liters per minute at 37° C, 760 mm Hg, and 100% relative humidity (body temperature and pressure, saturated, or BTPS conditions). A correction factor (0.826) can be used to convert BTPS to STPD conditions, and $\dot{V}_A$ can be multiplied by 1000 to convert $\dot{V}_A$ to milliliters per minute, as the following shows:

9. $$P_ACO_2 = \frac{\dot{V}CO_2(mL/min, STPD) \times (P_B - 47)}{\dot{V}_A(L/min, BTPS) \times 0.826 \times 1000}$$

Equation 9 can be rewritten as follows:

10. $$P_ACO_2 = \frac{\dot{V}CO_2 \times 713}{\dot{V}_A \times 0.826 \times 1000}$$

To simplify, 713 can be divided by (0.826 × 1000) to form the following equation:

11. $$P_ACO_2 = \frac{\dot{V}CO_2 \times 0.863}{\dot{V}_A}$$

Equation 11, known as the PCO_2 equation, also can be solved for $\dot{V}_A$:

12. $$\dot{V}_A = \frac{\dot{V}CO_2 \times 0.863}{P_ACO_2}$$

Because P_ACO_2 usually equals $PaCO_2$ in the absence of alveolar dead space, the clinical form of equation 12 uses $PaCO_2$ in the denominator:

13. $$\dot{V}_A = \frac{\dot{V}CO_2 \times 0.863}{PaCO_2}$$

This equation is useful for estimating $\dot{V}_A$; one can directly measure $\dot{V}CO_2$ and $PaCO_2$, but not $\dot{V}_A$.

CORRECTION FACTOR TO CONVERT BTPS TO STPD

This factor, used in equation 9, requires the use of the following combined gas law equation:

$$\frac{V_1P_1}{T_1} = \frac{V_2P_2}{T_2}$$

In this equation, V represents volume, P represents pressure, and T represents temperature. V_1, P_1, and T_1 represent STPD conditions, and V_2, P_2, and T_2 represent BTPS conditions. T is expressed in absolute degrees Kelvin ($0°$ C = $273°$ K). STPD and BTPS conditions are as follows:

STPD = 273° K, 760 mm Hg, P_{H2O} = 0
BTPS = 310° K, 760 mm Hg, P_{H2O} = 47 mm Hg

1. $$\frac{V_1 \times 760}{273} = \frac{V_2 \times (760 - 47)}{310}$$

Cross-multiplying:

2. $V_1 \times 760 \times 310 = V_2 \times 713 \times 273$

Solving for V_1:

3. $$V_1 = \frac{V_2 \times 713 \times 273}{760 \times 310}$$

4. $V_1 = V_2 \times 0.826$

Multiplying a volume obtained under BTPS conditions by 0.826 converts the volume to its value under STPD conditions.

V_D/V_T OR DEAD SPACE FRACTION

First, consider the following components of expired minute ventilation ($\dot{V}_E$):

1. $\dot{V}_E = \dot{V}_A + \dot{V}_D$

The amount of carbon dioxide in the expired minute volume is equal to the amount of carbon dioxide coming from the alveoli per minute. $\dot{V}_D$ cannot contribute carbon dioxide to expired gas because dead space is not in contact with pulmonary capillary blood. Therefore, the equation can be written as follows:

2. $\dot{V}_E \times F_{\bar{E}}CO_2 = \dot{V}_A \times F_ACO_2$

$F_{\bar{E}}CO_2$ represents the fraction of carbon dioxide in expired mixed gas obtained in 1 minute. (Both sides of equation 2 are equal to the total amount of expired carbon dioxide.) Equation 1 can be solved for $\dot{V}_A$ as follows:

3. $\dot{V}_A = \dot{V}_E - \dot{V}_D$

Substituting ($\dot{V}_E - \dot{V}_D$) for $\dot{V}_A$ in equation 2 is as follows:

4. $\dot{V}_E \times F_{\bar{E}}CO_2 = (\dot{V}_E - \dot{V}_D) \times F_ACO_2$

The reason for making this substitution is to introduce the term $\dot{V}_D$ into the equation. Expanding the equation produces the following:

5. $\dot{V}_E \times F_{\bar{E}}CO_2 = \dot{V}_E \times F_ACO_2 - \dot{V}_D \times F_ACO_2$

To collect both $\dot{V}_E$ terms on the same side of the equation, solve for ($\dot{V}_D \times F_ACO_2$) as follows:

6. $\dot{V}_D \times F_ACO_2 = \dot{V}_E \times F_ACO_2 - \dot{V}_E \times F_{\bar{E}}CO_2$

7. $\dot{V}_D \times F_ACO_2 = \dot{V}_E(F_ACO_2 - F_{\bar{E}}CO_2)$

Dividing both sides by ($\dot{V}_E \times F_ACO_2$) is as follows:

8. $$\frac{\dot{V}_D}{\dot{V}_E} = \frac{F_ACO_2 - F_{\bar{E}}CO_2}{F_ACO_2}$$

Because the fractional concentration of any gas is proportional to its partial pressure and because P_ACO_2 usually approximates $PaCO_2$, the final clinical form of the dead space equation is as follows:

9. $$\frac{\dot{V}_D}{\dot{V}_E} = \frac{PaCO_2 - P_{\bar{E}}CO_2}{PaCO_2}$$

On a single-breath basis, the equation is written as follows:

10. $$\frac{V_D}{V_T} = \frac{PaCO_2 - P_{\bar{E}}CO_2}{PaCO_2}$$

The numerator of this equation states that the magnitude of the difference between $PaCO_2$ and $P_{\bar{E}}CO_2$ is proportional to the amount of dead space volume present. Because dead space contributes carbon dioxide–free gas to the mixed expired stream, it dilutes the alveolar carbon dioxide concentration, lowering the $P_{\bar{E}}CO_2$. The V_D/V_T is the dead space fraction, or the fraction of the tidal volume composed of dead space. Multiplying this fraction by the $\dot{V}_E$ yields the volume of dead space ventilation. By subtraction, the alveolar ventilation can be computed as follows:

Given: $\dot{V}_E$ = 5 L/min and V_D/V_T = 0.4
$\dot{V}_D$ = 0.4(5 L/min) = 2.0 L/min
$\dot{V}_A$ = 5 L/min − 2 L/min = 3 L/min

Dubois Body Surface Area Chart

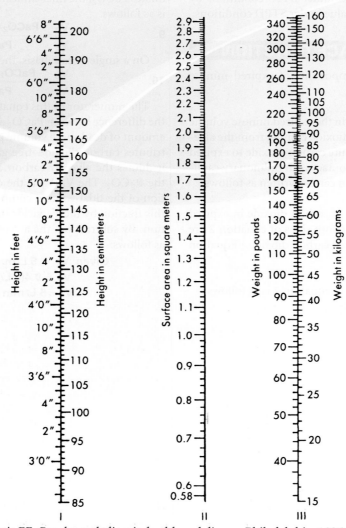

(From DuBois EF: *Basal metabolism in health and disease*, Philadelphia, 1936, Lea & Febiger.)

Index

Page numbers followed by *f* indicate figures; *t*, tables; *b*, boxes.